Diagnosis, Evaluation, and Management of Diseases during Pregnancy

Diagnosis, Evaluation, and Management of Diseases during Pregnancy

Editors

Marius L. Craina
Elena Bernad

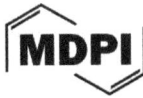

Basel • Beijing • Wuhan • Barcelona • Belgrade • Novi Sad • Cluj • Manchester

Editors
Marius L. Craina
"Victor Babes" University of Medicine
and Pharmacy from Timisoara
Timisoara
Romania

Elena Bernad
"Victor Babes" University of Medicine
and Pharmacy from Timisoara
Timisoara
Romania

Editorial Office
MDPI
St. Alban-Anlage 66
4052 Basel, Switzerland

This is a reprint of articles from the Special Issue published online in the open access journal *Medicina* (ISSN 1648-9144) (available at: https://www.mdpi.com/journal/medicina/special_issues/Pregnancy_Diseases).

For citation purposes, cite each article independently as indicated on the article page online and as indicated below:

Lastname, A.A.; Lastname, B.B. Article Title. *Journal Name* **Year**, *Volume Number*, Page Range.

ISBN 978-3-0365-9738-6 (Hbk)
ISBN 978-3-0365-9739-3 (PDF)
doi.org/10.3390/books978-3-0365-9739-3

© 2023 by the authors. Articles in this book are Open Access and distributed under the Creative Commons Attribution (CC BY) license. The book as a whole is distributed by MDPI under the terms and conditions of the Creative Commons Attribution-NonCommercial-NoDerivs (CC BY-NC-ND) license.

Contents

About the Editors ix

Preface xi

Soo Jung Kim, So-Yeon Shim, Hyun-Hae Cho, Mi-Hye Park and Kyung A. Lee
Prenatal Diagnosis of Fetal Obstructed Hemivagina and Ipsilateral Renal Agenesis (OHVIRA) Syndrome
Reprinted from: *Medicina* 2023, 59, 703, doi:10.3390/medicina59040703 1

Eirini Giovannopoulou, Ioannis Tsakiridis, Apostolos Mamopoulos, Ioannis Kalogiannidis, Ioannis Papoulidis, Apostolos Athanasiadis and Themistoklis Dagklis
Invasive Prenatal Diagnostic Testing for Aneuploidies in Singleton Pregnancies: A Comparative Review of Major Guidelines
Reprinted from: *Medicina* 2022, 58, 1472, doi:10.3390/medicina58101472 9

Andreea Roxana Florian, Gheorghe Cruciat, Georgiana Nemeti, Adelina Staicu, Cristina Suciu, Mariam Chaikh Sulaiman, et al.
Umbilical Cord Biometry and Fetal Abdominal Skinfold Assessment as Potential Biomarkers for Fetal Macrosomia in a Gestational Diabetes Romanian Cohort
Reprinted from: *Medicina* 2022, 58, 1162, doi:10.3390/medicina58091162 27

Jara Pascual-Mancho, Pilar Pintado-Recarte, Jorge C. Morales-Camino, Carlos Romero-Román, Concepción Hernández-Martin, Coral Bravo, et al.
Brain-Derived Neurotrophic Factor Levels in Cord Blood from Growth Restricted Fetuses with Doppler Alteration Compared to Adequate for Gestational Age Fetuses
Reprinted from: *Medicina* 2022, 58, 178, doi:10.3390/medicina58020178 37

Marina Dinu, Anne Marie Badiu, Andreea Denisa Hodorog, Andreea Florentina Stancioi-Cismaru, Mihaela Gheonea, Razvan Grigoras Capitanescu, et al.
Early Onset Intrauterine Growth Restriction—Data from a Tertiary Care Center in a Middle-Income Country
Reprinted from: *Medicina* 2023, 59, 17, doi:10.3390/medicina59010017 47

Felicia Fiat, Petru Eugen Merghes, Alexandra Denisa Scurtu, Bogdan Almajan Guta, Cristina Adriana Dehelean, Narcis Varan and Elena Bernad
The Main Changes in Pregnancy—Therapeutic Approach to Musculoskeletal Pain
Reprinted from: *Medicina* 2022, 58, 1115, doi:10.3390/medicina58081115 61

Irene Soto-Fernández, Sagrario Gómez-Cantarino, Benito Yáñez-Araque, Jorge Sánchez-Infante, Alejandra Zapata-Ossa and Mercedes Dios-Aguado
A Cross-Sectional Study Examining the Association between Physical Activity and Perinatal Depression
Reprinted from: *Medicina* 2022, 58, 1174, doi:10.3390/medicina58091174 83

Petra Völgyesi, Márta Radnai, Gábor Németh, Krisztina Boda, Elena Bernad and Tibor Novák
Maternal Periodontal Status as a Factor Influencing Obstetrical Outcomes
Reprinted from: *Medicina* 2023, 59, 621, doi:10.3390/medicina59030621 93

Nabila Sher, Murad A. Mubaraki, Hafsa Zafar, Rubina Nazli, Mashal Zafar, Sadia Fatima and Fozia Fozia
Effect of Lipid-Based Multiple Micronutrients Supplementation in Underweight Primigravida Pre-Eclamptic Women on Maternal and Pregnancy Outcomes: Randomized Clinical Trial
Reprinted from: *Medicina* 2022, 58, 1772, doi:10.3390/medicina58121772 101

Agne Marcinkeviciene, Diana Rinkuniene and Aras Puodziukynas
Long QT Syndrome Management during and after Pregnancy
Reprinted from: *Medicina* **2022**, *58*, 1694, doi:10.3390/medicina58111694 . . . . **111**

Lara Sánchez-Trujillo, Cielo García-Montero, Oscar Fraile-Martinez, Luis G. Guijarro, Coral Bravo, Juan A. De Leon-Luis, et al.
Considering the Effects and Maternofoetal Implications of Vascular Disorders and the Umbilical Cord
Reprinted from: *Medicina* **2022**, *58*, 1754, doi:10.3390/medicina58121754 . . . . **119**

Viviana Aursulesei Onofrei, Cristina Andreea Adam, Dragos Traian Marius Marcu, Radu Crisan Dabija, Alexandr Ceasovschih, Mihai Constantin, et al.
Infective Endocarditis during Pregnancy—Keep It Safe and Simple!
Reprinted from: *Medicina* **2023**, *59*, 939, doi:10.3390/medicina59050939 . . . . **135**

Tina-Ioana Bobei, Bashar Haj Hamoud, Romina-Marina Sima, Gabriel-Petre Gorecki, Mircea-Octavian Poenaru, Octavian-Gabriel Olaru and Liana Ples
The Impact of SARS-CoV-2 Infection on Premature Birth—Our Experience as COVID Center
Reprinted from: *Medicina* **2022**, *58*, 587, doi:10.3390/medicina58050587 . . . . **153**

Alina-Madalina Luca, Elena Bernad, Dragos Nemescu, Cristian Vaduva, Anamaria Harabor, Ana-Maria Adam, et al.
Unraveling the Efficacy of Therapeutic Interventions for Short Cervix: Insights from a Retrospective Study for Improved Clinical Management
Reprinted from: *Medicina* **2023**, *59*, 1018, doi:10.3390/medicina59061018 . . . . **161**

Miruna Samfireag, Cristina Potre, Ovidiu Potre, Lavinia-Cristina Moleriu, Izabella Petre, Ema Borsi, et al.
Assessment of the Particularities of Thrombophilia in the Management of Pregnant Women in the Western Part of Romania
Reprinted from: *Medicina* **2023**, *59*, 851, doi:10.3390/medicina59050851 . . . . **173**

Miruna Samfireag, Cristina Potre, Ovidiu Potre, Raluca Tudor, Teodora Hoinoiu and Andrei Anghel
Approach to Thrombophilia in Pregnancy—A Narrative Review
Reprinted from: *Medicina* **2022**, *58*, 692, doi:10.3390/medicina58050692 . . . . **187**

Viorel Dragos Radu, Ingrid-Andrada Vasilache, Radu-Cristian Costache, Ioana-Sadiye Scripcariu, Dragos Nemescu, Alexandru Carauleanu, et al.
Pregnancy Outcomes in a Cohort of Patients Who Underwent Double-J Ureteric Stenting—A Single Center Experience
Reprinted from: *Medicina* **2022**, *58*, 619, doi:10.3390/medicina58050619 . . . . **201**

Tiziana Filardi, Maria Cristina Gentile, Vittorio Venditti, Antonella Valente, Enrico Bleve, Carmela Santangelo and Susanna Morano
The Impact of Ethnicity on Fetal and Maternal Outcomes of Gestational Diabetes
Reprinted from: *Medicina* **2022**, *58*, 1161, doi:10.3390/medicina58091161 . . . . **211**

Eriko Fukuda, Takuya Misugi, Kohei Kitada, Megumi Fudaba, Yasushi Kurihara, Mie Tahara, et al.
The Hematopoietic Effect of Ninjinyoeito (TJ-108), a Traditional Japanese Herbal Medicine, in Pregnant Women Preparing for Autologous Blood Storage
Reprinted from: *Medicina* **2022**, *58*, 1083, doi:10.3390/medicina58081083 . . . . **219**

Robert Rednic, Iasmina Marcovici, Razvan Dragoi, Iulia Pinzaru, Cristina Adriana Dehelean, Mirela Tomescu, et al.
In Vitro Toxicological Profile of Labetalol-Folic Acid/Folate Co-Administration in H9c2(2-1) and HepaRG Cells
Reprinted from: *Medicina* 2022, 58, 784, doi:10.3390/medicina58060784 227

María Álvarez-González, Raquel Leirós-Rodríguez, Lorena Álvarez-Barrio and Ana F. López-Rodríguez
Perineal Massage during Pregnancy for the Prevention of Postpartum Urinary Incontinence: Controlled Clinical Trial
Reprinted from: *Medicina* 2022, 58, 1485, doi:10.3390/medicina58101485 239

Irina Pacu, Nikolaos Zygouropoulos, Alina Elena Cristea, Cristina Zaharia, George-Alexandru Rosu, Alexandra Matei, et al.
The Risk of Obstetrical Hemorrhage in Placenta Praevia Associated with Coronavirus Infection Antepartum or Intrapartum
Reprinted from: *Medicina* 2022, 58, 1004, doi:10.3390/medicina58081004 247

Andreea Taisia Tiron, Anca Filofteia Briceag, Liviu Moraru, Lavinia Alice Bălăceanu, Ion Dina and Laura Caravia
Management of Postpartum Extensive Venous Thrombosis after Second Pregnancy
Reprinted from: *Medicina* 2023, 59, 871, doi:10.3390/medicina59050871 261

Ciprian Ilea, Ovidiu-Dumitru Ilie, Olivia-Andreea Marcu, Irina Stoian and Bogdan Doroftei
The Very First Romanian Unruptured 13-Weeks Gestation Tubal Ectopic Pregnancy
Reprinted from: *Medicina* 2022, 58, 1160, doi:10.3390/medicina58091160 271

Dominyka Surgontaitė, Artūras Sukovas, Dalia Regina Railaitė, Tautvydas Jankauskas, Arnoldas Bartusevičius and Eglė Bartusevičienė
Trophoblastic Tissue Reimplantation below the Spleen Following Laparoscopic Bilateral Salpingectomy for Ectopic Tubal Pregnancy: A Case Report
Reprinted from: *Medicina* 2023, 59, 701, doi:10.3390/medicina59040701 281

Małgorzata Kampioni, Karolina Chmaj-Wierzchowska, Katarzyna Wszołek and Maciej Wilczak
Interstitial Ectopic Pregnancy—Case Reports and Medical Management
Reprinted from: *Medicina* 2023, 59, 233, doi:10.3390/medicina59020233 287

Alina-Sinziana Melinte-Popescu, Radu-Florin Popa, Valeriu Harabor, Aurel Nechita, AnaMaria Harabor, Ana-Maria Adam, Ingrid-Andrada Vasilache, Marian Melinte-Popescu, Cristian Vaduva and Demetra Socolov
Managing Fetal Ovarian Cysts: Clinical Experience with a Rare Disorder
Reprinted from: *Medicina* 2023, 59, 715, doi:10.3390/medicina59040715 297

Jinha Chung, Mi-Young Lee, Jin-Hoon Chung and Hye-Sung Won
Extremely Rare Case of Fetal Anemia Due to Mitochondrial Disease Managed with Intrauterine Transfusion
Reprinted from: *Medicina* 2022, 58, 328, doi:10.3390/medicina58030328 307

Ioana Rosca, Alina Turenschi, Alin Nicolescu, Andreea Teodora Constantin, Adina Maria Canciu, Alice Denisa Dica, et al.
Endocrine Disorders in a Newborn with Heterozygous Galactosemia, Down Syndrome and Complex Cardiac Malformation: Case Report
Reprinted from: *Medicina* 2023, 59, 856, doi:10.3390/medicina59050856 311

Roxana-Elena Bohîlțea, Bianca-Margareta Mihai, Elena Szini, Ileana-Alina Șucaliuc and Corin Badiu
Diagnosis and Management of Fetal and Neonatal Thyrotoxicosis
Reprinted from: *Medicina* **2023**, *59*, 36, doi:10.3390/medicina59010036 . . . . **319**

About the Editors

Marius L. Craina

Marius L. Craina is a professor at "Victor Babes" University of Medicine and Pharmacy in Timisoara (UMFVBT), Romania, where he has been coordinating educational and research activities. He was born in 1964 and graduated from the Faculty of Medicine at UMFVBT in 1990. He obtained the title of Doctor of Medicine in 2004 and followed his university career. He specialises in obstetrics and gynaecology. He is a senior physician with expertise in obstetric and gynaecological ultrasonography, laparoscopy and hysteroscopy at "Pius Brinzeu" Emergency County Hospital Timisoara, Romania. In the last few years, he has coordinated the administrative activity of several university and hospital structures.

He oversaw multiple administrative operations of the hospital and the university in the past few years. He participated in research initiatives and specialised studies, conducting extensive scientific research. His prolific publishing of books and numerous essays in publications with a global readership attested to his solid scientific pursuits. His outstanding organisational skills were demonstrated by his involvement in planning multiple well-attended national and international scientific meetings.

He earned his habilitation in 2007 and has been organising the activities of PhD students ever since. He belongs to numerous esteemed national and international medical groups and societies. He has prior expertise in evaluating studies by peers. He speaks and writes in English and German. He is not married. He likes to be surrounded by people willing to learn the secrets of obstetrics–gynaecology and research in the field.

Elena Bernad

Elena Bernad is an associate professor at "Victor Babes" University of Medicine and Pharmacy in Timisoara (UMFVBT), Romania, where she has been coordinating educational and research activities. She was born in 1969 and graduated from the Faculty of Medicine at UMFVBT in 1996. She obtained the title of Doctor of Medicine in 2004 and followed her university career. She completed her studies with two master's courses in Health Management (2010) and Embryology and Teratology (2012). At the same time, she specialises in obstetrics and gynaecology. She currently works as a senior physician with expertise in obstetric and gynaecological ultrasonography, laparoscopy, colposcopy, hysteroscopy, maternal–foetal medicine, and reproductive medicine. She is working at "Pius Brinzeu" Emergency County Hospital Timisoara, Romania, where, over the years, she has coordinated the administrative activity of several structures.

She has conducted intense scientific research by participating in research projects and specialised studies, and has had many articles published in international circulation journals and books. She has contributed to the organisation of several successful national and international scientific events, proving her exceptional organisational abilities.

In 2008, she obtained a habilitation degree; since then, she has coordinated PhD students' activities. She is a member of several prestigious national and international medical societies and associations. She has experience in the peer evaluation of research.

She speaks and writes in English, French and Hungarian. She is married and has a daughter and a son. She likes to be active, and strives to constantly face new challenges in all walks of life.

Preface

Pregnancy is a unique period in a woman's life. The physiological changes that occur help the mother's body to adapt to this transitional period. Ultrasonography is the most used imaging exploration method in pregnancy. It has broad applicability in prenatal diagnosis, both regarding the detection of foetal malformations and the evolution of the pregnancy. The pathologies that can be associated with pregnancy can lead to maternal and foetal complications that require medical interventions in order to complete the pregnancy in good conditions. This volume includes studies on the diagnosis, evaluation and management of pathologies diagnosed during pregnancy. The information provided in these pages will be helpful for specialists in the field of obstetrics and gynaecology, potentially improving case management. The authors of the articles included in this Special Issue aimed to present their personal achievements or structured information related to specific essential topics in the form of reviews, and we thank them for their efforts. We also thank the reviewers for their suggestions and recommendations, which increased the quality of the manuscripts. Additionally, the Editorial Office of *Medicine* provided us with excellent support, which significantly eased the Guest Editors' job. This volume is the result of the combined efforts of all involved.

Marius L. Craina and Elena Bernad
Editors

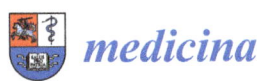

Case Report

Prenatal Diagnosis of Fetal Obstructed Hemivagina and Ipsilateral Renal Agenesis (OHVIRA) Syndrome

Soo Jung Kim [1], So-Yeon Shim [2], Hyun-Hae Cho [3], Mi-Hye Park [1] and Kyung A. Lee [1,*]

1. Department of Obstetrics and Gynecology, Ewha Womans University College of Medicine, Ewha Womans University Seoul Hospital, Seoul 07804, Republic of Korea; bossksj25@gmail.com (S.J.K.)
2. Department of Pediatrics, Ewha Womans University College of Medicine, Ewha Womans University Seoul Hospital, Seoul 07804, Republic of Korea
3. Department of Radiology, Ewha Womans University College of Medicine, Ewha Womans University Seoul Hospital, Seoul 07804, Republic of Korea
* Correspondence: leekyunga@gmail.com; Tel.: +82-6986-1749

Abstract: *Background*: Obstructed hemivagina and ipsilateral renal agenesis (OHVIRA) syndrome, also known as Herlyn-Werner-Wunderlich syndrome, is a rare syndrome characterized by the triad of uterus didelphys, obstructed hemivagina, and ipsilateral renal agenesis. Most cases of OHVIRA have been reported in adolescents or adults. Gartner duct cysts, including those manifesting as vaginal wall cysts, are also rare. Fetal OHVIRA syndrome and Gartner duct cysts are difficult to diagnose. *Case Presentation*: Here, the authors report a case of combined OHVIRA and Gartner duct cyst diagnosed prenatally by ultrasonography, along with a brief review of the relevant published reports. A 30-year-old nulliparous female was referred to our institution at 32 weeks' gestation for fetal right kidney agenesis. Detailed ultrasonographic examinations using 2D, 3D, and Doppler ultrasounds revealed hydrocolpometra, and uterus didelphys, with a normal anus and right kidney agenesis. *Conclusions*: When encountering female fetuses with ipsilateral renal agenesis or vaginal cysts, clinicians should be aware of OHVIRA syndrome and Gartner duct cysts and perform systematic ultrasonographic examinations for other genitourinary anomalies.

Keywords: Herlyn-Werner-Wunderlich syndrome; obstructed hemivagina and ipsilateral renal agenesis syndrome (OHVIRA); Gartner duct cyst; prenatal diagnosis

1. Introduction

Obstructed hemivagina and ipsilateral renal agenesis (OHVIRA) syndrome, also known as Herlyn-Werner-Wunderlich syndrome, is a rare syndrome characterized by the triad of uterus didelphys, obstructed hemivagina, and ipsilateral renal agenesis. In 1922, Purslow first reported this syndrome [1]. In 1971, Herlyn and Werner reported a case of renal agenesis with a blind hemivagina, and Wunderlich described the association of renal aplasia, a bicornuate uterus with a simple vagina, and an isolated hematocervix in 1976 [2].

OHVIRA syndrome is believed to be related to the abnormal development of the Müllerian ducts during the eighth week of gestation, but the exact pathogenesis is unclear. It is a rare congenital abnormality of the genitourinary system with an estimated incidence of 0.1–3.8% [3]. Most cases have been reported in adolescents or adults after menarche and have included progressive dysmenorrhea, abnormal pain, menstrual irregularities, and pelvic masses. The clinical presentation of OHVIRA syndrome can vary significantly, making it essential to consider differential diagnoses for unilateral kidney agenesis in adolescent women, including obstructive genital tract anomalies and Gartner duct cysts. An accurate diagnosis is crucial to preventing potential complications such as endometriosis, infertility, and abortion. As a result, timely follow-up and treatment, particularly during adolescence, can aid in preventing these long-term consequences. It is difficult to diagnose fetal OHVIRA syndrome.

Gartner duct cysts occur as a result of obstruction of the mesonephric duct system during fetal development and represent cystic remnants [4,5]. These cysts can be associated with an abnormal genitourinary system, such as in the context of OHVIRA syndrome, and they may be located submucosally along the anterior or lateral wall of the vagina [6]. Accurate diagnosis of Gartner duct cysts requires a combination of physical examination and imaging modalities such as ultrasound and MRI. The management options for Gartner duct cysts include aspiration, deroofing, or complete cyst removal via a vaginal approach. The appropriate timing for treatment is not yet clear, particularly in the case of newborns.

Recently, fetal cases have been diagnosed thanks to the development and use of prenatal ultrasound examinations. Here, the authors report a case of OHVIRA diagnosed prenatally by ultrasound examinations, with Gartner duct cysts detected after birth.

2. Case

A nulliparous woman, aged 30 years, was referred to our institution at 32 weeks of gestation for further investigation of fetal right kidney agenesis. The patient denied experiencing any symptoms and had no relevant family history or prior kidney issues. Prenatal screening tests, including the Sequential test, showed low risk, and the maternal oral glucose tolerance test was normal. Upon physical examination, no specific findings were noted, and the cervix was found to be closed.

A transabdominal ultrasound scan showed a normally growing female fetus with right kidney agenesis. On a transabdominal ultrasound scan, the estimated fetal weight and abdominal circumference were consistent with 32 weeks of gestation, with adequate amniotic fluid and no placental abnormalities observed. The fetal brain and heart were normal, and Doppler waveforms from the umbilical artery and middle cerebral artery were within acceptable ranges. Additionally, detailed ultrasonographic examinations using 2D and Doppler ultrasounds revealed right kidney agenesis, uterine didelphys, hydrocolpometra, and a vaginal cyst (Figure 1A,B). Based on the imaging, fetal OHVIRA syndrome was highly suspected.

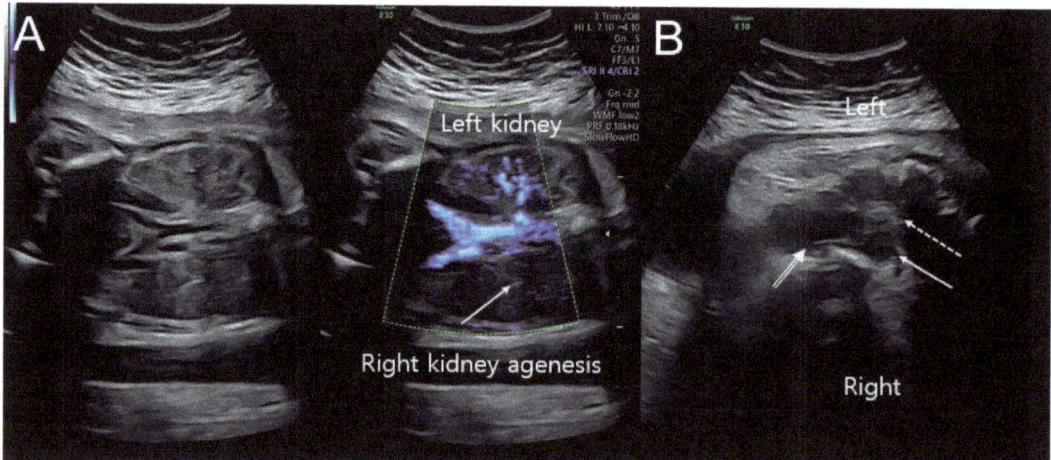

Figure 1. Ultrasonographic findings at prenatal examination. (**A**) Color Doppler ultrasound of the left kidney with the renal artery and right kidney agenesis (arrow) without the renal artery at 32 weeks of gestation. (**B**) Uterine didelphys with right hydrocolpometra (arrow), left uterus (dotted arrow), and vaginal cyst (double-lined arrow) at 37 weeks of gestation.

At 39 weeks and 3 days of gestation, the amniotic sac membrane ruptured; however, labor did not proceed, and an emergency cesarean delivery was performed at 39 weeks and 4 days of gestation. The patient delivered a healthy female newborn with a birth weight of

3190 g, a 1 min Apgar score of 8, and a 5 min Apgar score of 10. There were no problems during the postpartum period.

After birth, the newborn was admitted to the neonatal intensive care unit for evaluation of the genitourinary system for any malformations. The newborn's weight at birth, 3190 g, was appropriate for gestational age, and her height, head circumference, and chest circumference were 51.5 cm, 34 cm, and 33 cm, respectively. The neonate appeared healthy and active, with symmetric chest movements, normal breathing and respiratory patterns, and no evidence of pectus excavatum. On the second day after birth, an abdominal ultrasound revealed probable right kidney agenesis with underlying uterine didelphys, a small amount of fluid collected within the right side of the uterine fundus, and a fluid-filled dilated right hemivagina. Additionally, the abdominal ultrasound detected three simple cysts two days after birth.

Perineal inspection revealed a normal anus, a normally situated urethral meatus, a bulge at the vaginal introitus, and a cystic mass protruding between the labia minora (Figure 2A). The remainder of the physical examination was unremarkable.

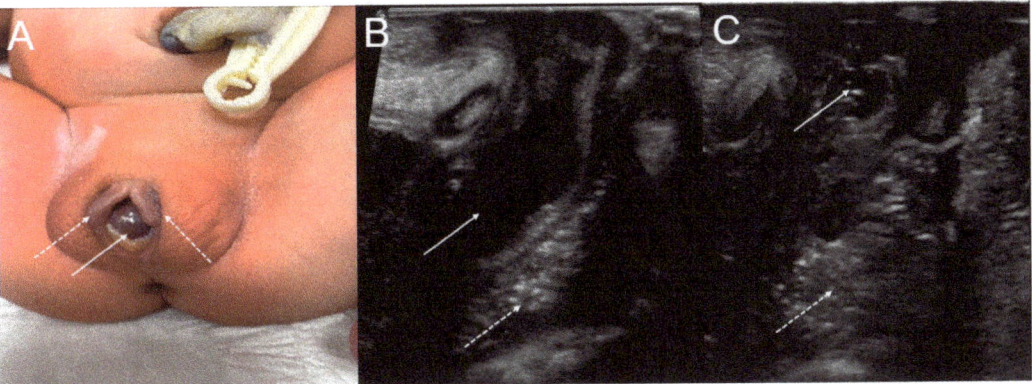

Figure 2. (**A**) The cystic bulging mass (arrow) arising from the right vaginal wall between the labia minora (dotted arrow) after birth. (**B**) On the initial ultrasound with a perineal approach, a fluid-filled cystic lesion (arrow) in the right pelvic cavity was noted anterior to the rectum (dotted arrow). (**C**) After aspiration, the previously observed cystic lesion collapsed (arrow).

When the baby was eight days old, an ultrasound-guided needle aspiration of the cystic mass protruding between the labia minora, not the vaginal septum, was performed, and yellow serous fluid was aspirated. The collapsed cystic lesion was observed after the needle aspiration, and its appearance was suggestive of a Gartner duct cyst diagnosis (Figure 2B,C).

A magnetic resonance imaging (MRI) scan of the baby's abdomen and pelvis was done to see how three cystic masses were related to the vaginal wall. The MRI, performed on the fourth day after birth, revealed agenesis of the right kidney with a compensatory hypertrophied left kidney (Figure 3A), uterine didelphys, an obstructed right hemivagina with hydrocolpometra, a non-obstructed left hemivagina, and three cystic lesions along the right hemivagina. These cystic lesions were thought to be tubulocystic anomalies (Figure 3B,C). Therefore, the diagnosis of OHVIRA syndrome and Gartner duct cyst was established (Figure 3D).

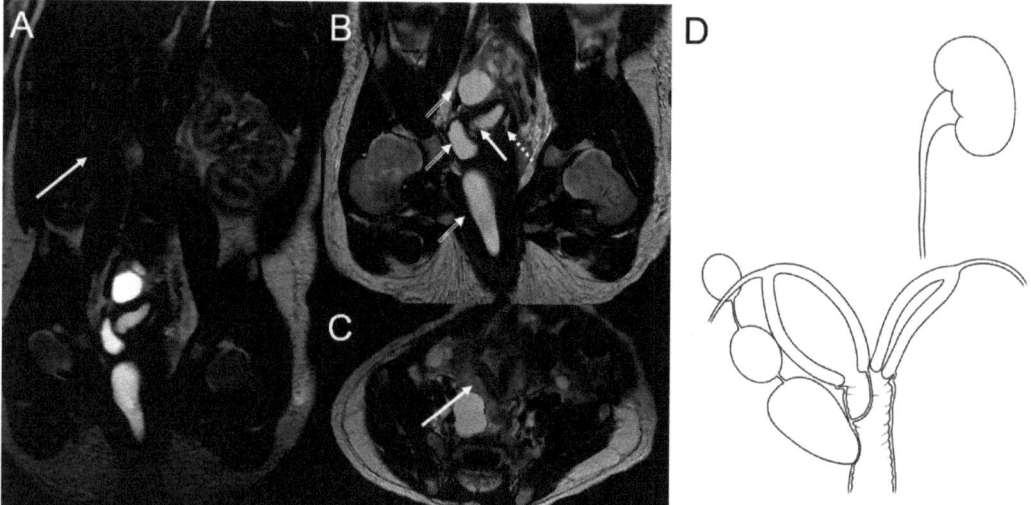

Figure 3. (**A**) Coronal T2-weighted abdominopelvic magnetic resonance image showing an absent right kidney (arrow) with compensatory left kidney hypertrophy. (**B**) Coronal T2-weighted image of the pelvic area showing uterine didelphys with an obstructed right hemivagina and hydrocolpometra (arrow) as well as the non-obstructed left hemivagina (dotted arrow). Three cystic lesions along the right hemivagina were thought to be tubulocystic anomalies, suggesting a diagnosis of Gartner duct cysts (double-lined arrows). (**C**) Axial T2-weighted images showing uterine didelphys (arrow). (**D**) Schematic diagram of OHVIRA syndrome and possible Gartner cysts.

The newborn was discharged on the eleventh day after birth and examined 3 weeks later, and there were no problems. The child is undergoing follow-up at an outpatient clinic by a pediatric nephrologist.

3. Discussion

The true incidence of OHVIRA syndrome is unknown, but it is estimated to be between 0.1% and 3.8% [3]. Biological sex is established at fertilization, but the fetus begins to attain sexual characteristics by the seventh week of gestation. The genital system is closely related to the urinary system, and the development of these two systems is closely linked. The development of the Müllerian ducts—the embryonic formation of the female reproductive tract—includes elongation, fusion, canalization, and septal resorption. OHVIRA syndrome is thought to result from abnormal development of the Müllerian ducts during the fetal period, but the exact pathogenetic mechanism is unclear [3,7].

There are many classification systems for Müllerian abnormalities. The American Fertility Society (AFS) classification has been most widely used since 1988. Recently, however, new anatomic variants have been discovered, so a new classification was needed. The American Society for Reproductive Medicine (ASRM) updated the AFS's 1988 classification with simple and descriptive terminology for identifying anomalies of the uterus, cervix, and vagina. The ASRM Müllerian Anomalies Classification 2021 (MAC 2021) classifies Müllerian anomalies into nine categories and provides guidance on diagnostic and treatment options. Anomalies are classified into different categories based on descriptive terminology, which include Müllerian agenesis, cervical agenesis, unicornuate uterus, uterus didelphys, bicornuate uterus, septate uterus, longitudinal vaginal septum, transverse vaginal septum, and complex anomalies [8].

The most common symptoms of OHVIRA syndrome are nonspecific, with patients complaining of lower abdominal and pelvic pain, progressive dysmenorrhea, or cystic masses in the vaginal wall after menarche [9]. Additionally, the obstructed vaginal septum affects the menstrual flow and causes urinary incontinence, endometriosis, and pelvic infections, such as abscesses, pyosalpinx, and peritonitis [10]. Endometriosis and subsequent pelvic adhesions may result in infertility or miscarriages [11]. The diagnosis of OHVIRA syndrome is often delayed until after the early reproductive years due to the normal external genitalia [12,13]. Moreover, ipsilateral anomalies of the urinary system, such as kidney agenesis, dysplastic or polycystic kidney, and ectopic or duplicated ureters, have been reported. Coexisting urologic anomalies can result in recurrent urinary tract infections [10].

Early diagnosis of OHVIRA syndrome is important for managing clinical symptoms and preventing complications. A speculum examination may reveal features suggestive of OHVIRA syndrome, but radiologic examinations are essential for the definitive diagnosis [12]. MRI is the gold standard for imaging and identifying Müllerian anomalies, as it provides details about uterine morphology and vaginal luminal continuity. MRI can also identify renal abnormalities [14]. Additionally, 3D transvaginal ultrasound and 3D computed tomography can provide accurate anatomical information about the uterine cavity's external contour and internal shape [10]. These results can help determine appropriate treatment methods.

OHVIRA is typically diagnosed during the peri-pubertal period after the manifestation of menstruation-related problems, including dysmenorrhea and pelvic pain. With advances in sonographic imaging, neonatal diagnosis is becoming more frequent and often occurs after the incidental identification of hydrocolpos or renal agenesis. On the other hand, prenatal diagnosis of OVHIRA is extremely rare, with only two reported cases in the literature to date. Han et al. described a case of prenatal diagnosis of OHVIRA at 37 weeks of gestation following visualization of an absent left kidney and a cystic mass in the retrovesical space [15]. Tuna et al. reported a case of prenatal diagnosis of OHVIRA at 36 weeks' gestation after the detection of right renal agenesis and hydrocolpos. An MRI was performed in both cases to confirm the diagnoses [2]. These cases emphasize the significance of conducting a comprehensive prenatal sonographic examination to facilitate timely identification of OHVIRA syndrome during the prenatal phase. It is important to possess knowledge about OHVIRA syndrome for early diagnosis and subsequent treatment to prevent potential complications such as endometriosis, infertility, and spontaneous abortion. There is no clear optimal treatment for OHVIRA syndrome; however, most clinicians agree that, in most cases, resection of the vaginal septum restores reproductive function [10]. The resection is usually not an emergency and should be performed around the pubertal period, except for rare cases where OHVIRA is complicated by infections, such as pelvic inflammatory disease and abscess formation [11,13]. Surgical treatment is important and is the optimal treatment to relieve obstruction and symptoms, prevent complications of retrograde flow, and preserve fertility [14,16]. OHVIRA with a didelphys uterus has not been associated with infertility or pregnancy complications, such as spontaneous miscarriage or preterm delivery. However, OHVIRA with a septate uterus is a known risk factor for infertility and a cause of pregnancy complications, and pregnancy outcomes can be markedly improved after resection of the uterine septum [16]. The presence of a thick vaginal septum may restrict the distal distension of the affected hemivagina, leading to retrograde menstrual bleeding into the peritoneal cavity, ultimately resulting in endometriosis. Patients with OHVIRA have been reported to have a prevalence of endometriosis as high as 23%. Treatment with gonadotropin-releasing hormone analogs may be a good option for maintaining amenorrhea and reducing pelvic pain associated with endometriosis [10,11].

Gartner duct cysts are extremely rare in fetuses and neonates. They result from obstruction of the mesonephric duct system during fetal development and have been reported to be caused by a failure of separation of the ureteric bud from the mesonephric duct, but this remains unclear [5]. Gartner duct cysts are located in the anterior or lateral wall of the vagina. The vaginal cysts are lined with stratified squamous epithelium as they originate from the Müllerian duct, while Gartner duct cysts are lined with cuboidal epithelium. The majority of cases are asymptomatic and detected incidentally. The association of Gartner duct cysts with ipsilateral renal agenesis or dysplasia is infrequent and results from the abnormal development of the ureter [6]. For an accurate diagnosis, a physical examination and imaging tests, such as an ultrasound and an MRI, should be performed. During the examination, the patient should be positioned in the frog-leg position, and the labia majora should be delicately grasped and laterally pulled to examine the introitus and vagina. The management options are aspiration, deroofing, and the removal of the entire cyst through a vaginal approach [6]. The optimal timing for the treatment of Gartner duct cysts remains uncertain, particularly in newborns. Nevertheless, the long-term prognosis is generally favorable.

4. Conclusions

It is common for individuals with OHVIRA syndrome to exhibit symptoms such as progressive dysmenorrhea, abnormal pain, menstrual irregularities, and pelvic masses after the onset of menarche. Therefore, it is recommended that appropriate medical attention and management, perhaps initiated during adolescence, be provided to individuals with OHVIRA syndrome in order to prevent complications such as endometriosis, infertility, and spontaneous abortion. OHVIRA syndrome is associated with a favorable prognosis, and severe complications can be avoided by early diagnosis and surgical intervention. Gartner duct cysts are rare, associated with renal anomalies, and have a favorable long-term prognosis. The novel aspect of this report is the presentation of a case accompanied by a Gartner duct cyst in addition to OHVIRA syndrome. Therefore, a differential diagnosis is crucial since other genitourinary anomalies, such as Gartner duct cysts, may coexist. Therefore, clinicians, especially obstetricians and pediatricians, should perform systematic ultrasound examinations to identify any other genitourinary anomalies when encountering female fetuses with ipsilateral renal agenesis or vaginal cysts.

Author Contributions: Conceptualization, M.-H.P.; formal analysis, S.J.K.; investigation, S.J.K.; resources, M.-H.P.; data curation, S.J.K. and H.-H.C.; writing—original draft preparation, S.J.K.; writing—review and editing, S.J.K.; visualization, S.J.K., S.-Y.S. and H.-H.C.; supervision, K.A.L.; project administration, K.A.L. All authors have read and agreed to the published version of the manuscript.

Funding: This research received no external funding.

Institutional Review Board Statement: The study was conducted in accordance with the Declaration of Helsinki and approved by the Institutional Review Board of Ewha Womans University Seoul Hospital (protocol code 2022-07-028 and date of approval: 15 July 2022).

Informed Consent Statement: Patient consent was waived for the following reasons: No informed consent was required as the study was written only with the previous medical records.

Data Availability Statement: The data presented in this study are available on request from the corresponding author. The data are not publicly available due to privacy and ethical concerns.

Conflicts of Interest: The authors declare no conflict of interest.

References

1. Purslow, C.E. A case of unilateral haematocolps, haematometria, and haematosalpinx. *J. Obstet. Gynaecol. Br. Emp.* **1992**, *29*, 643. [CrossRef]
2. Tuna, T.; Estevão-Costa, J.; Ramalho, C.; Fragoso, A.C. Herlyn-Werner-Wunderlich syndrome: Report of a prenatally recognised case and review of the literature. *Urology* **2019**, *125*, 205–209. [CrossRef] [PubMed]
3. Burgis, J. Obstructive Müllerian anomalies: Case report, diagnosis, and management. *Am. J. Obstet. Gynecol.* **2001**, *185*, 338–344. [CrossRef] [PubMed]
4. Sheih, C.; Li, Y.W.; Liao, Y.J.; Huang, T.S.; Kao, S.P.; Chen, W.J. Diagnosing the combination of renal dysgenesis, Gartner's duct cyst and ipsilateral Mullerian duct obstruction. *J. Urol.* **1998**, *159*, 217–221. [CrossRef] [PubMed]
5. Coleman, R.; Sanchez, O.; Ghattaura, H.; Green, K.; Chandran, H.; McCarthy, L.; Parashar, K. Tubulocystic anomalies of the mesonephric duct associated with ipsilateral renal dysgenesis. *J. Pediatr. Urol.* **2019**, *15*, 46.e1–46.e6. [CrossRef] [PubMed]

6. Tiwari, C.; Shah, H.; Desale, J.; Waghmare, M. Neonatal Gartner duct cyst: Two cases reports and literature review. *Dev. Period. Med.* **2017**, *21*, 35–37. [PubMed]
7. Feng, T.; Rao, X.; Yang, X.; Yu, X.; Xia, F.; Du, X. A rare variant of obstructed hemivagina and ipsilateral renal agenesis and its improvement of classification. *J. Obstet. Gynaecol. Res.* **2022**, *48*, 869–874. [CrossRef] [PubMed]
8. Pfeifer, S.M.; Attaran, M.; Goldstein, J.; Lindheim, S.R.; Petrozza, J.C.; Rackow, B.W.; Siegelman, E.; Troiano, R.; Winter, T.; Zuckerman, A.; et al. ASRM müllerian anomalies classification 2021. *Fertil. Steril.* **2021**, *116*, 1238–1252. [CrossRef] [PubMed]
9. Wdowiarz, K.; Skrajna, A.; Reinholz-Jaskólska, M. Diagnosis and treatment of Herlyn-Werner-Wunderlich syndrome: A case report. *Menopause Rev.* **2021**, *20*, 52–56. [CrossRef] [PubMed]
10. Miyazaki, Y.; Orisaka, M.; Nishino, C.; Onuma, T.; Kurokawa, T.; Yoshida, Y. Herlyn-Werner-Wunderlich syndrome with cervical atresia complicated by ovarian endometrioma: A case report. *J. Obstet. Gynaecol. Res.* **2020**, *46*, 347–351. [CrossRef] [PubMed]
11. Lee, J.M. Herlyn-Werner-Wunderlich syndrome: A mini-review. *Child. Kidney Dis.* **2018**, *22*, 12–16. [CrossRef]
12. Pittokopitou, S.; Kathopoulis, N.; Protopapas, A.; Domali, E. Herlyn–Werner–Wunderlich syndrome: Report of a delayed diagnosed case with video presentation of the operative technique of vaginal septum resection. *J. Obstet. Gynaecol. Res.* **2021**, *47*, 2242–2245. [CrossRef] [PubMed]
13. Kamio, M.; Nagata, C.; Sameshima, H.; Togami, S.; Kobayashi, H. Obstructed hemivagina and ipsilateral renal anomaly (OHVIRA) syndrome with septic shock: A case report. *J. Obstet. Gynaecol. Res.* **2018**, *44*, 1326–1329. [CrossRef] [PubMed]
14. Fachin, C.G.; Rocha, J.L.A.S.; Maltoni, A.A.; das Chagas Lima, R.L.; Zendim, V.A.; Agulham, M.A.; Tsouristakis, A.; dos Santos Dias, A.I.R. Herlyn-Werner-Wunderlich syndrome: Diagnosis and treatment of an atypical case and review of literature. *Int. J. Surg. Case Rep.* **2019**, *63*, 129–134. [CrossRef] [PubMed]
15. Han, B.H.; Park, S.B.; Lee, Y.J.; Lee, K.S.; Lee, Y.K. Uterus didelphys with blind hemivagina and ipsilateral renal agenesis (Herlyn-Werner-Wunderlich syndrome) suspected on the presence of hydrocolpos on prenatal sonography. *J. Clin. Ultrasound.* **2013**, *41*, 380–382. [CrossRef] [PubMed]
16. Yi, S.; Jiang, J. Clinical characteristics and management of patients with complete septate uterus, double cervix, obstructed hemivagina, and ipsilateral renal agenesis. *J. Obstet. Gynaecol. Res.* **2021**, *47*, 1497–1501. [CrossRef] [PubMed]

Disclaimer/Publisher's Note: The statements, opinions and data contained in all publications are solely those of the individual author(s) and contributor(s) and not of MDPI and/or the editor(s). MDPI and/or the editor(s) disclaim responsibility for any injury to people or property resulting from any ideas, methods, instructions or products referred to in the content.

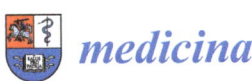

Review

Invasive Prenatal Diagnostic Testing for Aneuploidies in Singleton Pregnancies: A Comparative Review of Major Guidelines

Eirini Giovannopoulou [1], Ioannis Tsakiridis [1,*], Apostolos Mamopoulos [1], Ioannis Kalogiannidis [1], Ioannis Papoulidis [1,2], Apostolos Athanasiadis [1] and Themistoklis Dagklis [1]

[1] Third Department of Obstetrics and Gynaecology, School of Medicine, Faculty of Health Sciences, Aristotle University of Thessaloniki, 541 24 Thessaloniki, Greece
[2] Access to Genome—ATG, Clinical Laboratory Genetics, 551 34 Thessaloniki, Greece
* Correspondence: iotsakir@gmail.com; Tel.: +30-231-331-2120; Fax: +30-2310-992950

Abstract: Sophisticated screening protocols for genetic abnormalities constitute an important component of current prenatal care, aiming to identify high-risk pregnancies and offer appropriate counseling to parents regarding their options. Definite prenatal diagnosis is only possible by invasive prenatal diagnostic testing (IPDT), mainly including amniocentesis and chorionic villous sampling (CVS). The aim of this comparative review was to summarize and compare the existing recommendations on IPDT from the most influential guidelines. All the reviewed guidelines highlight that IPDT is indicated based on a positive screening test rather than maternal age alone. Other indications arise from medical history and sonography, with significant variations identified between the guidelines. The earlier time for amniocentesis is unequivocally set at ≥ 15 gestational weeks, whereas for CVS, the earlier limit varies from ≥ 10 to ≥ 11 weeks. Certain technical aspects and the overall approach demonstrate significant differences. Periprocedural management regarding Rhesus alloimmunization, virologic status and use of anesthesia or antibiotics are either inconsistent or insufficiently addressed. The synthesis of an evidence-based algorithm for IPDT is of crucial importance to healthcare professionals implicated in prenatal care to avoid unnecessary interventions without compromising optimal prenatal care.

Keywords: invasive prenatal diagnostic testing; chorionic villous sampling (CVS); amniocentesis; indications; technique; complications

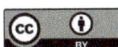

1. Introduction

Prenatal care involves providing a bundle of examinations and guidance to the pregnant woman, to promote education and awareness and prevent or ameliorate adverse outcomes [1]. Detection of genetic abnormalities and birth defects has been a main focus of prenatal screening policies, although screening has also expanded to include potentially preventable adverse outcomes, including preeclampsia, preterm birth and stillbirth [2]. Genetic or birth defects complicate about 3% of births; chromosomal abnormalities include aneuploidies, translocations, deletions and duplications [3]. Major chromosomal abnormalities affect up to 1 in 140 live births [4].

Prenatal screening protocols for common aneuploidies, especially trisomy 21, implement various sonographic and/or biochemical markers to produce a risk stratification [2]. During the past few decades, a substantial shift from maternal age alone-based screening to more sophisticated combined screening protocols evolved in clinical practice [5,6]. Different strategies of screening have been proposed in the literature, including integrated, stepwise sequential or contingency screening that are available in the first and/or second trimesters of pregnancy [7,8]. Aneuploidy screening has radically changed following the introduction of cell-free DNA (cfDNA) testing, which has been validated as a highly accurate screening tool, especially in singleton pregnancies [9].

According to its definition, screening provides only a risk estimate and does not constitute a diagnosis. Definite diagnosis is only achieved by cytogenetic analysis of cells obtained through invasive prenatal diagnostic testing (IPDT); the latter includes chorionic villous sampling (CVS) and amniocentesis as well as fetal blood sampling (FBS) under specific indications [10,11]. The first diagnostic amniocentesis for trisomy 21 dates back to 1968 [12], and the description of the technique preceded this by several years [13,14]. Amniocentesis became the gold standard of prenatal diagnosis during the 1970s, and CVS was introduced a decade later [15,16]. Since then, as experience in IPDT has accumulated, several alterations were implemented on indications, timing, technical aspects and cytogenetic analysis techniques; procedure-related complications were also described [11]. The choice of the procedure is affected by both the operator's expertise and the individual patient's preferences that are reflected in decision making. IPDT should be undertaken by appropriately trained healthcare professionals, taking into consideration the inter-operator variability, as well as the associated cost [17–19].

Several medical societies have developed guidelines to address the issues related to IPDT and guide clinical practice, which has substantially evolved during the past few decades. As there are considerable differences in recommended practices and approaches, usually affected by cost-effectiveness analyses and associated healthcare policies, we decided to undertake this review to summarize and compare the recommendations provided by influential medical societies with regard to IPDT for fetal genetic defects and underline potential agreements and disagreements.

2. Evidence Acquisition

The most recently published guidelines from seven medical societies on IPDT were retrieved, and a descriptive review was performed. We included recommendations from the National Society of Genetic Counselors (NSGC 2013) [7], the American College of Obstetricians and Gynecologists and the Society for Maternal-Fetal Medicine (ACOG-SMFM 2016) [20], the International Society of Ultrasound in Obstetrics and Gynecology (ISUOG 2016) [21], the Human Genetics Society of Australasia and the Royal Australian and New Zealand College of Obstetricians and Gynaecologists (HGSA—RANZCOG 2018) [22], as well as the Royal College of Obstetricians and Gynaecologists (RCOG 2021) [23].

An overview of recommendations is presented in Table 1 (indications for IPDT), Table 2 (amniocentesis), Table 3 (chorionic villus sampling) and Table 4 (periprocedural management). Of note, the RCOG guideline does not make any reference to the indications of IPDT.

Table 1. Summary of recommendations on the indications for invasive prenatal diagnostic testing.

	NSGC	ACOG-SMFM	ISUOG	HGSA-RANZCOG	RCOG
Issued	2013	2016	2016	2018	2021
Title	NSGC Practice Guideline: Prenatal Screening and Diagnostic Testing Options for Chromosome Aneuploidy.	Prenatal Diagnostic Testing for Genetic Disorders.	ISUOG Practice Guidelines: Invasive procedures for prenatal diagnosis.	Prenatal screening and diagnostic testing for fetal chromosomal and genetic conditions.	Amniocentesis and chorionic villus sampling.
Pages	12	14	13	35	15
References	44	74	106	47	55

Table 1. Cont.

	NSGC	ACOG-SMFM	ISUOG	HGSA-RANZCOG	RCOG
Issued	2013	2016	2016	2018	2021
Indications for IPDT	Positive screening result. Ultrasound findings (NT > 3.0 mm or >95th percentile).	Positive screening result. Ultrasound findings (not specified).	Positive screening result. Ultrasound findings (structural defects associated with chromosomal abnormalities).	Positive screening result.	Not discussed
Past History	Not discussed	Previous child or fetus with chromosomal aneuploidy. Known parental carrier status.	Previous child or fetus with chromosomal aneuploidy. Known parental carrier status.	Not discussed	Not discussed
Maternal request	Available to all women.	Available to all women.	Only under specific circumstances.	Available to all women.	Not discussed
Maternal age	Not discussed	Advanced maternal age does not justify invasive testing.	Advanced maternal age does not justify invasive testing.	Available to all women irrespective of age.	Not discussed
Assisted Reproduction Techniques (ART)	Not discussed	Not discussed	IVF or ICSI is not an indication for IPDT.	Not discussed	Not discussed
Cell-free DNA	A positive cfDNA result.	A positive cfDNA result.	A positive cfDNA result.	A positive or a "no call" cfDNA result.	Not discussed

ICSI: intracytoplasmic sperm injection; IVF: in vitro fertilization; IPDT: invasive prenatal genetic diagnosis; NT: nuchal translucency.

Table 2. Summary of recommendations on amniocentesis.

	NSGC	ACOG-SMFM	ISUOG	HGSA-RANZCOG	RCOG
Issued	2013	2016	2016	2018	2021
Timing	≥15 weeks	≥15 weeks	≥15 weeks	≥15 weeks Not recommended before 14 weeks.	≥15 weeks
Technique	Not discussed	Continuous ultrasound guidance. Sterile technique. Needle size 22 G.	Continuous ultrasound guidance. Aseptic technique. Maximum needle size 20–22 G. Avoid placenta and placental cord insertion site, especially in Rhesus-negative women.	Not discussed	Continuous ultrasound guidance. Aseptic technique.
Complications	Fetal loss, limb defects, membrane rupture.	Fetal loss, vaginal spotting, membrane rupture.	Fetal loss, chorioamnionitis, membrane rupture. Fetal injury, maternal complications (rare).	Not discussed	Fetal loss, severe infection, fetal injury, maternal visceral injury.
Maternal cell contamination	Not discussed	Discard the first 1–2 mL.	Discard the first 2 mL.	Not discussed	Risk 1–2%.

Table 3. Summary of recommendations on chorionic villus sampling.

	NSGC	ACOG-SMFM	ISUOG	HGSA-RANZCOG	RCOG
Issued	2013	2016	2016	2018	2021
Timing	Not discussed	≥10 weeks	≥10 weeks	≥11 weeks	≥10 weeks If possible after 11 completed weeks, when technically easier.

Table 3. Cont.

	NSGC	ACOG-SMFM	ISUOG	HGSA-RANZCOG	RCOG
Issued	2013	2016	2016	2018	2021
Technique	Not discussed	Transabdominal or transcervical approach. Continuous ultrasound guidance.	Transabdominal or transcervical approach. Continuous ultrasound guidance. Aseptic technique.	Not discussed	Continuous ultrasound guidance. Aseptic technique.
Complications	Fetal loss, limb defects (especially before 10 weeks). Procedure-related complications comparable with amniocentesis, only in experienced centers.	Fetal loss, vaginal bleeding, limb defects (especially before 10 weeks).	Fetal loss, vaginal bleeding, amniotic fluid leakage, chorioamnionitis.	Not discussed	Fetal loss, severe infection, fetal injury, maternal visceral injury.

Table 4. Summary of recommendations on periprocedural management at invasive prenatal diagnostic testing.

	NSGC	ACOG-SMFM	ISUOG	HGSA-RANZCOG	RCOG
Issued	2013	2016	2016	2018	2021
Periprocedural management	Not discussed	Not discussed	Provide a detailed report. Ultrasound check for fetal heart rate, hematoma and amniotic fluid after the procedure.	Not discussed	Need to have a written consent form before invasive testing.
Rhesus alloimmunization	Not discussed	Not discussed	Check Rhesus and alloantibodies. Administer anti-D immunoglobulin in Rhesus-negative women within 72 h, unless there is proof that the alleged father is Rhesus-negative.	Not discussed	Inform patients of aftercare, including Rhesus immunization in non-sensitized Rhesus-negative women.
Blood-borne viral diseases	Not discussed	Routine screening not recommended. Recommendations apply to known chronic infections.	Routine screening for transmittable viral diseases not recommended.	Not discussed	Universal screening for blood-borne viral disease is recommended and is performed by review of previous records.
HIV, HBV, HCV	Not discussed	Low incidence of HBV vertical transmission with low viral load. Risk for HCV vertical transmission presumably low. Low risk of HIV vertical transmission in women under antiretroviral therapy and undetectable viral load. Optimally postpone invasive testing until viral load is below detection cut-off. Data for CVS are limited.	Noninvasive testing is preferable to invasive procedures in known HCV-, HBV- or HIV-positive status. If invasive testing is performed, avoid the placenta. In cases of HBsAg (+)/HbeAg (−) or HIV (+) in HAART, the risk of vertical transmission is not increased.	Not discussed	HBV or HCV infection is not a contraindication for invasive testing. Minimal risk for vertical transmission for HBV and low viral load and no proven risk for HCV. Withhold invasive testing until HIV results available. In cases of HIV (+) under HAART, the risk is low. Optimally, postpone invasive testing until viral load is below detection cut-off.

Table 4. Cont.

	NSGC	ACOG-SMFM	ISUOG	HGSA-RANZCOG	RCOG
Issued	2013	2016	2016	2018	2021
Aseptic technique	Not discussed	Sterile technique. Details not specified.	Sterile gloves, gauzes, needles, forceps. Skin decontamination (chlorhexidine or iodine). Sterile drape. Sterile bag for ultrasound probe or probe disinfection. Sterile gel. Sterile speculum and disinfection of cervical and vaginal mucosa for transcervical CVS.	Not discussed	Skin decontamination. Sterile bag for ultrasound probe. Sterile gel.
Anesthesia	Not discussed	Not discussed	Local anesthesia not recommended for amniocentesis. There are no available data for transcervical CVS. Consider local anesthesia for transabdominal CVS to reduce discomfort and maternal movement.	Not discussed	Not discussed
Ultrasound evaluation	Not discussed	Not discussed	Pre-procedural (HR, GA, placenta, amniotic fluid). Post-procedural (HR. placenta, amniotic fluid). Check for complications immediately after or even days after.	Not discussed	Not discussed
Antibiotics	Not discussed	Not discussed	Antibiotic prophylaxis not recommended.	Not discussed	Consider antibiotic therapy in cases of purulent or cloudy amniotic aspirate or in the presence of clinical chorioamnionitis.
Thromboprophylaxis	Not discussed	Not discussed	Discontinuation of the regimen in women receiving thromboprophylaxis or low dose aspirin is not recommended.	Not discussed	Not discussed
Counseling	Refer for genetic counseling when there are concerns in decision making.	Offer pretest counseling. Nondirective counseling. Refer to genetic counseling after a suspected diagnosis of aneuploidy or in complex cases of mosaicism.	Offer pretest counseling. Genetic counseling in cases of sample mosaicism.	Offer individualized counseling. Genetic counseling in high-risk women	Pretest counseling by appropriately trained professionals.

HIV: human immunodeficiency virus; HBV: hepatitis-B virus; HCV: hepatitis-C virus; CVS: chorionic villus sampling; HAART: highly active antiretroviral therapy; HR: heart rate; GA: gestational age.

3. Indications for Invasive Prenatal Diagnostic Testing

It is well-documented that prenatal screening for fetal aneuploidies should be offered to all women [24]. Screening options are delineated by guidelines and local standards. However, as already mentioned, the result of a screening test does not constitute a definite diagnosis. Definite diagnosis requires IPDT, which is generally reserved for high-risk women.

3.1. High-Risk Groups for Fetal Aneuploidy

Several reviewed guidelines recommend offering IPDT when a screening test is positive or above predetermined cut-off values, including variable protocols for combined screening (NSGC, ACOG-SMFM, ISUOG, HGSA-RANZOG). Moreover, abnormal ultrasound findings represent another common indication for IPDT (NSGC, ACOG-SMFM, ISUOG); however, specific ultrasound findings that require diagnostic testing differ among these guidelines. In particular, ACOG-SMFM does not specify the ultrasound findings that should prompt investigation with IPDT. However, it is stated that the risk fluctuates based on the number and type of the anomalies. Wladimiroff et al. described the findings from karyotyping a total of 170 fetuses with specific structural defects or fetal growth restriction, polyhydramnios and fetal hydrops [25]. The majority of the cases included either one major defect (including cardiac defects, duodenal atresia, omphalocele or cystic hygroma), multiple minor defects or rare deficits; a chromosomal abnormality was detected in 20.5% of the analyzed cases [25]. ISUOG defines abnormal ultrasound findings as the recognition of a structural anomaly indicative of chromosomal abnormalities, but does not provide specific information on these abnormalities. Additionally, the NSGC states that a nuchal translucency (NT) measuring ≥ 3 mm or above the 95th percentile should be followed by IPDT. Souka et al., in a review on the association between increased NT and major fetal abnormalities in chromosomally normal fetuses, found that the prevalence of abnormalities increases with NT thickness (1.6% in NT < 95th percentile, 2.5% for NT between 95th and 99th percentiles, up to 45% for NT ≥ 6.5 mm) [26].

3.2. Past History

A personal history of a previous child or fetus diagnosed with chromosomal abnormality poses an independent indication for invasive testing (ACOG-SMFM, ISUOG). This is derived and supported by data reporting increased risk of recurrence in subsequent pregnancies [27]. Warburton et al. investigated the risk for trisomy recurrence combining the data from two large databases; the risk for trisomy 21 recurrence is higher than the expected based on maternal age, when the first occurrence was after 30 years of age [27]. Nevertheless, the risk of recurrence of a viable trisomy is multiplied by 1.6 to 1.8 after a previous history of trisomy 21, 18 or 13, independently of the viability of the fetus [27].

As far as parental status is concerned, known carrier status for a balanced chromosomal translocation or inversion or parental aneuploidy or mosaicism for aneuploidy justify further diagnostic testing according to ACOG-SMFM and ISUOG. Parental carrier status that has been diagnosed after a history of an affected child dramatically increases the risk for chromosomal abnormality in the current pregnancy, compared to cases incidentally diagnosed, with no previous history [28]. More specifically, the relevant risks are 5–30% compared to 0–5% for translocations and 5–10% compared to 1–3% for inversions [28].

3.3. Maternal Request

NSGC, ACOG-SMFM and HGSA-RANZCOG support offering the option of IPDT to all women, irrespective of age or other risk factors. According to ISUOG, however, IPDT is not justified based solely on maternal request and should be offered only after extensive counseling by an expert. The reasoning behind offering to all women the option of invasive testing is supported by the fact that using array comparative genomic hybridization (array-CGH) technology in pregnant women, irrespective of age, with normal ultrasound and karyotype, the risk of finding a pathogenic copy number variant is >1% [29,30]. Taking into consideration the distribution of maternal age, which gradually increases, the reduced complication rates of invasive procedures and the personal beliefs and expectations of each woman for their pregnancy, an individualized approach is encouraged to allow for informed decisions regarding invasive testing [31,32].

3.4. Maternal Age

ACOG-SMFM, ISUOG and HGSA-RANZCOG agree that maternal age as a standalone criterion is not an indication for invasive prenatal testing. The concept of maternal age-based strategies for IPDT has been re-evaluated in the past two decades [31]. There is a shift towards screening-based risk stratification and maternal age is co-evaluated among other factors, derived from screening protocols [32–35]. This shift is justified, as screening strategies are evolving to become more sensitive and intend to minimize procedure-related risks and costs, associated with invasive testing [31].

3.5. Assisted Reproduction Techniques

ISUOG recommends against routine IPDT following IVF or ICSI, in the absence of other risk factors; however, in the context of ICSI due to oligospermia, it recommends counseling of the couple for the higher risk of chromosomal abnormalities associated with infertility in the male offspring. Bonduelle et al. investigated 1586 fetuses conceived by ICSI and found a significantly higher rate of inherited chromosomal abnormalities in these cases, compared to the general population (1.4% vs. 0.3%) [36]. The majority were attributed to the male partner and associated with sperm quality, initially necessitating ICSI [36]. The other guidelines do not make any relevant recommendation.

3.6. Cell-Free DNA

cfDNA is based on the analysis of circulating fractions of fetal DNA in maternal serum to achieve prenatal screening for aneuploidies [37,38]. cfDNA is a screening and not diagnostic test and therefore should not substitute IPDT (NSGC). The role of cfDNA is either as a first-tier screening tool for fetal aneuploidy or as second-tier screening after a positive screening result (derived, for example, from combined first trimester screening) and before IPDT is undertaken (HGSA-RANZCOG). The latter approach may place some originally high-risk women at a low-risk level, and as they may avoid invasive testing, some cases with aneuploidy may be missed [39]. In any case, a positive result of a non-invasive prenatal test (NIPT) should be referred for IPDT (NSGC, ACOG-SMFM, ISUOG, HGSA-RANZCOG). Moreover, low fractions of cfDNA in maternal serum (less than 4%) may lead to an inconclusive test result, referred to as a "no call" result [24]. HGSA-RANZCOG suggests IPDT among other options (detailed ultrasound follow-up or combined screening if not already performed or even repeat cfDNA, on the grounds of a higher risk of aneuploidy). Pergament et al. analyzed cfDNA in 1051 pregnancies and found that in cases of aneuploidy, a percentage as high as 16% did not return a result; in half of these cases, the fetal fraction was below the 1.5th percentile compared to normal euploid samples [40]. Moreover, a "no-call" result due to a low fraction of cfDNA was associated with significantly higher odds for aneuploidy (OR: 5.7; 95% CI: 2.5–13.1), compared to samples within the normal range [40]. Several studies have demonstrated that fetal fraction is significantly higher in trisomy 21 and lower in trisomies 13, 18 and triploidies, compared to euploid pregnancies [41,42].

Of note, there may be additional contributing factors to a "no-call" result in the context of aneuploidy, other than low fetal fraction, that have not been extensively investigated or understood [43]. Particularly, variables such as maternal body mass index, maternal age, gestational age, medications, ethnicity and conception through assisted reproduction techniques may also interfere with the fraction of cfDNA, acting as significant confounders to the interpretation of the results [42,44,45]. Repeating the cfDNA test at a later gestational age in these cases is reasonable (as cfDNA fraction increases with advancing gestational age), but may delay definite diagnosis [43,45,46]. Previous screening results and ultrasound findings should be taken into account in the interpretation of noninformative results and clinical decision making [42].

Another concern is that confined placental mosaicism (CPM) is a common cause of a false positive cfDNA result associated with a normal euploid fetus [47]. On the other hand, CVS is associated with an incidence of about 2% of cell mosaicism, and only 13% of those cases correspond to true fetal mosaicism, as confirmed by amniocentesis [48]. Therefore, since CPM may per se be the reason for an abnormal cDNA result, there are thoughts about the potential superiority of amniocentesis over CVS to provide a definite diagnosis in such cases [49]; however, this issue is not addressed by the reviewed guidelines.

4. Available Techniques for Invasive Prenatal Diagnostic Testing
4.1. Amniocentesis
4.1.1. Timing

All guidelines agree that amniocentesis should be performed only after 15 completed gestational weeks. The reason for this recommendation is the well-documented higher risk of procedure-related complications in cases of early amniocentesis, including pregnancy loss, fetal congenital defects and membrane rupture at an earlier gestational age [50–53].

4.1.2. Technical Aspects

Amniocentesis involves the insertion of a needle system through the abdominal wall into the amniotic cavity to obtain amniotic fluid for genetic analysis [54]. The sample contains fetal exfoliated cells, transudate, fetal urine and secretions [54]. The maximum caliber of the needle for amniocentesis is a key technical aspect. ACOG-SMFM recommends a 22-gauge needle, whereas according to the ISUOG guidelines, either a 20 G or 22 G needle may be used; a larger caliber needle is associated with quicker fluid aspiration without increasing the risk of intrauterine bleeding [55]. Based on the findings of previous studies, transplacental needle passage increases the risk of contamination with blood [56–58]. Therefore, the passage of the needle through the placenta or at the placental cord insertion site should be avoided, unless it is the only alternative to safely access an adequate amniotic fluid pool. ACOG-SMFM and ISUOG further underline the importance of such an approach, especially for Rhesus-negative women, due to the potentially higher incidence of feto-maternal hemorrhage and alloimmunization [58]. ISUOG, ACOG-SMFM and RCOG highlight the necessity of continuous ultrasound visualization during the procedure. Of note, the other guidelines do not make any relevant recommendation.

4.1.3. Maternal Cell Contamination

ACOG-SMFM, ISUOG and RCOG are the only guidelines that comment on the possibility of maternal cell contamination in the sample retrieved from amniocentesis. The frequency of this condition greatly varies among different series and is higher in cases of transplacental passage, need for second needle insertion, operator's lack of experience and blood staining of the amniotic fluid [59–61]. In order to avoid maternal contamination, ACOG-SMFM and ISUOG encourage the disposal of the first 1–2 mL that are aspirated. RCOG states that the possibility of maternal contamination during amniocentesis is 1–2% but does not provide any further guidance on this matter.

4.1.4. Complications

Like any interventional procedure, amniocentesis is not without complications. In fact, this is a key issue in counseling, as parents need to decide based on the trade-off between the advantage of diagnosis and the associated risks. Fetal loss, postprocedural fluid leakage, fetal defects and chorioamnionitis are the main concerns following amniocentesis; the rate of estimated procedure-related complications varies among studies and, therefore, between different guidelines. According to ACOG-SMFM, amniocentesis has an overall complication rate of 0.1–0.3%, as suggested by recent studies [62–64]. Akolekar et al. conducted a systematic review and metanalysis on procedure-related fetal loss, including 42,716 women undergoing amniocentesis [62]. The procedure-related loss was estimated at 0.11%. Similarly, Odibo et al. provided data from a single-center retrospective analysis of 11,746 women subjected to amniocentesis, and the associated risk was estimated at 0.13% [63]. Moreover, Caughey et al. reported a fetal loss rate of 0.27% following amniocentesis [64].

NSGC agrees that fetal loss ranges between 0.1% and 0.3%, complying with the lower risk estimates [65]. On the other hand, ISUOG and RCOG refer to slightly higher miscarriage rates of 0.1–1% and <0.5%, respectively. A recent meta-analysis on procedure-related losses, including 64,901 amniocentesis and 19,000 CVS, updated the procedure-related fetal losses at 0.35% for both procedures [66]. According to ISUOG, fetal loss increases with multiple needle insertions, blood contamination of the amniotic fluid and the presence of an underlying fetal abnormality [67,68].

Rupture of membranes is another potential complication of amniocentesis, encountered in 1–2% of cases [53,69–71]. Congenital limb malformation is another concern; NSGC estimates the possibility of clubfoot to be less than 1% [53,69,72]. Post-procedural infection of the fetal membranes, clinically presenting as chorioamnionitis, is quite rare, with an incidence of <0.1%, as described by ISUOG. Other severe feto-maternal complications have been only occasionally reported and considered rare, such as sepsis, maternal visceral injury or fetal injury. Of note, experience, reflected on the number of procedures performed annually by each operator, also plays a critical role in the incidence of procedure-related complications [73–75]. Baker et al. retrospectively investigated the effect of multiple variables on procedure-related fetal losses after CVS and amniocentesis and found a positive association between increasing experience and lower procedure-related risks, highlighting that actual risks may be lower than those initially estimated and on which routine counseling is based [76]. Therefore, counseling should be accordingly reformed to incorporate the updated available evidence on associated risks.

4.2. Chorionic Villous Sampling

4.2.1. Timing

CVS is the only available diagnostic test during the first trimester (NSGC, ACOG-SMFM, ISUOG, HGSA-RANZCOG, RCOG), as early amniocentesis before 14 weeks is unanimously discouraged due to an unacceptably higher rate of complications [50–53]. However, the optimal gestational age after which CVS should be performed is not clear; NSGC, ACOG-SMFM, ISUOG and RCOG set the safe limit to perform CVS at 10 weeks, while HGSA-RANZOG recommends against CVS before 11 completed gestational weeks due to a higher risk of limb defects. RCOG also states that CVS should ideally be performed after 11 completed weeks, as the suboptimal development of the trophoblastic tissue increases the technical difficulty of the procedure at an earlier gestational age.

4.2.2. Technical Aspects

CVS includes the introduction of a needle system through the abdomen (transabdominal) or the cervix (transcervical) to retrieve chorionic tissue from the developing placenta for genetic analysis [19]. CVS can be safely carried out by either a transabdominal or transcervical approach by continuous US guidance (ISUOG, ACOG-SMFM, RCOG). ISUOG makes a recommendation on the needle size, recommending either a single needle of 17–20 G or a two-needle system with outer needle size of 17/19 G and inner needle size of 19/20 G. The variation in the technique and the needle size in clinical practice is highlighted by the study of Carlin et al. that reviewed the individual preferences in U.K. practice [77]. Like the amniocentesis technique, apart from ISUOG and RCOG, the other guidelines do not make any relevant recommendation.

4.2.3. Complications

Regarding the risk of pregnancy loss, CVS is comparable to mid-trimester amniocentesis, when performed by experienced operators. ACOG-SMFM reports a procedure-related loss of 0.22%, while ISUOG provides an estimate for fetal loss that greatly varies between 0.2% and 2% [62], underlining the absence of well-designed randomized controlled studies. In the systematic review and meta-analysis conducted by Akolekar et al., which included 8899 CVS procedures, the risk was estimated at 0.22% [62]. NSGC sets the risk between 0.5% and 1% and RCOG below 0.5%. Odibo et al. retrospectively evaluated the risk of pregnancy loss in 5148 CVS procedures and found a risk estimate of 0.2% and 0.5% for transabdominal and transcervical procedures, respectively [78]. Interestingly, the risk was not statistically different from the background risk in the control group [78]. CVS may also be associated with vaginal bleeding in 10% or even 30% of cases after a transcervical approach [79,80]. In addition, amniotic fluid leakage and intra-amniotic infection are encountered much less often (<0.5% and 1–2 per 3000 cases, respectively), according to ACOG-SMFM and ISUOG [79]. As far as maternal safety is concerned, no cases of severe maternal adverse outcomes have been described following CVS, or at worst, they are very rare [23].

4.2.4. Fetal Blood Sampling

FBS entails access to fetal circulation in order to obtain a blood sample for analysis. Fetal blood is obtained via puncture of the umbilical vein, and therefore, also referred to as "cordocentesis". The umbilical vein can be accessed either at the cord (cord insertion or independent loop) or even at its intrahepatic portion, according to placental location [81]. FBS is the first-line option for the hematologic assessment of the fetus in cases of severe anemia or thrombocytopenia. However, its role in prenatal genetic diagnosis is limited [81]. The only guideline that refers to FBS as a means of prenatal diagnosis is ISUOG. FBS is indicated in cases of mosaicism of the sample obtained from invasive testing, to exclude true fetal mosaicism. Concerning indications, the ISUOG guideline refers to investigation of mosaicism solely after amniocentesis with no referral to CVS. According to ISUOG, cordocentesis for FBS can be performed from 18 completed weeks [81], and the risk of procedure-related pregnancy loss is 1–2% [82]. However, this risk increases with gestational age under 24 weeks, possibly due to associated structural malformations or fetal growth restriction [83,84]. According to ISUOG, the optimal technique includes the use of a 20–22 G needle that is inserted to the cord, through the abdomen, under simultaneous ultrasound visualization.

5. Periprocedural Management

The optimal management of a woman who has an indication for invasive diagnosis is minutely delineated by the ISUOG and RCOG guidelines (ACOG-SMFM makes recommendations only for transmittable diseases).

a. Rhesus status

According to ISUOG, Rhesus status of the mother, along with the existence of alloantibodies in the maternal serum, is a prerequisite before the procedure, in order to administer immunoglobulin in Rhesus-negative women. Anti-D administration, when indicated, should not delay more than 72 h from the procedure (ISUOG). Additionally, according to ISUOG, immunization could be omitted, if the Rhesus status of the presumed father has been confirmed as negative. RCOG states that Rhesus-negative women should be provided appropriate aftercare for immunization but does not offer any further guidance.

b. Transmittable diseases

There is controversy regarding the need for screening for maternal blood-borne diseases before IPDT. In particular, ISUOG recommends against routine screening, based on available data indicating that vertical transmission is an unlikely event and may only affect pregnancies with high maternal viral load [85,86]. ISUOG also states that when invasive diagnosis is indicated, placental penetration should be avoided in women known to be HIV-, HBV- or HCV-positive [85]. On the other hand, RCOG emphasizes the need for universal screening or counseling for women who are unwilling to undergo virology testing, for the potential of vertical transmission during the procedure. Data mainly pertain to amniocentesis, as studies for vertical transmission of chronic infection in CVS are lacking.

5.1. HIV

ACOG-SMFM states that HIV transmission is not increased in women receiving antiretroviral therapy and whose viral load is undetectable. The ISUOG recommendation agrees that HIV-positive women on highly active antiretroviral therapy (HAART) are not at increased risk for vertical transmission [87], even if the viral load is high, as far as HAART is initiated at least two weeks before the procedure [88,89]. Postponement of the procedure until the viral load is undetectable is also suggested by ACOG-SMFM [85,90]. According to RCOG, IPDT should be withheld until HIV results are available. For HIV-positive women under HAART, therapy optimization to aim for undetectable viral load is reasonable before any intervention, to minimize the risk of vertical transmission [91].

5.2. HBV

ACOG-SMFM aligns with the low incidence of neonatal infection in HBV-infected mothers with low viral load but also underlines the relevant gap in the literature for exposed cases [92]. RCOG considers the risk for vertical transmission for HBV infection to be low unless the viral load exceeds the threshold of $\geq 7 \log_{10}$ copies/mL; individualized assessment of risk is thus recommended.

5.3. HCV

ACOG-SMFM comments on the paucity of knowledge regarding vertical transmission of HCV but states that the risk is presumably low [93]. ISUOG also underlines the importance of counseling about the limited data on fetal infection for CVS or FBS, compared to amniocentesis [85], while recommending that the option of non-invasive testing should be considered in women with transmittable diseases, in the absence of adequate high-quality evidence [69]. RCOG comments on the absence of evidence of HCV vertical transmission [93].

5.4. SARS-CoV-2

During the SARS-CoV-2 pandemic, another issue is dealing with pregnant women who tested positive and are in need of IPDT. Chronologically, the majority of the included guidelines (except RCOG) preceded the pandemic and hence, relevant recommendations are not available. The best available data, although limited, suggest that invasive testing is safe in COVID-19-positive pregnant women and the risk of vertical transmission is considered to be low [94].

c. Aseptic technique

To minimize the risk of infection, ACOG-SMFM, ISUOG and RCOG highlight the importance of a sterile technique. Of note, ISUOG and RCOG encourage the use of a sterile containment bag for the ultrasound probe and a separate sterile gel; decontamination of the ultrasound probe after each procedure is an alternative to the sterile bag (ISUOG). Moreover, both ISUOG and RCOG underline the significance of skin sterilization. ISUOG suggests skin decontamination with a chlorhexidine or iodine disinfectant solution and the use of sterile drape, and for transcervical CVS, the use of a sterile speculum and antisepsis of the cervical and vaginal mucosa.

d. Local anesthesia

Application of a local anesthetic is not recommended in amniocentesis [95,96] and is considered optional in transabdominal CVS by ISUOG [95–97]. Data for CVS through transcervical approach are not available. For FBS, the ISUOG recommendation follows that for transabdominal CVS [81]. The other guidelines do not make any relevant recommendation.

e. Other considerations

ISUOG explicitly states that ultrasound should be performed routinely both prior and after completion of invasive diagnosis. Pre-procedural ultrasound aims at confirming viability and gestational age and assessing the location of the placenta and the amount of amniotic fluid [97]. Post-procedural ultrasound should include fetal heart rate, assessment of the placenta and amniotic fluid to exclude complications associated with placental hematoma or post-procedural fluid leakage and may take place immediately after the procedure or even days later, based on routine practice [67].

Routine antibiotic prophylaxis or any other medical therapy are generally not recommended. However, RCOG states that if there are clinical signs of chorioamnionitis or a macroscopic appearance of the amniotic fluid consistent with microbial infection, analysis of the sample and initiation of antibiotic therapy is recommended.

Based on the results of studies investigating other invasive percutaneous procedures [98], women receiving thromboprophylaxis or prophylactic low-dose aspirin are not advised to discontinue the regimen, according to ISUOG.

f. Counseling

All guidelines underline the significance of proper genetic counseling in patients at high risk of aneuploidy provided by an appropriately trained healthcare professional. Pretest counseling should precede an invasive procedure to address the risks, the benefits, the technical aspects and the available options in a nondirective manner. In cases of mosaicism, genetic counseling is recommended to discuss the possibility of fetal involvement and allow for offering options (ACOG-SMFM, ISUOG). Counseling should be based on evidence regarding the possibility of true fetal mosaicism. Malvestiti et al. investigated the incidence of mosaicism in 60,437 CVS samples and found a percentage of 2%; of those, 1001 cases were subjected to amniocentesis [48].

6. Conclusions

Overall, the included guidelines all support the availability of definite diagnostic testing to every pregnant woman after appropriate counseling and recommend IPDT based on a positive screening result. Maternal age alone should not constitute an indication for IPDT. There is, however, controversy among these guidelines on the additional indications that may prompt diagnostic testing, such as patient history (personal or familial), known carrier status of either parent, conception via ART or specific ultrasound findings, leading to substantial differences in clinical practice.

There is general agreement on the appropriate timing for amniocentesis, which is set at 15 weeks, whereas CVS is mostly recommended from 10 weeks, with the exception of HGSA-RANZOG, which recommends that it is performed after 11 weeks. The recommendations regarding counseling on complications rates are based on different studies and thus there are certain differences. However, there is a clear trend to counsel patients that complications are nowadays rarer than initially reported, and a significant decrease with advancing operators' experience is highlighted. Data on periprocedural management such as Rhesus alloimmunization, virologic status, the role of anesthesia and antibiotic administration are either inconsistent or insufficiently addressed.

The major strength of this comparative review is the synthesis of the most influential guidelines on IPDT. However, there are certain limitations. First, we opted not to search for all available guidelines systematically, because we intended to compare recommendations only from major medical societies. Thus, we included five guidelines, published in the English language, in our comparisons. Finally, the publication dates of the guidelines differ; some discrepancies may be due to the fact that some of the guidelines were developed up to nine years before and therefore may be partially outdated.

Amniocentesis and CVS are common procedures. However, our study has demonstrated that current national guidelines are in many aspects contradictory and incomplete, while international guidelines may not be able to be fully implemented in all settings due to different cultural and economic conditions. Thus, the development of a standardized, evidenced-based model for the efficient and safe use of IPDT is of paramount importance. Such an approach should help reduce the heterogeneity in local practices and offer a high level of prenatal care to all women, irrespective of national boundaries. The present review aimed to identify similarities and dissimilarities on IPDT and also highlight potential fields for future research. As knowledge accumulates, it becomes evident that the enormous amount of information should be properly guided and communicated to healthcare professionals in prenatal care with the aim to promote the health and well-being of every mother and her fetus.

Author Contributions: Conceptualization, T.D. and I.T.; Methodology, I.T. and I.P.; Validation, A.M., I.K. and A.A.; Investigation, E.G.; Resources, E.G.; Data Curation, E.G.; Writing—Original Draft Preparation, E.G.; Writing—Review and Editing, I.T.; Visualization, T.D.; Supervision, T.D.; Project Administration, T.D. All authors have read and agreed to the published version of the manuscript.

Funding: This paper received no external funding.

Institutional Review Board Statement: Not applicable.

Informed Consent Statement: Not applicable.

Data Availability Statement: All the data used for this article are publicly available.

Conflicts of Interest: The authors declare that they have no conflict of interest.

References

1. World Health Organization. *WHO Recommendations on Antenatal Care for a Positive Pregnancy Experience*; World Health Organization: Geneva, Switzerland, 2016.
2. Cuckle, H.; Maymon, R. Development of prenatal screening—A historical overview. *Semin. Perinatol.* **2016**, *40*, 12–22. [CrossRef]
3. Centers for Disease Control and Prevention (CDC). Update on overall prevalence of major birth defects—Atlanta, Georgia, 1978–2005. *MMWR Morb. Mortal Wkly. Rep.* **2008**, *57*, 1–5.
4. Sago, H. Prenatal Diagnosis of Chromosomal Abnormalities through Amniocentesis. *J. Mamm. Ova Res.* **2004**, *21*, 18–21. [CrossRef]
5. Saltvedt, S.; Almström, H.; Kublickas, M.; Valentin, L.; Bottinga, R.; Bui, T.-H.; Cederholm, M.; Conner, P.; Dannberg, B.; Malcus, P.; et al. Screening for Down syndrome based on maternal age or fetal nuchal translucency: A randomized controlled trial in 39 572 pregnancies. *Ultrasound Obstet. Gynecol.* **2005**, *25*, 537–545. [CrossRef] [PubMed]
6. Santorum, M.; Wright, D.; Syngelaki, A.; Karagioti, N.; Nicolaides, K.H. Accuracy of first-trimester combined test in screening for trisomies 21, 18 and 13. *Ultrasound Obstet. Gynecol.* **2017**, *49*, 714–720. [CrossRef]
7. Wilson, K.L.; Czerwinski, J.L.; Hoskovec, J.M.; Noblin, S.J.; Sullivan, C.M.; Harbison, A.; Campion, M.W.; Devary, K.; Devers, P.; Singletary, C. NSGC Practice Guideline: Prenatal Screening and Diagnostic Testing Options for Chromosome Aneuploidy. *J. Genet. Couns.* **2012**, *22*, 4–15. [CrossRef]
8. Malone, F.D.; Canick, J.A.; Ball, R.H.; Nyberg, D.A.; Comstock, C.H.; Bukowski, R.; Berkowitz, R.L.; Gross, S.J.; Dugoff, L.; Craigo, S.D.; et al. First-Trimester or Second-Trimester Screening, or Both, for Down's Syndrome. *N. Engl. J. Med.* **2005**, *353*, 2001–2011. [CrossRef]
9. Audibert, F.; De Bie, I.; Johnson, J.-A.; Okun, N.; Wilson, R.D.; Armour, C.; Chitayat, D.; Kim, R. RETIRED: No. 348-Joint SOGC-CCMG Guideline: Update on Prenatal Screening for Fetal Aneuploidy, Fetal Anomalies, and Adverse Pregnancy Outcomes. *J. Obstet. Gynaecol. Can.* **2017**, *39*, 805–817. [CrossRef]
10. Li, S.; Shi, Y.; Han, X.; Chen, Y.; Shen, Y.; Hu, W.; Zhao, X.; Wang, Y. Prenatal Diagnosis of Chromosomal Mosaicism in Over 18,000 Pregnancies: A Five-Year Single-Tertiary-Center Retrospective Analysis. *Front. Genet.* **2022**, *13*, 876887. [CrossRef]
11. Evans, M.I.; Wapner, R.J. Invasive Prenatal Diagnostic Procedures. *Semin. Perinatol.* **2005**, *29*, 215–218. [CrossRef]
12. Valenti, C.; Schutta, E.; Kehaty, T. Prenatal Diagnosis of Down's Syndrome. *Lancet* **1968**, *292*, 220. [CrossRef]
13. Serr, D.M.; Sachs, L.D.M. The diagnosis of sex before birth using cells from the amniotic fluid (a preliminary report). *Bull. Res. Counc. Isr.* **1955**, *5B*, 137–138.
14. Carlson, L.M.; Vora, N.L. Prenatal diagnosis: Screening. *Physiol. Behav.* **2017**, *176*, 139–148. [CrossRef]
15. Kuliev, A.M.; Modell, B.; Jackson, L.; Simpson, J.L.; Brambati, B.; Rhoads, G.; Froster, U.; Verlinsky, Y.; Smidt-Jensen, S.; Holzgreve, W.; et al. Risk evaluation of CVS. *Prenat. Diagn.* **1993**, *13*, 197–209. [CrossRef] [PubMed]
16. Olney, R.S.; Moore, C.A.; Khoury, M.J.; Erickson, J.D.; Edmonds, L.D.; Botto, L.D.; Atrash, H.K.; Centers for Disease Control and Prevention. Chorionic villus sampling and amniocentesis: Recommendations for prenatal counseling. *MMWR Recomm. Rep.* **1995**, *44*, 1–12.
17. Pajkrt, E.; Mol, B.W.J.; Boer, K.; Drogtrop, A.P.; Bossuyt, P.M.M.; Bilardo, C.M. Intra- and interoperator repeatability of the nuchal translucency measurement. *Ultrasound Obstet. Gynecol.* **2000**, *15*, 297–301. [CrossRef]
18. Ramirez-Abarca, T.G.; Gallardo-Gaona, J.M.; Lumbreras-Marquez, M.I.; Seifert, S.M.; Rodriguez-Sibaja, M.J.; Velazquez-Torres, B.; Ramirez-Calvo, J.A.; Acevedo-Gallegos, S. Amniocentesis learning curve using a low-cost simulation model to teach maternal–fetal medicine fellows. *Int. J. Gynecol. Obstet.* **2020**, *153*, 95–99. [CrossRef]
19. Young, C.; Von Dadelszen, P.; Alfirevic, Z. Instruments for chorionic villus sampling for prenatal diagnosis. *Cochrane Database Syst. Rev.* **2013**, *2013*, CD000114. [CrossRef]
20. Prenatal Diagnostic Testing for Genetic Disorders. ACOG. Available online: https://www.acog.org/clinical/clinical-guidance/practice-bulletin/articles/2016/05/prenatal-diagnostic-testing-for-genetic-disorders (accessed on 18 August 2022).

21. Ghi, T.; Sotiriadis, A.; Calda, P.; Costa, F.D.S.; Raine-Fenning, N.; Alfirevic, Z.; McGillivray, G. International Society of Ultrasound in Obstetrics and Gynecology (ISUOG) ISUOG Practice Guidelines: Invasive procedures for prenatal diagnosis. *Ultrasound Obstet. Gynecol.* **2016**, *48*, 256–268. [CrossRef]
22. RANZCOG. *Prenatal Screening and Diagnostic Testing for Fetal Chromosomal and Genetic Conditions*; The Royal Australian and New Zealand College of Obstetricians and Gynaecologists: Melbourne, Australia, 2018; pp. 1–35.
23. Navaratnam, K.; Alfirevic, Z.; Royal College of Obstetricians and Gynaecologists. Amniocentesis and chorionic villus sampling: Green-top Guideline no. 8. *BJOG Int. J. Obstet. Gynaecol.* **2022**, *129*, e1–e15. [CrossRef]
24. Rink, B.D.; Norton, M.E. Screening for fetal aneuploidy. *Semin. Perinatol.* **2016**, *40*, 35–43. [CrossRef] [PubMed]
25. Wladimiroff, J.W.; Sachs, E.S.; Reuss, A.; Stewart, P.A.; Pijpers, L.; Niermeijer, M.F.; Reynolds, J.F. Prenatal diagnosis of chromosome abnormalities in the presence of fetal structural defects. *Am. J. Med. Genet.* **1988**, *29*, 289–291. [CrossRef] [PubMed]
26. Souka, A.P.; von Kaisenberg, C.S.; Hyett, J.A.; Sonek, J.D.; Nicolaides, K.H. Increased nuchal translucency with normal karyotype. *Am. J. Obstet. Gynecol.* **2005**, *192*, 1005–1021. [CrossRef] [PubMed]
27. Warburton, D.; Dallaire, L.; Thangavelu, M.; Ross, L.; Levin, B.; Kline, J. Trisomy Recurrence: A Reconsideration Based on North American Data. *Am. J. Hum. Genet.* **2004**, *75*, 376–385. [CrossRef] [PubMed]
28. Gardner, R.M.; Sutherland, G.R.; Shaffer, L.G. *Chromosome Abnormalities and Genetic Counseling*, 3rd ed.; Oxford University Press (OUP): New York, NY, USA, 2011.
29. Wapner, R.J.; Martin, C.L.; Levy, B.; Ballif, B.C.; Eng, C.M.; Zachary, J.M.; Savage, M.; Platt, L.D.; Saltzman, D.; Grobman, W.A.; et al. Chromosomal Microarray versus Karyotyping for Prenatal Diagnosis. *N. Engl. J. Med.* **2012**, *367*, 2175–2184. [CrossRef] [PubMed]
30. Evans, M.I.; Wapner, R.; Berkowitz, R.L. Noninvasive prenatal screening or advanced diagnostic testing: Caveat emptor. *Am. J. Obstet. Gynecol.* **2016**, *215*, 298–305. [CrossRef]
31. Carroll, J.C.; Rideout, A.; Wilson, B.J.; Allanson, J.; Blaine, S.; Esplen, M.J.; Farrell, S.; Graham, G.E.; MacKenzie, J.; Meschino, W.S.; et al. Maternal age-based prenatal screening for chromosomal disorders: Attitudes of women and health care providers toward changes. *Can. Fam. Physician* **2013**, *59*, e39–e47.
32. Kuppermann, M.; Norton, M.E. Prenatal Testing Guidelines: Time for a new approach. *Gynecol. Obstet. Investig.* **2005**, *60*, 6–10. [CrossRef]
33. Hodges, R.J.; Wallace, E.M. Testing for Down syndrome in the older woman: A risky business? *Aust. N. Z. J. Obstet. Gynaecol.* **2005**, *45*, 486–488. [CrossRef]
34. Berkowitz, R.L.; Roberts, J.; Minkoff, H. Challenging the Strategy of Maternal Age–Based Prenatal Genetic Counseling. *JAMA* **2006**, *295*, 1446–1448. [CrossRef]
35. Chitayat, D.; Langlois, S.; Wilson, R.D.; Audibert, F.; Blight, C.; Brock, J.-A.; Cartier, L.; Carroll, J.; Désilets, V.A.; Gagnon, A.; et al. Prenatal Screening for Fetal Aneuploidy in Singleton Pregnancies. *J. Obstet. Gynaecol. Can.* **2011**, *33*, 736–750. [CrossRef]
36. Bonduelle, M.; Van Assche, E.; Joris, H.; Keymolen, K.; Devroey, P.; Van Steirteghem, A.; Liebaers, I. Prenatal testing in ICSI pregnancies: Incidence of chromosomal anomalies in 1586 karyotypes and relation to sperm parameters. *Hum. Reprod.* **2002**, *17*, 2600–2614. [CrossRef] [PubMed]
37. Wang, J.-W.; Lyu, Y.-N.; Qiao, B.; Li, Y.; Zhang, Y.; Dhanyamraju, P.K.; Bamme, Y.; Yu, M.D.; Yang, D.; Tong, Y.-Q. Cell-free fetal DNA testing and its correlation with prenatal indications. *BMC Pregnancy Childbirth* **2021**, *21*, 585. [CrossRef] [PubMed]
38. Liu, S.; Yang, F.; Chang, Q.; Jia, B.; Xu, Y.; Wu, R.; Li, L.; Chen, W.; Yin, A.; Huang, F.; et al. Positive predictive value estimates for noninvasive prenatal testing from data of a prenatal diagnosis laboratory and literature review. *Mol. Cytogenet.* **2022**, *15*, 29. [CrossRef] [PubMed]
39. Committee on Practice Bulletins—Obstetrics, Committee on Genetics, and the Society for Maternal-Fetal Medicine Practice Bulletin No. *Obstet. Gynecol.* **2016**, *127*, e123–e137. [CrossRef]
40. Pergament, E.; Cuckle, H.; Zimmermann, B.; Banjevic, M.; Sigurjonsson, S.; Ryan, A.; Hall, M.P.; Dodd, M.; Lacroute, P.; Stosic, M.; et al. Single-Nucleotide Polymorphism–Based Noninvasive Prenatal Screening in a High-Risk and Low-Risk Cohort. *Obstet. Gynecol.* **2014**, *124 Pt 1*, 210–218. [CrossRef]
41. Palomaki, G.E.; Kloza, E.M.; Lambert-Messerlian, G.M.; Boom, D.V.D.; Ehrich, M.; Deciu, C.; Bombard, A.T.; Haddow, J.E. Circulating cell free DNA testing: Are some test failures informative? *Prenat. Diagn.* **2015**, *35*, 289–293. [CrossRef]
42. Revello, R.; Sarno, L.; Ispas, A.; Akolekar, R.; Nicolaides, K.H. Screening for trisomies by cell-free DNA testing of maternal blood: Consequences of a failed result. *Ultrasound Obstet. Gynecol.* **2016**, *47*, 698–704. [CrossRef]
43. American College of Obstetricians and Gynecologists. Committee Opinion Summary No. 640: Cell-Free DNA Screening for Fetal Aneuploidy. *Obstet. Gynecol.* **2015**, *126*, 691–692. [CrossRef]
44. Hou, Y.; Yang, J.; Qi, Y.; Guo, F.; Peng, H.; Wang, D.; Wang, Y.; Luo, X.; Li, Y.; Yin, A. Factors affecting cell-free DNA fetal fraction: Statistical analysis of 13,661 maternal plasmas for non-invasive prenatal screening. *Hum. Genom.* **2019**, *13*, 62. [CrossRef]
45. Kypri, E.; Ioannides, M.; Achilleos, A.; Koumbaris, G.; Patsalis, P.; Stumm, M. Non-invasive prenatal screening tests—Update. *LaboratoriumsMedizin* **2022**, *46*, 311–320. [CrossRef]
46. Willems, P.; Dierickx, H.; Vandenakker, E.; Bekedam, D.; Segers, N.; Deboulle, K.; Vereecken, A. The first 3,000 Non-Invasive Prenatal Tests (NIPT) with the Harmony test in Belgium and the Netherlands. *Facts Views Vis. Obgyn.* **2014**, *6*, 7–12.

47. Zhang, H.; Gao, Y.; Jiang, F.; Fu, M.; Yuan, Y.; Guo, Y.; Zhu, Z.; Lin, M.; Liu, Q.; Tian, Z.; et al. Non-invasive prenatal testing for trisomies 21, 18 and 13: Clinical experience from 146 958 pregnancies. *Ultrasound Obstet. Gynecol.* **2015**, *45*, 530–538. [CrossRef] [PubMed]
48. Malvestiti, F.; Agrati, C.; Grimi, B.; Pompilii, E.; Izzi, C.; Martinoni, L.; Gaetani, E.; Liuti, M.R.; Trotta, A.; Maggi, F.; et al. Interpreting mosaicism in chorionic villi: Results of a monocentric series of 1001 mosaics in chorionic villi with follow-up amniocentesis. *Prenat. Diagn.* **2015**, *35*, 1117–1127. [CrossRef] [PubMed]
49. Mardy, A.; Wapner, R.J. Confined placental mosaicism and its impact on confirmation of NIPT results. *Am. J. Med. Genet. Part C Semin. Med. Genet.* **2016**, *172*, 118–122. [CrossRef] [PubMed]
50. Saura, R.; Taine, L.; Guyon, F.; Mangione, R.; Horovitz, J. Safety and fetal outcome of early and midtrimester amniocentesis. *Lancet* **1998**, *351*, 1434–1435. [CrossRef]
51. Farrell, S.A.; Summers, A.M.; Dallaire, L.; Singer, J.; Johnson, J.A.M.; Wilson, R.D. Club foot, an adverse outcome of early amniocentesis: Disruption or deformation? *J. Med. Genet.* **1999**, *36*, 843–846. [CrossRef]
52. Alfirevic, Z.; Navaratnam, K.; Mujezinovic, F. Amniocentesis and chorionic villus sampling for prenatal diagnosis. *Cochrane Database Syst. Rev.* **2017**, *2017*, CD003252. [CrossRef]
53. Wilson, R.D.; Johnson, J.M.; Dansereau, J.; Singer, J.; Drinnan, S.L.; Winsor, E.J.T.; Soanes, S.; Kalousek, D.; Hillier, J.; Ho, M.F.; et al. Randomised trial to assess safety and fetal outcome of early and midtrimester amniocentesis. *Lancet* **1998**, *351*, 242–247. [CrossRef]
54. Cruz-Lemini, M.; Parra-Saavedra, M.; Borobio, V.; Bennasar, M.; Goncé, A.; Martínez, J.M.; Borrell, A. How to perform an amniocentesis. *Ultrasound Obstet. Gynecol.* **2014**, *44*, 727–731. [CrossRef]
55. Athanasiadis, A.P.; Pantazis, K.; Goulis, D.G.; Chatzigeorgiou, K.; Vaitsi, V.A.; Tzevelekis, F.; Tsalikis, T. Comparison between 20G and 22G needle for second trimester amniocentesis in terms of technical aspects and short-term complications. *Prenat. Diagn.* **2009**, *29*, 761–765. [CrossRef] [PubMed]
56. Marthin, T.; Liedgren, S.; Hammar, M. Transplacental needle passage and other risk-factors associated with second trimester amniocentesis. *Acta Obstet. Gynecol. Scand.* **1997**, *76*, 728–732. [CrossRef]
57. Bombard, A.T.; Powers, J.F.; Carter, S.; Schwartz, A.; Nitowsky, H.M. Procedure-related fetal losses in transplacental versus nontransplacental genetic amniocentesis. *Am. J. Obstet. Gynecol.* **1995**, *172*, 868–872. [CrossRef]
58. Giorlandino, C.; Mobili, L.; Bilancioni, E.; D'Alessio, P.; Carcioppolo, O.; Gentili, P.; Vizzone, A. Transplacental amniocentesis: Is it really a higher-risk procedure? *Prenat. Diagn.* **1994**, *14*, 803–806. [CrossRef] [PubMed]
59. Hockstein, S.; Chen, P.X.; Thangavelu, M.; Pergament, E. Factors associated with maternal cell contamination in amniocentesis samples as evaluated by fluorescent in situ hybridization. *Obstet. Gynecol.* **1998**, *92*, 551–556. [CrossRef] [PubMed]
60. Brebaum, D.; Grond-Ginsbach, C. Maternal cell contamination in amniotic fluid samples as a consequence of the sampling technique. *Qual. Life Res.* **1994**, *93*, 121–124. [CrossRef]
61. Welch, R.A.; Salem-Elgharib, S.; Wiktor, A.E.; Van Dyke, D.L.; Blessed, W.B. Operator experience and sample quality in genetic amniocentesis. *Am. J. Obstet. Gynecol.* **2006**, *194*, 189–191. [CrossRef]
62. Akolekar, R.; Beta, J.; Picciarelli, G.; Ogilvie, C.; D'Antonio, F. Procedure-related risk of miscarriage following amniocentesis and chorionic villus sampling: A systematic review and meta-analysis. *Ultrasound Obstet. Gynecol.* **2014**, *45*, 16–26. [CrossRef]
63. Odibo, A.O.; Gray, D.L.; Dicke, J.M.; Stamilio, D.M.; Macones, G.A.; Crane, J.P. Revisiting the Fetal Loss Rate After Second-Trimester Genetic Amniocentesis: A single center's 16-year experience. *Obstet. Gynecol.* **2008**, *111*, 589–595. [CrossRef]
64. Caughey, A.B.; Hopkins, L.M.; Norton, M.E. Chorionic Villus Sampling Compared with Amniocentesis and the Difference in the Rate of Pregnancy Loss. *Obstet. Gynecol.* **2006**, *108*, 612–616. [CrossRef]
65. Eddleman, K.A.; Malone, F.D.; Sullivan, L.; Dukes, K.; Berkowitz, R.L.; Kharbutli, Y.; Porter, T.F.; Luthy, D.A.; Comstock, C.H.; Saade, G.R.; et al. Pregnancy Loss Rates After Midtrimester Amniocentesis. *Obstet. Gynecol.* **2006**, *108*, 1067–1072. [CrossRef] [PubMed]
66. Beta, J.; Lesmes-HereDia, C.; Bedetti, C.; Akolekar, R. Risk of miscarriage following amniocentesis and chorionic villus sampling: A systematic review of the literature. *Minerva Ginecol.* **2018**, *70*, 215–219. [CrossRef] [PubMed]
67. Kähler, C.; Gembruch, U.; Heling, K.-S.; Henrich, W.; Schramm, T. DEGUM guidelines for amniocentesis and chorionic villus sampling. *Ultraschall Med.* **2013**, *34*, 435–440. [CrossRef]
68. Hess, L.W.; Anderson, R.L.; Golbus, M.S. Significance of opaque discolored amniotic fluid at second-trimester amniocen-tesis. *Obstet. Gynecol.* **1986**, *67*, 44–46. [PubMed]
69. American College of Obstetricians and Gynecologists. ACOG Practice Bulletin No. 88: Invasive Prenatal Testing for Aneuploidy. *Obstet. Gynecol.* **2007**, *110*, 1459–1467. [CrossRef]
70. Philip, J.; Silver, R.K.; Wilson, R.D.; Thom, E.A.; Zachary, J.M.; Mohide, P.; Mahoney, M.J.; Simpson, J.L.; Platt, L.D.; Pergament, E.; et al. Late First-Trimester Invasive Prenatal Diagnosis: Results of an International Randomized Trial. *Obstet. Gynecol.* **2004**, *103*, 1164–1173. [CrossRef]
71. Wilson, J.; Johnson, J.; Windrim, R.; Dansereau, J.; Singer, J.; Winsor, E.; Kalousek, D. The Early Amniocentesis Study: A Randomized Clinical Trial of Early Amniocentesis and Midtrimester Amniocentesis. *Fetal Diagn. Ther.* **1997**, *12*, 97–101. [CrossRef] [PubMed]
72. Sundberg, K.; Bang, J.; Smidt-Jensen, S.; Brocks, V.; Lundsteen, C.; Parner, J.; Keiding, N.; Philip, J. Randomised study of risk of fetal loss related to early amniocentesis versus chorionic villus sampling. *Lancet* **1997**, *350*, 697–703. [CrossRef]

73. Shulman, L.P.; Elias, S. Amniocentesis and chorionic villus sampling. *West. J. Med.* **1993**, *159*, 260–268.
74. Blessed, W.B.; Lacoste, H.; Welch, R.A. Obstetrician-gynecologists performing genetic amniocentesis may be misleading themselves and their patients. *Am. J. Obstet. Gynecol.* **2001**, *184*, 1340–1344. [CrossRef]
75. Anandakumar, C.; Wong, Y.; Annapoorna, V.; Arulkumaran, S.; Chia, D.; Bongso, A.; Ratnam, S.S. Amniocentesis and Its Complications. *Aust. N. Z. J. Obstet. Gynaecol.* **1992**, *32*, 97–99. [CrossRef] [PubMed]
76. Bakker, M.; Birnie, E.; De Medina, P.R.; Sollie, K.M.; Pajkrt, E.; Bilardo, C.M. Total pregnancy loss after chorionic villus sampling and amniocentesis: A cohort study. *Ultrasound Obstet. Gynecol.* **2017**, *49*, 599–606. [CrossRef] [PubMed]
77. Carlin, A.J.; Alfirevic, Z. Techniques for chorionic villus sampling and amniocentesis: A survey of practice in specialist UK centres. *Prenat. Diagn.* **2008**, *28*, 914–919. [CrossRef] [PubMed]
78. Odibo, A.O.; Dicke, J.M.; Gray, D.L.; Oberle, B.; Stamilio, D.M.; Macones, G.A.; Crane, J.P. Evaluating the Rate and Risk Factors for Fetal Loss After Chorionic Villus Sampling. *Obstet. Gynecol.* **2008**, *112*, 813–819. [CrossRef]
79. Brambati, B.; Lanzani, A.; Tului, L. Transabdominal and transcervical chorionic villus sampling: Efficiency and risk evaluation of 2411 cases. *Am. J. Med. Genet.* **1990**, *35*, 160–164. [CrossRef]
80. Papp, C.; Beke, A.; Mezei, G.; Tóth-Pál, E.; Papp, Z. Chorionic Villus Sampling: A 15-Year Experience. *Fetal Diagn. Ther.* **2002**, *17*, 218–227. [CrossRef]
81. Berry, S.M.; Stone, J.; Norton, M.E.; Johnson, D.; Berghella, V. Fetal blood sampling. *Am. J. Obstet. Gynecol.* **2013**, *209*, 170–180. [CrossRef]
82. Tongsong, T.; Wanapirak, C.; Kunavikatikul, C.; Sirirchotiyakul, S.; Piyamongkol, W.; Chanprapaph, P. Fetal loss rate associated with cordocentesis at midgestation. *Am. J. Obstet. Gynecol.* **2001**, *184*, 719–723. [CrossRef] [PubMed]
83. Liao, C.; Wei, J.; Li, Q.; Li, L.; Li, J.; Li, D. Efficacy and safety of cordocentesis for prenatal diagnosis. *Int. J. Gynecol. Obstet.* **2006**, *93*, 13–17. [CrossRef]
84. Antsaklis, A.; Daskalakis, G.; Papantoniou, N.; Michalas, S. Fetal blood sampling—Indication-related losses. *Prenat. Diagn.* **1998**, *18*, 934–940. [CrossRef]
85. Gagnon, A.; Davies, G.; Wilson, R.D.; Audibert, F.; Brock, J.-A.; Campagnolo, C.; Carroll, J.; Chitayat, D.; Johnson, J.-A.; MacDonald, W.; et al. RETIRED: Prenatal Invasive Procedures in Women with Hepatitis B, Hepatitis C, and/or Human Immunodeficiency Virus Infections. *J. Obstet. Gynaecol. Can.* **2014**, *36*, 648–653. [CrossRef]
86. Yi, W.; Pan, C.Q.; Hao, J.; Hu, Y.; Liu, M.; Li, L.; Liang, D. Risk of vertical transmission of hepatitis B after amniocentesis in HBs antigen-positive mothers. *J. Hepatol.* **2013**, *60*, 523–529. [CrossRef]
87. Mandelbrot, L.; Jasseron, C.; Ekoukou, D.; Batallan, A.; Bongain, A.; Pannier, E.; Blanche, S.; Tubiana, R.; Rouzioux, C.; Warszawski, J. Amniocentesis and mother-to-child human immunodeficiency virus transmission in the Agence Nationale de Recherches sur le SIDA et les Hépatites Virales French Perinatal Cohort. *Am. J. Obstet. Gynecol.* **2009**, *200*, 160.e1–160.e9. [CrossRef]
88. Shapiro, D.E.; Sperling, R.S.; Mandelbrot, L.; Britto, P.; Cunningham, B.E. Risk factors for perinatal human immunodeficiency virus transmission in patients receiving zidovudine prophylaxis. Pediatric AIDS Clinical Trials Group protocol 076 Study Group. *Obstet. Gynecol.* **1999**, *94*, 897–908. [CrossRef]
89. Somigliana, E.; Bucceri, A.M.; Tibaldi, C.; Alberico, S.; Ravizza, M.; Savasi, V.; Marini, S.; Matrone, R.; Pardi, G. Early invasive diagnostic techniques in pregnant women who are infected with the HIV: A multicenter case series. *Am. J. Obstet. Gynecol.* **2005**, *193*, 437–442. [CrossRef]
90. Recommendations for Use of Antiretroviral Drugs in Pregnant HIV-1-Infected Women for Maternal Health and Interventions to Reduce Perinatal HIV Transmission in the United States. National Prevention Information Network. Connecting Public Health Professionals with Trusted Information and Each Other. Available online: https://npin.cdc.gov/publication/recommendations-use-antiretroviral-drugs-pregnant-hiv-1-infected-women-maternal-health (accessed on 18 August 2022).
91. Simões, M.; Marques, C.M.O.; Gonçalves, A.; Pereira, A.P.; Correia, J.; Castela, J.; Guerreiro, C. Amniocentesis in HIV Pregnant Women: 16 Years of Experience. *Infect. Dis. Obstet. Gynecol.* **2013**, *2013*, 914272. [CrossRef] [PubMed]
92. Davies, G.; Wilson, R.D.; Désilets, V.; Reid, G.J.; Shaw, D.; Summers, A.; Wyatt, P.; Young, D.; Canada, S.O.O.A.G.O. RETIRED: Amniocentesis and Women with Hepatitis B, Hepatitis C, or Human Immunodeficiency Virus. *J. Obstet. Gynaecol. Can.* **2003**, *25*, 145–148. [CrossRef]
93. Delamare, C.; Carbonne, B.; Heim, N.; Berkane, N.; Petit, J.C.; Uzan, S.; Grangé, J.-D. Detection of hepatitis C virus RNA (HCV RNA) in amniotic fluid: A prospective study. *J. Hepatol.* **1999**, *31*, 416–420. [CrossRef]
94. Di Mascio, D.; Buca, D.; Berghella, V.; Khalil, A.; Rizzo, G.; Odibo, A.; Saccone, G.; Galindo, A.; Liberati, M.; D'Antonio, F. Counseling in maternal–fetal medicine: SARS-CoV-2 infection in pregnancy. *Ultrasound Obstet. Gynecol.* **2021**, *57*, 687–697. [CrossRef]
95. Mujezinovic, F.; Alfirevic, Z. Analgesia for amniocentesis or chorionic villus sampling. *Cochrane Database Syst. Rev.* **2011**, *11*, CD008580. [CrossRef]
96. Van Schoubroeck, D.; Verhaeghe, J. Does local anesthesia at mid-trimester amniocentesis decrease pain experience? A randomized trial in 220 patients. *Ultrasound Obstet. Gynecol.* **2000**, *16*, 536–538. [CrossRef] [PubMed]

97. Wilson, R.D.; Davies, G.; Gagnon, A.; Desilets, V.; Reid, G.J.; Summers, A.; Wyatt, P.; Allen, V.M.; Langlois, S. Genetics Committee of the Society of Obstetricians and Gynaecologists of Canada RETIRED: Amended Canadian Guideline for Prenatal Diagnosis (2005) Change to 2005-Techniques for Prenatal Diagnosis. *J. Obstet. Gynaecol. Can.* **2005**, *27*, 1048–1054. [CrossRef] [PubMed]
98. Patel, I.J.; Davidson, J.C.; Nikolic, B.; Salazar, G.M.; Schwartzberg, M.S.; Walker, T.G.; Saad, W.A. Consensus Guidelines for Periprocedural Management of Coagulation Status and Hemostasis Risk in Percutaneous Image-guided Interventions. *J. Vasc. Interv. Radiol.* **2012**, *23*, 727–736. [CrossRef] [PubMed]

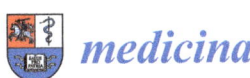

Article

Umbilical Cord Biometry and Fetal Abdominal Skinfold Assessment as Potential Biomarkers for Fetal Macrosomia in a Gestational Diabetes Romanian Cohort

Andreea Roxana Florian [1], Gheorghe Cruciat [1,*], Georgiana Nemeti [1,*], Adelina Staicu [1], Cristina Suciu [1], Mariam Chaikh Sulaiman [1], Iulian Goidescu [1], Daniel Muresan [1] and Florin Stamatian [2]

[1] Obstetrics and Gynecology I, Mother and Child Department, University of Medicine and Pharmacy "Iuliu Hatieganu", 400006 Cluj-Napoca, Romania
[2] Imogen Clinical Research Centre, 400006 Cluj-Napoca, Romania
* Correspondence: cruciat@yahoo.com (G.C.); georgiana_nemeti@yahoo.com (G.N.)

Abstract: *Background and Objectives:* Gestational diabetes mellitus (GDM) is a pregnancy-associated pathology commonly resulting in macrosomic fetuses, a known culprit of obstetric complications. We aimed to evaluate the potential of umbilical cord biometry and fetal abdominal skinfold assessment as screening tools for fetal macrosomia in gestational diabetes mellitus pregnant women. *Materials and methods:* This was a prospective case–control study conducted on pregnant patients presenting at 24–28 weeks of gestation in a tertiary-level maternity hospital in Northern Romania. Fetal biometry, fetal weight estimation, umbilical cord area and circumference, areas of the umbilical vein and arteries, Wharton jelly (WJ) area and abdominal fold thickness measurements were performed. *Results:* A total of 51 patients were enrolled in the study, 26 patients in the GDM group and 25 patients in the non-GDM group. There was no evidence in favor of umbilical cord area and WJ amount assessments as predictors of fetal macrosomia ($p > 0.05$). However, there was a statistically significant difference in the abdominal skinfold measurement during the second trimester between macrosomic and normal-weight newborns in the GDM patient group ($p = 0.016$). The second-trimester abdominal circumference was statistically significantly correlated with fetal macrosomia at term in the GDM patient group with a p value of 0.003, as well as when considering the global prevalence of macrosomia in the studied populations, 0.001, when considering both populations. *Conclusions:* The measurements of cord and WJ could not be established as predictors of fetal macrosomia in our study populations, nor differentiate between pregnancies with and without GDM. Abdominal skinfold measurement and abdominal circumference measured during the second trimester may be important markers of fetal metabolic status in pregnancies complicated by GDM.

Keywords: gestational diabetes mellitus; fetal macrosomia; umbilical cord area; abdominal skinfold; Wharton jelly

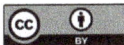

1. Introduction

Gestational diabetes mellitus (GDM) is defined as glucose intolerance newly diagnosed during pregnancy. Alongside type 1 and 2 diabetes mellitus, GDM prevalence has increased dramatically worldwide in the past decades [1]. Associated perinatal maternal–fetal consequences arise mostly from hyperglycemia per se but also due to complications such as excessive maternal weight gain, miscarriage, fetal anomalies, pre-eclampsia and fetal macrosomia.

Fetal macrosomia impacts both the fetal and maternal obstetric outcomes. Macrosomic fetuses have an increased risk of perinatal death, birth trauma due instrumental delivery and maneuvers required to address shoulder dystocia, neonatal hypoglycemia, hyperbilirubinemia, neonatal respiratory distress syndrome and longer neonatal intensive care unit admission intervals. In adulthood, these children are prone to developing impaired glucose tolerance, metabolic syndrome and cardiovascular diseases. Maternal effects range from complicated labor, higher rates of instrumental and operative deliveries and an increased risk of postpartum hemorrhage sometimes requiring transfusion of blood products to perineal trauma of different degrees, increased rates of caesarean deliveries and an augmented long-term risk of genital organ prolapse [2,3].

Despite the advances in ultrasound equipment technology, standards and guidance for fetal biometry measurements and better training of professionals, fetal macrosomia continues to represent a diagnostic issue. Overestimation of fetal weight leads to many unnecessary cesarean deliveries [4]. Contrarily, even correctly diagnosed, the outcome of vaginal delivery cannot be accurately predicted except for extremely macrosomic fetuses.

The umbilical cord (UC), which connects the fetus and placenta, has been extensively studied in recent years, anatomically, morphologically and by ultrasonography. It contains the umbilical vessels (normally, two umbilical arteries and one vein) and the remnant of the allantois, embedded in Wharton's jelly (WJ)—a network of glycoprotein microfibrils, collagen fibers and hyaluronic acid—surrounded by a single layer of amnion [5]. Wharton's jelly ensures a normal blood flow through the umbilical cord, preventing the collapse or knotting of the cord and therefore the disruption of vascular flow through the blood vessels. Various umbilical cord anomalies in size, vessel number, course and connection, structure and configuration have been described, with sometimes no impact on the course of pregnancy, but other times associated with various pregnancy conditions.

The umbilical cord is a vital structure for fetal development, and its detailed analysis can provide valuable information to allow the estimation of neonatal outcomes in various pregnancy-related pathologies. Changes in the amount of Wharton's jelly have been linked to the occurrence of pregnancy-associated pathologies such as pregnancy-induced hypertensive disease, gestational diabetes mellitus and stillbirth [6]. Decreases in WJ quantity, changes in its protein structure and variations in the size of the umbilical vessel area have been associated with the development of pre-eclampsia [7,8]. The link between increased umbilical cord diameter and the development of GDM and the relationship between IUGR and the reduced cord diameter with decreased WJ are subjects of debate [7,9–11]. An increased diameter of the UC has been found in cases of fetal macrosomia and aneuploidy [12–14].

The main objective of our study was to determine whether the ultrasound measurement of umbilical cord anthropometric parameters (umbilical cord area, umbilical cord vessel area, the amount of Wharton's jelly) and fetal abdominal skinfold assessment can be used as diagnostic or prognostic tools for fetal macrosomia in a selected population of Romanian patients.

2. Materials and Methods

This was a prospective case–control study conducted between January 2021 and June 2021 in the Obstetrics-Gynecology I Outpatient Department of the Emergency Cluj-Napoca County Hospital, Romania.

All procedures performed were in accordance with the national and European legislation (Declaration of Helsinki 1964), the enrollment of patients being carried out following counseling and obtaining their informed consent.

Inclusion criteria for the study group were represented by pregnant women with singleton pregnancies, during 24–28 weeks of gestation (WG), whose pregnancies were monitored in the Outpatient Department of the Emergency Cluj-Napoca County Hospital, with a planned delivery in the Obstetrics and Gynecology I maternity hospital.

The following represented study exclusion criteria: pre-existing type 1 or type 2 diabetes mellitus, the coexistence of pregnancy-associated pathologies, single umbilical artery, patients whose pregnancies were not monitored in the Outpatient Department of the ECCN, patient refusal to participate in the study.

All patients were evaluated and examined at the 24–28 WG pregnancy follow-up visit. Upon presentation, they were counseled about the check-up protocol and study implications and accepted or declined enrollment. Gestational diabetes mellitus screening by oral glucose tolerance test (OGTT) was performed in the morning, followed by ultrasound as the second step of evaluation. Patient family, medical, surgical and obstetric history, as well as current pregnancy history, maternal and fetal outcome data, were collected from medical records.

Screening for GDM was carried out according to IADPSG (International Association of the Diabetes and Pregnancy Study Groups) recommendations, by performing the OGTT with a 75 mg glucose load and 3 glycemia measurements: fasting, one hour and two hours following glucose ingestion. Gestational diabetes was diagnosed when one of the three values taken was altered: fasting blood glucose > 92 mg/dL (5.1 mmol/L), 1 h glycemia level > 180 mg/dL (10 mmol/L), 2 h glycemia level > 153 mg/dL (8.5 mmol/L) [15]

Fetal biometry, fetal weight estimation based on the formula C of Hadlock et al. (Hadlock C; log(10) BW = 1.335 − 0.0034(abdominal circumference (AC))(femur length (FL)) + 0.0316(biparietal diameter) + 0.0457(AC) + 0.1623(FL)) [16] umbilical cord area and circumference, areas of the umbilical vein and arteries, WJ area and abdominal fold thickness measurements were performed in all patients enrolled in the study by two examiners specializing in maternal–fetal medicine who performed examinations alternatively. All measurements were carried out using a GE VolusonE8 Expert with RAB6-D, 2–7 MHz convex abdominal probe. Ultrasonographers were blinded regarding the diagnosis of GDM (OGTT test results) in the respective pregnancy so as not to influence measurements.

Umbilical cord measurements were performed at the level of a free cord loop no more than 2 cm away from the fetal abdominal wall [9]. The umbilical cord diameter was meared circumferentially, outside the umbilical cord, using the "ellipse" measurement function of the ultrasound machine followed by the automatic calculation of the measured area (Figure 1A). Cord vessels and vessel area were similarly measured. The Wharton jelly area was calculated by subtracting the areas of the umbilical vein and arteries from the entire cross-sectional area of the cord. Fetal abdominal skinfold was identified as an external hyperechogenic surface on the standard transverse plane for the assessment of the abdominal circumference, the level at which measurements were performed. Fold thickness was measured by placing one caliper precisely between the fetal skin and adjacent amniotic fluid, with the second caliper being placed between the subcutaneous fat layer and the anterior abdominal wall (Figure 1B) [17].

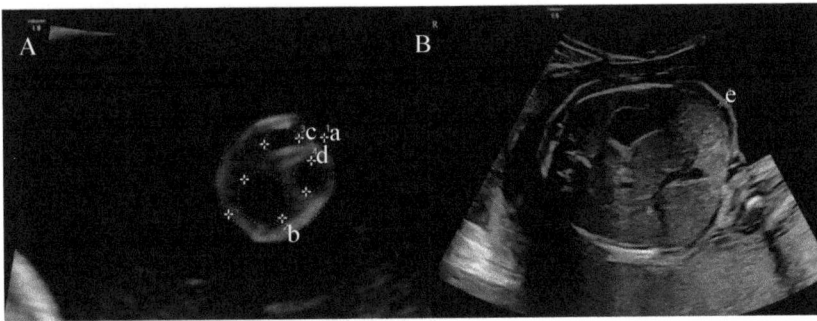

Figure 1. (**A**). Umbilical cord biometry ultrasound landmarks: a. umbilical cord area; b. umbilical cord vein; c,d. umbilical cord artery; (**B**). Fetal transverse abdominal plane: e. fetal abdominal skinfold.

Macrosomia was defined as estimated fetal weight above the 95th centile for any gestational age, at any point during pregnancy, or birth weight equal to or more than 4000 g [18].

Statistical Analysis

Analysis was performed using MedCalc Statistical Software version 19.1.5 (MedCalc Software, Ostend, Belgium; https://www.medcalc.org; Accessed on 25 May 2020). Continuous variables were tested for normality of distribution (Shapiro–Wilk test) and were described by means ± standard deviation. Nominal data are characterized by means of frequencies and percentages. Comparisons between groups were performed using the Mann–Whitney or chi-square test, whenever appropriate. The model included the variables that achieved a *p* value < 0.05 in the univariate analysis. A *p* value < 0.05 was considered statistically significant.

3. Results

The study group consisted of 51 pregnant patients who presented for the 24–28 WG follow-up visit and agreed to take part in the study. According to the OGTT test results, patients were divided into two groups, the GDM patient group (26 patients) and the non-GDM group, consisting of 25 patients.

The demographic characteristics of the study population are presented in Table 1.

Table 1. Demographic data of the study populations.

	GDM Patients Study Group (n = 26)	Non-GDM Patients Study Group (n = 25)	*p*-Value
	arithmetic mean ± SD *		
Age (years)	32.5 ± 4.95	29.96 ± 3.72	0.044
Pre-gestational BMI	23.23 ± 4.00	22.22 ± 3.41	0.340
Pregnancy weight gain (kg)	13.35 ± 4.65	14.52 ± 5.26	0.402
Final BMI	28.13 ± 4.13	27.71 ± 4	0.718
	number (%)		
Provenance ** Urban area	20 (76.9%)	17 (68.0%)	0.689
Rural area	6 (23.1%)	8 (32.0%)	
Family history of diabetes mellitus	5 (19.23%)	3 (12%)	0.703
Smoking habit	3 (11.5%)	4 (16%)	0.703

* Standard deviation. ** According to the Organization for Economic Cooperation and Development (OECD)—OECD Regional Outlook 2016—Productive Regions for Inclusive Societies, OECD Publishing, Paris, https://doi.org/10.1787/9789264260245-en (accessed on 27 July 2022).

Biometry evaluation for estimated fetal weight, as well as corresponding centiles for gestational age, measurement of UC parameters and abdominal skinfold assessment comparative results for the two groups are presented in Table 2.

Table 2. Fetal biometry, umbilical cord and abdominal skinfold measurement of the study populations performed during the second trimester.

	GDM Patients Study Group (n = 26)	Non-GDM Patients Study Group (n = 25)	*p* Value
Fetal estimated weight 2nd trimester (g)	951.96 ± 145.08	975.96 ± 233.07	0.659
Fetal weight 2nd trimester (centiles)	59.36 ± 11.44	55.92 ± 10.31	0.265
Umbilical cord area (cm^2)	2.03 ± 0.48	1.86 ± 0.41	0.189
Umbilical cord circumference (cm)	5.05 ± 0.66	4.82 ± 0.57	0.201
Umbilical cord vein (cm^2)	0.37 ± 0.13	0.32 ± 0.11	0.121
Umbilical cord artery 1 (cm^2)	0.09 ± 0.11	0.07 ± 0.02	0.363
Umbilical cord artery 2 (cm^2)	0.09 ± 0.13	0.07 ± 0.02	0.329
Wharton jelly (cm^2)	1.46 ± 0.42	1.39 ± 0.35	0.517
Abdominal skin fold (cm)	0.32 ± 0.07	0.22 ± 0.07	0.000
Abdominal circumference (cm)	22.14 ± 1.28	22.16 ± 1.93	0.970
Abdominal circumference (%)	60.18 ± 23.74	53.76 ± 23.53	0.337

The characteristics of the study group patients from the perspective of obstetric outcome, delivery and neonatal weight are presented comparatively in Table 3.

Table 3. Pregnancy outcome parameters of the study group patients compared to the control group patients.

	GDM Patients Study Group (n = 26)	Non-GDM Patients Study Group (n = 25)	p Value
	number (%)		
Parity			
Nulliparous	12 (46.2%)	15 (60%)	0.605
Multiparous	14 (54.8%)	10 (40%)	
Route of delivery			
Vaginal	10 (38.5%)	11 (44%)	0.907
C-section	16 (61.5%)	14 (56%)	
	arithmetic mean ± SD *		
Birthweight (g)	3487.31 ± 435.75	3388 ± 548.54	0.477
Birthweight (centiles)	74.62 ± 22.89	71.72 ± 24.72	0.666
Macrosomia (>95 centile)	8 (30.8%)	8 (32%)	1.000

* standard deviation.

When considering the parity and route of delivery, in the GDM study group, most patients were multiparous and gave birth via C-section.

The caesarean section indications were previous caesarean delivery (37.5% GDM, 42.8% non-GDM group), failed induction (25% GDM), breech presentation (6.25% GDM; 14.28 non-GDM), maternal pathology (31.25% GDM; 14.28% non-GDM) and placental insufficiency (21.42% non-GDM).

Table 4 depicts the correlation between fetal ultrasound parameters and maternal weight gain during pregnancy and term macrosomia.

Table 4. The correlations of fetal ultrasound measurements during the second trimester and fetal macrosomia in both the entire group and the GDM population sample.

	Mean ± SD *		p Value
Correlations in the entire population sample (51 patients)			
2nd-trimester estimated fetal weight—birthweight (%)			0.007
2nd-trimester estimated fetal weight (%)	57.67 ± 1.53		
Birthweight (%)	73.20 ± 3.31		
	Normal weight fetuses (n = 35)	Macrosomic fetuses (n = 16)	
Abdominal skinfold 2nd (cm)—term macrosomia	0.256 ± 0.012	0.295 ± 0.028	0.135
2nd-trimester estimated fetal weight (%)—term macrosomia	54.25 ± 1.63	65.16 ± 2.51	0.001
2nd-trimester abdominal circumference(%)—term macrosomia	49.83 ± 3.84	72.81 ± 4.34	0.001
Excessive maternal weight gain (kg)—term macrosomia	12.74 ± 0.69	16.50 ± 1.44	0.010
Correlations in the GDM group (26 patients)			
2nd-trimester estimated fetal weight—birthweight (%)			0.012
2nd-trimester estimated fetal weight (%)	59.36 ± 2.24		
Birthweight (%)	74.62 ± 4.49		
	Normal-weight fetuses (n = 18)	Macrosomic fetuses (n = 8)	
Abdominal skinfold 2nd-trimester (cm)—term macrosomia	0.269 ± 0.011	0.369 ± 0.034	0.016
2nd-estimated fetal weight (%)term macrosomia	54.52 ± 2.36	70.25 ± 1.91	0.000
2nd-trimester abdominal circumference (%)—term macrosomia	51.58 ± 5.18	79.55 ± 5.25	0.003
Excessive maternal weight gain (kg)—term macrosomia	13.06 ± 1.07	14.00 ± 1.18	0.643

* standard deviation.

In the GDM patient group, there was a statistically significant correlation between the second-trimester fetal weight and birthweight ($p = 0.012$), while no such correlation could be established in the non-GDM pregnancy group.

Umbilical cord area and WJ amount assessment could not be established as predictors of fetal macrosomia.

However, there was a statistically significant difference between the abdominal skinfold measurement during the second trimester between macrosomic and normal-weight newborns in the GDM patient group ($p = 0.016$). This confirms abdominal skinfold measurement during the second-trimester ultrasound evaluation as a potential predictor of fetal macrosomia at term in GDM pregnancies.

There was a statistically significant difference between the macrosomic and normal weighted fetuses at term in the GDM patient group when considering the second-trimester estimated fetal weight ($p = 0.000$), but also when considering the global prevalence of macrosomia in the studied populations ($p = 0.001$). The same was true for the measurement of the abdominal circumference during the second trimester with a p value of 0.003 for the GDM group, respectively 0.001 when considering both populations.

We also found a statistically significant difference between the fetal macrosomia status at term regarding the maternal weight gain during pregnancy when calculating for both patient groups globally ($p = 0.010$), but not when considering only the GDM patient sample ($p = 0.643$).

4. Discussion

The delivery of a macrosomic neonate leads to important maternal–fetal short- and long-term consequences. Diagnosis and prevention of fetal macrosomia thus represent obstetric priorities for reducing maternal and fetal morbidity. Several studies have suggested that ultrasound evaluation of umbilical cord biometry parameters and abdominal skinfold measurement could be a powerful adjunct in the prediction of term macrosomia [18,19]. Our purpose was to test the utility of these measurements as predictive and diagnostic tools for fetal macrosomia in a Romanian population.

Measurement of umbilical cord parameters at the time of GDM screening, prior to the initiation of dietary and therapeutic interventions, was targeted in our research. Ultrasound measurements of the umbilical cord parameters and fetal abdomen showed higher values in fetuses from mothers diagnosed with GDM, such as umbilical cord area, WJ area, abdominal circumference and abdominal skinfold. Umbilical cord area and Wharton jelly could not be established as predictors of fetal macrosomia in our study. Abdominal skinfold and the abdominal circumference measurements in the second trimester were significantly higher in the fetuses from GDM pregnancies compared to fetuses from non-GDM pregnancies. The fetal abdominal skinfold, the abdominal circumference, estimated second-trimester fetal weight and maternal weight gain during pregnancy were also statistically significantly correlated with fetal macrosomia at term.

It has been reported that umbilical cord cross-sectional measurement and estimation of umbilical cord components correlate with fetal size [20]. Our study demonstrated a statistically significant relationship between estimated second-trimester fetal weight, maternal weight gain during pregnancy and macrosomia at term/delivery.

A study conducted by Pietryga et al. evaluated umbilical cord and WJ areas in GDM and non-GDM patients between 22 and 40 WG and concluded that there were no differences between the parameters measured in the two groups and supported the limited value of cord biometry as a predictor of macrosomia at birth in GDM patients [21].

In our study, we found no statistically significant correlations between umbilical cord area umbilical cord area, the amount of cross-sectional WJ and birthweight, respectively, in GDM and non-GDM patients. The explanation for this may be that in pregnancies with GDM, treatment and diet applied after diagnosis prevent the development of fetal macrosomia as well as the umbilical cord and WJ biometry. This conclusion was also reached by Naylor et al., who showed that fetal birthweight is normal in GDM pregnancies because of timely and proper treatment [22].

Structural or volume changes in the umbilical cord and the amount of Wharton's jelly have been shown to signal unfavorable maternal and fetal outcomes. These parameters may provide information on the efficiency of management in various pregnancy-related pathologies, such as pre-eclampsia, intrauterine growth restriction, stillbirth and intrapartum fetal distress [14]. Based on these premises, attempts have been made to incorporate cord area measurement into fetal biometry assessment to improve detection of either macrosomia or growth-restricted fetuses. Nomograms for gestational-age specific cord parameter values have been calculated. It appears that umbilical cord area and WJ area gradually increase up to 30 WG, reach a maximum value around 34 WG and then remain constant [20,23,24].

Weissman et al. confirmed the finding of increased cord areas in pregnancies complicated by GDM on account of increased WJ measurements [25]. This is presumably due to hemorrhage in the umbilical artery walls, increased permeability and subsequent plasma extravasation [26]. The authors speculated that differences in WJ may be useful to discriminate between constitutional macrosomia from macrosomia in GDM-complicated pregnancies. However, in our study, there was no statistically significant difference between the measurement of cord area and WJ between GDM and non-GDM pregnancies.

Several authors obtained similar results to ours regarding the correlation between fetal weight at 24–28 WG and birthweight. A similar highly significant correlation between fetal weight estimation at 26–28 WG and neonatal macrosomia at delivery was recorded by Togni et al. This comes as proof of the correspondence between fetal biometry estimation before 33–34 WG, the amount of WJ and excessive fetal weight at birth. It was also postulated that, after 34 WG, the amount of WJ decreases progressively and its measurement is no longer useful in estimating fetal weight [27]. A more recent study assessed the value of abdominal circumference and estimated fetal weight growth velocity in the prediction of macrosomia but established they do not improve detection as compared to the standard third trimester estimation using the Hadlock formula [28]. The amount of fat in the fetal body and therefore the thickness of the abdominal fold is influenced by numerous factors, such as race, maternal BMI, maternal weight gain during pregnancy, family factors, maternal hypertensive pathology or GDM [17,29,30].

Maternal hyperglycemia and subsequent fetal hyperglycemia lead to hyperactivation of the pancreas with excessive insulin production. The endpoint of these physiopathologic processes is a macrosomic fetus due to increased fat and protein stores.

Jain et al. found a highly significant statistical correlation between serial fetal abdominal circumference measurements at 30–32 and 36–38 WG, respectively, and increased birth weight. In the same study, statistically significant differences were recorded at 30–32 WG between fetal abdominal circumference values in GDM and non-GDM patients [31].

The finding of increased fetal abdominal skinfold in GDM patients resulting from our research was also reported by de Santis et al., who noted an exponential increase with gestational age and a higher developmental curve in fetuses from mothers with GDM compared to control fetuses from non-GDM pregnancies [32]. Bernstein et al. studied changes in fetal fat mass during pregnancy and found that it increased approximately tenfold between 19 and 40 WG [33].

An increased pre-pregnancy BMI and excessive maternal weight gain in pregnancy have been recognized as prerequisites for fetal macrosomia by many researchers [34–37]. Even a protective effect of low pre-pregnancy BMI in non-diabetic women has been described [38,39]. In our study groups, maternal pre-pregnancy obesity did not correlate with macrosomia, while excessive pregnancy weight gain correlated with large fetuses only when considering both groups and not the GDM category solely. This might be due to the limited patient number studied.

The delivery route of GDM patients in our study group was clearly balanced towards operative deliveries. Caesarean section accounted for 61.5% of the total number of deliveries, similar to the value of 73.2% reported by Naylor, and this occurred when not all the fetuses were macrosomic [22]. The high percentage of caesarean section deliveries, even with a normal weight fetus, was due to the large number of patients with obstetric indications, failed induction and patient refusal of induction.

There are several limitations to our study. Firstly, the size of the study groups, which does not allow the generalization of results. Another potential limitation/aspect is related to the technique of measuring cord parameters at the level of a single free cord loop. As this is not yet standardized, further studies are needed to establish the optimal number and points of measurement, considering that the thickness of the umbilical cord may vary along its length. Further research on larger groups of patients could help clinicians to achieve a better selection of patients at risk of developing GDM and may open new horizons in terms of early therapeutic management. Large-scale studies are needed to assess the clinical value of including fetal adnexal measurements in fetal weight estimation formulas. This is an easily reproducible technique, with a short learning curve, which could easily be implemented as a screening tool for fetal macrosomia. Another limitation of the current study is the lack of neonatal follow-up, which could allow the assessment of postpartum complications. At the same time, a more detailed study regarding the prediction of macrosomia might include the evaluation of maternal anthropometric parameters and a second cord biometry measurement at term. The adjunct of these parameters could enhance macrosomia detection.

5. Conclusions

In conclusion, in our study populations, the measurements of the cord and WJ could not be established as predictors of fetal macrosomia, nor differentiate between pregnancies with and without GDM. On the other hand, fetal abdominal skinfold measurement, fetal abdominal circumference, estimated second-trimester fetal weight and maternal weight gain during pregnancy may be important markers of fetal metabolic status in pregnancies complicated by GDM.

Author Contributions: A.R.F. and G.C. were the main coordinators of the project and were responsible for the study design. M.C.S., C.S. and G.N. drafted the manuscript of the present paper. I.G. was involved in the supervising of data collection and stratification. A.S. contributed to data assembly and analysis. D.M. and F.S. contributed to manuscript revision and corrections. All authors have read and agreed to the published version of the manuscript.

Funding: This research received no external funding.

Institutional Review Board Statement: The study was conducted in accordance with the Declaration of Helsinki and approved by the Bioethics Commission of the "Iuliu Hatieganu" University of Medicine and Pharmacy in Cluj-Napoca, Romania (Nr.247/08.06.2017). Patients who participated in this research had complete clinical data. Signed informed consents were obtained from the patients or the guardians.

Informed Consent Statement: Informed consent was obtained from all subjects involved in the study.

Data Availability Statement: The data presented in this study are available on request from the corresponding author. The data are not publicly available being part of the ECCN Cluj-Napoca, Romania archives.

Conflicts of Interest: The authors declare no conflict of interest.

References

1. Choudhury, A.A.; Devi Rajeswari, V. Gestational diabetes mellitus—A metabolic and reproductive disorder. *Biomed. Pharmacother.* **2021**, *143*, 112183. [CrossRef] [PubMed]
2. Committee ADAPP. 15. Management of Diabetes in Pregnancy: Standards of Medical Care in Diabetes—2022. *Diabetes Care* **2021**, *45* (Suppl. S1), S232–S243. [CrossRef]
3. Beta, J.; Khan, N.; Khalil, A.; Fiolna, M.; Ramadan, G.; Akolekar, R. Maternal and neonatal complications of fetal macrosomia: Systematic review and meta-analysis. *Ultrasound Obstet. Gynecol.* **2019**, *54*, 308. [CrossRef]
4. Chauhan, S.P.; Grobman, W.A.; Gherman, R.A.; Chauhan, V.B.; Chang, G.; Magann, E.F.; Hendrix, N.W. Suspicion and treatment of the macrosomic fetus: A review. *Am. J. Obstet. Gynecol.* **2005**, *193*, 332–346. [CrossRef] [PubMed]
5. Wang, H.-S.; Hung, S.-C.; Peng, S.-T.; Huang, C.-C.; Wei, H.-M.; Guo, Y.-J.; Fu, Y.-S.; Lai, M.-C.; Chen, C.-C. Mesenchymal stem cells in the Wharton's jelly of the human umbilical cord. *Stem Cells* **2004**, *22*, 1330–1337. [CrossRef]
6. Bańkowski, E.; Sobolewski, K.; Romanowicz, L.; Chyczewski, L.; Jaworski, S. Collagen and glycosaminoglycans of Wharton's jelly and their alterations in EPH-gestosis. *Eur. J. Obstet. Gynecol. Reprod. Biol.* **1996**, *66*, 109–117. [CrossRef]
7. Ghezzi, F.; Raio, L.; Di Naro, E.; Franchi, M.; Buttarelli, M.; Schneider, H. First-trimester umbilical cord diameter: A novel marker of fetal aneuploidy. *Soc. Ultrasound Obstet. Gynecol.* **2002**, *19*, 235–239. [CrossRef]

8. Bańkowski, E.; Pałka, J.; Jaworski, S. Preeclampsia is associated with alterations in insulin-like growth factor (IGF)-1 and IGF-binding proteins in Wharton's jelly of the umbilical cord. *Clin. Chem. Lab. Med.* **2000**, *38*, 603–608. [CrossRef]
9. Raio, L.; Ghezzi, F.; di Naro, E.; Gomez, R.; Franchi, M.; Mazor, M.; Brühwiler, H. Sonographic measurement of the umbilical cord and fetal anthropometric parameters. *Eur. J. Obstet. Gynecol. Reprod. Biol.* **1999**, *83*, 131–135. [CrossRef]
10. Qureshi, F.; Jacques, S.M. Marked segmental thinning of the umbilical cord vessels. *Arch. Pathol. Lab. Med.* **1994**, *118*, 826–830.
11. Ghezzi, F.; Raio, L.; Günter Duwe, D.; Cromi, A.; Karousou, E.; Dürig, P. Sonographic umbilical vessel morphometry and perinatal outcome of fetuses with a lean umbilical cord. *J. Clin. Ultrasound* **2005**, *33*, 18–23. [CrossRef] [PubMed]
12. Predanic, M.; Perni, S.C.; Chasen, S.; Chervenak, F.A. Fetal aneuploidy and umbilical cord thickness measured between 14 and 23 weeks' gestational age. *J. Ultrasound Med.* **2004**, *23*, 1177–1183. [CrossRef] [PubMed]
13. Raio, L.; Ghezzi, F.; Di Naro, E.; Franchi, M.; Bolla, D.; Schneider, H. Altered sonographic umbilical cord morphometry in early-onset preeclampsia. *Obstet. Gynecol.* **2002**, *100*, 311–316.
14. Cromi, A.; Ghezzi, F.; Naro, E.D.I.; Siesto, G.; Bergamini, V.; Raio, L. Large cross-sectional area of the umbilical cord as a predictor of fetal macrosomia. *Ultrasound Obstet. Gynecol.* **2007**, *30*, 861–866. [CrossRef]
15. Shang, M.; Lin, L. IADPSG criteria for diagnosing gestational diabetes mellitus and predicting adverse pregnancy outcomes. *J. Perinatol.* **2014**, *34*, 100–104. [CrossRef] [PubMed]
16. Hadlock, F.P.; Harrist, R.B.; Sharman, R.S.; Deter, R.L.; Park, S.K. Estimation of fetal weight with the use of head, body, and femur measurements-a prospective study. *Am. J. Obstet. Gynecol.* **1985**, *151*, 333–337. [CrossRef]
17. Rigano, S.; Ferrazzi, E.; Radaelli, T.; Cetin, E.T.; Pardi, G. Sonographic measurements of subcutaneous fetal fat in pregnancies complicated by gestational diabetes and in normal pregnancies. *Croat. Med. J.* **2000**, *41*, 240–244.
18. Silasi, M. Fetal macrosomia. In *Obstetric Imaging: Fetal Diagnosis and Care*, 2nd ed.; Elsevier Inc.: Philadelphia, PA, USA, 2017; pp. 460–462. [CrossRef]
19. Stanirowski, P.J.; Majewska, A.; Lipa, M.; Bomba-Opoń, D.; Wielgoś, M. Ultrasound evaluation of the fetal fat tissue, heart, liver and umbilical cord measurements in pregnancies complicated by gestational and type 1 diabetes mellitus: Potential application in the fetal birth-weight estimation and prediction of the fetal macrosomia. *Diabetol. Metab. Syndr.* **2021**, *13*, 22. [CrossRef]
20. Rostamzadeh, S.; Kalantari, M.; Shahriari, M.; Shakiba, M. Sonographic measurement of the umbilical cord and its vessels and their relation with fetal anthropometric measurements. *Iran J Radiol.* **2015**, *12*, e12230. [CrossRef]
21. Pietryga, M.; Brązert, J.; Wender-Ożegowska, E.; Zawiejska, A.; Brązert, M.; Dubiel, M.; Gudmundsson, S. Ultrasound measurements of umbilical cord transverse area in normal pregnancies and pregnancies complicated by diabetes mellitus. *Ginekol. Pol.* **2014**, *85*, 810–814. [CrossRef]
22. Naylor, C.D.; Sermer, M.; Chen, E.; Sykora, K. Cesarean delivery in relation to birth weight and gestational glucose tolerance: Pathophysiology or practice style? Toronto Trihospital Gestational Diabetes Investigators. *JAMA* **1996**, *275*, 1165–1170. [CrossRef] [PubMed]
23. Raio, L.; Ghezzi, F.; Di Naro, E.; Franchi, M.; Maymon, E.; Mueller, M.D.; Brühwiler, H. Prenatal diagnosis of a lean umbilical cord: A simple marker for the fetus at risk of being small for gestational age at birth. *Ultrasound Obstet. Gynecol* **1999**, *13*, 176–180. [CrossRef] [PubMed]
24. Weissman, A.; Jakobi, P.; Bronshtein, M.; Goldstein, I. Sonographic measurements of the umbilical cord and vessels during normal pregnancies. *J. Ultrasound Med.* **1994**, *13*, 11–14. [CrossRef] [PubMed]
25. Weissman, A.; Jakobi, P. Sonographic measurements of the umbilical cord in pregnancies complicated by gestational diabetes. *J. Ultrasound Med.* **1997**, *16*, 691–694. [CrossRef] [PubMed]
26. Singh, S.D. Gestational diabetes and its effect on the umbilical cord. *Early Hum Dev.* **1986**, *14*, 89–98. [CrossRef]
27. Togni, F.A.; Júnior, E.A.; Moron, A.F.; Vasques, F.A.; Torloni, M.R.; Nardozza, L.M.; Filho, H.A. Reference intervals for the cross sectional area of the umbilical cord during gestation. *J. Perinat. Med.* **2007**, *35*, 130–134. [CrossRef]
28. Roeckner, J.T.; Odibo, L.; Odibo, A.O. The value of fetal growth biometry velocities to predict large for gestational age (LGA) infants. *J. Matern. Neonatal Med.* **2022**, *35*, 2099–2104. [CrossRef]
29. Buchanan, T.A.; Xiang, A.H.; Kjos, S.L.; Trigo, E.; Lee, W.P.; Peters, R.K. Antepartum predictors of the development of type 2 diabetes in Latino women 11-26 months after pregnancies complicated by gestational diabetes. *Diabetes* **1999**, *48*, 2430–2436. [CrossRef]
30. Chen, L.; Wu, J.J.; Chen, X.H.; Cao, L.; Wu, Y.; Zhu, L.J.; Lv, K.T.; Ji, C.B.; Guo, X.R. Measurement of fetal abdominal and subscapular subcutaneous tissue thickness during pregnancy to predict macrosomia: A pilot study. *PLoS ONE* **2014**, *9*, e93077. [CrossRef]
31. Jain, N.; Singh, A. Original Article Estimation of Sonographic Umbilical Cord Area and Its Correlation with Birth Weight in Gestational Diabetes Mellitus. *Ann. Appl. Bio-Sci.* **2016**, *3*, A-122–A-127.
32. de Santis, M.S.N.; Taricco, E.; Radaelli, T.; Spada, E.; Rigano, S.; Ferrazzi, E.; Milani, S.; Cetin, I. Growth of fetal lean mass and fetal fat mass in gestational diabetes. *Ultrasound Obstet. Gynecol.* **2010**, *36*, 328–337. [CrossRef]
33. Bernstein, I.M.; Goran, M.I.; Amini, S.B.; Catalano, P.M. Differential growth of fetal tissues during the second half of pregnancy. *Am. J. Obstet. Gynecol.* **1997**, *176*, 28–32. [CrossRef]
34. Cui, D.; Yang, W.; Shao, P.; Li, J.; Wang, P.; Leng, J.; Wang, S.; Liu, E.; Chan, J.C.; Yu, Z.; et al. Interactions between Prepregnancy Overweight and Passive Smoking for Macrosomia and Large for Gestational Age in Chinese Pregnant Women. *Obes. Facts* **2021**, *14*, 520–530. [CrossRef]

35. Tela, F.G.; Bezabih, A.M.; Adhanu, A.K.; Tekola, K.B. Fetal macrosomia and its associated factors among singleton live-births in private clinics in Mekelle city, Tigray, Ethiopia. *BMC Pregnancy Childbirth* **2019**, *19*, 219. [CrossRef]
36. Woltamo, D.D.; Meskele, M.; Workie, S.B.; Badacho, A.S. Determinants of fetal macrosomia among live births in southern Ethiopia: A matched case-control study. *BMC Pregnancy Childbirth* **2022**, *22*, 465. [CrossRef] [PubMed]
37. Song, X.; Shu, J.; Zhang, S.; Chen, L.; Diao, J.; Li, J.; Li, Y. Pre-Pregnancy Body Mass Index and Risk of Macrosomia and Large for Gestational Age Births with Gestational Diabetes Mellitus as a Mediator: A Prospective Cohort Study in Central China. *Nutrients* **2022**, *14*, 1072. [CrossRef] [PubMed]
38. Li, G.; Xing, Y.; Wang, G.; Zhang, J.; Wu, Q.; Ni, W.; Jiao, N.; Chen, W.; Liu, Q.; Gao, L.; et al. Differential effect of pre-pregnancy low BMI on fetal macrosomia: A population-based cohort study. *BMC Med.* **2021**, *19*, 175. [CrossRef] [PubMed]
39. Sun, Y.; Zhang, M.; Liu, R.; Wang, J.; Yang, K.; Wu, Q.; Yue, W.; Yin, C. Protective Effect of Maternal First-Trimester Low Body Mass Index Against Macrosomia: A 10-Year Cross-Sectional Study. *Front. Endocrinol.* **2022**, *13*, 805636. [CrossRef]

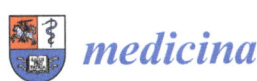

Article

Brain-Derived Neurotrophic Factor Levels in Cord Blood from Growth Restricted Fetuses with Doppler Alteration Compared to Adequate for Gestational Age Fetuses

Jara Pascual-Mancho [1,2,3,4], Pilar Pintado-Recarte [1,2,3], Jorge C. Morales-Camino [5], Carlos Romero-Román [5], Concepción Hernández-Martin [1,2,3], Coral Bravo [1,2,3], Julia Bujan [6,7], Melchor Alvarez-Mon [6,7,8], Miguel A. Ortega [6,7,*] and Juan De León-Luis [1,2,3]

1. Department of Public and Maternal and Child Health, School of Medicine, Complutense University of Madrid, 28040 Madrid, Spain; japasma@gmail.com (J.P.-M.); ppintadorec@yahoo.es (P.P.-R.); concepcion.hernadez@salud.madrid.org (C.H.-M.); cbravoarribas@gmail.com (C.B.); jaleon@ucm.es (J.D.L.-L.)
2. Department of Obstetrics and Gynecology, University Hospital Gregorio Marañón, 28009 Madrid, Spain
3. Health Research Institute Gregorio Marañón, Unidad de Investigación Materno Infantil Familia Alonso (UDIMFFA), 28009 Madrid, Spain
4. Department of Obstetrics, Prenatal Diagnosis, Miguel Servet University Hospital, 50009 Zaragoza, Spain
5. Laboratory of Clinical Biochemistry, Albacete Hospital, 02006 Albacete, Spain; jorgcmorales@hotmail.com (J.C.M.-C.); crroman@sescam.jccm.es (C.R.-R.)
6. Ramón y Cajal Institute of Healthcare Research (IRYCIS), 28034 Madrid, Spain; mjulia.bujan@uah.es (J.B.); mademons@gmail.com (M.A.-M.)
7. Department of Medicine and Medical Specialties, Faculty of Medicine and Health Sciences, University of Alcalá, Alcalá de Henares, 28801 Madrid, Spain
8. Immune System Diseases-Rheumatology and Internal Medicine Service, Center for Biomedical Research Network for Liver and Digestive Diseases (CIBEREHD), University Hospital Príncipe de Asturias, Alcalá de Henares, 28801 Madrid, Spain
* Correspondence: miguel.angel.ortega92@gmail.com; Tel.: +34-91-885-45-40; Fax: +34-91-885-48-85

Abstract: *Background and Objectives*: Fetal growth restriction (FGR) is a severe obstetric disease characterized by a low fetal size entailing a set of undesired consequences. For instance, previous studies have noticed a worrisome association between FGR with an abnormal neurodevelopment. However, the precise link between FGR and neurodevelopmental alterations are not yet fully understood yet. Brain-derived neurotrophic factor (BDNF) is a critical neurotrophin strongly implicated in neurodevelopmental and other neurological processes. In addition, serum levels of BDNF appears to be an interesting indicator of pathological pregnancies, being correlated with the neonatal brain levels. Therefore, the aim of this study is to analyze the blood levels of BDNF in the cord blood from fetuses with FGR in comparison to those with weight appropriate for gestational age (AGA). *Materials and Methods*: In this study, 130 subjects were recruited: 91 in group A (AGA fetuses); 39 in group B (16 FGR fetuses with exclusively middle cerebral artery (MCA) pulsatility index (PI) < 5th percentile and 23 with umbilical artery (UA) PI > 95th percentile). Serum levels of BDNF were determined through ELISA reactions in these groups. *Results*: Our results show a significant decrease in cord blood levels of BDNF in FGR and more prominently in those with UA PI >95th percentile in comparison to AGA. FGR fetuses with exclusively decreased MCA PI below the 5th percentile also show reduced levels of BDNF than AGA, although this difference was not statistically significant. *Conclusions*: Overall, our study reports a potential pathophysiological link between reduced levels of BDNF and neurodevelopmental alterations in fetuses with FGR. However, further studies should be conducted in those FGR subjects with MCA PI < 5th percentile in order to understand the possible implications of BDNF in this group.

Keywords: FGR; BDNF; umbilical Doppler; brain sparing; cord blood

Citation: Pascual-Mancho, J.; Pintado-Recarte, P.; Morales-Camino, J.C.; Romero-Román, C.; Hernández-Martin, C.; Bravo, C.; Bujan, J.; Alvarez-Mon, M.; Ortega, M.A.; De León-Luis, J. Brain-Derived Neurotrophic Factor Levels in Cord Blood from Growth Restricted Fetuses with Doppler Alteration Compared to Adequate for Gestational Age Fetuses. *Medicina* **2022**, *58*, 178. https://doi.org/10.3390/medicina58020178

Academic Editors: Marius Craina and Elena Bernad

Received: 15 December 2021
Accepted: 21 January 2022
Published: 25 January 2022

Publisher's Note: MDPI stays neutral with regard to jurisdictional claims in published maps and institutional affiliations.

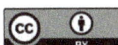

Copyright: © 2022 by the authors. Licensee MDPI, Basel, Switzerland. This article is an open access article distributed under the terms and conditions of the Creative Commons Attribution (CC BY) license (https://creativecommons.org/licenses/by/4.0/).

1. Introduction

Fetal growth restriction (FGR) is a severe complication in pregnancy. It monopolizes great resources of maternal fetal research, and though clearly stated in some guidelines [1], inconsistency in terminology and definition hampers interpretation and comparison of studies. Some define fetal growth as a statistical definition of fetal size below a certain centile, referring to different thresholds for diagnosis. This also adds the possibility of including normally grown fetuses as growth restricted as well as the opposite, as it is difficult to predict the growth potential of a certain fetus [2]. The relationship between FGR and abnormal neurodevelopment has been reflected in numerous studies where the prenatal influence of poor growth on motor and executive functions in children has been explored [3,4]. Antenatal surveillance of growth-restricted fetuses is based, amongst others, on Doppler assessment [1]. The progression of FGR has been previously described and undergoes several hemodynamic phases, passing through a decrease in the estimated fetal weight centile below 10, followed by decreased pulsatility index (PI) in MCA and later, an elevation of the umbilical PI until reaching the final phase that is the alteration of the ductus venosus [5]. These stages have been related to postnatal neurodevelopment [6]. A condition deserving a highlight is the fetal Doppler adaptation to growth restriction named "brain sparing". This phenomenon of cerebral vasodilation has been interpreted as an adaptive mechanism, but more recent studies associate it with poor results in later neurodevelopment and reviews have stated poor cognitive function and lower IQ scores [7,8].

The etiology of the neurodevelopmental alterations in FGR is not completely known. It is based on abnormal feto–maternal exchange and fetal hypoxia because of a chronic decrease in umbilical flow due to placental insufficiency [9]. Oxidative stress, neurotoxicity, apoptotic degeneration and microglial-mediated neuroinflammation are the main mechanisms related to brain injury in these fetuses [10–12].

On account of the difficulty of accessing the human brain in vivo, studies focused on various animal models of hypoxia have attempted to identify these intermediate mechanisms, studying neuronal growth, proliferation and survival after injury [13], the different modifications depending on the brain area studied and the severity of the growth restriction [14]. Furthermore, initial investigations on non-invasive human proton magnetic resonance spectroscopy have been ignited, showing higher lactate peaks on severely growth restricted fetal brains [15] and on not so severely restricted fetuses, as in the Sanz-Cortes study where late FGR and small for gestational age fetuses showed lower N-acetylaspartate to choline ratios, attributable to either a delay in maturational processes or to neuronal injury [16].

Other in vivo studies have tried to identify those intermediate steps centered on proteins with an important role on prenatal neurodevelopment, such as reelin on fetuses with FGR [17]. These studies try to find objective and reproductive data, easy to obtain as cord blood, to set associations to prenatal conditions, such as FGR.

Although many molecules have been described as neurotrophic biomarkers, playing important roles in neurodevelopment, neurotrophins are one of the most important actors in brain development. They are involved in neuronal differentiation and synaptic plasticity, also playing a central role in neuronal survival. Brain-derived neurotrophic factor (BDNF) is one of the most studied neurotrophins and it is closely related to neuroinflammation through its role as a modulator of neuroglia [18]. In animal models of intrauterine growth restriction, it has been widely seen that BDNF is decreased especially in the hippocampus [19,20], which is the brain region with the main expression of this neurotrophin, enhancing neuronal plasticity and relating it to memory and learning [11]. Furthermore, in vivo models have shown that the lack of microglia after cerebral ischemia increases cytokine levels, findings consistent with the protective role of microglia in the removal of waste products that indirectly relates BDNF to neuroinflammation and neuroplasticity [21].

BDNF alterations in neonates have also been studied as indicators of FGR, infection, pre-eclampsia [22], hours of rupture of membranes, corticosteroid maturation and magnesium sulfate treatment [23,24]. The largest study to date, related low levels of BDNF in dry blood tests (blood spots) taken on the first day of life in newborns with intrauterine growth restriction [25]. Furthermore, there are studies that link lower levels of BDNF with neonatal periventricular hemorrhage secondary to hypoxic-ischemic lesions [26]. Likewise, as a therapeutic approach, BDNF is being studied for neuroprotection, reducing cell apoptosis in the face of external insults, promoting specific populations of neurons in both central and peripheral nervous systems as well as after hypoxic or inflammatory brain injuries [27–29]. On the other hand, since the origin of neonatal BDNF in cord blood is believed to be a reflection of brain levels in animal studies [30], there are publications in the medical literature that assess BDNF levels as a predictor of behavior diseases [31] and its role in major depression, autism spectrum disorders and degenerative diseases [32,33].

Hence, due to the important role of BDNF in neurodevelopment as well as the extensive published literature on the influence of prenatal variables on their levels in newborns, this neurotrophin is a candidate for the study of intermediate processes that may relate to the prenatal insult reflected as restricted intrauterine growth and impaired postnatal neurodevelopment. Therefore, this study focuses on BDNF behavior from FGR fetuses cord blood compared to fetuses with weight appropriate for gestational age (AGA).

2. Materials and Methods

2.1. Patients Selection and Fetal Growing Assessment

Pregnant patients were prospectively recruited during their visit at the Maternity Unit of the Gregorio Marañón University Hospital. These pregnancies were dated using the cranio–caudal length at their first trimester ultrasound. Cases were selected after estimating fetal weight (EFW) by ultrasound using the Hadlock 4 formula and plotting the EFW on our own population reference tables. When the EFW was below the 10th percentile, in accordance with the ISUOG FGR criteria [1], a Doppler study was performed, assessing the pulsatility index of the umbilical artery (UA PI), the PI of the middle cerebral artery (MCA PI) and the mean PI of the uterine arteries (UtA PI) according to Ciobanu [34] and Gomez [35] reference charts, respectively, with a maximum of 7 days prior to delivery. In fetuses with adequate for gestational age weight, a Doppler study was not performed. The birth weight was obtained at the delivery room for all fetuses except for 9 FGR who were weighed within the first 12 h at the neonatal intensive care unit. Birth weights were plotted to our neonatal birth weight reference. Exclusion criteria were fetus with known congenital anomalies diagnosed prenatally or immediately postnatally, including genetic conditions, clinical chorioamnionitis, use of illicit drugs or alcohol during pregnancy or poor gestational control defined as first appointment beyond first trimester or less than 4 visits to the clinic [36]. Maternal data were withdrawn from the medical records during hospital stays, such as for preeclampsia.

To carry out the BDNF nálisis according to FGR severity, the study subjects were divided in two groups. Group A contained fetuses with weight appropriate for gestational age (AGA) birth weight $\geq$ 10th percentile. Group B was made up of FGR fetuses (birth weight < 10th percentile) with abnormal umbilical or cerebral Doppler study. Further detailed Doppler assessment in FGR fetuses was performed in order to assess the effect of brain vasodilation on BDNF levels. For that reason, we divided group B into two subgroups: fetuses with decreased MCA PI < 5th percentile and fetuses with increased UA PI > 95th percentile in order to assess the effect of cerebral vasodilation on BDNF levels.

2.2. Sample Collection, Initial Processing and Storage

Samples were collected at the time of delivery, prior to placenta evacuation and deposited into standard clinical tubes containing lithium heparin. The blood was centrifuged within the first hour of birth at the Biochemistry department, by the on-call laboratory technicians. Eppenddorf aliquots, a minimum of one and a maximum of three, coded with the study identifier were stored in racks in a Thermo Scientific Fisher Forma freezer at −86 °C. Thawing was carried out at room temperature and on only one occasion, no subsequent freezing was performed.

2.3. Determination of BDNF in Umbilical Vein by ELISA Methodology

BDNF determination was achieved by the Quantikine Human BDNF Immunoassay assay (R&D Systems) according to the manufacturer's instructions. This is a sandwich-type solid phase ELISA. Anti-BDNF antibodies are immobilized on the surface of the wells of the microplate. These antibodies capture the BDNF contained in the samples, controls and calibrators and after washing a second antiBDNF, peroxidase enzyme-conjugated antibody is added, leading to a colorimetric reaction by adding the substrate (3, 3', 5, 5'-Tetramethylbenzidine), emitting a signal proportional to the BDNF concentration. The absorbance of each sample is read spectrophotometrically at a wavelength of 450 nm. Generation of a standard curve allows for identification of the protein concentration. The intra assay and inter assay coefficients of variation for the ELISA were 5 and 9, respectively. All samples were assayed in duplicate.

2.4. Statistical Analysys

For the statistical analysis, IBM SPSS Statistics V21.0 was used. Differences between the groups of study were assessed using chi-square or non-parametric Mann-Whitney test, based on the normal distribution of the variables in these different groups. When assessing the influence of FGR on BDNF levels a multivariable linear regression model was performed in order to adjust for fetal variables.

3. Results

Our sample consisted of 130 subjects: 91 in group A (AGA fetuses); 39 in group B (16 FGR fetuses with MCA PI < 5th percentile and 23 with UA PI > 95th percentile). Fetal Doppler measurement was performed a mean of 3 days before delivery.

Obstetric and neonatal characteristics of the two groups are shown in Table 1. The characteristics surrogated to severity of FGR, such as cesarean section, admission to neonatal care unit and intraventricular hemorrhage were higher in group B. Birth weight, weight centile and gestational age were higher in group A compared to group B. Other variables, such as preeclampsia and increased PI UtA, also had different frequencies. Conversely, inflammatory markers were controlled by leukocytosis and there were no significant differences observed.

Table 1. Bivariate analysis of maternal and neonatal clinical characteristics of the study groups.

	GROUP A AGA $N = 91$	GROUP B FGR $N = 39$	p
Maternal age (years) M (IQR)	32 (7)	34 (5)	NS
Gestational age (weeks) M (IQR)	38 (4)	35 (5)	<0.001
Fetal sex (female) n (%)	49 (54)	15 (38)	NS
MgSO$_4$ n (%)	0	9 (23)	<0.001
Lung maturation n (%)	1 (1)	16 (41)	<0.001
Cesarean section n (%)	11 (12)	25 (64)	<0.001
UtA PI > p95 n (%)	N/A	18 (46)	N/A
Preeclampsia n (%)	1 (1)	6 (15)	0.005
Birth weight (g) M (IQR)	3290 (650)	1750 (870)	<0.001
Weight centile M (IQR)	65 (45)	0 (1)	<0.001
pH AU M (IQR)	7.29 (0.11)	7.26 (0.09)	NS
Cord blood leukocytes (number/uL) M (IQR)	15,600 (6500)	12,700 (7500)	NS
Neonatal care admission n (%)	6 (6.6)	25 (64)	<0.001
Intraventricular hemorrhage n (%)	0	4 (10)	0.007
BDNF (pg/mL) M (IQR)	6980 (3735)	4838 (4724)	0.001

AGA: adequate for gestational age weight. FGR: fetal growth restriction; UtA PI: uterine artery pulsatility index PROM: premature rupture of membranes; IQR: interquartile range; M: median; NS: no significative. N/A: not applicable.

The FGR group had 41% of fetuses who required corticosteroids for lung maturation and 23% neuroprotection with MgSO$_4$ due to prematurity. The four cases of intraventricular hemorrhage diagnosed during admission to neonatal care were limited to the germinal matrix.

Figure 1 shows the BDNF values according to the groups under study. We found significant BDNF differences between medians in groups with non-parametric U Mann–Whitney test (p = 0.002). As fetuses with impaired growth were more likely to be preterm, we adjusted for gestational age to see the stability of the association with a linear regression (p = 0.034).

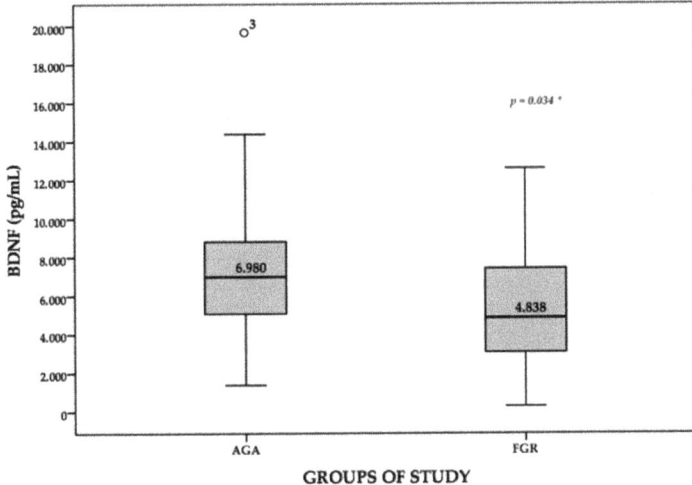

Figure 1. BDNF Box plot across study groups. p * is adjusted for gestational age with linear regression.

Subgroup analysis to assess the effect of decreased MCA PI on BDNF was performed. Clinical characteristics and differences between both groups are shown in Table 2. BDNF levels showed a downward trend, but no differences were found. AGA fetuses and FGR fetuses with decreased MCA PI showed similar BDNF levels. Within FGR fetuses, no differences were found between fetuses with decreased MCA PI and FGR fetuses with UA PI > 95th percentile (Figure 2).

Table 2. Bivariate analysis of maternal and perinatal features between clinical subgroups.

	AGA N = 91	FGR with MCA PI < 5th Exclusively N = 16	p
Maternal age (years) M (SD)	32 (28–35)	34 (31–35)	NS
Gestational age (weeks) M (IQR)	38 (36–40)	36 (35–38)	0.027
Fetal sex (female) n (%)	49 (54)	9 (56)	NS
MgSO$_4$ n (%)	0	3 (19)	0.003
Lung maturation n (%)	1 (1)	3 (19)	0.01
Cesarean section n (%)	11 (12)	10 (63)	<0.001
UtA PI > p95 n (%)	N/A	4 (25)	N/A
Preeclampsia n (%)	1 (1.3)	4 (25)	NS
Birth weight (g) m (SD)	3302 (442)	2069 (412)	<0.001
Weight centile M (IQR)	65 (43–88)	1 (1–3)	<0.001
pH AU M (IQR)	7.29 (0.11)	7.27 (0.08)	NS
Cord blood leukocytes (number/uL) M (IQR)	15,600 (6500)	14,700 (7225)	NS
Neonatal care admission n (%)	6 (6.6)	6 (37.5)	0.002
Intraventricular hemorrhage n (%)	0	0	NS
BDNF (pg/mL) m (SD)	6980 (3735)	6268 (3539)	NS

PROM: premature rupture of membranes; AGA: adequate for gestational age weight. IQR: interquartile range; SD: standard deviation. NS: no significative. N/A: not applicable.

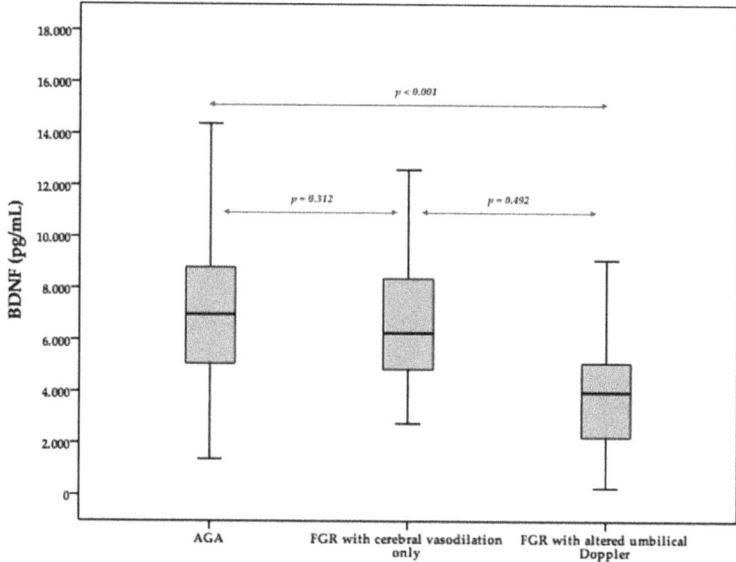

Figure 2. BDNF Box plot with subgroup of fetuses with brain sparing. p adjusted for gestational age with linear regression.

4. Discussion

So far, this study is the first to demonstrate a decrease in BDNF on FGR fetuses with a fetal Doppler alteration. This difference was mainly due to the low BDNF levels in the subgroup of fetuses most severely affected with an increased umbilical Doppler PI, as it is shown in Figure 2. BDNF concentration in FGR fetuses with decreased MCA PI exclusively did not differ from the other fetuses, either AGA or FGR, with UA PI > 95th percentile. Perinatal variables from FGR fetuses were different from AGA in those variables subrogated to the growth restriction environment. Preeclampsia and increased uterine artery PI are risk factors for growth restriction due to impaired placentation, and prematurity is common amongst those fetuses as the optimal time of delivery is still under discussion [37]. This explains why perinatal variables linked to gestational age, such as lung maturation and neuroprotection with $MgSO_4$ as well as preeclampsia rate and pathological UtA PI linked to impaired placentation, were more likely on FGR group. Other variables also linked to either prematurity and FGR, such as intraventricular hemorrhage, cesarean section rate and neonatal care admission, were more frequent in the FGR group.

Studies in humans have also demonstrated decreased levels of BDNF in FGR fetuses [25,38,39], regardless of adaptive fetal Doppler status. However, not all studies are consistent with our findings. Malamitsi-Putchner observed there were no differences in BDNF between growth-restricted and adequate newborns [40]. These study groups had no differences in fetal Doppler; in fact, it was a recommendation that they carried out future studies. Other studies from the same group evaluated fetal BDNF behavior in diabetic mothers, seeing that the levels were lower than the healthy controls in the latter, regardless of the FGR degree they had [38]. A decreased neonatal BDNF level in diabetic mothers has been observed [41,42], and this effect could mask the one caused by the growth defect since it was diagnosed by a birth weight centile lower than 5 exclusively without Doppler evaluation. Another recent study found no differences between very low birth weight FGR and very low birth weight AGA fetuses when assessing trophic biomarkers as BDNF or vascular endothelial growth factor (VEGF). FGR criteria was again only a birth centile threshold of 10th centile [43] without any examination of Doppler status. Paradoxically, these groups had no birth weight differences. With this in mind, our study cohort had strict selection criteria, besides a birth weight centile classification for FGR condition; we also applied Doppler criteria, either umbilical or cerebral. This condition ensures a sample where healthy fetuses that are small for gestational age are not included, thereby overcoming one of the difficulties in the design of FGR studies.

Besides a rigorous selection of FGR fetuses, these studies have to deal with confounding factors. Brain injury is sometimes overcome by prematurity in severe FGR; for that reason, an adjustment for gestational age is advised. In our study, the association of the severity of growth restriction with decreased BDNF persisted after adjustment for gestational age. Another study from our group observed on healthy term newborns that BDNF cord blood levels decrease as gestational age at delivery increases (unpublished data). This fact would also confirm a low BDNF on FGR despite its lower gestational age. In order to cope with the prematurity confounding factor, Antonakopoulos et al. performed a BDNF analysis on amniotic fluid on ongoing pregnancies. They found higher levels of BDNF on amniotic fluid from small for gestational age (SGA) fetuses assessed early in the second trimester. They did not study Doppler nor fetal growth status at the time of amniocentesis as it was performed for other reasons, finding BDNF levels on large for gestational age and SGA fetuses [44].

Another factor to consider is the treatment with corticoids, as it has been related to high BDNF levels [23]. In our study, the FGR group had a higher proportion of antenatal steroids for lung maturation (41%) but despite that fact, this group had the lowest concentrations still after gestational age adjustment.

FGR fetuses have a described mechanism of adaptation to preserve important body functions called "brain sparing". In general, it has been observed that brain vasodilation is associated with lower scores on cognitive neurodevelopmental scales at 2 years [45]; however, regarding motor alterations or low scores on early scales, no differences have been seen when comparing to newborns without brain redistribution. This probably reflects cognitive alteration rather than motor function, as attributed to the frontal cortex [7]. Regarding our fetuses with decreased MCA PI exclusively, we noted the finding of a decrease in BDNF concentration although this was not statistically significant, especially after gestational age adjustment. When the target is set to study the consequences of "brain sparing", early and late FGR is an important factor as many of these fetuses with late onset FGR will have a slower clinical progression and might be more likely to reach term [6]. Studies with larger numbers should focus on this group of patients and long-term neurodevelopment assessment is encouraged in matched case-control studies.

However, our study has some limitations, not only in the number recruited, but also the possible confusion in the face of variables associated with the severity of FGR. Ventricular hemorrhage occurred, although it was limited to germinal matrix, and intraventricular hemorrhage can be associated with lower levels of BDNF [26]. Although we controlled for prenatal malformations, known genetic conditions at birth and infectious diseases, one of the variables that has been observed to modulate BDNF expression is maternal obesity and we lacked this data [41]. Moreover, we did not perform Doppler exam on AGA fetuses; this group might include fetuses who did not reach their growth potential, although the interquartile range was from 43 to 88. Regarding prematurity, we tried to overcome this bias through linear regression and gestational age adjustment. This handicap is present in many studies focused on FGR. Assessing brain development, neurotrophic factors and postnatal neurodevelopment with age matched controlled studies is of paramount importance but also difficult to achieve as growth restriction is linked to prematurity and healthy preterm fetuses are difficult to identify [37].

Even considering these BDNF differences in FGR, due to the fundamental role of this neurotrophin in prenatal neurodevelopment, our study lacks postnatal follow-up. Future studies of BDNF levels on growth restricted fetuses and linking to the evaluation of subsequent neurodevelopment are necessary to elucidate the intermediate mechanisms that cause such postnatal alteration. These should also serve to identify individuals at increased neurological risk and assess future intervention actions as it has already been studied in hypoxic brain injuries in postnatal Noxa [46].

5. Conclusions

We have observed a significant decrease in cord blood BDNF in FGR with Doppler alteration compared to AGA fetuses. This difference was greater between AGA and FGR fetuses with UA PI > 95th percentile. Decreased MCA PI in FGR fetuses needs further study as we could not find statistical differences on BDNF cord blood concentration when compared to AGA fetuses, although lower levels were observed.

Author Contributions: Conceptualization, J.P.-M., P.P.-R. and J.D.L.-L.; methodology, J.P.-M., M.A.-M., M.A.O. and J.D.L.-L.; software, J.P.-M. and C.R.-R.; validation, M.A.-M. and J.D.L.-L.; formal analysis, J.P.-M.; investigation, J.P.-M., P.P.-R., J.C.M.-C., C.R.-R., C.H.-M., C.B., J.B., M.A.-M., M.A.O. and J.D.L.-L.; resources, J.P.-M., M.A.-M. and J.D.L.-L.; data curation, J.P.-M., M.A.O. and J.D.L.-L.; writing—original draft preparation, J.P.-M., P.P.-R., J.C.M.-C., C.R.-R., C.H.-M., C.B., J.B., M.A.-M., M.A.O. and J.D.L.-L.; writing—review and editing, J.P.-M., P.P.-R., J.C.M.-C., C.R.-R., C.H.-M., C.B., J.B., M.A.-M., M.A.O. and J.D.L.-L.; visualization, J.B., M.A.-M. and J.D.L.-L.; supervision, M.A.-M. and J.D.L.-L.; project administration, J.B., M.A.-M. and J.D.L.-L.; funding acquisition, J.B., M.A.-M. and J.D.L.-L. All authors have read and agreed to the published version of the manuscript.

Funding: This study (FIS-PI18/00912) has been supported by the Instituto de Salud Carlos III (Plan Estatal de I + D + i 2013–2016) and co-financed by the European Regional Development Fund "A Road to Europe" (ERDF) and B2017/BMD-3804 MITIC-CM and Halekulani S.L. and Maternal-fetal medicine research grant (Santiago Dexeus Font Foundation).

Institutional Review Board Statement: The study was conducted according to the guidelines of the Declaration of Helsinki, and approved by the Institutional Review Board of Clinical Research Ethics Committee 28 May 2009 (89/09).

Informed Consent Statement: Informed consent was obtained from all subjects involved in the study.

Data Availability Statement: The data used to support the findings of the present study are available from the corresponding author upon request.

Conflicts of Interest: The authors declare no conflict of interest.

References

1. Lees, C.C.; Stampalija, T.; Baschata, A.A.; Da Silva Costa, F.; Ferrazzi, E.; Figueras, F.; Hecher, K.; Kingdom, J.; Poon, L.C.; Salomon, L.J.; et al. ISUOG Practice Guidelines: Diagnosis and management of small-for-gestational-age fetus and fetal growth restriction. *Ultrasound Obstet. Gynecol.* **2020**, *56*, 298–312. [CrossRef] [PubMed]
2. Gordijn, S.J.; Beune, I.M.; Ganzevoort, W. Building consensus and standards in fetal growth restriction studies. *Best Pract. Res. Clin. Obstet. Gynaecol.* **2018**, *49*, 117–126. [CrossRef] [PubMed]
3. Sacchi, C.; Marino, C.; Nosarti, C.; Vieno, A.; Visentin, S.; Simonelli, A. Association of Intrauterine Growth Restriction and Small for Gestational Age Status with Childhood Cognitive Outcomes. *JAMA Pediatr.* **2020**, *174*, 772. [CrossRef] [PubMed]
4. Arcangeli, T.; Thilaganathan, B.; Hooper, R.; Khan, K.S.; Bhide, A. Neurodevelopmental delay in small babies at term: A systematic review. *Ultrasound Obstet. Gynecol.* **2012**, *40*, 267–275. [CrossRef]
5. Baschat, A.A.; Gembruch, U.; Harman, C.R. The sequence of changes in Doppler and biophysical parameters as severe fetal growth restriction worsens. *Ultrasound Obstet. Gynecol.* **2001**, *18*, 571–577. [CrossRef]
6. Baschat, A.A. Neurodevelopment after Fetal Growth Restriction. *Fetal Diagn. Ther.* **2014**, *36*, 136–142. [CrossRef]
7. Meher, S.; Hernandez-Andrade, E.; Basheer, S.N.; Lees, C. Impact of cerebral redistribution on neurodevelopmental outcome in small for gestational age or growth restricted babies: A systematic review. *Ultrasound Obstet. Gynecol.* **2015**, *46*, 398–404. [CrossRef]
8. Benítez-Marín, M.J.; Marín-Clavijo, J.; Blanco-Elena, J.A.; Jiménez-López, J.; González-Mesa, E. Brain Sparing Effect on Neurodevelopment in Children with Intrauterine Growth Restriction: A Systematic Review. *Children* **2021**, *8*, 745. [CrossRef]
9. Baschat, A.A. Neurodevelopment following fetal growth restriction and its relationship with antepartum parameters of placental dysfunction. *Ultrasound Obstet. Gynecol.* **2011**, *37*, 501–514. [CrossRef]
10. Rees, S.; Harding, R.; Walker, D. The biological basis of injury and neuroprotection in the fetal and neonatal brain. *Int. J. Dev. Neurosci.* **2011**, *29*, 551–563. [CrossRef]
11. Basilious, A.; Yager, J.; Fehlings, M.G. Neurological outcomes of animal models of uterine artery ligation and relevance to human intrauterine growth restriction: A systematic review. *Dev. Med. Child Neurol.* **2015**, *57*, 420–430. [CrossRef] [PubMed]

12. Wixey, J.A.; Chand, K.K.; Colditz, P.B.; Bjorkman, S.T. Review: Neuroinflammation in intrauterine growth restriction. *Placenta* **2017**, *54*, 117–124. [CrossRef] [PubMed]
13. Koehler, R.C.; Yang, Z.-J.; Lee, J.K.; Martin, L.J. Perinatal hypoxic-ischemic brain injury in large animal models: Relevance to human neonatal encephalopathy. *J. Cereb. Blood Flow Metab.* **2018**, *38*, 2092–2111. [CrossRef] [PubMed]
14. Ruff, C.A.; Faulkner, S.D.; Rumajogee, P.; Beldick, S.; Foltz, W.; Corrigan, J.; Basilious, A.; Jiang, S.; Thiyagalingam, S.; Yager, J.Y.; et al. The extent of intrauterine growth restriction determines the severity of cerebral injury and neurobehavioural deficits in rodents. *PLoS ONE* **2017**, *12*, e0184653. [CrossRef] [PubMed]
15. Cetin, I.; Barberis, B.; Brusati, V.; Brighina, E.; Mandia, L.; Arighi, A.; Radaelli, T.; Biondetti, P.; Bresolin, N.; Pardi, G.; et al. Lactate detection in the brain of growth-restricted fetuses with magnetic resonance spectroscopy. *Am. J. Obstet. Gynecol.* **2011**, *205*, 350.e1–350.e7. [CrossRef] [PubMed]
16. Sanz-Cortés, M.; Simoes, R.V.; Bargalló, N.; Masoller, N.; Figueras, F.; Gratacos, E. Proton magnetic resonance spectroscopy assessment of fetal brain metabolism in late-onset 'small for gestational age' versus "intrauterine growth restriction" fetuses. *Fetal Diagn. Ther.* **2014**, *37*, 108–116. [CrossRef]
17. Pascual Mancho, J.; Pintado-Recarte, P.; Romero-Román, C.; Morales-Camino, J.C.; Hernández-Martin, C.; Bujan, J.; Ortega, M.A.; De León-Luis, J. Influence of Cerebral Vasodilation on Blood Reelin Levels in Growth Restricted Fetuses. *Diagnostics* **2021**, *11*, 1036. [CrossRef]
18. Giacobbo, B.L.; Doorduin, J.; Klein, H.C.; Dierckx, R.A.J.O.; Bromberg, E.; Vries, E.F.J. Brain-Derived Neurotrophic Factor in Brain Disorders: Focus on Neuroinflammation. *Mol. Neurobiol.* **2019**, *56*, 3295–3312. [CrossRef]
19. Ninomiya, M.; Numakawa, T.; Adachi, N.; Furuta, M.; Chiba, S.; Richards, M.; Shibata, S.; Kunugi, H. Cortical neurons from intrauterine growth retardation rats exhibit lower response to neurotrophin BDNF. *Neurosci. Lett.* **2010**, *476*, 104–109. [CrossRef]
20. Coupé, B.; Dutriez-Casteloot, I.; Breton, C.; Lefèvre, F.; Mairesse, J.; Dickes-Coopman, A.; Silhol, M.; Tapia-Arancibia, L.; Lesage, J.; Vieau, D. Perinatal undernutrition modifies cell proliferation and brain-derived neurotrophic factor levels during critical time-windows for hypothalamic and hippocampal development in the male rat. *J. Neuroendocrinol.* **2009**, *21*, 40–48. [CrossRef]
21. Calabrese, F.; Rossetti, A.C.; Racagni, G.; Gass, P.; Riva, M.A.; Molteni, R. Brain-derived neurotrophic factor: A bridge between inflammation and neuroplasticity. *Front. Cell. Neurosci.* **2014**, *8*, 430. [CrossRef] [PubMed]
22. D'Souza, V.A.; Kilari, A.S.; Joshi, A.A.; Mehendale, S.S.; Pisal, H.M.; Joshi, S.R. Differential regulation of brain-derived neurotrophic factor in term and preterm preeclampsia. *Reprod. Sci.* **2014**, *21*, 230–235. [CrossRef] [PubMed]
23. Rao, R.; Mashburn, C.B.; Mao, J.; Wadhwa, N.; Smith, G.M.; Desai, N.S. Brain-derived neurotrophic factor in infants. *Pediatr. Res.* **2009**, *65*, 548–552. [CrossRef] [PubMed]
24. Bachnas, M.A.; Mose, J.C.; Effendi, J.S.; Andonotopo, W. Influence of antenatal magnesium sulfate application on cord blood levels of brain-derived neurotrophic factor in premature infants. *J. Perinat. Med.* **2014**, *42*, 129–134. [CrossRef]
25. Leviton, A.; Allred, E.N.; Yamamoto, H.; Fichorova, R.N.; Kuban, K.; O'Shea, T.M.; Dammann, O.; ELGAN Study Investigators. Antecedents and correlates of blood concentrations of neurotrophic growth factors in very preterm newborns. *Cytokine* **2017**, *94*, 21–28. [CrossRef]
26. Chouthai, N.S.; Sampers, J.; Desai, N.; Smith, G.M. Changes in Neurotrophin Levels in Umbilical Cord Blood from Infants with Different Gestational Ages and Clinical Conditions. *Pediatr. Res.* **2003**, *53*, 965–969. [CrossRef]
27. Harris, N.M.; Ritzel, R.; Mancini, N.S.; Jiang, Y.; Yi, X.; Manickam, D.S.; Banks, W.A.; Kabanov, A.V.; McCullough, L.D.; Verma, R. Nano-particle delivery of brain derived neurotrophic factor after focal cerebral ischemia reduces tissue injury and enhances behavioral recovery. *Pharmacol. Biochem. Behav.* **2016**, *150*, 48–56. [CrossRef]
28. Chen, H.; Dang, Y.; Liu, X.; Ren, J.; Wang, H. Exogenous brain-derived neurotrophic factor attenuates neuronal apoptosis and neurological deficits after subarachnoid hemorrhage in rats. *Exp. Ther. Med.* **2019**, *18*, 3837–3844. [CrossRef]
29. Husson, I.; Rangon, C.-M.; Lelièvre, V.; Bemelmans, A.-P.; Sachs, P.; Mallet, J.; Kosofsky, B.E.; Gressens, P. BDNF-induced white matter neuroprotection and stage-dependent neuronal survival following a neonatal excitotoxic challenge. *Cereb. Cortex* **2005**, *15*, 250–261. [CrossRef]
30. Karege, F.; Schwald, M.; Cisse, M. Postnatal developmental profile of brain-derived neurotrophic factor in rat brain and platelets. *Neurosci. Lett.* **2002**, *328*, 261–264. [CrossRef]
31. Ghassabian, A.; Sundaram, R.; Chahal, N.; McLain, A.C.; Bell, E.; Lawrence, D.A.; Yeung, E.H. Determinants of neonatal brain-derived neurotrophic factor and association with child development. *Dev. Psychopathol.* **2017**, *29*, 1499–1511. [CrossRef] [PubMed]
32. Chen, S.; Jiang, H.; Liu, Y.; Hou, Z.; Yue, Y.; Zhang, Y.; Zhao, F.; Xu, Z.; Li, Y.; Mou, X.; et al. Combined serum levels of multiple proteins in tPA-BDNF pathway may. *Sci. Rep.* **2017**, *7*, 6871.
33. Adachi, N. New insight in expression, transport, and secretion of brain-derived neurotrophic factor: Implications in brain-related diseases. *WJBC* **2014**, *5*, 409. [CrossRef] [PubMed]
34. Ciobanu, A.; Wright, A.; Syngelaki, A.; Wright, D.; Akolekar, R.; Nicolaides, K.H. Fetal Medicine Foundation reference ranges for umbilical artery and middle cerebral artery pulsatility index and cerebroplacental ratio. *Ultrasound Obstet. Gynecol.* **2019**, *53*, 465–472. [CrossRef]
35. Gómez, O.; Figueras, F.; Fernández, S.; Bennasar, M.; Martínez, J.M.; Puerto, B.; Gratacós, E. Reference ranges for uterine artery mean pulsatility index at 11–41 weeks of gestation. *Ultrasound Obstet. Gynecol.* **2008**, *32*, 128–132. [CrossRef]

36. Grupo de trabajo de la Guia de práctica clñinica de atención en el embarazo y puerperio, Ministerio de Sanidad, Servicios Sociales e Igualdad. Agencia de Evaluación de Tecnologías Sanitarias de Andalucía 2014. Guías de Práctica Clínica en el SNS. AETSA 2011/10. 2014, pp. 1–494. Available online: https://portal.guiasalud.es/wp-content/uploads/2018/12/GPC_533_Embarazo_AETSA_compl.pdf (accessed on 14 December 2021).
37. Fleiss, B. Knowledge Gaps and Emerging Research Areas in Intrauterine Growth Restriction-Associated Brain Injury. *Front. Endocrinol.* **2019**, *10*, 188. [CrossRef]
38. Briana, D.D.; Papastavrou, M.; Boutsikou, M.; Marmarinos, A.; Gourgiotis, D.; Malamitsi-Puchner, A. Differential expression of cord blood neurotrophins in gestational diabetes: The impact of fetal growth abnormalities. *J. Matern. Fetal Neonatal Med.* **2018**, *31*, 278–283. [CrossRef]
39. Matoba, N.; Ouyang, F.; Mestan, K.K.L.; Porta, N.F.M.; Pearson, C.M.; Ortiz, K.M.; Bauchner, H.C.; Zuckerman, B.S.; Wang, X. Cord blood immune biomarkers in small for gestational age births. *J. Dev. Orig. Health Dis.* **2011**, *2*, 89–98. [CrossRef]
40. Malamitsi-Puchner, A.; Nikolaou, K.E.; Economou, E.; Boutsikou, M.; Boutsikou, T.; Kyriakakou, M.; Puchner, K.; Hassiakos, D. Intrauterine growth restriction and circulating neurotrophin levels at term. *Early Hum. Dev.* **2007**, *83*, 465–469. [CrossRef]
41. Prince, C.S.; Maloyan, A.; Myatt, L. Maternal obesity alters brain derived neurotrophic factor (BDNF) signaling in the placenta in a sexually dimorphic manner. *Placenta* **2017**, *49*, 55–63. [CrossRef]
42. Su, C.-H.; Liu, T.-Y.; Chen, I.T.; Ou-Yang, M.-C.; Huang, L.-T.; Tsai, C.-C.; Chen, C.-C. Correlations between serum BDNF levels and neurodevelopmental outcomes in infants of mothers with gestational diabetes. *Pediatr. Neonatol.* **2021**, *62*, 298–304. [CrossRef] [PubMed]
43. Yue, S.L.; Eke, A.C.; Vaidya, D.; Northington, F.J.; Everett, A.D.; Graham, E.M. Perinatal blood biomarkers for the identification of brain injury in very low birth weight growth-restricted infants. *J. Perinatol.* **2021**, *41*, 2252–2260. [CrossRef] [PubMed]
44. Antonakopoulos, N.; Iliodromiti, Z.; Mastorakos, G.; Iavazzo, C.; Valsamakis, G.; Salakos, N.; Papageorghiou, A.; Margeli, A.; Kalantaridou, S.; Creatsas, G.; et al. Association between Brain-Derived Neurotrophic Factor (BDNF) Levels in 2nd Trimester Amniotic Fluid and Fetal Development. *Mediat. Inflamm.* **2018**, *2018*, 8476217. [CrossRef] [PubMed]
45. Eixarch, E.; Meler, E.; Iraola, A.; Illa, M.; Crispi, F.; Hernandez-Andrade, E.; Gratacos, E.; Figueras, F. Neurodevelopmental outcome in 2-year-old infants who were small-for-gestational age term fetuses with cerebral blood flow redistribution. *Ultrasound Obstet. Gynecol.* **2008**, *32*, 894–899. [CrossRef]
46. Novak, I. Emergent Prophylactic, Reparative and Restorative Brain Interventions for Infants Born Preterm with Cerebral Palsy. *Front. Physiol.* **2019**, *10*, 15.

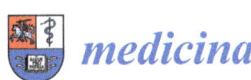

Article

Early Onset Intrauterine Growth Restriction—Data from a Tertiary Care Center in a Middle-Income Country

Marina Dinu [1], Anne Marie Badiu [2], Andreea Denisa Hodorog [3], Andreea Florentina Stancioi-Cismaru [4], Mihaela Gheonea [1,4], Razvan Grigoras Capitanescu [1,4], Ovidiu Costinel Sirbu [1,4], Florentina Tanase [1,4], Elena Bernad [5,6,*] and Stefania Tudorache [1,4]

1. 8th Department, Faculty of Medicine, University of Medicine and Pharmacy of Craiova, 200349 Craiova, Romania
2. 1st Department, Faculty of Medicine, University of Medicine and Pharmacy of Craiova, 200349 Craiova, Romania
3. Obstetrics and Gynecology Department, Mioveni City Hospital, 115400 Mioveni, Romania
4. Obstetrics and Gynecology Department, Emergency County Hospital, 200349 Craiova, Romania
5. Obstetrics and Gynecology Department, Faculty of Medicine, "Victor Babes" University of Medicine and Pharmacy, 300041 Timisoara, Romania
6. Obstetrics and Gynecology Department, "Pius Brinzeu" County Clinical Emergency Hospital, 300723 Timisoara, Romania
* Correspondence: bernad.elena@umft.ro

Abstract: *Background and Objectives:* In this study, we aimed to describe the clinical and ultrasound (US) features and the outcome in a group of patients suspected of or diagnosed with early onset intrauterine growth restriction (IUGR) requiring iatrogenic delivery before 32 weeks, having no structural or genetic fetal anomalies, managed in our unit. A secondary aim was to report the incidence of the condition in the population cared for in our hospital, data on immediate postnatal follow-up in these cases and to highlight the differences required in prenatal and postnatal care. *Materials and Methods:* We used as single criteria for defining the suspicion of early IUGR the sonographic estimation of fetal weight < p10 using the Hadlock 4 technique at any scan performed before 32 weeks' gestation (WG). We used a cohort of patients having a normal evolution in pregnancy and uneventful vaginal births as controls. Data on pregnancy ultrasound, characteristics and neonatal outcomes were collected and analyzed. We hypothesized that the gestational age (GA) at delivery is related to the severity of the condition. Therefore, we performed a subanalysis in two subgroups, which were divided based on the GA at iatrogenic delivery (between 27+0 WG and 29+6 WG and 30+0–32+0 WG, respectively). *Results:* The prospective cohort study included 36 pregnancies. We had three cases of intrauterine fetal death (8.3%). The incidence was 1.98% in our population. We confirmed that severe cases (very early diagnosed and delivered) were associated with a higher number of prenatal visits and higher uterine arteries (UtA) pulsatility index (PI) centile in the third trimester—TT (compared with the early diagnosed and delivered). In the very early suspected IUGR subgroup, the newborns required significantly more NICU days and total hospitalization days. *Conclusions:* Patients with isolated very early and early IUGR—defined as ultrasound (US) estimation of fetal weight < p10 using the Hadlock 4 technique requiring iatrogenic delivery before 32 weeks' gestation—require closer care prenatally and postnatally. These patients represent an economical burden for the health system, needing significantly longer hospitalization intervals, GA at birth and UtA PI centiles being related to it.

Keywords: early onset intrauterine growth restriction; ultrasound; uterine artery pulsatility index; tertiary care center; middle-income country; number of prenatal visits

Citation: Dinu, M.; Badiu, A.M.; Hodorog, A.D.; Stancioi-Cismaru, A.F.; Gheonea, M.; Grigoras Capitanescu, R.; Sirbu, O.C.; Tanase, F.; Bernad, E.; Tudorache, S. Early Onset Intrauterine Growth Restriction—Data from a Tertiary Care Center in a Middle-Income Country. *Medicina* 2023, *59*, 17. https://doi.org/10.3390/medicina59010017

Academic Editors: Themistoklis Dagklis and Simone Ferrero

Received: 25 October 2022
Revised: 12 December 2022
Accepted: 16 December 2022
Published: 21 December 2022

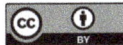

Copyright: © 2022 by the authors. Licensee MDPI, Basel, Switzerland. This article is an open access article distributed under the terms and conditions of the Creative Commons Attribution (CC BY) license (https://creativecommons.org/licenses/by/4.0/).

1. Introduction

Severe early-onset intrauterine growth restriction (IUGR) complicates around 0.4% of pregnancies [1–3] and is associated with poor and very poor pregnancy outcome due to high morbidity and mortality. This is related primarily to premature iatrogenic delivery both for fetal and for maternal indications [4]. Placental disease is associated with a low volume of uteroplacental blood flow and a spectrum of hypertensive disorders. Thus, these cases are often referred to tertiary centers.

The neonatal intensive care unit (NICU) stay is required in most cases and the long-term neurodevelopmental sequelae are important, affecting more than two-thirds of these babies. Survival rates for extremely early born growth-restricted babies (<28 weeks' gestation—WG) vary from 7% to 33% [4–6]. Neonatal morbidity is gestational age (GA) related [7] and related to the severity of IUGR also [8].

The costs of this population of fetuses/neonates include the cost of increased antenatal surveillance (with or without hospitalization days), caesarean delivery, NICU care, routine post-NICU follow-up, and specialized neurodevelopmental assessments and interventions. Such costs represent an important economic burden, especially in developing and middle-income countries. Safe pregnancy prolongation implies a higher number of prenatal consultations [9].

Doppler waveform analysis in pregnancies complicated by IUGR helps in confirming/ruling out the compromise of uteroplacental circulation and placental hypoperfusion. Currently, there are no specific evidence-based therapies for placental insufficiency and for early-onset severe IUGR. Bed rest and hospital admission for surveillance are not scientifically supported by randomized controlled trials. Many management strategies were proposed and studied, including medical interventions, such as Sildenafil citrate [2,3].

IUGR remained the second leading cause of perinatal mortality following prematurity [10]. It has significant consequences on neonatal, childhood and adult morbidity [11]. Currently, there have been scarce reports regarding early-onset IUGR in populations in Romania. This study aimed to assess the prevalence at birth of early-onset IUGR requiring preterm birth before 32 WG in a tertiary center and its associated factors. The end-target is to follow up long-term this population of newborns.

2. Materials and Methods

We performed a nested cohort prospective study. It was designed and conducted in the Prenatal Diagnosis Unit of the Emergency County Hospital of Craiova, which is a tertiary referral university-affiliated Hospital in the south-west region of Romania.

The study included singleton pregnancies having an estimated fetal weight less than the 10th percentile (<p10) at any scan between 22 and 32 WG and no known structural or genetic abnormality. We used the Hadlock 4 technique [12] for the US estimation of fetal weight (EFW). The cases falling under p10 (thus defined as suspected of having early IUGR) were enrolled consecutively between 22- and 31+6 WG.

The study was carried out over a period of three years (1 September 2019–1 September 2022). We report data on 36 pregnancies with prenatal and postnatal care provided in our hospital (complete follow-up, delivery, and postnatal care).

We used a poststudy selected control group. In this group, we included 56 cases of normal pregnancies. The cases were retrospectively selected, consecutively, from the population completely followed up and delivered in our hospital following the study beginning date, September the 1st 2019: healthy mothers having singleton normal fetuses (in terms of structure and growth curve) with pregnancies resulting in normal vaginal term uncomplicated births.

Even if included in a low-risk pregnancy group at registration, all women having prenatal care in our unit are offered and scheduled for the end of the first trimester (detailed anomaly and "genetic" scan [13,14]), for a second trimester (structural survey—anomaly scan) and a third trimester (well-being) US scan. If the prenatal exams (dating and FT anomaly and genetic scan) lead to completely normal data, for the ST scan, the GA offered is 20–23 weeks, and for the TT, it is 29–33 weeks.

In the study group, we included cases requiring hospitalization and/or followed up as outpatients.

We included exclusively pregnancies with a known gestational age (GA) confirmed by US during the first trimester (before 13 weeks 6 days). Patients with fetal structural/chromosomal anomalies, uncertain gestational age and/or unavailable complete data were excluded from the analysis.

We used for all cases a Voluson E10 (GE Medical Systems, Chicago, IL, USA) ultrasound machine equipped with a 4–8 MHz curvilinear transducer. When using color Doppler, the mechanical and thermal indices were kept as low as possible (ALARA principle) [15], and safety guidelines were followed [16].

All scans were performed by the author (obstetrician sonographer M.D.) and—in selected cases—repeated by a senior consultant (S.T.). The study protocol was approved by the university ethics committee, and informed consent was obtained from all participants prior to enrolment.

Internal policy adjusted to current guidelines [17,18] was applied regarding the administration of antenatal steroids for fetal lung maturity and magnesium sulfate for fetal neuroprotection.

We used for the uterine arteries (UtA) [14,19], umbilical artery (UmbA) [14,20], middle cerebral artery (MCA) [14,21] and ductus venosus (DV) Doppler [14,22] assessment the technique previously recommended. We also calculated the cerebroplacental ratio (CPR) as previously described [14,23].

We chose to report separately the Doppler indices for each uterine artery instead of reporting the median of both. The observer diagnosed lateral placenta if more than half of the placenta was seen on US on one side of the uterine cavity only. The corresponding (right or left) uterine artery was named "placental". The other one was named "non-placental" uterine artery on the US form.

The timing of delivery was customized based on the gestational age, the severity of the disease—depending on the results of fetal surveillance, the parents' decisions, and a team of senior consultants, including neonatologists. If the internal policy was not changed by the attending physician (increasing or decreasing the intensity of prenatal care and the frequency of medical visits) or on parental desire (e.g., transfer to another unit or fetal abandonment), we proceeded as follows:

o In prestage I (defined as EFW between 10th centile and the 3rd centile), we used weekly US monitoring regardless of the GA—amniotic fluid volume assessment (using the deepest vertical pocket technique—DVP [24]), fetal biophysical profile (BPP) [25] and Doppler interrogation at the two fetal sites (UmbA and MCA), the CPR, both UtA and pulsatility index (PI); in this stage, we used US for EFW every two weeks. If the BPP and Dopplers were normal, expectance was proposed until 32 WG, and the case was discarded from the study. If the BPP was abnormal, the case was followed up daily. If there was a persistent abnormal BPP (below 5, two days consecutively), we performed elective C-section before 32 WG, regardless of the Doppler results.

o In stage I by Figueras [26] (EFW < 3rd centile or CPR < 5th centile or any UtA PI > 95th centile), we offered the same weekly monitoring protocol and the same management. If the BPP was normal, we monitored until we registered the case as advancing toward stage II or until progressing over 32 WG. If the BPP was abnormal, the case was followed up daily. If the BPP was persistently abnormal (below 5, two days consecutively), we added the DV assessment, and we performed an elective C-section before 32 WG regardless of the Doppler results.

o In stage II by Figueras [26]—defined as UmbA absent end-diastolic velocity (AEDV)—we offered hospitalization. If the parents declined admittance, we re-examined twice a week. Inpatients were also offered twice-weekly additional cardiotocography (CTG) and DV assessment daily. In this stage, we performed an elective C-section before 32 WG in all cases.

- In stage III by Figueras [26]—defined as UmbA reversed end-diastolic velocity (REDV), we monitored cases by US daily. In surviving fetuses, we offered delivery by cesarean section before 30 weeks based on the DV assessment.
- In stage IV by Figueras [26]—defined as reversed flow ductus venosus (DV), we offered immediate delivery after 27 weeks by caesarean section to all couples. Benefits and expectations were extensively explained to the parents in these cases.

Demographic data and maternal baseline characteristics, as well as data regarding the course of pregnancy and newborn outcomes, were collected prospectively for the study group and retrospectively (using the institution's computerized database containing the patient's antenatal/intra/postnatal records) for the control group.

In the study group, all US data were collected more than once, according to the study design. The statistical analysis was performed on the values at the beginning of the specific trimester (the second or the third). Therefore, the processed values were the ones obtained at 22 weeks' or at the first prenatal visit in our unit—in all cases enrolled in the ST. The data entering in the final analysis were obtained at 28 weeks' gestation (in all cases already enrolled) or at the first prenatal visit (at enrollment) in cases enrolled or referred to our unit in the TT.

We collected maternal data and demographics, pregnancy complications, prenatal care, US prenatal features, and postnatal data in newborns.

We perform routine screening for gestational diabetes mellitus (GDM). We use the one-step approach: oral glucose tolerance test (OGTT) at 24–28 WG (without prior plasma or serum glucose screening). We use a 75 g glucose load, and the glucose threshold values are: for fasting—95 mg/dL, at 1 h—180 mg/dL and at 2 h later—155 mg/dL. We classified the patient as positive in this study if two or more of the venous plasma concentrations were met or exceeded [27].

Maternal blood pressure was measured automatically with a calibrated OMRON M6 Confort device, according to standard procedure. Blood pressure was measured in one arm (right or left) without distinction, while women were seated and after a 5 min rest. We defined gestational hypertension as a systolic blood pressure of 140 mmHg or more or a diastolic blood pressure of 90 mmHg or more, or both, on two occasions at least 4 h apart after 20 weeks of gestation in a woman with a previously normal blood pressure [28]. We defined preeclampsia as a systolic blood pressure of 140 mm Hg or more or a diastolic blood pressure of 90 mm Hg or more with 300 mg or more of proteinuria. In the absence of proteinuria, new-onset hypertension was determined with the new onset of any of the following: thrombocytopenia: less than $100.000/mm^3$; renal insufficiency; impaired liver function: elevated liver transaminases to twice normal concentration; pulmonary edema; new-onset headache [28]. We defined HELLP syndrome as hemolysis, elevated liver enzymes and low platelet count [29].

We tested for hereditary thrombophilia and defined positive cases if Factor V Leiden homozygote mutation, antithrombin deficiency or protein C or protein S deficiency were found [30].

We performed C-section in all cases, either elective or in emergency circumstances.

We collected data on the newborns during the postpartum hospitalization.

We defined neonatal resuscitation as the set of interventions at the time of birth to support the establishment of breathing and circulation [31]. Respiratory distress was diagnosed if the newborn presented apnea, cyanosis, grunting, inspiratory stridor, nasal flaring, poor feeding, and tachypnoea (more than 60 breaths per minute), retractions in the intercostal, subcostal, or supracostal spaces and if the newborn received surfactant in the therapeutic scheme. Bronchopulmonary dysplasia was diagnosed if fibrotic opacities and cystic changes on the chest imaging X-ray (and on the computed tomography—CT scan) were found. The systemic blood pressure was measured noninvasively in all cases (by means of oscillometric technique, using appropriately sized cuffs). A specific case was reported as positive for hypotension if the abnormal values of systemic blood pressure were documented in the newborn's file and corrected by volume expansion, inotropes and corticosteroids. Persistent ductus arteriosus (PDA) was suspected on heart murmur and diagnosed by means of postnatal echocardiography. All cases were offered serial transfontanellar ultrasound (on days 3, 7, 14 and at discharge). All newborns benefited from additional heat (warmers and/or incubators). The immature gastro-intestinal (GI) system diagnosis was achieved after excluding other conditions, in babies having feeding intolerances: vomiting, stomach bile, or both; abdominal distension, reduced or absent bowel sounds and reduced or absent stool. All cases received empirical antibiotic treatment. Cases with clinical symptoms and/or with abnormal results on laboratory tests (abnormal white blood cell count, acidosis, hyperglycemia, lethargy, diminished responsiveness, fever, abnormal breathing, and circulatory disorders) were classified as neonatal infection.

We report exclusively data on cases requiring delivery between 27 and 32 completed weeks. By the internal unit's policy, in cases of severely early restricted fetuses needing iatrogenic delivery before 27 weeks, the parents are repeatedly counselled in multidisciplinary teams, and in utero transfer to superior centers is offered. Cases not requiring ending the pregnancy before 32 completed weeks (those continuing the pregnancy later than 32 weeks) were excluded from the analysis.

Statistical Analysis

Statistical analysis was performed using Minitab 17 Statistical Software. The distributions of the continuous variables were tested for normal values by using the Anderson–Darling test. Data with a normal distribution were presented as a mean value ± standard deviation (SD); the data that did not have a normal distribution were presented as a median and interquartile rate (IQR). To determine the statistical significance of the differences between the two groups for non-normal data, we used the Mann–Whitney test, comparing the medians (p value < 0.05), and for categorical data, we used the Chi-Square Test for Association (p value < 0.05).

3. Results

We performed the observational study during a three-year interval, and we summarized the workflow in Figure 1.

We had 30.5% self-presented cases and 69.4% referrals for sonography in our case series. Most cases (83.3%) had fetal indications for C-section, and the remaining ones had combined indications (fetal and maternal).

The general characteristics of pregnant women in the study are presented in Table 1. Cases were significantly more likely to be smokers or ex-smokers than controls ($p < 0.01$) and tended to be older ($p = 0.053$).

Among the 36 reported cases, we found in 30 cases exclusively laterally located placentas. In the remaining six cases, with the placenta located rather centrally, the operator decided on subjective criteria the assignment of the uterine arteries.

Both uterine arteries (placental and non-placental) assessed by means of spectral Doppler in the ST and in the TT were abnormal in all cases in the study group.

CPR percentiles were abnormal in the TT in the study group.

The mean gestational age at delivery was 30.7 (27–32) weeks in the study group and 39 weeks (37–41) of gestation in the control group.

In the study group, we had three cases of intrauterine fetal death (incidence 8.3%).

The numbers of prenatal medical follow-up visits (the total number and the third trimester number) in pregnant women included in the study are listed and compared (Table 2).

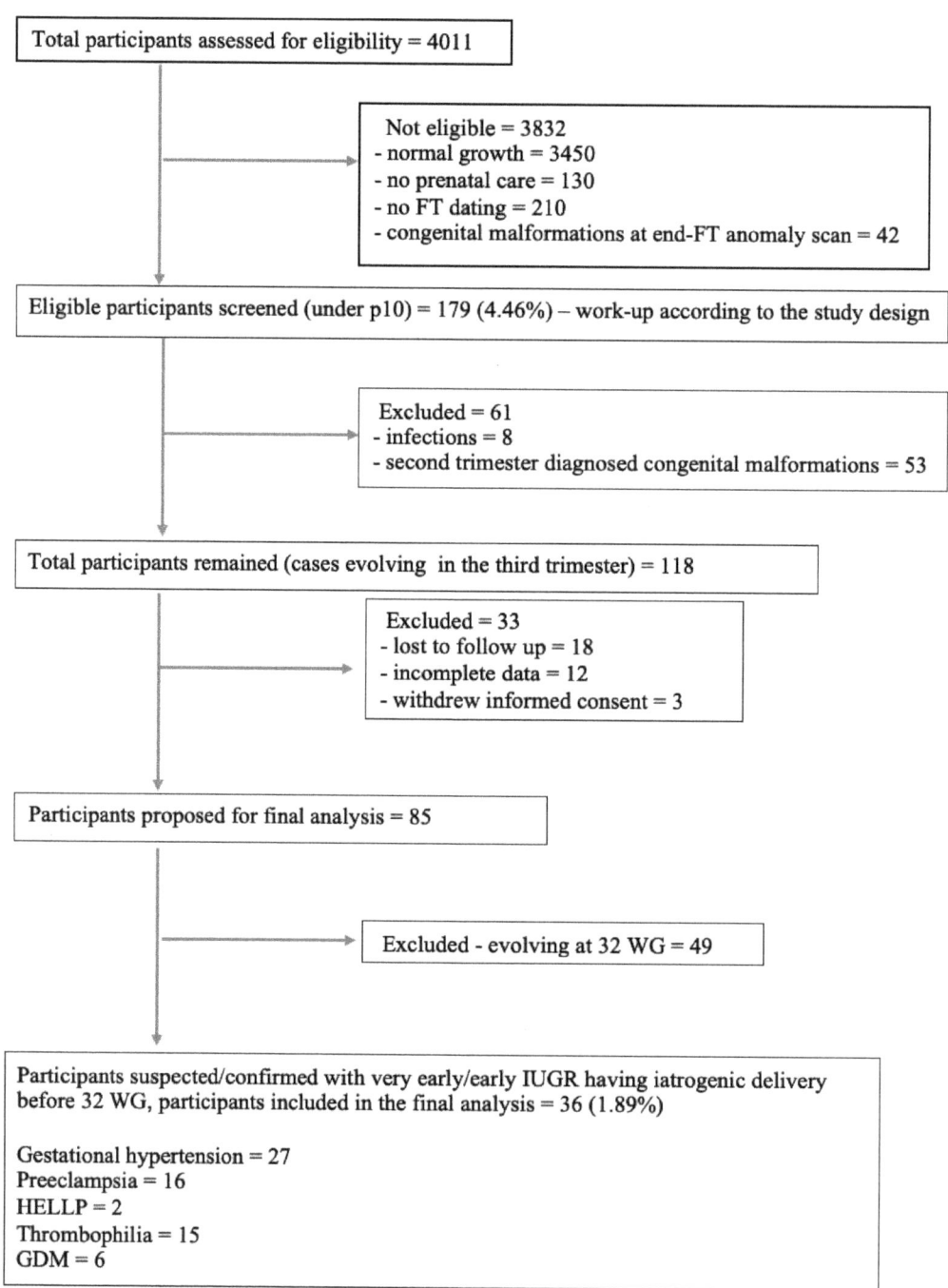

Figure 1. Flow chart diagram.

Table 1. Demographic maternal characteristics in pregnancies with suspected early IUGR and control group.

Characteristics	susp Early IUGR	Control	p
Smoking/former smoker	66.67%	21.4%	<0.01
Age	29.17 (19–37)	27.17 (18–35)	0.053
BMI	24.5 (19–27)	27.0 (17–31)	0.374

Abbreviations: IUGR intrauterine growth restriction, BMI body mass index. Age and BMI are expressed as median.

Table 2. Number of prenatal visits in pregnancy and in the third trimester in the study IUGR group versus the control group.

Variable	susp Early IUGR	Control	p
Nr of prenatal visits	11.5 (10–30)	5 (5–6)	<0.01
Nr of prenatal visits in the TT	6 (5–15)	2 (1–3)	<0.01

Abbreviations: TT the third trimester, IUGR intrauterine growth restriction, Nr number.

The newborn data in the study group is summarized below (Table 3).

Table 3. Newborn data in pregnancies complicated with early IUGR.

Characteristic/Complications	susp Early IUGR	Controls	p
Hospitalization days	36 (22–90)	3.8 (2–5)	<0.01
Apgar Score	5.5 (1–8)		
Resuscitation	17 (47.2%)		
Birth percentile	1% (1–10%)		
NICU days	10.5 (0–60)		
Respiratory Distress Syndrome	20 (55.5%)		
Bronchopulmonary Dysplasia	1 (2.7%)		
Transient Apnea	36 (100%)		
Hypotension	4 (11.1%)		
PDA	15 (41.6%)		
IVH	6 (16.6%)		
PVL	2 (5.5%)		
Hypothermia	0		
Immature GI System	32 (88.8%)		
NEC	1 (2.7%)		
Anemia	36 (100%)		
Jaundice	10 (27.7%)		
Transient Hypoglycaemia	16 (44.4%)		
Infection	9 (25%)		

Abbreviations: NICU Neonatal intensive care unit, PDA Persistent ductus arteriosus, IVH intraventricular hemorrhage, PVL periventricular leukomalacia, GI gastro-intestinal, NEC necrotizing enterocolitis.

As expected, the number of postnatal hospitalization days was significantly higher in the suspected early IUGR group vs. the control group. The Apgar score and the number of NICU days are expressed as median. Resuscitation measures were required at birth in almost half of the population. During hospitalization, all newborns presented one or more episodes of transient apnea. In very few cases, hypotension occurred. Persistent ductus arteriosus (PDA) was diagnosed frequently and was treated with anti-inflammatory non-steroid drugs, fluid restriction and/or diuretic drugs. No case required surgical treatment for PDA. All cases of intraventricular hemorrhage were mild. We had no case of large brain bleeding, which was expected to induce permanent brain injury. No newborn developed clinical signs of hypothermia. The single case of necrotizing enterocolitis received surgical treatment in the third day of life. All neonates in the study group had various degree of anemia, and all received blood products or transfusions. All neonates developed jaundice, but most of them had minor forms. Transient hypoglycemia was present in almost half of the cases immediately after birth. We had no case of severe persistent hypoglycemia. Despite the routine empirical antibiotic treatment, we had nine severe cases of neonatal infection. One only case had an early-onset form, while the remaining eight cases were diagnosed with late onset infection.

To describe better the severity and the continuum of the disease in the study group, we chose to perform a subanalysis and to compare the antenatal and the postnatal data in 12 pregnancies with very early IUGR (requiring iatrogenic delivery between 27 and 29.6 weeks of gestation) and 24 pregnancies in which the delivery was delayed until 30–32 weeks of gestation.

The ultrasound data regarding the UtA centile in the TT in these two subgroups is graphically represented and compared (Figure 2). In the extremely early suspected IUGR group, we found a higher median than in the early suspected IUGR. The boxplot of umbilical artery percentile revealed that in the very early suspected IUGR group, we found a higher median than in the early IUGR group. Based on the Kruskal–Wallis test, the differences between medians are statistically significant ($p < 0.01$).

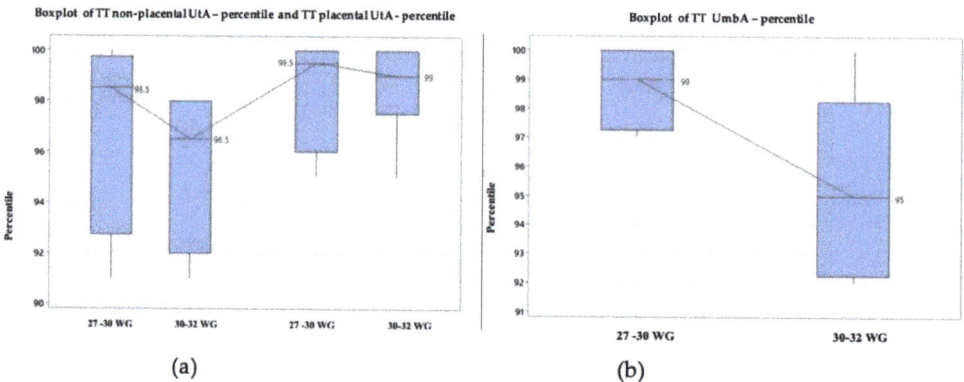

Figure 2. Doppler indices compared in the two subgroups: very early IUGR (requiring iatrogenic delivery between 27 and 29.6 weeks of gestation) and pregnancies which allowed continuing the pregnancy until 30–32 weeks of gestation. (**a**) The boxplot of placental and non-placental uterine artery assessed in the TT; (**b**) The boxplot of umbilical artery percentile. Abbreviations: TT third trimester, UtA uterine artery, WG weeks' gestation, Umb A umbilical artery.

Total prenatal visits in pregnancy and of TT visits revealed an increased number of medical visits in the very early suspected IUGR subgroup (Figure 3). Based on the Kruskal–Wallis test, the differences between medians are statistically significant ($p < 0.01$).

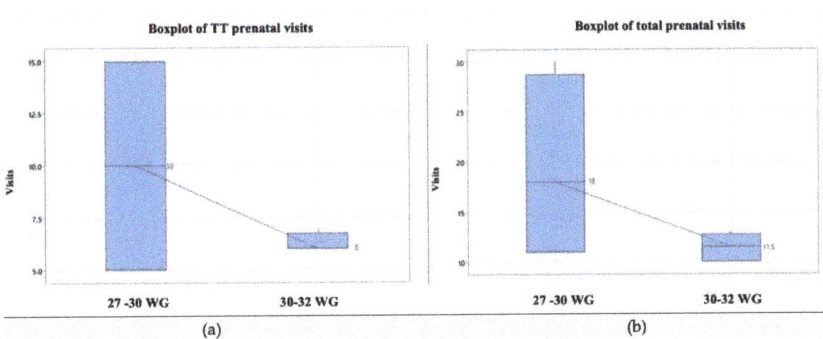

Figure 3. (a) The boxplot of TT prenatal visits; (b) The boxplot of total number of scheduled medical appointments. Abbreviations: WG weeks' gestation, TT—third trimester.

In the very early suspected IUGR subgroup, we had higher median values for NICU and total hospitalization days (21.5 days and 49 days, respectively) compared to the early suspected IUGR subgroup (Figure 4). Based on the Kruskal–Wallis test, the differences between medians are statistically significant ($p < 0.01$).

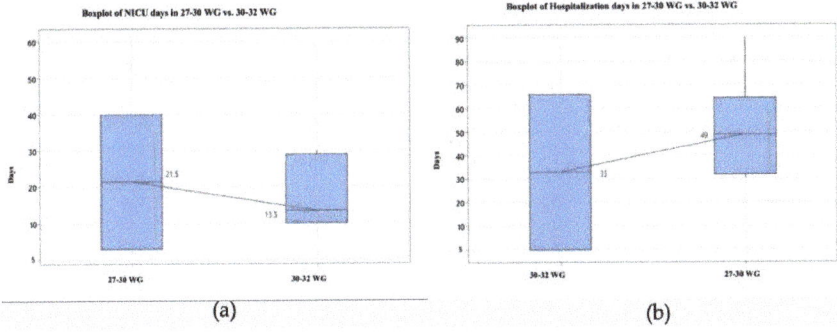

Figure 4. (a) The boxplot of NICU days in very early suspected IUGR subgroup vs. in the early suspected IUGR subgroup; (b) The boxplot of hospitalization days in the very early suspected IUGR subgroup vs. in early suspected IUGR subgroup. Abbreviations: GA gestational age, NICU neonatal Intensive Care Unit, WG weeks' gestation.

There were statistically significant differences between all US parameters in the very early suspected IUGR subgroup compared with the early suspected IUGR subgroup.

4. Discussion

IUGR reflects an abnormal adaptive fetal growth in a deleterious environment. Among all the modalities we have available to assess a fetus—we still do not know how each of them (EFW, Doppler velocities, BPP score), isolated or in combination, will perform in IUGR diagnosis and/or in deciding the time of the delivery [32]. Our data may be used in forthcoming logistic and linear repression analyses needed to prove the independent predictors for long-term outcome.

Our study targeted a very limited population of IUGR fetuses requiring early iatrogenic birth before 32 weeks. We confirmed the known association with hypertensive disorders in pregnancy [33], which is present in 70% in this case series. We searched for associations with non-modifiable (hereditary thrombophilia [34]) and modifiable risk factors (smoking) [35,36].

Early-onset IUGR has significant risks for major and minor neonatal morbidity [37]. We confirmed that the neonatal care is influenced by the severity of prematurity. The NICU days were significantly higher in the very early suspected/diagnosed and delivered group.

We also confirmed the recent reported high overall survival rates in IUGR suspected before 32 WG [37]. We registered three fetal deaths in the study group, having an overall in utero mortality of 8.3%. Among them, two fetuses did not benefit from medical management (fetal abandonment was decided by the parents). One fetus had the EFW < p3 at 26 WG, and the fetal demise occurred between two consecutive follow-up visits, at 29 WG. We registered one only neonatal death in our cohort. Previous reports [38] showed 6% mortality in the IUGR group and 24% severe morbidity.

We have no treatment for IUGR. The sole intervention having some treatment-like effect is the early iatrogenic termination of pregnancy [39]. Yet, the antenatal detection of inadequate fetal growth leads to increased surveillance and reduces the risk of fetal death [40]. According to some results, the prenatal diagnosis may also improve perinatal morbidity [41], although the scientific proof of this statement is still debated [42]. In our case series, the intensity of prenatal care was amplified in early and very early suspicion of IUGR. The total number of prenatal visits in pregnancy and the total number of TT visits was significantly higher in the very early suspected IUGR subgroup. Both sets of figures are much higher than the number recommended by the current guidelines in low-risk pregnancies [43–45]. Defensive medicine may play a role in these results, but it cannot be weighted from these data.

We did not report the CPR centiles to describe this population of fetuses, although CPR proved to be superior to the UmbA Doppler assessment in the prediction of adverse perinatal outcome [46,47] and in the prediction of long-term developmental problems [48]. Currently, there are no clinical trials investigating the effectiveness of the CPR in guiding clinical management in IUGR, and it is still unclear to which subgroup of pregnant women this applies best. In our case series, this parameter was abnormal in all cases in the TT. Regarding the maternal interface, we confirmed [49] that all searched parameters were abnormal in both trimesters.

A cost-analysis to follow our report may be appropriate due to the high number of US scans, NICU and total hospitalization days needed in this high-risk population. Our results have the potential to help local authorities in the healthcare system plan an adequate strategy (primary care, medical education, audit, merged databases in university centers, funding), adjusted for emergency state hospitals. Results may lead to appropriate centralization to improve the neonatal outcome.

As limitations, we provide no long-term data on the neonates included in the study.

In this study, the US expertise of the primary referring doctors was not investigated. In Romania, obstetricians ultrasonographers are the main healthcare provider responsible for the assessment of fetal growth in low-risk pregnancies, and TT scan is optional. The primary doctors' skills are important for identifying impaired fetal growth and referring the mother to a customized prenatal care. Unless placed in an at-risk category, the pregnancy will not be monitored appropriately.

In IUGR, an impressive amount of recent research was published. Definitions of IUGR and significant predictors varied largely throughout the last decades: AC < p10 and UmbA PI > p95 [38] (consensus amongst 20 European experts in perinatology), AC < p10 or EFW < p5 and UmbA PI > p95 [50] (very wide GA considered). We defined "suspected IUGR" as the US EFW less than the 10th centile prior to delivery. We are aware that most researchers define IUGR as two components associated: small size and functional evidence of placental impairment (abnormal Dopplers). We acknowledge the risk of including a certain proportion of small for gestational age healthy fetuses (small sized and having normal results on Doppler interrogation). Yet, we may assume that this population was very limited, since we excluded all pregnancies continuing at 32 WA, and we had no case of pregnancy with normal fetal BPP and normal velocities iatrogenically interrupted, regardless the pEFW.

It has been shown that multivariable Integrative models (using additionally maternal characteristics and maternal biochemical markers) offer only modest improvement in the detection of IUGR when compared with screening based on EFW centile alone [51].

We did not assess the data immediate before delivery. This might have an impact on results due to the dynamic of US parameters [52].

We centered the study in a state hospital, having issues in subsidizing some of the already known strategies to improve the IUGR detection in the antenatal period: FT maternal serum placental growth factor (PlGF) and soluble forms-like tyrosine kinase-1 (sFLT) [51,53].

In our view, this report has also some advantages: we provided data on the characteristics of the mother, US features and the type of prenatal surveillance, covering three years, in a single tertiary center in an upper middle-income country.

Data obtained by a single operator using a single US equipment and a standardized technique for Doppler interrogation assured homogeneity in this study. This has the potential to lead to consistent results, given the considerable methodological heterogeneity in studies reporting reference ranges for UmbA and MCA Doppler indices and CPR. Using different references has important implications for clinical practice [51]

We did not use CTG and short-term variation of fetal heart rate in this population of fetuses suspected of early-onset IUGR, as scientific proof for its benefits is still missing [53].

We had the opportunity to use the hospital's electronic records, which improved the retrospective collection of data in the control group.

In our view, the contextual factors should be considered. Our study interval overlapped the pandemics, and this heavily impacted the internal policy of the unit, the continuity of care and the rate of admittance. This resulted most probably in biasing the population selection, budgets, staffing, workload, safety, the practice climate, and the management decisions. On the other hands, the attempt to use the same guidelines in different countries without local validation may be difficult, given the differences in the prevalence of adverse pregnancy outcomes in different settings. The prevalence and the severity of a disease influences the diagnostic performance; thus, context-specific guidance is necessary. Given the local reporting gaps about the predictive ability of antenatal Doppler for adverse pregnancy outcomes and for the pregnancy care costs, our data on a very high-risk fetal population may prove informative.

5. Conclusions

Fetuses with isolated very early and early fetal growth restriction—defined as ultrasound estimation of fetal weight < p10 using the Hadlock 4 technique and requiring delivery before 32 weeks' gestation—are likely to be scanned more frequently, and newborns have longer hospitalizations. GA at iatrogenic birth and UtA PI centiles are related to the latter. In developing and middle-income countries, cost-analysis studies should be developed in the future due to the high number of prenatal visits, scans performed by experts, NICU and total hospitalization days. This would help local authorities in the healthcare system plan an adequate strategy (primary care, medical education, audit, centralization and funding) to improve outcome in these cases.

Author Contributions: Conceptualization, M.D. and A.D.H.; methodology M.D. and M.G.; validation S.T. and R.G.C.; investigation F.T., O.C.S. and A.F.S.-C.; data collection M.D., A.D.H. and A.M.B.; writing—original draft M.D.; preparation M.D. and A.D.H.; visualization E.B., S.T.; writing—review and editing S.T., R.G.C. and O.C.S.; supervision S.T. All authors have read and agreed to the published version of the manuscript.

Funding: This work was supported by a grant from the University of Medicine and Pharmacy Craiova, project number 26/812/3: "US parameters and sFlt-1/PlGF ratio in predicting preeclampsia and maternal/fetal complications".

Institutional Review Board Statement: The study was conducted in accordance with the Declaration of Helsinki and approved by the Ethics Committee of University of Medicine and Pharmacy of Craiova (protocol code 206/24.10.2019).

Informed Consent Statement: Informed consent was obtained from all subjects involved in the study.

Conflicts of Interest: The authors declare no conflict of interest.

References

1. Gordijn, S.J.; Beune, I.M.; Thilaganathan, B.; Papageorghiou, A.; Baschat, A.A.; Baker, P.N.; Silver, R.M.; Wynia, K.; Ganzevoort, W. Consensus definition of fetal growth restriction: A Delphi procedure. *Ultrasound Obstet. Gynecol.* **2016**, *48*, 333–339. [CrossRef] [PubMed]
2. Ganzevoort, W.; Alfirevic, Z.; von Dadelszen, P.; Kenny, L.; Papageorghiou, A.; van Wassenaer-Leemhuis, A.; Gluud, C.; Mol, B.W.; Baker, P.N. STRIDER: Sildenafil Therapy In Dismal prognosis Early-onset intrauterine growth Restriction—A protocol for a systematic review with individual participant data and aggregate data meta-analysis and trial sequential analysis. *Syst. Rev.* **2014**, *3*, 23. [CrossRef] [PubMed]
3. von Dadelszen, P.; Dwinnell, S.; Magee, L.A.; Carleton, B.C.; Gruslin, A.; Lee, B.; Lim, K.I.; Liston, R.M.; Miller, S.P.; Rurak, D.; et al. Sildenafil citrate therapy for severe early-onset intrauterine growth restriction. *BJOG* **2011**, *118*, 624–628. [CrossRef] [PubMed]
4. Lee, M.J.; Conner, E.L.; Charafeddine, L.; Woods, J.R., Jr.; Del Priore, G. A critical birth weight and other determinants of survival for infants with severe intrauterine growth restriction. *Ann. N. Y. Acad. Sci.* **2001**, *943*, 326–339. [CrossRef]
5. Batton, D.G.; DeWitte, D.B.; Espinoza, R.; Swails, T.L. The impact of fetal compromise on outcome at the border of viability. *Am. J. Obstet. Gynecol.* **1998**, *178*, 909–915. [CrossRef]
6. Petersen, S.G.; Wong, S.F.; Urs, P.; Gray, P.H.; Gardener, G.J. Early onset, severe fetal growth restriction with absent or reversed end-diastolic flow velocity waveform in the umbilical artery: Perinatal and long-term outcomes. *Aust. N. Z. J. Obstet. Gynaecol.* **2009**, *49*, 45–51. [CrossRef]
7. Ganzevoort, W.; Rep, A.; de Vries, J.I.; Bonsel, G.J.; Wolf, H.; PETRA-Investigators. Prediction of maternal complications and adverse infant outcome at admission for temporizing management of early-onset severe hypertensive disorders of pregnancy. *Am. J. Obstet. Gynecol.* **2006**, *195*, 495–503. [CrossRef]
8. Guellec, I.; Lapillonne, A.; Renolleau, S.; Charlaluk, M.L.; Roze, J.C.; Marret, S.; Vieux, R.; Monique, K.; Ancel, P.Y.; Group, E.S. Neurologic outcomes at school age in very preterm infants born with severe or mild growth restriction. *Pediatrics* **2011**, *127*, e883–e891. [CrossRef] [PubMed]
9. Carter, E.B.; Tuuli, M.G.; Caughey, A.B.; Odibo, A.O.; Macones, G.A.; Cahill, A.G. Number of prenatal visits and pregnancy outcomes in low-risk women. *J. Perinatol.* **2016**, *36*, 178–181. [CrossRef]
10. Peleg, D.; Kennedy, C.M.; Hunter, S.K. Intrauterine growth restriction: Identification and management. *Am. Fam. Physician* **1998**, *58*, 453–460, 466–467.
11. Cosmi, E.; Fanelli, T.; Visentin, S.; Trevisanuto, D.; Zanardo, V. Consequences in infants that were intrauterine growth restricted. *J. Pregnancy* **2011**, *2011*, 364381. [CrossRef] [PubMed]
12. Hadlock, F.P.; Harrist, R.B.; Carpenter, R.J.; Deter, R.L.; Park, S.K. Sonographic estimation of fetal weight. The value of femur length in addition to head and abdomen measurements. *Radiology* **1984**, *150*, 535–540. [CrossRef] [PubMed]
13. Iliescu, D.; Tudorache, S.; Comanescu, A.; Antsaklis, P.; Cotarcea, S.; Novac, L.; Cernea, N.; Antsaklis, A. Improved detection rate of structural abnormalities in the first trimester using an extended examination protocol. *Ultrasound Obstet. Gynecol.* **2013**, *42*, 300–309. [CrossRef] [PubMed]
14. Tudorache, S.; Cara, M.; Iliescu, D.G.; Novac, L.; Cernea, N. First trimester two- and four-dimensional cardiac scan: Intra- and interobserver agreement, comparison between methods and benefits of color Doppler technique. *Ultrasound Obstet. Gynecol.* **2013**, *42*, 659–668. [CrossRef]
15. Strauss, K.J.; Kaste, S.C. The ALARA (as low as reasonably achievable) concept in pediatric interventional and fluoroscopic imaging: Striving to keep radiation doses as low as possible during fluoroscopy of pediatric patients—A white paper executive summary. *Pediatr. Radiol.* **2006**, *36* (Suppl. S2), 110–112. [CrossRef] [PubMed]
16. Bhide, A.; Acharya, G.; Baschat, A.; Bilardo, C.M.; Brezinka, C.; Cafici, D.; Ebbing, C.; Hernandez-Andrade, E.; Kalache, K.; Kingdom, J.; et al. ISUOG Practice Guidelines (updated): Use of Doppler velocimetry in obstetrics. *Ultrasound Obstet. Gynecol.* **2021**, *58*, 331–339. [CrossRef]
17. Shennan, A.; Suff, N.; Jacobsson, B.; FIGO Working Group for Preterm Birth. FIGO good practice recommendations on magnesium sulfate administration for preterm fetal neuroprotection. *Int. J. Gynecol. Obstet.* **2021**, *155*, 31–33. [CrossRef]
18. Norman, J.; Shennan, A.; Jacobsson, B.; Stock, S.J.; FIGO Working Group for Preterm Birth. FIGO good practice recommendations on the use of prenatal corticosteroids to improve outcomes and minimize harm in babies born preterm. *Int. J. Gynaecol. Obstet.* **2021**, *155*, 26–30. [CrossRef]
19. Gomez, O.; Figueras, F.; Fernandez, S.; Bennasar, M.; Martinez, J.M.; Puerto, B.; Gratacos, E. Reference ranges for uterine artery mean pulsatility index at 11–41 weeks of gestation. *Ultrasound Obstet. Gynecol.* **2008**, *32*, 128–132. [CrossRef]

20. Acharya, G.; Wilsgaard, T.; Berntsen, G.K.; Maltau, J.M.; Kiserud, T. Reference ranges for serial measurements of umbilical artery Doppler indices in the second half of pregnancy. *Am. J. Obstet. Gynecol.* **2005**, *192*, 937–944. [CrossRef]
21. Figueras, F.; Fernandez, S.; Eixarch, E.; Gomez, O.; Martinez, J.M.; Puerto, B.; Gratacos, E. Middle cerebral artery pulsatility index: Reliability at different sampling sites. *Ultrasound Obstet. Gynecol.* **2006**, *28*, 809–813. [CrossRef]
22. Kessler, J.; Rasmussen, S.; Hanson, M.; Kiserud, T. Longitudinal reference ranges for ductus venosus flow velocities and waveform indices. *Ultrasound Obstet. Gynecol.* **2006**, *28*, 890–898. [CrossRef] [PubMed]
23. Ciobanu, A.; Wright, A.; Syngelaki, A.; Wright, D.; Akolekar, R.; Nicolaides, K.H. Fetal Medicine Foundation reference ranges for umbilical artery and middle cerebral artery pulsatility index and cerebroplacental ratio. *Ultrasound Obstet. Gynecol.* **2019**, *53*, 465–472. [CrossRef] [PubMed]
24. Magann, E.F.; Chauhan, S.P.; Washington, W.; Whitworth, N.S.; Martin, J.N.; Morrison, J.C. Ultrasound estimation of amniotic fluid volume using the largest vertical pocket containing umbilical cord: Measure to or through the cord? *Ultrasound Obstet. Gynecol.* **2002**, *20*, 464–467. [CrossRef]
25. Manning, F.A.; Platt, L.D.; Sipos, L. Antepartum fetal evaluation: Development of a fetal biophysical profile. *Am. J. Obstet. Gynecol.* **1980**, *136*, 787–795. [CrossRef] [PubMed]
26. Figueras, F.; Gratacos, E. Update on the diagnosis and classification of fetal growth restriction and proposal of a stage-based management protocol. *Fetal Diagn. Ther.* **2014**, *36*, 86–98. [CrossRef] [PubMed]
27. American Diabetes, A. Gestational diabetes mellitus. *Diabetes Care* **2003**, *26* (Suppl. S1), S103–S105. [CrossRef]
28. American College of Obstetricians and Gynecologists. Gestational Hypertension and Preeclampsia: ACOG Practice Bulletin, Number 222. *Obstet. Gynecol.* **2020**, *135*, e237–e260. [CrossRef]
29. Haram, K.; Svendsen, E.; Abildgaard, U. The HELLP syndrome: Clinical issues and management. A Review. *BMC Pregnancy Childbirth* **2009**, *9*, 8. [CrossRef]
30. American College of Obstetricians and Gynecologists' Committee on Practice Bulletins–Obstetrics. ACOG Practice Bulletin No. 197: Inherited Thrombophilias in Pregnancy. *Obstet. Gynecol.* **2018**, *132*, e18–e34. [CrossRef]
31. Lee, A.C.; Cousens, S.; Wall, S.N.; Niermeyer, S.; Darmstadt, G.L.; Carlo, W.A.; Keenan, W.J.; Bhutta, Z.A.; Gill, C.; Lawn, J.E. Neonatal resuscitation and immediate newborn assessment and stimulation for the prevention of neonatal deaths: A systematic review, meta-analysis and Delphi estimation of mortality effect. *BMC Public Health* **2011**, *11* (Suppl. S3), S12. [CrossRef] [PubMed]
32. Romero, R.; Kalache, K.D.; Kadar, N. Timing the delivery of the preterm severely growth-restricted fetus: Venous Doppler, cardiotocography or the biophysical profile? *Ultrasound Obstet. Gynecol.* **2002**, *19*, 118–121. [CrossRef] [PubMed]
33. Bilardo, C.M.; Hecher, K.; Visser, G.H.A.; Papageorghiou, A.T.; Marlow, N.; Thilaganathan, B.; Van Wassenaer-Leemhuis, A.; Todros, T.; Marsal, K.; Frusca, T.; et al. Severe fetal growth restriction at 26–32 weeks: Key messages from the TRUFFLE study. *Ultrasound Obstet. Gynecol.* **2017**, *50*, 285–290. [CrossRef] [PubMed]
34. Mirzaei, F.; Farzad-Mahajeri, Z. Association of hereditary thrombophilia with intrauterine growth restriction. *Iran. J. Reprod. Med.* **2013**, *11*, 275–278.
35. Jaddoe, V.W.; Verburg, B.O.; de Ridder, M.A.; Hofman, A.; Mackenbach, J.P.; Moll, H.A.; Steegers, E.A.; Witteman, J.C. Maternal smoking and fetal growth characteristics in different periods of pregnancy: The generation R study. *Am. J. Epidemiol.* **2007**, *165*, 1207–1215. [CrossRef]
36. Quinton, A.E.; Cook, C.M.; Peek, M.J. The relationship between cigarette smoking, endothelial function and intrauterine growth restriction in human pregnancy. *BJOG* **2008**, *115*, 780–784. [CrossRef]
37. Pels, A.; Beune, I.M.; van Wassenaer-Leemhuis, A.G.; Limpens, J.; Ganzevoort, W. Early-onset fetal growth restriction: A systematic review on mortality and morbidity. *Acta Obstet. Gynecol. Scand.* **2020**, *99*, 153–166. [CrossRef]
38. Lees, C.; Marlow, N.; Arabin, B.; Bilardo, C.M.; Brezinka, C.; Derks, J.B.; Duvekot, J.; Frusca, T.; Diemert, A.; Ferrazzi, E.; et al. Perinatal morbidity and mortality in early-onset fetal growth restriction: Cohort outcomes of the trial of randomized umbilical and fetal flow in Europe (TRUFFLE). *Ultrasound Obstet. Gynecol.* **2013**, *42*, 400–408. [CrossRef]
39. Unterscheider, J.; Cuzzilla, R. Severe early-onset fetal growth restriction: What do we tell the prospective parents? *Prenat. Diagn.* **2021**, *41*, 1363–1371. [CrossRef]
40. Gardosi, J.; Giddings, S.; Buller, S.; Southam, M.; Williams, M. Preventing stillbirths through improved antenatal recognition of pregnancies at risk due to fetal growth restriction. *Public Health* **2014**, *128*, 698–702. [CrossRef]
41. Verlijsdonk, J.W.; Winkens, B.; Boers, K.; Scherjon, S.; Roumen, F. Suspected versus non-suspected small-for-gestational age fetuses at term: Perinatal outcomes. *J. Matern. Fetal Neonatal Med.* **2012**, *25*, 938–943. [CrossRef] [PubMed]
42. Ewigman, B.G.; Crane, J.P.; Frigoletto, F.D.; LeFevre, M.L.; Bain, R.P.; McNellis, D. Effect of prenatal ultrasound screening on perinatal outcome. RADIUS Study Group. *N. Engl. J. Med.* **1993**, *329*, 821–827. [CrossRef] [PubMed]
43. Lees, C.C.; Stampalija, T.; Baschat, A.; da Silva Costa, F.; Ferrazzi, E.; Figueras, F.; Hecher, K.; Kingdom, J.; Poon, L.C.; Salomon, L.J.; et al. ISUOG Practice Guidelines: Diagnosis and management of small-for-gestational-age fetus and fetal growth restriction. *Ultrasound Obstet. Gynecol.* **2020**, *56*, 298–312. [CrossRef]
44. American College of Obstetricians and Gynecologists' Committee on Practice Bulletins—Obstetrics and the Society for Maternal-Fetal Medicine. ACOG Practice Bulletin No. 204: Fetal Growth Restriction. *Obstet. Gynecol.* **2019**, *133*, e97–e109. [CrossRef] [PubMed]
45. Grivell, R.M.; Wong, L.; Bhatia, V. Regimens of fetal surveillance for impaired fetal growth. *Cochrane Database Syst. Rev.* **2012**, *2012*, CD007113. [CrossRef]

46. Vollgraff Heidweiller-Schreurs, C.A.; De Boer, M.A.; Heymans, M.W.; Schoonmade, L.J.; Bossuyt, P.M.M.; Mol, B.W.J.; De Groot, C.J.M.; Bax, C.J. Prognostic accuracy of cerebroplacental ratio and middle cerebral artery Doppler for adverse perinatal outcome: Systematic review and meta-analysis. *Ultrasound Obstet. Gynecol.* **2018**, *51*, 313–322. [CrossRef] [PubMed]
47. Oros, D.; Ruiz-Martinez, S.; Staines-Urias, E.; Conde-Agudelo, A.; Villar, J.; Fabre, E.; Papageorghiou, A.T. Reference ranges for Doppler indices of umbilical and fetal middle cerebral arteries and cerebroplacental ratio: Systematic review. *Ultrasound Obstet. Gynecol.* **2019**, *53*, 454–464. [CrossRef] [PubMed]
48. Meher, S.; Hernandez-Andrade, E.; Basheer, S.N.; Lees, C. Impact of cerebral redistribution on neurodevelopmental outcome in small-for-gestational-age or growth-restricted babies: A systematic review. *Ultrasound Obstet. Gynecol.* **2015**, *46*, 398–404. [CrossRef]
49. Cnossen, J.S.; Morris, R.K.; ter Riet, G.; Mol, B.W.; van der Post, J.A.; Coomarasamy, A.; Zwinderman, A.H.; Robson, S.C.; Bindels, P.J.; Kleijnen, J.; et al. Use of uterine artery Doppler ultrasonography to predict pre-eclampsia and intrauterine growth restriction: A systematic review and bivariable meta-analysis. *CMAJ* **2008**, *178*, 701–711. [CrossRef]
50. Unterscheider, J.; Daly, S.; Geary, M.P.; Kennelly, M.M.; McAuliffe, F.M.; O'Donoghue, K.; Hunter, A.; Morrison, J.J.; Burke, G.; Dicker, P.; et al. Optimizing the definition of intrauterine growth restriction: The multicenter prospective PORTO Study. *Am. J. Obstet. Gynecol.* **2013**, *208*, 290.e1-6. [CrossRef]
51. Gaccioli, F.; Aye, I.; Sovio, U.; Charnock-Jones, D.S.; Smith, G.C.S. Screening for fetal growth restriction using fetal biometry combined with maternal biomarkers. *Am. J. Obstet. Gynecol.* **2018**, *218*, S725–S737. [CrossRef] [PubMed]
52. Hecher, K.; Bilardo, C.M.; Stigter, R.H.; Ville, Y.; Hackeloer, B.J.; Kok, H.J.; Senat, M.V.; Visser, G.H. Monitoring of fetuses with intrauterine growth restriction: A longitudinal study. *Ultrasound Obstet. Gynecol.* **2001**, *18*, 564–570. [CrossRef] [PubMed]
53. Miranda, J.; Rodriguez-Lopez, M.; Triunfo, S.; Sairanen, M.; Kouru, H.; Parra-Saavedra, M.; Crovetto, F.; Figueras, F.; Crispi, F.; Gratacos, E. Prediction of fetal growth restriction using estimated fetal weight vs a combined screening model in the third trimester. *Ultrasound Obstet. Gynecol.* **2017**, *50*, 603–611. [CrossRef] [PubMed]

Disclaimer/Publisher's Note: The statements, opinions and data contained in all publications are solely those of the individual author(s) and contributor(s) and not of MDPI and/or the editor(s). MDPI and/or the editor(s) disclaim responsibility for any injury to people or property resulting from any ideas, methods, instructions or products referred to in the content.

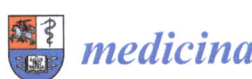

Review

The Main Changes in Pregnancy—Therapeutic Approach to Musculoskeletal Pain

Felicia Fiat [1,†], Petru Eugen Merghes [2,†], Alexandra Denisa Scurtu [3,4,*], Bogdan Almajan Guta [5,*], Cristina Adriana Dehelean [3,4], Narcis Varan [2] and Elena Bernad [1]

[1] Department of Obstetrics-Gynecology II, Faculty of Medicine, "Victor Babes" University of Medicine and Pharmacy, Eftimie Murgu Square, No. 2, 300041 Timisoara, Romania
[2] Department of Physical Education and Sport, Banat's University of Agricultural Sciences and Veterinary Medicine "King Mihai I of Romania" from Timisoara, Calea Aradului 119, 300645 Timisoara, Romania
[3] Department of Toxicology and Drug Industry, Faculty of Pharmacy, "Victor Babes" University of Medicine and Pharmacy, Eftimie Murgu Square, No. 2, 300041 Timisoara, Romania
[4] Research Centre for Pharmaco-Toxicological Evaluation, "Victor Babes" University of Medicine and Pharmacy, Eftimie Murgu Square, No. 2, 300041 Timisoara, Romania
[5] Department of Physical Therapy and Special Motor Skills, Faculty of Physical Education and Sport, West University of Timisoara, Vasile Parvan Boulevard, No. 4, 300223 Timisoara, Romania
* Correspondence: alexandra.scurtu@umft.ro (A.D.S.); bogdan.almajan@e-uvt.ro (B.A.G.)
† These authors contributed equally to this work.

Abstract: *Background and Objectives*: During pregnancy, women undergo various physiological and anatomical changes that are accentuated as the pregnancy progresses, but return to their previous state a few weeks/months after the pregnancy. However, a targeted therapeutic approach is needed. Most of the time, during this period, these changes precipitate the appearance of pain, musculoskeletal pain being the most common. Pregnant women should avoid treating musculoskeletal pain with medication and should choose alternative and complementary methods. Exercise along with rest is the basis for treating chronic musculoskeletal pain. Side effects of physical therapy are rare and, in addition, it is not contraindicated in pregnant women. The benefits of this type of treatment in combating pain far outweigh the risks, being an easy way to improve quality of life. The objective of this article is to discuss the management of musculoskeletal pain during pregnancy, to identify the main musculoskeletal pain encountered in pregnant women along with drug treatment, and to expose the beneficial effects of alternative and complementary methods in combating pain. *Materials and Methods*: A literature search was conducted using medical databases, including PubMed, Google Scholar, and ScienceDirect, using the keywords "changes of pregnancy", "musculoskeletal pain", "pregnancy pain", "pain management", "pharmacological approach", "alternative and complementary treatment" and specific sites. Information was collected from studies whose target population included pregnant women who complained of musculoskeletal pain during the 9 months of pregnancy; pregnant women with other pathologies that could increase their pain were not included in this review. *Results*: The articles related to the most common non-obstetric musculoskeletal pain in pregnancy along with pharmacological treatment options and alternative and complementary methods for musculoskeletal pain management during pregnancy were selected. *Conclusions*: The results were used to guide information towards the safest methods of therapy but also to raise awareness of the treatment criteria in order to compare the effectiveness of existing methods. Treatment must consider the implications for the mother and fetus, optimizing non-pharmacological therapeutic options.

Keywords: pregnancy; changes of pregnancy; musculoskeletal pain; treatment

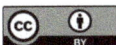

1. Introduction

During pregnancy, a woman's body undergoes various changes, both physiological and anatomical, necessary to meet the increased metabolic needs in order to support the growing fetus, for its harmonious development and also to prepare the body for birth [1,2]. It has been observed that the first changes appear in the first trimester of pregnancy and intensify once the final term is reached and return to normal a few weeks after birth [2]. The physiological changes produced by pregnancy are generally well tolerated by healthy women, but certain changes are still likely to aggravate different pathologies or give rise to a variety of disorders, especially musculoskeletal, which is the most common in pregnancy [3]. A woman's body undergoes major changes during pregnancy in all organs to support both the mother and the fetus.

A proper diet is important at any time of life, especially during pregnancy. The diet of the pregnant woman must provide nutrients and energy to support both the normal requirements of the mother and the needs of the developing fetus. The recommended diet for pregnant women does not differ much from the diet of an adult, necessarily comprising a healthy, balanced and varied diet. For pregnant women, it is recommended to use foods rich in minerals and vitamins, especially iron, vitamin D and folate [4]. Additionally, at the time of conception, a balanced diet is required, and it is preferable for the woman to have a healthy body weight with a body mass index of 20–25, since lower or higher values can influence the fertility and harmonious growth of the fetus [5]. Excessive weight gain during pregnancy has countless negative effects on the health of the mother and child, including high blood pressure, diabetes, birth trauma and asphyxia. This weight gain in pregnant women is associated with a higher risk of long-term obesity but also with the precipitation of musculoskeletal pain [6]. Moreover, aside from diet, the evolution of pregnancy is influenced by a multitude of factors, including age, previous experiences and family history, as well as stress, smoking and excessive alcohol or coffee consumption [7]. Both extremes of age considered appropriate for the conception of the child can cause unwanted effects on pregnancy. Young mothers have a high risk of low birth weight, premature birth and fetal death resulting from biological immaturity, lack of access to prenatal care to socioeconomic factors. However, the mother's advanced age is more strongly associated with complications at birth [8]. There is a close relationship between healthy mothers and healthy newborns, and proper nutrition and physical activity are key factors that contribute to its achievement; factors that can prevent and combat musculoskeletal pain encountered during pregnancy. Special attention was paid to physiotherapy in pregnancy with the help of the American College of Obstetrics and Gynecologists guidelines in 2002 [9], which led to studies focusing on the beneficial effects of exercise during pregnancy.

New detailed clinical trials are currently needed regarding the treatment of the most common pain in pregnancy, adapted to current times with socio-economic or dietary modifications; a treatment that must be correlated with physiological and anatomical changes that normally occur in pregnant women. In the foreground should be non-pharmacological treatment; physiotherapy being a method more easily accepted by pregnant women. This paper provides a comprehensive look at the physiological and anatomical changes in pregnancy, the main musculoskeletal problems and the treatment that can be addressed, pharmacological treatment and especially non-pharmacological treatment, based on alternative and complementary methods.

2. Physiological and Anatomical Changes of Pregnancy

2.1. The Main Changes That Occur at the Organ Level

Regarding the cardiovascular system, during pregnancy heart rate can increase by up to 60% with the highest values registered from week 20 until birth. Cardiac output is required to increase and to maintain normal blood pressure. Initially, the increase in cardiac output is achieved by an increase in stroke volume, followed at the end of the third trimester by an increase in heart rhythm [2,10]. The highest increase in cardiac output is achieved in the kidneys, uterus and skin to control the mother's temperature and to produce nutrients needed for the fetus and to eliminate fetal and maternal waste [11–13]. The presence of the pregnant uterus leads to the lateral movement of the heart. In the first weeks of pregnancy, the pregnant uterus begins to cause the mechanical compression of the inferior vena cava and the descending aorta. Thus, a reduction in cardiac output and venous return is observed, resulting in maternal hypotension and fetal acidemia. To correct and compensate for compression, heart rate and sympathetic tone increase. In many pregnant women, these mechanisms may be insufficient to support blood pressure and aortocaval compression syndrome may set in. This hypotensive syndrome is accompanied by symptoms such as pallor, dizziness, sweating and tachycardia, followed by bradycardia and hypotension in the supine position, while the severe form can cause death [14,15].

During pregnancy, in the gastrointestinal tract, gastric motility is most affected. High levels of hormones, especially progesterone, cause smooth muscle relaxation and decreased bowel motility, thus prolonging gastric emptying time, leading to constipation [16]. Likewise, the progesterone-mediated relaxation of the lower esophageal sphincter induces a decrease in its tone manifested as gastroesophageal reflux disease [17]. Additionally, high hormone levels cause vomiting and nausea, known as morning sickness, which occur at any time of the day in more than 70% of pregnant women. However, if these conditions increase after week 20 or lead to ketosis with a massive weight loss, hyperemesis gravidarum can be reached and intravenous vitamins and fluids may be needed [18].

Respiratory changes also occur in pregnant women. The diaphragm rises by about 2 cm, which leads to a 5% decrease in lung capacity. The current volume increases by up to 40% leading to a decrease in the expiratory reserve volume by 20% and an increase in ventilation per minute (VM). The increase in VM determines an increase in the level of arterial (PaO_2) and alveolar (PAO_2) pressure but also a decrease in the partial pressure of arterial carbon dioxide ($PaCO_2$). The decrease in $PaCO_2$ produces an increased gradient of carbon dioxide (CO_2) between mother and fetus, helping to deliver oxygen to the fetus and eliminate CO_2. Elevated progesterone levels create this gradient, with progesterone being a respiratory stimulant that sensitizes CO_2 receptors [19–21]. Dyspnea in pregnancy, which occurs in about 70% of pregnant women is due to these low levels of $PaCO_2$ as well as decreased total lung capacity and increased VM. Thus, most often in the third trimester, the pregnant woman may experience a feeling of shortness of breath [1].

In addition, renal changes were observed; renal plasma flow and glomerular filtration rate were increased. This increase in glomerular filtration rate maintains plasma sodium levels, which increase because of the activation the renin–angiotensin–aldosterone system, and also lowers serum creatine and urea nitrogen in the blood [20]. At the renal level, elevated progesterone levels work to reduce peristalsis, urethral tone and contraction pressure, producing renal vasodilation. Furthermore, hormone levels, but also external mechanical compression and changes in the urethral wall, can cause hydronephrosis and hydroureter in the pregnant woman. Urinary tract infections, urinary incontinence and nocturia are common in pregnancy. All changes that occur during this period return to the previous state up to 6 weeks after birth [13].

Additionally, during pregnancy, plasma volume increases by up to 50% and erythrocyte volume by up to 30%. These significant changes can lead to physiological anemia and decreased hematocrit, an effect that reduces blood viscosity and resistance to blood flow. Regarding the number of leukocytes, they increase and can reach very high values during labor, which can often explain the severity of the infection; however, these values do not make the pregnant woman more prone to infections [22]. In general, the concentration of platelets is maintained at normal values, but there are some cases in which their number decreases (gestational thrombocytopenia) due to the increase in plasma volume, which disappears after birth [23]. Fibrinolytic and coagulation pathways also undergo changes, and venous stasis leads to an increased risk of thromboembolism, beginning in the first trimester of pregnancy and lasting up to 3 months after birth [20].

In pregnant woman, high levels of estrogen stimulate the production of the thyroid-binding globulin, leading to an increase in the total levels of triiodothyronine (T3) and thyroxine (T4) by about 50%, while free T3 and T4 levels remain constant or slightly altered. It also increases the production of hormones by the adrenal glands. Low blood pressure and vascular resistance stimulate the renin–angiotensin–aldosterone system, resulting in an up to 10-fold increase in aldosterone at the end of the third trimester of pregnancy. Moreover, there is an increase in the level of cortisol and adrenocorticotropic hormone, a corticosteroid-binding globulin, which leads to a state of hypercortisol. On the other hand, the high levels of estradiol in pregnancy result in an increase in prolactin that induces growth in the pituitary gland [1,2,20].

2.2. Musculoskeletal Changes

Over time, it has been observed that many physiological and anatomical changes occur in pregnant women that can affect the essential organs, but the most common are those at the musculoskeletal level. Weight gain, the enlargement of the uterus with a shift in the center of gravity and hormonal and vascular changes cause a number of musculoskeletal problems. Changing the center of gravity causes lumbar lordosis with the flexion of the neck and the drooping of the shoulders [24,25].

Mechanical pressure, elevated progesterone and relaxin levels increase joint laxity and prepare a woman's body for childbirth. Additionally, in pregnant women, fluid retention causes the compression of soft tissues. All these changes that occur make the pregnant woman susceptible to musculoskeletal disorders. Most pregnant women complain of musculoskeletal disorders, and some of them show signs of disability. The majority conditions have been described as spinal pain, pain in the upper and lower extremities, peripheral neuropathy and muscle cramps. In addition, carpal tunnel syndrome, which results from compression of the median nerve, is quite common in pregnant women [19,20,26]. Major changes that occur in the body of pregnant women at different system level are shown in Figure 1.

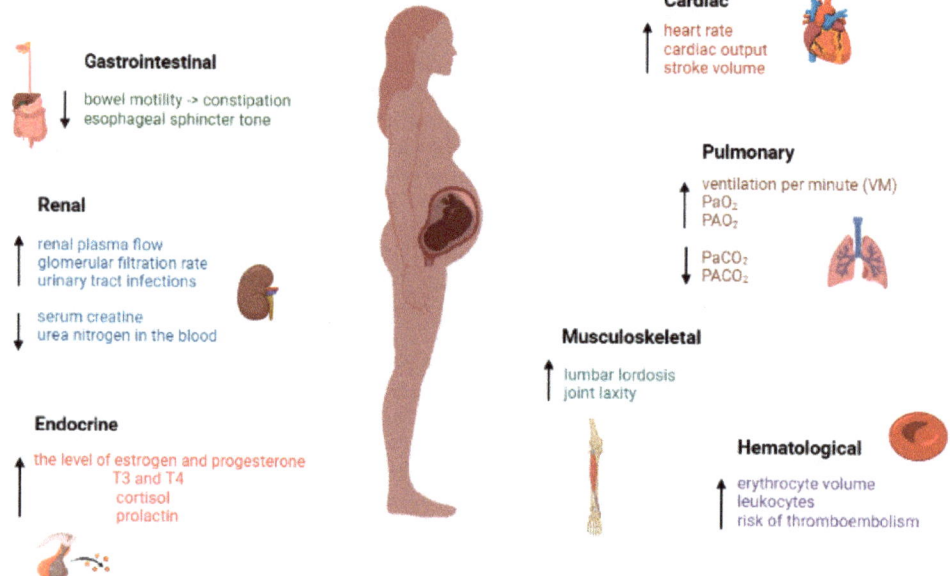

Figure 1. The main physiological and anatomical changes of pregnancy. (↑—increase, ↓—decrease).

These musculoskeletal disorders cause disabilities and loss of work capacity in pregnant women [27]. Pain during pregnancy can be of various causes and is not limited only to labor pain. The non-obstetric causes of pain in pregnancy are common, from acute conditions, such as infection or injury, to secondary pain from underlying medical conditions. Pregnancy manifests physiological effects on a woman's body, likewise influencing the endocrine, cardiovascular and renal systems as well as the musculoskeletal system. Additionally, weight gain during pregnancy and the presence of the pregnant uterus put pressure on the skeletal system. During the nine months of pregnancy, various changes occur in the body. These physiological and anatomical changes precipitate the onset of pain or may exacerbate pre-existing painful disorders.

Next, some aspects of the main imaging investigations for the diagnosis of musculoskeletal disorders will be presented.

X-rays are among the oldest types of imaging available, which use electromagnetic waves to produce an image. Bone lesions can be highlighted by radiography, but in order to diagnose muscle disorders more advanced imaging explorations are needed. The possibility that an X-ray taken during pregnancy will produce serious effects on the fetus is very small. However, the risk of affecting the child depends on the amount of radiation exposure and its gestational age. Thus, the exposure to high doses of radiation in the first two weeks after conception can cause a miscarriage; exposure up to eight weeks can increase the risk of congenital malformations; and up to week 16, high doses of radiation can lead to intellectual disability. The dose of a single exposure to radiation is far lesser than the doses associated with these risks. Another method of diagnosing musculoskeletal disorders is computed tomography (CT), which investigates bone and muscle injuries. This method offers a more detailed examination of body compared to radiography. It is not proven that the fetus is affected by the amount of radiation used in CT. However, its use on the abdomen or pelvic area is to be avoided in order to exclude any risk of developing cancer in childhood. If the examination of both the mother and the fetus is necessary, other imaging tests, such as ultrasound or magnetic resonance imaging (MRI), are used. Ultrasound uses sound waves to photograph the inside of the body. Ultrasound captures images of soft tissues, muscles and ligaments and can also diagnose musculoskeletal conditions along with MRI. Ultrasound can easily detect the signs of inflammation at the muscle and joint level. This imaging method is the most used for pregnant women, but if the images obtained do not provide a clear answer, an MRI examination can be resorted to. MRI is a method that uses radio waves and magnetic fields to capture images of the inside of the body. MRI can capture images of the body's soft tissues, even muscles, unlike X-ray imaging. In addition, MRI can capture joint injuries, such as torn ligaments or cartilage. There are no proven adverse effects due to the MRI either in the pregnant woman nor in the fetus, and is a frequently used method today [28,29].

The main musculoskeletal pains encountered during pregnancy can be classified into lumbar, pelvic and joint pain.

2.2.1. Lower Back Pain

Lower back pain occurs in about half of pregnant women and is considered a normal pain during pregnancy [30]. A higher risk of lower back pain is associated with age, the presence of pain before pregnancy and especially during menstruation, and ethnicity, particularly in African American and Caucasian individuals; although individuals of Hispanic ethnicity do not show strong associations with lower back pain during pregnancy, nor do factors such as caffeine, tobacco, oral contraceptive medication, parity and exercise [31,32]. Additionally, other factors that can contribute to lower back pain are the mechanical compressions of the pregnant uterus that modifies the center of gravity and increases the force applied to the spine, as well as the pelvic ligament laxity and vascular compression.

In addition, lower back pain encountered at night during pregnancy may be due to venous engorgement in the pelvis. The growing uterus presses on the vena cava and combined with fluid retention in pregnancy causes venous congestion and hypoxia in the lumbar spine [33]. Some women experience this pain from the first trimester when the mechanical pressure is not high, in this case the hormonal level being the factor that influences the appearance of the musculoskeletal disorder [31]. Most women recover easily in the first months after birth, of which only 50% seek professional medical assistance. The rapid identification of pain and the application of specific methods of treatment according to the particularities of each individual ultimately leads to total recovery. However, pregnant women who have gained more weight have a higher risk of postpartum lower back pain [34].

The most affected musculoskeletal structures during pregnancy and postpartum are the pubic symphysis and the sacroiliac joints. Most of the time it is difficult to establish the exact cause of the pain based only on the anamnesis, and detailed imaging investigations are required. Non-inflammatory causes of back pain, such as mechanical stress on the pelvic area caused by pregnancy, can cause subchondral bone marrow edema that cannot be differentiated from axial spondyloarthritis [35].

Bone marrow edema (BME) is a condition encountered in radiology described as a nonspecific lesion pattern, characterized by a change in marrow signal intensity at the level of the femoral head suggesting marrow infiltration through interstitial edema. Many aspects can lead to bone marrow changes, especially at the level of the sacroiliac joints, it is not yet clear whether postpartum bone marrow changes, which are mechanically induced, are different from inflammatory sacroiliitis seen on MRI. From an imaging point of view, spondyloarthropathy is characterized by BME around the sacroiliac joint (sacroiliitis) and structural changes, such as the fatty replacement of the bone marrow at the sites of inflammation, subchondral erosions and sclerosis [36].

The scientific team led by Agten compared the MRI results of the sacroiliac joints subjected to mechanical stress due to pregnancy with those of a group of women known to have spondyloarthritis to make the differential diagnosis. It was found that mechanical pressure on the joints can lead to bone marrow edema, only inflammatory changes being present, while in the group with spondyloarthritis, structural changes and erosions were also evident. Thus, these findings may provide guidance to differentiate mechanically- and hormonally-induced bone marrow changes and inflammatory sacroiliitis [37].

2.2.2. Pelvic Pain

Pelvic pain is described by pregnant women as a burning sensation, stabbing in the sacral area or as pain in the pubic symphysis. This pain may radiate to the groin or posterior thigh. The first symptoms appear during week 18 and reach a maximum intensity in week 36 [38]. Pelvic girdle pains are not pains that normally occur in pregnancy, so it is necessary to intervene as soon as possible in their treatment, otherwise they can lead to severe pain. If timely therapeutic measures are taken, recovery is rapid. Up to 22% of pregnant women may suffer from pelvic pain and up to 8% may experience severe symptoms [39]. The causes of pelvic pain in pregnancy are multifactorial. Increased movement of the pelvic girdle causes pain due to increased ligament laxity caused by high levels of relaxin and estrogen. These high concentrations of hormones lead to enlargement of the pubic symphysis, which results in pain due to the increased mobility of the joints. Pelvic pain is amplified by mechanical exertion, anterior back pain or anterior pelvic trauma [26,40].

Furthermore, it has been shown that high body mass index, multiparity, mental stress, physical exhaustion and smoking are factors that can accelerate the onset of pelvic pain in pregnancy [41].

Lumbar disc herniation is considered the most common pathology of the spine in pregnant women; however, the condition is very rare in pregnant women compared to pelvic pain, with an estimated occurrence of 1 in 10,000 women. In recent years, an increase in the average age of women who become pregnant has been observed, a consideration that may increase the incidence of lumbar disc herniation among pregnant women. The most frequent symptoms were represented by radicular pain, along with the weakness of the muscles innervated by the root of a spinal nerve, the reduced sensation in the sensory distribution of a spinal nerve but also urinary incontinence. According to data from the literature, no more than 15% of patients suffering from this disorder develop severe neurological deficits. In terms of therapeutic management, it has been observed that the majority of lumbar disc herniation sufferers do not require surgery [42].

2.2.3. Joint Pain

Pregnant women may experience joint pain, which often raises the suspicion of inflammatory diseases, such as rheumatoid arthritis or systemic lupus erythematosus. However, the development of new-onset inflammatory arthritis is rare during pregnancy, and there is evidence that pregnancy protects against new-onset rheumatoid arthritis [43]. Soft tissue swelling as well as joint laxity are physiological changes considered predisposing factors for the development of joint pain. In addition, hormonal changes with increased levels of progesterone, estrogen, relaxin and cortisol are associated with joint symptoms, stiffness and even arthralgia [44]. A study by Choi et al. aimed to establish the incidence of arthritis and arthralgia among pregnant women. Thus, of the 155 healthy pregnant women in the study, 9% developed arthritis and 16% had arthralgia. These conditions intensified in the third trimester of pregnancy, but the prognosis was generally good, with most of the disorders improving rapidly, concluding that the proximal interphalangeal joint of the hand was the most affected [45].

Another common condition is carpal tunnel syndrome, which occurs in the third trimester of pregnancy and affects the wrist. Due to water retention during pregnancy, the median nerve is subject to high compression. The symptoms are characterized by pain, paresthesia and tingling in the distribution area of the median nerve, which intensify after repeated movements and during the night [46]. Carpal tunnel syndrome developed in pregnancy has a benign course, most symptoms disappear after birth. However, a study of 45 pregnant women found that 49% still had symptoms 3 years postpartum [47]. Pregnant women undergo changes in every part of the body, and Figure 2 presents the most representative changes in terms of posture.

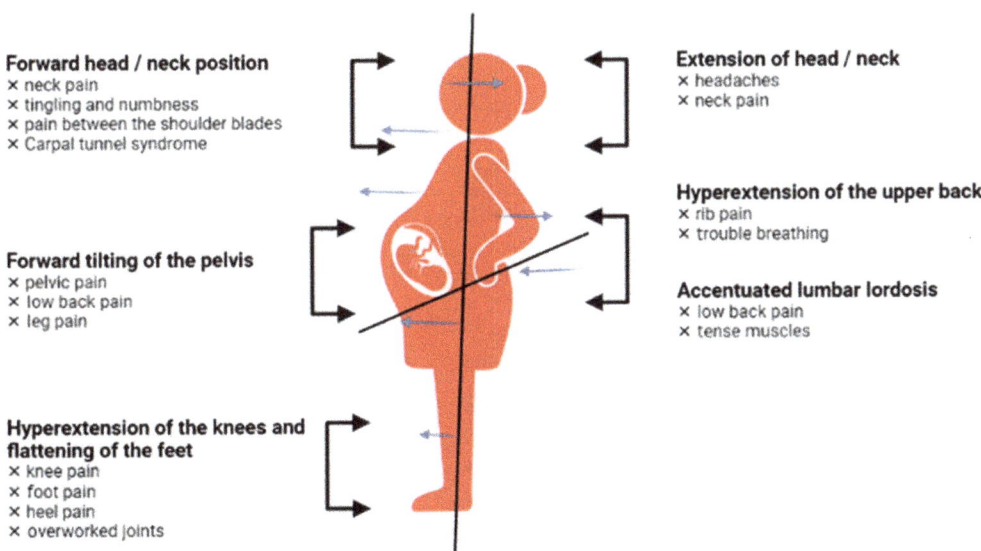

Figure 2. Postural changes in pregnant women.

3. Treatment of Musculoskeletal Pain with Medication

The treatment of musculoskeletal pain should include a structured approach, combining non-pharmacological and pharmacological options, while surgery is only desired in extreme situations, such as for acute disc herniation [48]. For the treatment of pregnant women, the basic principle that must be observed is to reduce the use of drug therapy as much as possible, taking into account that it can have harmful effects on the fetus, the mother and the harmonious development of pregnancy. Many aspects need to be considered when setting up a treatment for a pregnant woman. A major limitation in the administration of drugs in pregnancy is the presence of potential embryotoxic and teratogenic effects of the therapeutic agent.

Liposolubility, molecular weight, maternal metabolism speed and the binding to plasma proteins are the main parameters on which the presence of drugs in the fetal and placental circulation depends. Most therapeutic agents reach the placental circulation to a greater or lesser extent, with the exception of large molecules, such as insulin and heparin. The stage with the highest teratogenic risk is the one between weeks 4 and 10 during the development of the organs. After this period, the action of drugs that cross the placental barrier can reduce the amount of amniotic fluid, can delay the birth of the fetus or can trigger certain pathologies [49]. A proportion of 3% of newborns have an obvious congenital malformation at birth, of which only 25% develop genetic malformations, the rest representing different causes, including the excess of drugs in pregnancy. On the other hand, an impediment in the investigation of the teratogenic effect of therapeutic agents is the specificity of the species. A well-known example is the administration of thalidomide, which caused severe malformations of the limbs of newborns, although studies on non-primates have not shown a teratogenic effect [50].

In the late 1970s, the Food and Drug Administration (FDA) implemented a cataloging system that assesses the potential risks of pregnancy-administered drugs. This system, based on scientific evidence, has classified drugs into five broad categories (Table 1). However, despite knowledge of these aspects, the risks of using pain medication during pregnancy are incomplete, and the benefit/risk balance must be analyzed in detail before initiating drug treatment in the pregnant woman [51].

Table 1. The FDA's classification of drugs used in pain management regarding pregnancy risk.

Classification	Definition	Examples	References
Category A	Controlled studies in pregnant women have not shown a risk to the fetus.	-	
Category B	Animal studies have not shown toxic effects on the fetus, but there are no controlled clinical trials in humans. Animal studies have shown toxic effects but have not been confirmed in studies in pregnant women.	Acetaminophen Oxycodone Lidocaine Dexamethasone	[52–55]
Category C	Animal studies have shown teratogenic risk, but no controlled studies have been performed in pregnant women.	Piroxicam Codeine Hydrocodone Diclofenac Ibuprofen Naloxone Ketoprofen Celecoxib Naproxen Tramadol	[56–65]
Category D	Positive evidence of fetal risk but their use is accepted, the benefit of the mother outweighs the risk of the fetus.	Acetyl salicylic acid	[66]
Category X	Studies in both animals and humans have shown fetal malformations or no evidence. The risks outweigh the benefits, they are contraindicated in pregnancy.	Ergot derivatives	[67]

3.1. Non-Opioid Medications

3.1.1. Paracetamol (Acetaminophen)

Paracetamol is the most widely used analgesic in pregnancy. It has an analgesic potency similar to aspirin, being considered an effective and safe therapeutic agent at standard therapeutic doses throughout pregnancy. Acetaminophen is the main active substance used by pregnant women to combat mild to moderate pain and fever, due to its painkiller and antipyretic effects [68]. There are no studies showing congenital side effects. A study of thousands of pregnant women has shown the safety profile of acetaminophen, with no risk of malformations or other adverse effects of pregnancy [69,70]. Paracetamol has been reported to possibly present a high risk of attention deficit hyperactivity disorder when administered for more than 6 weeks, but according to the FDA these data are inconclusive [71]. Finally, several studies have evaluated the relationship between acetaminophen exposure in pregnancy and abnormalities. Various observational studies have investigated the effect of paracetamol on the reproductive and urogenital systems in thousands of mother–child pairs. Some of these studies have suggested that prenatal exposure to acetaminophen poses a high risk of cryptorchidism [72,73] and short anogenital distance (AGD), which is an indicator of genital masculinity [74,75]. In addition, another study found a possible link between paracetamol exposure and early puberty in females [76]. However, other studies have shown that there is no major risk of hypospadias after exposure to paracetamol in pregnancy [77–79].

Moreover, regarding the effects observed at the genital level following prenatal paracetamol exposure, possible neurological side effects have been identified. Observational studies have reported several associations between the occurrence of neurological disorders and the administration of acetaminophen during pregnancy, disorders such as autism [80–82], attention deficit hyperactivity disorder, decreased IQ (intelligence quotient) and speech/language delays, with exposure time having a significant influence [83–90]. Although paracetamol is considered a safe medication, based on the information gathered on the implications for the pregnant woman, it is recommended to be administrated with caution at the lowest effective dose and for the shortest period of time. These possible anomalies are summarized in Figure 3.

3.1.2. Non-Steroidal Anti-Inflammatory Agents

The activity of NSAIDs (non-steroidal anti-inflammatory drugs) on the fetus is mediated by inhibiting the production of prostaglandins, which stimulate blood circulation in the organs. The effects of nonsteroidal anti-inflammatory drugs on the fetus differ depending on the period of pregnancy in which the mother used them [91]. In general, nonsteroidal anti-inflammatory agents are divided into groups according to their chemical structure and selectivity as follows: derivatives of salicylic acid (aspirin), propionic acid (naproxen, ibuprofen), acetic acid (diclofenac, indomethacin), enolic acid (piroxicam, metamizole) and selective cyclooxygenase-2 (COX-2) inhibitors (celecoxib). Figure 4 shows the chemical structures of the most used substances from the NSAID class by pregnant women. NSAIDs should be avoided during pregnancy, in the first trimester there is a risk of miscarriage [92,93] and in the third trimester, these drugs may have a negative effect on fetal circulation due to premature closure of the arterial canal and may present a risk of oligohydramnios [94]. Treatment with NSAIDs can cause reversible infertility in humans, as the inhibition of cyclooxygenases prevents normal reproductive processes. This therapeutic class is frequently used by young women for the treatment of various pathologies, even in the treatment of unruptured luteinized ovarian follicles. After stopping the administration of NSAIDs, ovulation returns to normal. However, this effect can be used in the planning of in vitro fertilization treatments. A representative that has demonstrated this action in several studies is indomethacin. Indomethacin has been shown to prevent follicular rupture and reduce premature ovulation, showing an increase in the recovery rate of immature eggs [95]. In addition, the administration of NSAIDs in the third trimester of pregnancy can narrow the arterial channel by inhibiting COX-2 and can cause pulmonary hypertension in the newborn. Diclofenac is the representative of the class that shows the greatest power to inhibit prostaglandin E2 (PGE2) production both in vitro and in vivo. Diclofenac is a low molecular weight molecule that easily crosses membranes, with an average maternal/fetus drug ratio < 1, concluding that over time it can accumulate in the fetal tissue [96,97]. Metamizole sodium, withdrawn from the US but still available in Europe and Latin America, has been studied for its toxic effect on the fetus. In Brazil, studies thereof have not been associated with birth defects, intrauterine death or premature birth [98–100]. On the other hand, there are studies that associate the administration of dipyrone with the appearance of Wilms tumors in children and in addition associate this drug with general class side effects, such as oligohydramnios, by decreasing renal perfusion in the fetus [101]. Likewise, NSAIDs are drugs associated with increased labor duration and onset of labor. Many pregnant women are exposed to this class of drugs, such as ibuprofen or naproxen, because they are released without a prescription. Aspirin, at doses up to 80 mg/day, has not been shown to pose a major risk to the mother and fetus, but when given in high doses, it can cause intracranial hemorrhage in premature babies born before week 35 [102]. The administration of low-dose aspirin (LDA) between 80 and 150 mg/day is currently one of the key interventions for the prevention of preeclampsia, along with optimal calcium intake and an appropriate lifestyle. Preeclampsia can cause severe complications for both the mother and the fetus. Most guidelines recommend LDA as prophylaxis for women at high risk of preeclampsia, but the method of identifying women at this risk has not been clearly established [103].

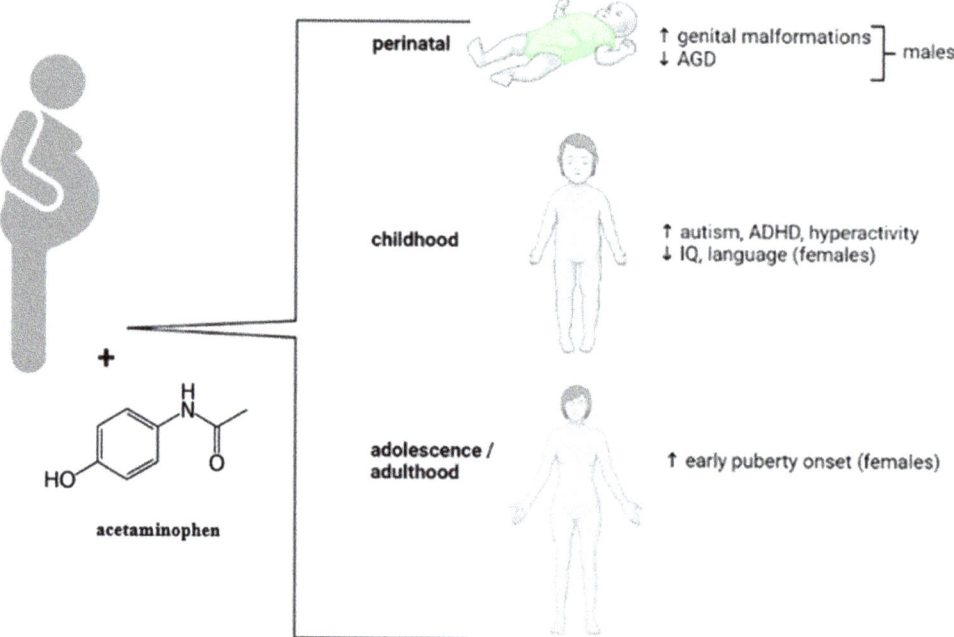

Figure 3. Acetaminophen exposure in potential pregnancy-associated effects observed in human studies. (↑—increase, ↓—decrease).

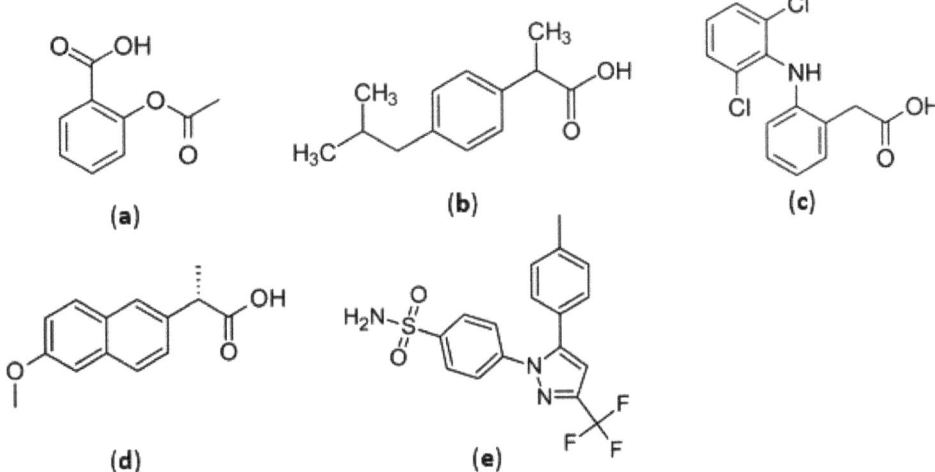

Figure 4. Chemical structures of non-steroidal anti-inflammatory agents: (**a**) aspirin, (**b**) ibuprofen, (**c**) diclofenac, (**d**) naproxen and (**e**) celecoxib.

3.2. Opioid Medications

According to the FDA classification, codeine and most opioid compounds are in category C with potentially toxic to the fetus. The main compounds in this class are morphine-like agonists (hydromorphone, hydrocodone, codeine, oxycodone), meperidine-like agonists, and synthetic opioid compounds (tramadol). A study of 563 pregnant women showed that mothers' exposure to codeine (Figure 5a) in the first trimester could lead to the birth of children with respiratory problems, with eight cases reported in this study [50].

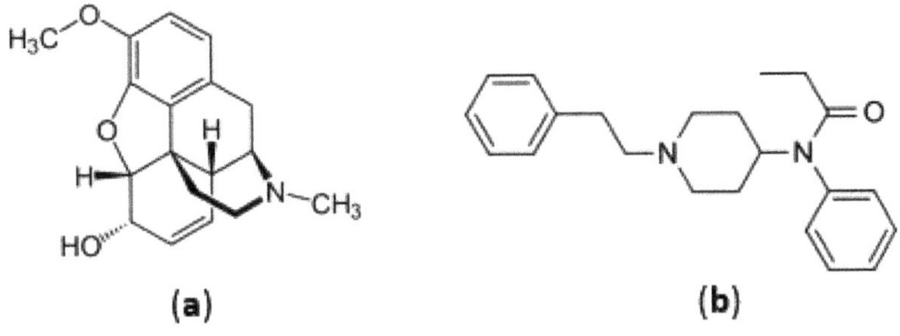

Figure 5. Chemical structure of opioids: (**a**) codeine and (**b**) fentanyl.

In the case of pregnant women undergoing chronic opioid treatment, it is recommended that the lowest dose be used or, if possible, that the therapeutic agent be discontinued gradually, initially being replaced with the methadone of buprenorphine, to prevent withdrawal symptoms [104]. It has been observed that buprenorphine is an opioid medicine, which has some advantages, namely that it rarely causes withdrawal symptoms after stopping the administration and, in addition, mothers who receive treatment with this substance give birth to children with higher weight and who need shorter hospitalization times compared to other opioids [105]. Meperidine is not recommended for repeated use due to its metabolite, normeperidine, which accumulates in the body and produces exciting effects on the CNS (Central Nervous System). Whenever it is necessary to resort to opioid treatment, it is recommended to administer opioids without active metabolites [106]. Fentanyl (Figure 5b) patches are recommended as a treatment during pregnancy and even during breastfeeding; however, in this case also, great attention must be paid to the withdrawal symptoms [107].

3.3. Transdermal Therapies

Capsaicin and lidocaine in the form of topical treatment can be used to treat lower back pain. Topical lidocaine 5% inhibits fast sodium channels in neuronal membranes, stopping nociceptive activity potentials. While capsaicin acts as an agonist for the transient receptor potential vanilloid subtype 1 (TRPV1) channel at the level of nociceptors. Their adverse effects generally consist of localized erythema and skin rash [108].

According to the FDA, patches with 5% lidocaine are classified in category B regarding the potential risk following administration to pregnant women. There are no studies on the human species that affirm the safety of the drug, but in studies on rats, the transdermal application of lidocaine in a dose of 30 mg/kg did not produce adverse reactions in the fetus. In the Collaborative Perinatal Project, in the 293 children born to mothers exposed to lidocaine in the first trimester of pregnancy, no increase in the frequency of congenital anomalies was observed. The safety of topical capsaicin during pregnancy or breastfeeding has not been established in humans. Animal studies have not shown fetal teratogenicity in the development of the fetus, and knowing that small amounts are absorbed through the skin, it is not considered to cause adverse reactions in humans [109].

4. Treatment of Musculoskeletal Pain by Alternative and Complementary Methods

Exercise and rest are the basis for treating chronic musculoskeletal pain. The main goals of physical activity are to regain strength, endurance, flexibility and, especially, to reduce chronic pain by modulating the biochemical processes in the body [110]. The side effects of physical therapy are rare and are limited to musculoskeletal injuries, increased pain, dehydration, hypo or hyperthermia and, in more severe cases, respiratory and cardiac problems [111]. Physical therapy is not contraindicated for pregnant women. The benefits of this type of treatment in combating pain far outweigh the risks, being an easy way to improve quality of life. However, it is important to note that in the special condition of pregnancy, physical therapy is recommended to be performed only under the strict supervision of a person authorized in this field [48]. There are various physical therapy programs that differ in intensity, frequency, design and area of action. In order to relieve lower back pain, relaxation exercises and the correction of the sleeping position are recommended. Exercise in water is used by pregnant women to combat the pain caused by the mechanical pressure placed by the pregnant uterus on the muscles [112,113].

Non-invasive therapy is most often preferred over drug treatment, and surgery is not considered an option during pregnancy. Specialists in this field use several treatment techniques for pregnancy-associated lower back pain, including passive treatments, such as rest, but especially active treatments, such as exercise [40].

4.1. Physical Exercises and Water Gymnastics

The effects of exercise during pregnancy and postpartum have been evaluated in several randomized controlled trials [114–125]. In most studies, exercise has been associated with other methods of physiotherapy, such as manual therapy, pelvic girdle strengthening and physical therapy. In most cases where these physiotherapy techniques have been used, positive effects on pain in pregnancy have been reported compared to control groups or those undergoing only standard care [114,116,122,125]. However, one study found that the group receiving acupuncture treatment had lower pain intensity and increased physical activity than standard physical therapy treatment, home exercise, pelvic girdle exercises, and massage [115]. Exercise-only therapy is an insufficient method of relieving or combating pain in pregnancy, but it is still more successful than not intervening at all [126].

No significant side effects of the stabilization exercises were reported, with the exception of three women who reported a high intensity of pain during the exercises [127]. Some clinical trials conducted in this regard have highlighted preventive exercises. In a randomized clinical trial conducted in two groups, it was observed that pregnant women in the group who exercised for 12 weeks (aerobic and strengthening exercises) both at home and in joint sessions requested a lower proportion of medical leave due to pelvic pain than women in the group that received only standard care associated with adequate information from a specialist [119]. Furthermore, another study found that exercise decreased the incidence of lower back pain at the end of pregnancy, with increased physical function [128]. Another study compared lumbopelvic pain experienced by pregnant women exercising in water and on land. It was observed that after performing the exercises in the water, the pain was less intense and less medical leave was needed compared to the group who performed exercises on land [129].

In another study, water gymnastics proved effective. Specifically, performing exercises in the water once a week in the second half of pregnancy has significantly reduced back and back pain, with no risk of urinary or vaginal infections following this therapy. Therefore, the reduction of back pain has also reduced the need for medical leave because of this [111].

4.2. Manual Therapy

Massage therapy and chiropractic care are effective treatment options for pregnant women suffering from lower back and pelvic pain. Regarding side effects, very few were reported, not affecting the baby, lumbar spine or pelvis [130,131].

With the development of pregnancy, especially in the third trimester, the center of gravity of the pregnant woman moves to the anterior and there is an increase in lumbar lordosis, which has the effect of hyperactivity of the pelvic muscles and the hypermobility of the joints. In this case, a chiropractor can intervene to help the pregnant woman reduce the mechanical pain, and even giving advice about special pillows can significantly reduce these problems in the pregnant woman. In addition, high pressure is exerted on the lower limbs, requiring proper footwear, orthoses or massage to provide the necessary comfort [132]. Massage therapy has been shown to be effective in combating chronic and subacute back pain in the general population [133]. Evidence for the effectiveness of manual therapy in relieving pain in pregnant women is limited. A randomized clinical trial investigated craniosacral therapy. It was reported that this therapy in combination with standard therapy reduced the intensity of pain in the morning, with a slight impairment of function compared to standard therapy alone [134]. Another study evaluated manual therapy, and osteopathic therapy showed a decrease in pain intensity and disability compared to general therapy without or with sham-ultrasound [135]. Osteopathic therapy approaches the whole body, using classic techniques of light pressure, stretching and resistance [136]. Pregnancy produces major changes in the musculoskeletal system, from the straining of ligaments and the decrease in range of motion to an increase in muscle tension, causing pain. The main aim of osteopathic treatment for pregnant women is to relieve pain and support general function. Treatment includes soft tissue massage and the targeted mobilization of affected muscles and joints. Gentle exercises at home are recommended to manage symptoms but also to prepare the mother for the birth and for the life that follows. In addition, osteopathic manipulative treatment is defined as a manually guided force therapy by an osteopathic physician to support homeostasis and improve physiological function that has been affected by somatic dysfunction [137].

4.3. Pelvic Belt

Another method of treatment for the removal of musculoskeletal pain in pregnant women is the use of the pelvic girdle.

Randomized clinical trials have shown that using this method in women with pelvic girdle pain reduced their disability and pain intensity compared to women who only exercised or received general treatment information [117].

Another randomized study in women with symphyseal pain showed that wearing a stiff belt decreased pain in all patients, as well as in the group of those who exercised, but the combination of the two methods did not show an improvement in reducing pain intensity [138]. Moreover, in another study, lumbopelvic pain was reduced with the help of two non-rigid belts, one of which showed greater efficacy, although there were no significant differences between the two [139].

4.4. Acupuncture

Acupuncture is another technique for treating pain. Studies in this direction have shown that needle therapy used in pregnant women has significantly reduced pain and increased function [114,115,140,141]. One study found that the effectiveness of acupuncture is similar to that of therapy by combining training, stretching for postpartum pain regression with manual therapy [142]. In addition, acupuncture did not cause serious adverse reactions in either mother or fetus [127,143]. The main treatment methods used to combat musculoskeletal pain are shown in Figure 6.

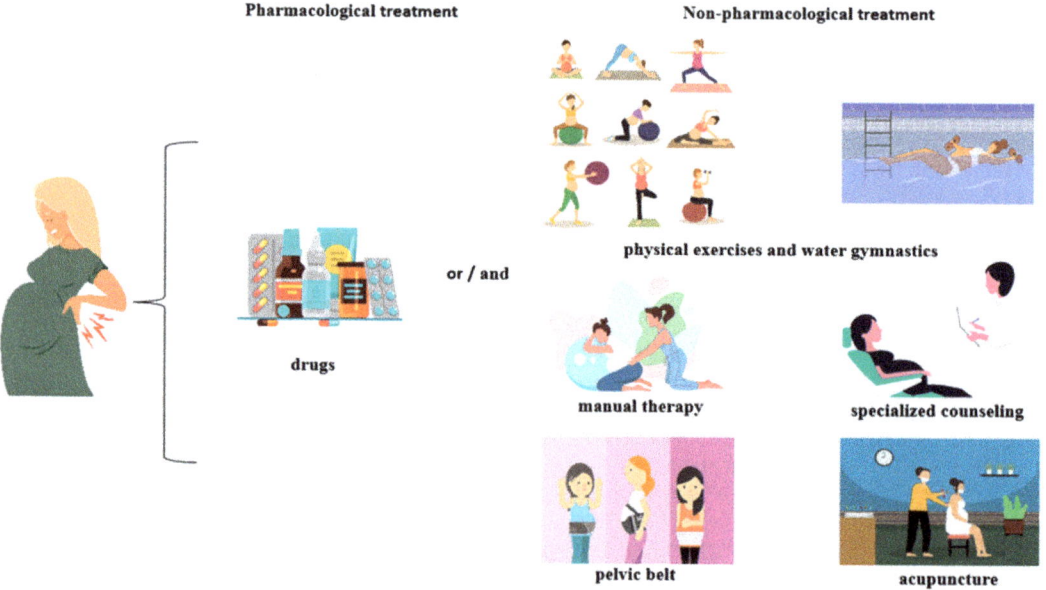

Figure 6. Pharmacological and non-pharmacological treatment of pain in pregnant women.

4.5. Electrotherapy

Exercise and manual therapy should be the main treatment methods for relieving pelvic and lower back pain during pregnancy. However, if these techniques are not enough or are limited due to pregnancy, electrotherapy can be used [144]. TENS (transcutaneous electrical nerve stimulation) is a non-pharmacological method that uses a low-intensity electrical current to inhibit the transmission of pain information to the central nervous system [145]. The effectiveness of TENS was evaluated in a randomized clinical trial. The results showed a decrease in pain intensity and an increase in function in pregnant women who used this therapy compared to groups who used exercise or who received paracetamol [146]. Evidence is limited, requiring more clinical trials.

Likewise, TENS can be used to reduce pain during labor, it has been shown to be a safe technique for both mother and newborn [147].

4.6. The Benefits of Physiotherapy

Exercise is recommended for pregnant women to limit weight gain but also to maintain cardiovascular function and to prevent chronic diseases. Exercises on land or in the water, as well as manual therapy, acupuncture and electrotherapy, have been shown to be beneficial in combating muscle pain during pregnancy, as presented. Furthermore, exercise has beneficial effects on other levels. Significant weight gain during pregnancy increases the risk of many pathologies, from gestational diabetes to pregnancy-induced hypertension. Thus, it has been found that frequent exercise during pregnancy reduces the risk of obesity and the association with a healthy diet is the best method of weight control [148]. Another positive finding of physiotherapy in pregnancy is the benefit regarding gestational diabetes. A study conducted by Barakat and his team found that moderate exercise improves maternal glucose tolerance without any signs of gestational diabetes [149]. Moreover, exercise in women with gestational diabetes has reduced the need for insulin [150]. During pregnancy, the woman undergoes various anatomical and physiological changes that can even lead to an increased rate of urinary stress incontinence. In this regard, there have been studies that have shown the benefits of pelvic floor exercises in preventing and treating this problem in pregnancy [151,152].

However, one aspect that should not be overlooked is the psychological impact of physiotherapy. Clinical studies have concluded that exercise is an ameliorating factor in pregnancy and postpartum depression, improving the quality of life and the perception of pain and general health [153–155].

5. Conclusions

Many women experience musculoskeletal problems during pregnancy, which often limit their daily activities, so therapeutic intervention is needed to prevent or combat pain. The information collected showed that alternative and complementary methods decrease the intensity of pain and in addition help to improve musculoskeletal function. Although there is clear evidence of the effectiveness of exercise therapy in combating lower back and pelvic pain in pregnancy, it is not possible to specify exactly what kind of exercises are suitable for each pregnant woman, the exercises being different in the studies. To be able to compare the effectiveness of existing therapies, it is necessary to select groups according to the same set of criteria. Further studies are needed to strengthen the effectiveness of physical activity, as well as more robust data on the effectiveness of electrotherapy and craniosacral and osteopathic therapy, as data are limited in this direction. An optimal level of intensity of physical activities must be established to maintain the safety of the woman and the fetus, and more detailed studies are required to determine the relationship between the type of exercise, its dose, intensity, and desired response of preventing or treating a problem.

Author Contributions: Conceptualization, C.A.D. and E.B.; writing—original draft preparation, F.F., P.E.M., A.D.S., B.A.G. and N.V.; writing—review and editing, F.F., P.E.M., A.D.S., B.A.G. and N.V.; supervision, C.A.D. and E.B. All authors have read and agreed to the published version of the manuscript.

Funding: This research was financed by "Victor Babes" University of Medicine and Pharmacy, 2, Eftimie Murgu Square, 300041 Timisoara, Romania.

Institutional Review Board Statement: Not applicable.

Informed Consent Statement: Not applicable.

Data Availability Statement: The data supporting the findings of the study are available within the article.

Conflicts of Interest: The authors declare no conflict of interest.

References

1. Pascual, Z.N.; Langaker, M.D. Physiology, pregnancy. In *StatPearls*; StatPearls Publishing: Treasure Island, FL, USA, 2022.
2. Bhatia, P.; Chhabra, S. Physiological and anatomical changes of pregnancy: Implications for anaesthesia. *Indian J. Anaesth.* **2018**, *62*, 651–657. [CrossRef] [PubMed]
3. Kesikburun, S.; Güzelküçük, Ü.; Fidan, U.; Demir, Y.; Ergün, A.; Tan, A.K. Musculoskeletal pain and symptoms in pregnancy: A descriptive study. *Ther. Adv. Musculoskelet. Dis.* **2018**, *10*, 229–234. [CrossRef] [PubMed]
4. Williamson, C.S. Nutrition in pregnancy. *Nutr. Bull.* **2006**, *31*, 28–59. [CrossRef]
5. Zaadstra, B.M.; Seidell, J.C.; Van Noord, P.A.; te Velde, E.R.; Habbema, J.D.; Vrieswijk, B.; Karbaat, J. Fat and female fecundity: Prospective study of effect of body fat distribution on conception rates. *BMJ* **1993**, *306*, 484–487. [CrossRef]
6. Vanstone, M.; Kandasamy, S.; Giacomini, M.; DeJean, D.; McDonald, S.D. Pregnant women's perceptions of gestational weight gain: A systematic review and meta-synthesis of qualitative research. *Matern. Child Nutr.* **2017**, *13*, e12374. [CrossRef]
7. Bang, S.W.; Lee, S.S. The factors affecting pregnancy outcomes in the second trimester pregnant women. *Nutr. Res. Pract.* **2009**, *3*, 134–140. [CrossRef]
8. Londero, A.P.; Rossetti, E.; Pittini, C.; Cagnacci, A.; Driul, L. Maternal age and the risk of adverse pregnancy outcomes: A retrospective cohort study. *BMC Pregnancy Childbirth* **2019**, *19*, 261. [CrossRef]
9. Artal, R.; O'Toole, M. Guidelines of the American College of Obstetricians and Gynecologists for exercise during pregnancy and the postpartum period. *Br. J. Sports Med.* **2003**, *37*, 6–12. [CrossRef]
10. Robson, S.C.; Hunter, S.; Boys, R.J.; Dunlop, W. Serial study of factors influencing changes in cardiac output during human pregnancy. *Am. J. Physiol.* **1989**, *256*, H1060–H1065. [CrossRef]
11. Palmer, S.K.; Zamudio, S.; Coffin, C.; Parker, S.; Stamm, E.; Moore, L.G. Quantitative estimation of human uterine artery blood flow and pelvic blood flow redistribution in pregnancy. *Obstet. Gynecol.* **1992**, *80*, 1000–1006.
12. Katz, M.; Sokal, M.M. Skin perfusion in pregnancy. *Am. J. Obstet. Gynecol.* **1980**, *137*, 30–33. [CrossRef]
13. Cheung, K.L.; Lafayette, R.A. Renal physiology of pregnancy. *Adv. Chronic Kidney Dis.* **2013**, *20*, 209–214. [CrossRef]
14. Kinsella, S.M.; Lohmann, G. Supine hypotensive syndrome. *Obstet. Gynecol.* **1994**, *83*, 774–788.
15. Lanni, S.M.; Tillinghast, J.; Silver, H.M. Hemodynamic changes and baroreflex gain in the supine hypotensive syndrome. *Am. J. Obstet. Gynecol.* **2002**, *187*, 1636–1641. [CrossRef]
16. Whitehead, E.M.; Smith, M.; Dean, Y.; O'Sullivan, G. An evaluation of gastric emptying times in pregnancy and the puerperium. *Anaesthesia* **1993**, *48*, 53–57. [CrossRef]
17. Shah, S.; Nathan, L.; Singh, R.; Fu, Y.S.; Chaudhuri, G. E_2 and not P_4 increases NO release from NANC nerves of the gastrointestinal tract: Implications in pregnancy. *Am. J. Physiol.-Regul. Integr. Comp. Physiol.* **2001**, *280*, R1546–R1554. [CrossRef]
18. Hu, H.; Pasca, I. Management of complex cardiac issues in the pregnant patient. *Crit. Care Clin.* **2016**, *32*, 97–107. [CrossRef]
19. Gaiser, R. Physiologic changes of pregnancy. In *Chestnut's Obstetric Anesthesia: Principles and Practice*, 5th ed.; Chestnut, D.H., Wng, C.A., Tsen, L.C., Ngan Kee, W.D., Beilin, Y., Mhyre, J.M., Eds.; Elsevier Saunders: Philadelphia, PA, USA, 2014; pp. 15–38.
20. Soma-Pillay, P.; Nelson-Piercy, C.; Tolppanen, H.; Mebazaa, A. Physiological changes in pregnancy. *Cardiovasc. J. Afr.* **2016**, *27*, 89–94. [CrossRef]
21. LoMauro, A.; Aliverti, A. Respiratory physiology of pregnancy: Physiology masterclass. *Breathe* **2015**, *11*, 297–301. [CrossRef]
22. Stirrat, G.M. Pregnancy and immunity. *BMJ* **1994**, *308*, 1385–1386. [CrossRef]
23. Burrows, R.F.; Kelton, J.G. Incidentally detected thrombocytopenia in healthy mothers and their infants. *N. Engl. J. Med.* **1988**, *319*, 142–145. [CrossRef] [PubMed]
24. Thabah, M.; Ravindran, V. Musculoskeletal problems in pregnancy. *Rheumatol. Int.* **2015**, *35*, 581–587. [CrossRef] [PubMed]
25. Smith, M.W.; Marcus, P.S.; Wurtz, L.D. Orthopedic issues in pregnancy. *Obstet. Gynecol. Surv.* **2008**, *63*, 103–111. [CrossRef] [PubMed]
26. Borg-Stein, J.; Dugan, S.A. Musculoskeletal disorders of pregnancy, delivery and postpartum. *Phys. Med. Rehabil. Clin. N. Am.* **2007**, *18*, 459–476. [CrossRef]
27. Sumilo, D.; Kurinczuk, J.J.; Redshaw, M.E.; Gray, R. Prevalence and impact of disability in women who had recently given birth in the UK. *BMC Pregnancy Childbirth* **2012**, *12*, 31. [CrossRef]
28. Imaging Tests for Musculoskeletal Disorders and Muscle Damage. Available online: https://www.envrad.com/imaging-tests-musculoskeletal-disorders-muscle-damage/ (accessed on 26 July 2022).
29. Test and Treatment Topics. Available online: https://www.radiologyinfo.org/en/test-treatment (accessed on 26 July 2022).
30. Mack, K.A.; Jones, C.M.; Paulozzi, L.J. Vital signs: Overdoses of prescription opioid pain relievers and other drugs among women—United States, 1999–2010. *Morb. Mortal. Wkly. Rep.* **2013**, *62*, 537–542.
31. Fast, A.; Shapiro, D.; Ducommun, E.J.; Friedmann, L.W.; Bouklas, T.; Floman, Y. Low-back pain in pregnancy. *Spine* **1987**, *12*, 368–371. [CrossRef]
32. Wang, S.M.; Dezinno, P.; Maranets, I.; Berman, M.R.; Caldwell-Andrews, A.A.; Kain, Z.N. Low back pain during pregnancy: Prevalence, risk factors, and outcomes. *Obstet. Gynecol.* **2004**, *104*, 65–70. [CrossRef]
33. Sabino, J.; Grauer, J.N. Pregnancy and low back pain. *Curr. Rev. Musculoskelet. Med.* **2008**, *1*, 137–141. [CrossRef]
34. Katonis, P.; Kampouroglou, A.; Aggelopoulos, A.; Kakavelakis, K.; Lykoudis, S.; Makrigiannakis, A.; Alpantaki, K. Pregnancy-related low back pain. *Hippokratia* **2011**, *15*, 205–210.

35. Germann, C.; Kroismayr, D.; Brunner, F.; Pfirrmann, C.W.A.; Sutter, R.; Zubler, V. Influence of pregnancy/childbirth on long-term bone marrow edema and subchondral sclerosis of sacroiliac joints. *Skeletal. Radiol.* **2021**, *50*, 1617–1628. [CrossRef]
36. Šimac, D.V.; Vujaklija, D.V.; Mirić, F.; Novak, S. Transitory bone marrow oedema of the hip in pregnant patient with antiphospholipid syndrome: A case report. *Egypt. Rheumatol.* **2021**, *43*, 209–212. [CrossRef]
37. Agten, C.A.; Zubler, V.; Zanetti, M.; Binkert, C.A.; Kolokythas, O.; Prentl, E.; Buck, F.M.; Pfirrmann, C.W.A. Postpartum bone marrow edema at the sacroiliac joints may mimic sacroiliitis of axial spondyloarthritis on MRI. *Am. J. Roentgenol.* **2018**, *211*, 1306–1312. [CrossRef]
38. Wu, W.H.; Meijer, O.G.; Uegaki, K.; Mens, J.M.A.; van Dieen, J.H.; Wuisman, P.I.J.M.; Ostgaard, H.C. Pregnancy-related pelvic girdle pain (PPP), I: Terminology, clinical presentation, and prevalence. *Eur. Spine J.* **2004**, *13*, 575–589. [CrossRef]
39. Keriakos, R.; Bhatta, S.R.; Morris, F.; Mason, S.; Buckley, S. Pelvic girdle pain during pregnancy and puerperium. *J. Obstet. Gynaecol.* **2011**, *31*, 572–780. [CrossRef]
40. Vleeming, A.; Albert, H.B.; Östgaard, H.C.; Sturesson, B.; Stuge, B. European guidelines for the diagnosis and treatment of pelvic girdle pain. *Eur. Spine J.* **2008**, *17*, 794–819. [CrossRef]
41. Walters, C.; West, S.; Nippita, T.A. Pelvic girdle pain in pregnancy. *Aust. J. Gen. Pract.* **2018**, *47*, 439–443. [CrossRef]
42. Paslaru, F.G.; Giovani, A.; Iancu, G.; Panaitescu, A.; Peltecu, G.; Gorgan, R.M. Methods of delivery in pregnant women with lumbar disc herniation: A narrative review of general management and case report. *J. Med. Life* **2020**, *13*, 517–522. [CrossRef]
43. Silman, A.; Kay, A.; Brennan, P. Timing of pregnancy in relation to the onset of rheumatoid arthritis. *Arthritis Rheum.* **1992**, *35*, 152–155. [CrossRef]
44. Shah, S.; Banh, E.T.; Koury, K.; Bhatia, G.; Nandi, R.; Gulur, P. Pain management in pregnancy: Multimodal approaches. *Pain Res. Treat.* **2015**, *2015*, 987483. [CrossRef]
45. Choi, H.J.; Lee, J.C.; Lee, Y.J.; Lee, E.B.; Shim, S.S.; Park, J.S.; Jun, J.K.; Song, Y.W. Prevalence and clinical features of arthralgia/arthritis in healthy pregnant women. *Rheumatol. Int.* **2008**, *28*, 1111–1115. [CrossRef]
46. Descatha, A.; Dale, A.M.; Franzblau, A.; Coomes, J.; Evanoff, B. Comparison of research case definitions for carpal tunnel syndrome. *Scand. J. Work Environ. Health* **2011**, *37*, 298–306. [CrossRef]
47. Mondelli, M.; Rossi, S.; Monti, E.; Aprile, I.; Caliandro, P.; Pazzaglia, C.; Romano, C.; Padua, L. Long term follow-up of carpal tunnel syndrome during pregnancy: A cohort study and review of the literature. *Electromyogr. Clin. Neurophysiol.* **2007**, *47*, 259–271.
48. Zaghw, A.; Koronfel, M.; Podgorski, E.; Siddiqui, S.; Valliani, A.; Karmakar, A.; Khan, J. Pain management for pregnant women in the opioid crisis era. In *Pain Management in Special Circumstances*; Shallik, N.A., Ed.; IntechOpen: London, UK, 2018. [CrossRef]
49. Roberto Díaz, R.; Lopera Rivera, A. Manejo del dolor no obstétrico durante el embarazo. Artículo de revisión. *Rev. Colomb. Anestesiol.* **2012**, *40*, 213–223. [CrossRef]
50. Rathmell, J.P.; Viscomi, C.M.; Ashburn, M.A. Management of nonobstetric pain during pregnancy and lactation. *Anesth. Analg.* **1997**, *85*, 1074–1087. [CrossRef] [PubMed]
51. Food and Drug Administration. Content and format of labeling for human prescription drug and biological products; requirements for pregnancy and lactation labeling. Final rule. *Fed. Regist.* **2014**, *79*, 72063–72103.
52. Acetaminophen Information. Available online: https://www.fda.gov/drugs/information-drug-class/acetaminophen-information (accessed on 16 May 2022).
53. Purdue Pharma, L.P. OxyContin. Prescribing Information. Available online: www.accessdata.fda.gov/drugsatfda_docs/label/2010/022272lbl.pdf (accessed on 16 May 2022).
54. APP Pharmaceuticals, LLC. Xylocaine. Prescribing Information. Available online: www.accessdata.fda.gov/drugsatfda_docs/label/2010/006488s074lbl.pdf (accessed on 16 May 2022).
55. Pfizer Laboratories Div Pfizer Inc. Dexamethasone Sodium Phosphate. Available online: http://www.drugs.com/pro/dexamethasone-sodium-phosphate.html (accessed on 16 May 2022).
56. Roxane Laboratories, Inc. Codeine Sulfate. Prescribing Information. Available online: http://www.drugs.com/pro/codeine-sulfate.html (accessed on 16 May 2022).
57. Abbott Laboratories. Vicodin. Prescribing Information. Available online: http://www.drugs.com/pro/vicodin.html# (accessed on 16 May 2022).
58. TEVA Pharmaceuticals USA Inc. Diclofenac. Prescribing Information. Available online: http://www.drugs.com/pro/diclofenac.html (accessed on 16 May 2022).
59. Polygen Pharmaceuticals LLC. Ibuprofen. Prescribing Information. Available online: http://www.drugs.com/pro/ibuprofen.html (accessed on 16 May 2022).
60. Hospira, I. Naloxone. Prescribing Information. Available online: http://www.drugs.com/pro/naloxone.html (accessed on 16 May 2022).
61. H.J. Harkins Company, Inc. Ketoprofen Prescribing Information. Available online: http://www.drugs.com/pro/ketoprofen.html (accessed on 16 May 2022).
62. Pfizer. Celecoxib, Capsules. Medication Guide. Available online: www.fda.gov/downloads/Drugs/DevelopmentApprovalProcess/DevelopmentResources/UCM162532.pdf (accessed on 16 May 2022).
63. Roxane Laboratories, Inc. Naproxen. Prescribing Information. Available online: http://www.drugs.com/pro/naproxen.html (accessed on 16 May 2022).

64. Lachman Consultant Services, Inc. Tramadol. Attachment, C. Available online: www.fda.gov/ohrms/dockets/dailys/04/sep04/090804/04p-0405-cp00001-04-Attachment-C-vol1.pdf (accessed on 16 May 2022).
65. Teva Pharmaceuticals USA, Inc. Piroxicam. Prescribing Information. Available online: http://www.drugs.com/pro/piroxicam.html (accessed on 16 May 2022).
66. Himprit Pharmachem Pvt, Ltd. Aspirine. Prescribing Information. Available online: http://www.drugs.com/pro/aspirin.html (accessed on 16 May 2022).
67. West-Ward Pharmaceutical Corp. Ergotamine and Caffeine. Prescribing Information. Available online: http://www.drugs.com/pro/ergotamine-and-caffeine.html (accessed on 16 May 2022).
68. Bauer, A.Z.; Swan, S.H.; Kriebel, D.; Liew, Z.; Taylor, H.S.; Bornehag, C.G.; Andrade, A.M.; Olsen, J.; Jensen, R.H.; Mitchell, R.T.; et al. Paracetamol use during pregnancy—A call for precautionary action. *Nat. Rev. Endocrinol.* **2021**, *17*, 757–766. [CrossRef]
69. Rebordosa, C.; Kogevinas, M.; Horváth-Puhó, E.; Nørgård, B.; Morales, M.; Czeizel, A.E.; Vilstrup, H.; Sørensen, H.T.; Olsen, J. Acetaminophen use during pregnancy: Effects on risk for congenital abnormalities. *Am. J. Obstet. Gynecol.* **2008**, *198*, 178.e1–178.e7. [CrossRef]
70. Rebordosa, C.; Kogevinas, M.; Bech, B.H.; Sørensen, H.T.; Olsen, J. Use of acetaminophen during pregnancy and risk of adverse pregnancy outcomes. *Int. J. Epidemiol.* **2009**, *38*, 706–714. [CrossRef]
71. Cooper, M.; Langley, K.; Thapar, A. Antenatal acetaminophen use and attention-deficit/hyperactivity disorder: An interesting observed association but too early to infer causality. *JAMA Pediatr.* **2014**, *168*, 306–307. [CrossRef]
72. Kristensen, D.M.; Hass, U.; Lesné, L.; Lottrup, G.; Jacobsen, P.R.; Desdoits-Lethimonier, C.; Boberg, J.; Petersen, J.H.; Toppari, J.; Jensen, T.K.; et al. Intrauterine exposure to mild analgesics is a risk factor for development of male reproductive disorders in human and rat. *Hum. Reprod.* **2011**, *26*, 235–244. [CrossRef] [PubMed]
73. Snijder, C.A.; Kortenkamp, A.; Steegers, E.A.; Jaddoe, V.W.; Hofman, A.; Hass, U.; Burdorf, A. Intrauterine exposure to mild analgesics during pregnancy and the occurrence of cryptorchidism and hypospadia in the offspring: The Generation R Study. *Hum. Reprod.* **2012**, *27*, 1191–1201. [CrossRef] [PubMed]
74. Lind, D.V.; Main, K.M.; Kyhl, H.B.; Kristensen, D.M.; Toppari, J.; Andersen, H.R.; Andersen, M.S.; Skakkebæk, N.E.; Jensen, T.K. Maternal use of mild analgesics during pregnancy associated with reduced anogenital distance in sons: A cohort study of 1027 mother-child pairs. *Hum. Reprod.* **2017**, *32*, 223–231. [CrossRef] [PubMed]
75. Fisher, B.G.; Thankamony, A.; Hughes, I.A.; Ong, K.K.; Dunger, D.B.; Acerini, C.L. Prenatal paracetamol exposure is associated with shorter anogenital distance in male infants. *Hum. Reprod.* **2016**, *31*, 2642–2650. [CrossRef]
76. Ernst, A.; Brix, N.; Lauridsen, L.L.B.; Olsen, J.; Parner, E.T.; Liew, Z.; Olsen, L.H.; Ramlau-Hansen, C.H. Acetaminophen (paracetamol) exposure during pregnancy and pubertal development in boys and girls from a nationwide puberty cohort. *Am. J. Epidemiol.* **2019**, *188*, 34–46. [CrossRef]
77. Feldkamp, M.L.; Meyer, R.E.; Krikov, S.; Botto, L.D. Acetaminophen use in pregnancy and risk of birth defects: Findings from the National Birth Defects Prevention Study. *Obstet. Gynecol.* **2010**, *115*, 109–115. [CrossRef]
78. Lind, J.N.; Tinker, S.C.; Broussard, C.S.; Reefhuis, J.; Carmichael, S.L.; Honein, M.A.; Olney, R.S.; Parker, S.E.; Werler, M.M.; National Birth Defects Prevention Study. Maternal medication and herbal use and risk for hypospadias: Data from the National Birth Defects Prevention Study, 1997–2007. *Pharmacoepidemiol. Drug Saf.* **2013**, *22*, 783–793. [CrossRef]
79. Interrante, J.D.; Ailes, E.C.; Lind, J.N.; Anderka, M.; Feldkamp, M.L.; Werler, M.M.; Taylor, L.G.; Trinidad, J.; Gilboa, S.M.; Broussard, C.S.; et al. Risk comparison for prenatal use of analgesics and selected birth defects, National Birth Defects Prevention Study 1997–2011. *Ann. Epidemiol.* **2017**, *27*, 645–653. [CrossRef]
80. Avella-Garcia, C.B.; Julvez, J.; Fortuny, J.; Rebordosa, C.; García-Esteban, R.; Galán, I.R.; Tardón, A.; Rodríguez-Bernal, C.L.; Iñiguez, C.; Andiarena, A.; et al. Acetaminophen use in pregnancy and neurodevelopment: Attention function and autism spectrum symptoms. *Int. J. Epidemiol.* **2016**, *45*, 1987–1996. [CrossRef]
81. Liew, Z.; Ritz, B.; Virk, J.; Olsen, J. Maternal use of acetaminophen during pregnancy and risk of autism spectrum disorders in childhood: A Danish national birth cohort study. *Autism Res.* **2016**, *9*, 951–958. [CrossRef]
82. Ji, Y.; Azuine, R.E.; Zhang, Y.; Hou, W.; Hong, X.; Wang, G.; Riley, A.; Pearson, C.; Zuckerman, B.; Wang, X. Association of cord plasma biomarkers of in utero acetaminophen exposure with risk of attention-deficit/hyperactivity disorder and autism spectrum disorder in childhood. *JAMA Psychiatry* **2020**, *77*, 180–189. [CrossRef]
83. Thompson, J.M.; Waldie, K.E.; Wall, C.R.; Murphy, R.; Mitchell, E.A.; ABC study group. Associations between acetaminophen use during pregnancy and ADHD symptoms measured at ages 7 and 11 years. *PLoS ONE* **2014**, *9*, e108210. [CrossRef]
84. Leppert, B.; Havdahl, A.; Riglin, L.; Jones, H.J.; Zheng, J.; Smith, G.D.; Tilling, K.; Thapar, A.; Reichborn-Kjennerud, T.; Stergiakouli, E. Association of maternal neurodevelopmental risk alleles with early-life exposures. *JAMA Psychiatry* **2019**, *76*, 834–842. [CrossRef]
85. Ystrom, E.; Gustavson, K.; Brandlistuen, R.E.; Knudsen, G.P.; Magnus, P.; Susser, E.; Davey Smith, G.; Stoltenberg, C.; Surén, P.; Håberg, S.E.; et al. Prenatal exposure to acetaminophen and risk of ADHD. *Pediatrics* **2017**, *140*, e20163840. [CrossRef]
86. Ji, Y.; Riley, A.W.; Lee, L.C.; Hong, X.; Wang, G.; Tsai, H.J.; Mueller, N.T.; Pearson, C.; Thermitus, J.; Panjwani, A.; et al. Maternal biomarkers of acetaminophen use and offspring attention deficit hyperactivity disorder. *Brain Sci.* **2018**, *8*, 127. [CrossRef]
87. Tovo-Rodrigues, L.; Schneider, B.C.; Martins-Silva, T.; Del-Ponte, B.; Loret de Mola, C.; Schuler-Faccini, L.; Vianna, F.S.L.; Munhoz, T.N.; Entiauspe, L.; Silveira, M.F.; et al. Is intrauterine exposure to acetaminophen associated with emotional and hyperactivity problems during childhood? Findings from the 2004 Pelotas birth cohort. *BMC Psychiatry* **2018**, *18*, 368. [CrossRef]

88. Liew, Z.; Kioumourtzoglou, M.A.; Roberts, A.L.; O'Reilly, É.J.; Ascherio, A.; Weisskopf, M.G. Use of negative control exposure analysis to evaluate confounding: An example of acetaminophen exposure and attention-deficit/hyperactivity disorder in Nurses' Health Study II. *Am. J. Epidemiol.* **2019**, *188*, 768–775. [CrossRef]
89. Chen, M.-H.; Pan, T.-L.; Wang, P.-W.; Hsu, J.-W.; Huang, K.-L.; Su, T.-P.; Li, C.-T.; Lin, W.-C.; Tsai, S.-J.; Chen, T.-J.; et al. Prenatal exposure to acetaminophen and the risk of attention-deficit/hyperactivity disorder: A nationwide study in Taiwan. *J. Clin. Psychiatry* **2019**, *80*, 18m12612. [CrossRef]
90. Baker, B.H.; Lugo-Candelas, C.; Wu, H.; Laue, H.E.; Boivin, A.; Gillet, V.; Aw, N.; Rahman, T.; Lepage, J.-F.; Whittingstall, K.; et al. Association of prenatal acetaminophen exposure measured in meconium with risk of attention-deficit/hyperactivity disorder mediated by frontoparietal network brain connectivity. *JAMA Pediatr.* **2020**, *174*, 1073–1081. [CrossRef]
91. Ofori, B.; Oraichi, D.; Blais, L.; Rey, E.; Bérard, A. Risk of congenital anomalies in pregnant users of non-steroidal antiinflammatory drugs: A nested case-control study. *Birth Defects Res. Part B Dev. Reprod. Toxicol.* **2006**, *77*, 268–279. [CrossRef]
92. Nielsen, G.L.; Sørensen, H.T.; Larsen, H.; Pedersen, L. Risk of adverse birth outcome and miscarriage in pregnant users of non-steroidal anti-inflammatory drugs: Population based observational study and case-control study. *BMJ* **2001**, *322*, 266–270. [CrossRef] [PubMed]
93. Li, D.K.; Liu, L.; Odouli, R. Exposure to non-steroidal anti-inflammatory drugs during pregnancy and risk of miscarriage: Population based cohort study. *BMJ* **2003**, *327*, 368. [CrossRef] [PubMed]
94. Hardy, J.B. The collaborative perinatal project: Lessons and legacy. *Ann. Epidemiol.* **2003**, *13*, 303–311. [CrossRef]
95. Livshits, A.; Seidman, D.S. Role of non-steroidal anti-inflammatory drugs in gynecology. *Pharmaceuticals* **2010**, *3*, 2082–2089. [CrossRef]
96. Le Duc, K.; Gilliot, S.; Baudelet, J.B.; Mur, S.; Boukhris, M.R.; Domanski, O.; Odou, P.; Storme, L. Case report: Persistent pulmonary hypertension of the newborn and narrowing of the ductus arteriosus after topical use of non-steroidal anti-inflammatory during pregnancy. *Front. Pharmacol.* **2021**, *12*, 756056. [CrossRef]
97. Shintaku, K.; Hori, S.; Satoh, H.; Tsukimori, K.; Nakano, H.; Fujii, T.; Taketani, Y.; Ohtani, H.; Sawada, Y. Prediction and evaluation of fetal toxicity induced by NSAIDs using transplacental kinetic parameters obtained from human placental perfusion studies. *Br. J. Clin. Pharmacol.* **2012**, *73*, 248–256. [CrossRef]
98. Arruza Gómez, L.; Corredera Sánchez, A.; Montalvo Montes, J.; de Marco Guilarte, E.; Moro Serrano, M. Cierre intrauterino del conducto arterial en probable relación con la ingesta materna de metamizol durante el tercer trimestre de gestación [Intrauterine closure of the ductus arteriosus probably associated with the taking of metamizole during the third trimester]. *An. Pediatr.* **2008**, *68*, 626–627. [CrossRef]
99. da Silva Dal Pizzol, T.; Schüler-Faccini, L.; Mengue, S.S.; Fischer, M.I. Dipyrone use during pregnancy and adverse perinatal events. *Arch. Gynecol. Obstet.* **2009**, *279*, 293–297. [CrossRef]
100. Bar-Oz, B.; Clementi, M.; Di Giantonio, E.; Greenberg, R.; Beer, M.; Merlob, P.; Arnon, J.; Ornoy, A.; Zimmerman, D.M.; Berkovitch, M. Metamizol (dipyrone, optalgin) in pregnancy, is it safe? A prospective comparative study. *Eur. J. Obstet. Gynecol. Reprod. Biol.* **2005**, *119*, 176–179. [CrossRef]
101. Sharpe, C.R.; Franco, E.L.; Brazilian Wilms' Tumor Study Group. Use of dipyrone during pregnancy and risk of Wilms' tumor. *Epidemiology* **1996**, *7*, 533–535. [CrossRef]
102. Ives, T.J.; Tepper, R.S. Drug use in pregnancy and lactation. *Prim. Care* **1990**, *17*, 623–645. [CrossRef]
103. van Montfort, P.; Scheepers, H.C.J.; van Dooren, I.V.A.; Meertens, L.J.E.; Zelis, M.; Zwaan, I.M.; Spaanderman, M.E.A.; Smits, L.J.M. Low-dose-aspirin usage among women with an increased preeclampsia risk: A prospective cohort study. *Acta Obstet. Gynecol. Scand.* **2020**, *99*, 875–883. [CrossRef]
104. American Society of Anesthesiologists Task Force on Chronic Pain Management; American Society of Regional Anesthesia and Pain Medicine. Practice guidelines for chronic pain management: An updated report by the American Society of Anesthesiologists Task Force on Chronic Pain Management and the American Society of Regional Anesthesia and Pain Medicine. *Anesthesiology* **2010**, *112*, 810–833. [CrossRef]
105. Kakko, J.; Heilig, M.; Sarman, I. Buprenorphine and methadone treatment of opiate dependence during pregnancy: Comparison of fetal growth and neonatal outcomes in two consecutive case series. *Drug Alcohol Depend.* **2008**, *96*, 69–78. [CrossRef]
106. Hagmeyer, K.O.; Mauro, L.S.; Mauro, V.F. Meperidine-related seizures associated with patient-controlled analgesia pumps. *Ann. Pharmacother.* **1993**, *27*, 29–32. [CrossRef]
107. Cohen, R.S. Fentanyl transdermal analgesia during pregnancy and lactation. *J. Hum. Lact.* **2009**, *25*, 359–361. [CrossRef]
108. Peck, J.; Urits, I.; Peoples, S.; Foster, L.; Malla, A.; Berger, A.A.; Cornett, E.M.; Kassem, H.; Herman, J.; Kaye, A.D.; et al. Comprehensive review of over the counter treatment for chronic low back pain. *Pain Ther.* **2021**, *10*, 69–80. [CrossRef]
109. Lalkhen, A.; Grady, K. Non-obstetric pain in pregnancy. *Rev. Pain* **2008**, *1*, 10–14. [CrossRef]
110. Geneen, L.J.; Moore, R.A.; Clarke, C.; Martin, D.; Colvin, L.A.; Smith, B.H. Physical activity and exercise for chronic pain in adults: An overview of Cochrane Reviews. *Cochrane Database Syst. Rev.* **2017**, *4*, CD011279. [CrossRef]
111. Thompson, P.D.; Franklin, B.A.; Balady, G.J.; Blair, S.N.; Corrado, D.; Estes, N.M., III; Fulton, J.E.; Gordon, N.F.; Haskell, W.L.; Link, M.S. Exercise and acute cardiovascular events placing the risks into perspective: A scientific statement from the American Heart Association Council on Nutrition, Physical Activity, and Metabolism and the Council on Clinical Cardiology. *Circulation* **2007**, *115*, 2358–2368. [CrossRef]

112. Mogren, I.M. Previous physical activity decreases the risk of low back pain and pelvic pain during pregnancy. *Scand. J. Public Health* **2005**, *33*, 300–306. [CrossRef]
113. Kihlstrand, M.; Stenman, B.; Nilsson, S.; Axelsson, O. Water-gymnastics reduced the intensity of back/low back pain in pregnant women. *Acta Obstet. Gynecol. Scand.* **1999**, *78*, 180–185.
114. Elden, H.; Ladfors, L.; Olsen, M.F.; Ostgaard, H.C.; Hagberg, H. Effects of acupuncture and stabilising exercises as adjunct to standard treatment in pregnant women with pelvic girdle pain: Randomised single blind controlled trial. *BMJ* **2005**, *330*, 761. [CrossRef]
115. Wedenberg, K.; Moen, B.; Norling, A. A prospective randomized study comparing acupuncture with physiotherapy for low-back and pelvic pain in pregnancy. *Acta Obstet. Gynecol. Scand.* **2000**, *79*, 331–335.
116. George, J.W.; Skaggs, C.D.; Thompson, P.A.; Nelson, D.M.; Gavard, J.A.; Gross, G.A. A randomized controlled trial comparing a multimodal intervention and standard obstetrics care for low back and pelvic pain in pregnancy. *Am. J. Obstet. Gynecol.* **2013**, *208*, 295. [CrossRef] [PubMed]
117. Kordi, R.; Abolhasani, M.; Rostami, M.; Hantoushzadeh, S.; Mansournia, M.A.; Vasheghani-Farahani, F. Comparison between the effect of lumbopelvic belt and home based pelvic stabilizing exercise on pregnant women with pelvic girdle pain; a randomized controlled trial. *J. Back Musculoskelet. Rehabil.* **2013**, *26*, 133–139. [CrossRef] [PubMed]
118. Nilsson-Wikmar, L.; Holm, K.; Oijerstedt, R.; Harms-Ringdahl, K. Effect of three different physical therapy treatments on pain and activity in pregnant women with pelvic girdle pain: A randomized clinical trial with 3, 6, and 12 months follow-up postpartum. *Spine* **2005**, *30*, 850–856. [CrossRef] [PubMed]
119. Stafne, S.N.; Salvesen, K.A.; Romundstad, P.R.; Stuge, B.; Morkved, S. Does regular exercise during pregnancy influence lumbopelvic pain? A randomized controlled trial. *Acta Obstet. Gynecol. Scand.* **2012**, *91*, 552–559. [CrossRef] [PubMed]
120. Kashanian, M.; Akbari, Z.; Alizadeh, M.H. The effect of exercise on back pain and lordosis in pregnant women. *Int. J. Gynaecol. Obstet.* **2009**, *107*, 160–161. [CrossRef]
121. Eggen, M.H.; Stuge, B.; Mowinckel, P.; Jensen, K.S.; Hagen, K.B. Can supervised group exercises including ergonomic advice reduce the prevalence and severity of low back pain and pelvic girdle pain in pregnancy? A randomized controlled trial. *Phys. Ther.* **2012**, *92*, 781–790. [CrossRef]
122. Kluge, J.; Hall, D.; Louw, Q.; Theron, G.; Grove, D. Specific exercises to treat pregnancy-related low back pain in a South African population. *Int. J. Gynaecol. Obstet.* **2011**, *113*, 187–191. [CrossRef]
123. Gutke, A.; Sjodahl, J.; Oberg, B. Specific muscle stabilizing as home exercises for persistent pelvic girdle pain after pregnancy: A randomized, controlled clinical trial. *J. Rehabil. Med.* **2010**, *42*, 929–935. [CrossRef]
124. Chaudry, S.; Rashid, F.; Shah, S.I.H. Effectiveness of core stabilization exercises along with postural correction in postpartum back pain. *Rawal Med. J.* **2013**, *38*, 256–259.
125. Garshasbi, A.; Faghih Zadeh, S. The effect of exercise on the intensity of low back pain in pregnant women. *Int. J. Gynaecol. Obstet.* **2005**, *88*, 271–275. [CrossRef]
126. Gutke, A.; Betten, C.; Degerskär, K.; Pousette, S.; Olsén, M.F. Treatments for pregnancy-related lumbopelvic pain: A systematic review of physiotherapy modalities. *Acta Obstet. Gynecol. Scand.* **2015**, *94*, 1156–1167. [CrossRef]
127. Elden, H.; Ostgaard, H.C.; Fagevik-Olsen, M.; Ladfors, L.; Hagberg, H. Treatments of pelvic girdle pain in pregnant women: Adverse effects of standard treatment, acupuncture and stabilising exercises on the pregnancy, mother, delivery and the fetus/neonate. *BMC Complement. Altern. Med.* **2008**, *8*, 34. [CrossRef]
128. Mens, J.M.; Snijders, C.J.; Stam, H.J. Diagonal trunk muscle exercises in peripartum pelvic pain: A randomized clinical trial. *Phys. Ther.* **2000**, *80*, 1164–1173. [CrossRef]
129. Granath, A.B.; Hellgren, M.S.; Gunnarsson, R.K. Water aerobics reduces sick leave due to low back pain during pregnancy. *J. Obstet. Gynecol. Neonatal Nurs.* **2006**, *35*, 465–471. [CrossRef]
130. Khorsan, R.; Hawk, C.; Lisi, A.J.; Kizhakkeveettil, A. Manipulative therapy for pregnancy and related conditions: A systematic review. *Obs. Gynecol. Surv.* **2009**, *64*, 416–427. [CrossRef]
131. Stuber, K.J.; Wynd, S.; Weis, C.A. Adverse events from spinal manipulation in the pregnant and postpartum periods: A critical review of the literature. *Chiropr. Man. Ther.* **2012**, *20*, 8. [CrossRef]
132. Aldabe, D.; Milosavljevic, S.; Bussey, M.D. Is pregnancy related pelvic girdle pain associated with altered kinematic, kinetic and motor control of the pelvis? A systematic review. *Eur. Spine J.* **2012**, *21*, 1777–1787. [CrossRef] [PubMed]
133. Brosseau, L.; Wells, G.A.; Poitras, S.; Tugwell, P.; Casimiro, L.; Novikov, M.; Loew, L.; Sredic, D.; Clément, S.; Gravelle, A.; et al. Ottawa Panel evidence-based clinical practice guidelines on therapeutic massage for low back pain. *J. Bodyw. Mov.* **2012**, *16*, 424–455. [CrossRef] [PubMed]
134. Elden, H.; Ostgaard, H.C.; Glantz, A.; Marciniak, P.; Linner, A.C.; Olsen, M.F. Effects of craniosacral therapy as adjunct to standard treatment for pelvic girdle pain in pregnant women: A multicenter, single blind, randomized controlled trial. *Acta Obstet. Gynecol. Scand.* **2013**, *92*, 775–782. [CrossRef]
135. Licciardone, J.C.; Buchanan, S.; Hensel, K.L.; King, H.H.; Fulda, K.G.; Stoll, S.T. Osteopathic manipulative treatment of back pain and related symptoms during pregnancy: A randomized controlled trial. *Am. J. Obstet. Gynecol.* **2010**, *202*, 43. [CrossRef] [PubMed]
136. American Osteopathic Association. Osteopathic Medicine and Your Health. Available online: http://www.osteopathic.org/osteopathic-health/treatment/Pages/default.aspx (accessed on 22 May 2022).

137. Hensel, K.L.; Buchanan, S.; Brown, S.K.; Rodriguez, M.; Cruser, D.A. Pregnancy research on osteopathic manipulation optimizing treatment effects: The PROMOTE study. *Am. J. Obstet. Gynecol.* **2015**, *212*, 108. [CrossRef] [PubMed]
138. Depledge, J.; McNair, P.J.; Keal-Smith, C.; Williams, M. Management of symphysis pubis dysfunction during pregnancy using exercise and pelvic support belts. *Phys. Ther.* **2005**, *85*, 1290–1300. [CrossRef]
139. Kalus, S.M.; Kornman, L.H.; Quinlivan, J.A. Managing back pain in pregnancy using a support garment: A randomised trial. *BJOG Int. J. Obstet. Gynaecol.* **2007**, *115*, 68–75. [CrossRef]
140. Kvorning, N.; Holmberg, C.; Grennert, L.; Aberg, A.; Akeson, J. Acupuncture relieves pelvic and low-back pain in late pregnancy. *Acta Obstet. Gynecol. Scand.* **2004**, *83*, 246–250. [CrossRef]
141. Wang, S.M.; Dezinno, P.; Lin, E.C.; Lin, H.; Yue, J.J.; Berman, M.R.; Braveman, F.; Kain, Z.N. Auricular acupuncture as a treatment for pregnant women who have low back and posterior pelvic pain: A pilot study. *Am. J. Obstet. Gynecol.* **2009**, *201*, 271. [CrossRef]
142. Elden, H.; Hagberg, H.; Olsen, M.F.; Ladfors, L.; Ostgaard, H.C. Regression of pelvic girdle pain after delivery: Follow-up of a randomised single blind controlled trial with different treatment modalities. *Acta Obstet. Gynecol. Scand.* **2008**, *87*, 201–208. [CrossRef]
143. Ternov, N.K.; Grennert, L.; Aberg, A.; Algotsson, L.; Akeson, J. Acupuncture for lower back and pelvic pain in late pregnancy: A retrospective report on 167 consecutive cases. *Pain Med.* **2001**, *2*, 204–207. [CrossRef]
144. Oxford Health NHS. TENS Machine in Pregnancy. Available online: https://www.oxfordhealth.nhs.uk/wp-content/uploads/2014/08/OP-100.15-TENS-machine-in-pregnancy.pdf (accessed on 17 June 2022).
145. Behailu Kribet. Transcutaneous Electrical Nerve Stimulation during Pregnancy: The Electric Field in the Fetal Brain. Available online: https://bkibret.com/tens-during-pregnancy (accessed on 17 June 2022).
146. Keskin, E.A.; Onur, O.; Keskin, H.L.; Gumus, I.I.; Kafali, H.; Turhan, N. Transcutaneous electrical nerve stimulation improves low back pain during pregnancy. *Gynecol. Obstet. Investig.* **2012**, *74*, 76–83. [CrossRef]
147. Njogu, A.; Qin, S.; Chen, Y.; Hu, L.; Luo, Y. The effects of transcutaneous electrical nerve stimulation during the first stage of labor: A randomized controlled trial. *BMC Pregnancy Childbirth* **2021**, *21*, 164. [CrossRef]
148. Nascimento, S.L.; Surita, F.G.; Cecatti, J.G. Physical exercise during pregnancy. *Curr. Opin. Obstet. Gynecol.* **2012**, *24*, 387–394. [CrossRef]
149. Barakat, R.; Cordero, Y.; Coteron, J.; Luaces, M.; Montejo, R. Exercise during pregnancy improves maternal glucose screen at 24–28 weeks: A randomised controlled trial. *Br. J. Sports Med.* **2012**, *46*, 656–661. [CrossRef]
150. de Barros, M.C.; Lopes, M.A.; Francisco, R.P.; Sapienza, A.D.; Zugaib, M. Resistance exercise and glycemic control in women with gestational diabetes mellitus. *Am. J. Obstet. Gynecol.* **2010**, *203*, 556. [CrossRef]
151. Mason, L.; Roe, B.; Wong, H.; Davies, J.; Bamber, J. The role of antenatal pelvic floor muscle exercises in prevention of postpartum stress incontinence: A randomised controlled trial. *J. Clin. Nurs.* **2010**, *19*, 2777–2786. [CrossRef]
152. Ko, P.C.; Liang, C.C.; Chang, S.D.; Lee, J.T.; Chao, A.S.; Cheng, P.J. A randomized controlled trial of antenatal pelvic floor exercises to prevent and treat urinary incontinence. *Int. Urogynecol. J.* **2011**, *22*, 17–22. [CrossRef]
153. Robledo-Colonia, A.F.; Sandoval-Restrepo, N.; Mosquera-Valderrama, Y.F.; Escobar-Hurtado, C.; Ramírez-Vélez, R. Aerobic exercise training during pregnancy reduces depressive symptoms in nulliparous women: A randomised trial. *J. Physiother.* **2012**, *58*, 9–15. [CrossRef]
154. Vallim, A.L.; Osis, M.J.; Cecatti, J.G.; Baciuk, É.P.; Silveira, C.; Cavalcante, S.R. Water exercises and quality of life during pregnancy. *Reprod. Health* **2011**, *8*, 14. [CrossRef]
155. Barakat, R.; Pelaez, M.; Montejo, R.; Luaces, M.; Zakynthinaki, M. Exercise during pregnancy improves maternal health perception: A randomized controlled trial. *Am. J. Obstet. Gynecol.* **2011**, *204*, 402. [CrossRef] [PubMed]

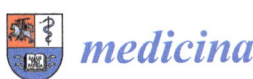

Article

A Cross-Sectional Study Examining the Association between Physical Activity and Perinatal Depression

Irene Soto-Fernández [1], Sagrario Gómez-Cantarino [2], Benito Yáñez-Araque [3,*], Jorge Sánchez-Infante [4], Alejandra Zapata-Ossa [5] and Mercedes Dios-Aguado [6]

1. Faculty of Physiotherapy and Nursing, University of Castilla-La Mancha, 45004 Toledo, Spain
2. Department of Nursing, Physiotherapy and Occupational Therapy, Faculty of Physiotherapy and Nursing, University of Castilla-La Mancha, 45004 Toledo, Spain
3. Department of Business Administration, Faculty of Law and Social Science, University of Castilla-La Mancha, 45071 Toledo, Spain
4. Performance and Sport Rehabilitation Laboratory, Faculty of Sport Sciences, University of Castilla-La Mancha, 45071 Toledo, Spain
5. Department of Physical Activity and Sports Sciences, Faculty of Sports Sciences, University of Castilla-La Mancha, Av. Carlos III, s/n, 45071 Toledo, Spain
6. Yepes Health Center, Health Service of Castilla-La Mancha, Av. Santa Reliquia 26, 45313 Toledo, Spain
* Correspondence: benito.yanez@uclm.es

Abstract: *Background and Objectives:* International organisations recommend that women without illness should have regular moderate-intensity physical exercise throughout their pregnancy and postpartum period as a measure to prevent possible pathologies in both the mother and the newborn. Physical activity during pregnancy reduces the likelihood of depression during pregnancy and after childbirth, benefiting both the pregnant woman and the foetus. However, most pregnant women are known to be inactive. The Pregnancy Physical Activity Questionnaire (PPAQ) analyses the level of physical activity of pregnant women. These data are correlated with the variable depression, for which the Edinburgh Postnatal Depression Scale (EPDS) during pregnancy was used. *Materials and Methods:* The research employed a cross sectional study design on ninety-nine pregnant women. *Results:* The data on physical activity in relation to depression in those pregnant women who had not previously suffered from depression were 719.29 METS min/wk compared with 624.62 METS min/wk in those who had. And for pregnant women who suffered from depression at the time of the study, their physical activity was 698.25 METS min/wk, while those who did not suffer from depression reached 826.57 METS. *Conclusions:* Pregnant women without depression are much more active. A favourable employment situation or a high level of education is directly related to higher physical activity. Physical activity and higher energy expenditure occur at home, as opposed to activity carried out as transport, exercise or at work.

Keywords: gestational depression; maternal and child health; physical activity; pregnancy

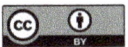

1. Introduction

International and national organisations recommend that pregnant women without illness should have regular moderate-intensity physical exercise throughout pregnancy and during the puerperium [1,2] as around 60% of pregnant women are inactive [3]. Hence, the need to prescribe the duration and intensity of physical exercise that a pregnant woman should do [4], since physical exercise is known to prevent diabetes and hypertension [5]. Not forgetting that the practice of physical activity in turn has an impact on child health [6].

The World Health Organisation (WHO) warns that one in four people in their lifetime may suffer from a mental illness, with depression being a very common disorder that can cause sadness, feelings of guilt or shame, loss or interruption of appetite, fatigue and/or lack of concentration [7]. On the one hand, there are studies that support that pregnancy and the postpartum period are protective periods for women against depression due to the lower suicide rate [8], and a recent study conducted during the pandemic underlines the idea that pregnancy has decreased depressive symptoms in this period compared to nonpregnant women [9]. Research carried out in the United States warns that between 8% and 16% of women of reproductive age are affected by this mental pathology [10]. On the other hand, other investigations affirm that the postpartum period increases the risk of MDD (Major Depressive Disorder) [11]. Other studies indicate that women are 70% more likely to suffer from this pathology than men, due to hormonal and/or psychosocial changes experienced by women throughout their lives [12]. However, knowledge is scarce regarding the mechanisms that give rise to mood disorders. Furthermore, studies have not concluded whether increased oestrogen and progesterone affect mood [13,14], or whether it is oestradiol and progesterone that influence levels of the neurotransmitters serotonin, noradrenaline and dopamine that may influence depression [15,16]. In contrast, perinatal mood alterations and psychological factors thought to influence fatigue during gestation have been recognised for more than a century [17,18].

However, some studies show that physical activity during pregnancy reduces the likelihood of depression during pregnancy, and regular physical activity during pregnancy improves the mother's mood, reduces maternal fatigue and reduces uncertainty about her baby's health [19–22]. In addition, yoga-based exercises have been found to have beneficial effects on maternal mood and depression [23].

The aim of the present study was to analyse the level of physical activity performed by pregnant women not only as physical exercise, but also when travelling, at home and at work, using the Pregnancy Physical Activity Questionnaire (PPAQ). In addition, the data correlate with the variable depression, so, it was interesting to know whether the depression was pregestational or emerged during pregnancy. The analysis of the variable will be carried out by means of the Edinburgh Postnatal Depression Scale (EPDS) during pregnancy.

2. Materials and Methods

2.1. Study Population and Design

The research employed a descriptive, correlational and cross-sectional method [24]. The overall research sample consisted of a total of 99 pregnant women, with a mean age of 32.9 years and a standard deviation of 4.38, who received care throughout their pregnancy at the Health Centre, in a health area of the province of Toledo (Castilla-La Mancha, Spain). In this health area in 2020, according to the municipal census, there were 2570 women, of whom 1040 were of childbearing age (15–49 years). Taking as a reference the 341,315 births in Spain in 2020, the sampling error was 9.85% (confidence level = 95%; $z = 1.96$; $p = q = 0.50$; $\alpha = 0.05$). The research was carried out between January 2019 and March 2020. The inclusion criteria were women over 18 years of age, with a singleton pregnancy and who voluntarily agreed to participate in the study. Exclusion criteria were women with pregestational pathologies, such as hypertension, preeclampsia in previous pregnancies or gestational diabetes.

In addition, the following dependent variables were used for the study: depression before and during pregnancy, age, trimester of pregnancy, level of education, marital status, not having offspring, economic resources and employment status. The independent variables were physical activity at home, physical activity in transport, physical activity at work and total physical activity.

2.2. Measuring Instruments

Two scales were used throughout the research, the first being the semiquantitative questionnaire, Pregnancy Physical Activity Questionnaire (PPAQ) [25]. It is a specific questionnaire of physical activity during pregnancy in which the amount of time the woman is active is recorded. The measurement can be divided into days and reflects the gestational trimester.

The PPAQ is made up of 36 questions, 32 of which refer to the activities carried out by the pregnant woman, including home and/or care of others (13 activities), occupational (5 activities), sports and/or exercise (8 activities), transport (3 activities) and inactivity (3 activities). The Likert scale is used as a response tool, where the response options range from 0 to 5, where 0 means no physical activity at all, 1 less than half an hour a day, 2 from half an hour to almost an hour, 3 from one hour to almost two hours, 4 from two to almost three hours a day and 5 three or more hours a day.

The PPAQ questionnaire is an easy-to-use measurement tool, as it assigns a value to each activity, expressed in METS, per hour during the week. Thus, according to the intensity of each activity, it is classified as follows: Sedentary (1.5 METs), Light (1.5–3.0 METs), Moderate (3.0–6.0 METs) and High (>6 METS) [26]. The results were analysed following the Guidelines for data processing and analysis of international Physical Activity Questionnaire (IPAQ) [27].

The second scale used was the Edinburgh Postnatal Depression Scale (EPDS) during pregnancy [28,29]. The questionnaire is a validated screening instrument for the detection of depressive symptoms during pregnancy, which consists of 10 items measuring depressive symptoms on a Likert scale, where the scoring options for each item range from 0 to 4. Thus, 0 means not at all, 1 infrequent, 2 sometimes and 3 frequently. So, at the end of the questionnaire, the total response score can range from 0 to 30 points. This means that higher scores indicate a higher probability of suffering from depression. Therefore, this scale is a valid and sensitive instrument for predicting depressive disorders not only in the postnatal but also in the prenatal period.

2.3. Statistical Analysis

The data collected were all quantitative, and the statistical package SPSS/PC ver. 25.0 (IBM, Chicago, IL, USA) was used for the analysis. After data collection, the data were transferred to SPSS to create the database needed to study the information collected. Once the database was created, women who did not meet the previously defined inclusion criteria and requirements were removed from the database. Therefore, in turn, a nonparametric correlational study with crosstabulations was carried out.

Median, mean, standard deviation (SD) or interquartile range (IR) were used to describe the parameters used. Differences in parameter distributions were analysed using Student's t-test, ANOVA or Mann–Whitney U test if the distribution deviated from normality. For categorical data, the chi-square test was used, and relationships between variables were established with Pearson's or Spearman's correlation coefficients.

2.4. Ethical Considerations

The research was conducted according to the highest ethical standards in accordance with the Declaration of Helsinki, the Guidelines of the International Conference on Harmonisation of Good Clinical Practice and national ethical and legal requirements. All participants signed an informed consent form prior to inclusion in the study, which could be revoked at any time. The Clinical Research Ethics Committee of the Toledo Hospital, Castilla-La Mancha Public Health Service (SESCAM), REC no. 125.

3. Results

3.1. Characteristics of the Sample

The descriptive analysis of the data reveals the following percentages of age of the pregnant women: 5 (5.1%) of them were between 20–25 years old; 60 (60.6%) were between 26 and 35 years old, and 34 (34.3%) were between 36 and 40 years old. In relation to their gestational trimester, 85 (85.9%) were in the first trimester, and 14 (14.1%) were in the second trimester. Regarding marital status, 80 (80.8%) of the pregnant women reported being married, and 19 (19.2%) reported being single. In terms of offspring, 50 (50.5%) of the participating women have offspring compared to 49 (49.5%) who do not have any. According to the level of studies, 44 (44.4%) of the women in the sample have university studies; 38 (38.4%) have secondary studies, such as baccalaureate or vocational training, and 17 (17.2%) have only primary studies. As far as economic resources are concerned, 74 (74.7%) of the pregnant women said they were unemployed; 15 (15.2%) said they were on sick leave, and 10 (10.1%) were working.

3.2. Physical Activity Carried out by the Pregnant Women in the Study

In order to analyse the physical activity of the women in the sample, the pregnant women were divided into three age groups: (a) 20 to 25, (b) 26 to 35 and (c) 36 to 40 (Table 1).

Table 1. MET scores by activity block and age group.

		N	Mean	Standard Deviation	Standard Error	95% Confidence Interval for the Mean	
						Lower Limit	Upper Limit
MET Home	20 to 25 years old	5	597.38	276.86	123.82	253.61	941.15
	26 to 35 years old	60	433.16	146.98	19.14	394.86	471.46
	36 to 40 years old	34	417.61	173.99	29.84	356.90	478.32
	Total	99	436.50	166.04	16.69	403.40	469.61
MET Transport	20 to 25 years old	5	49.00	31.30	14.00	10.13	87.87
	26 to 35 years old	60	34.88	18.04	2.35	30.18	39.58
	36 to 40 years old	34	33.97	14.64	2.51	28.86	39.08
	Total	99	35.21	17.76	1.79	31.67	38.75
MET Exercise	20 to 25 years old	5	234.08	160.15	71.62	35.23	432.93
	26 to 35 years old	60	145.74	140.80	18.33	109.05	182.44
	36 to 40 years old	34	158.57	79.69	13.67	130.77	186.38
	Total	99	153.84	123.96	12.46	129.12	178.57
MET Work	20 to 25 years old	5	119.14	102.09	45.66	−7.62	245.90
	26 to 35 years old	60	79.53	76.61	9.97	59.56	99.49
	36 to 40 years old	34	82.09	45.21	7.87	66.06	98.12
	Total	99	82.14	68.54	6.92	68.40	95.88
PPAQ	20 to 25 years old	5	999.60	476.29	213.00	408.21	1590.99
	26 to 35 years old	60	693.31	315.25	41.04	611.15	775.46
	36 to 40 years old	34	689.83	187.55	32.16	624.39	755.27
	Total	99	706.86	290.82	29.23	648.85	764.86

Once the groups were selected, women in the 20–25 age group had the highest MET score. However, when correlating physical activity and level of education, in all the crosstabulations, it was women with a university education who were more physically active, irrespective of their age group.

However, when crossing the data with the variable employment status, in the first two age groups, women who were working scored higher in METS, while women in the third group scored higher for those who were on sick leave. According to the maximum and minimum scores recorded by the women in the sample in relation to their employment status, the highest scores in all blocks were obtained by working pregnant women, as shown in Table 1.

However, when relating the results of physical activity with age and gestational trimester, in all subgroups, the pregnant women in the second gestational trimester obtained the highest scores: (a) 489.90 METS, (b) 38.50 METS and (c) 161.60.

However, when crossing the data with the variable of having offspring, it was in the 20 to 25 and 26 to 35 age groups that the pregnant women were most active, with the women without offspring achieving the highest figures: group (a) 455.63 METS and group (b) 165.42 METS.

3.3. Depression and Physical Activity

Of the 99 women in the sample, 85.13% reported not having suffered from depression before becoming pregnant, and 14.87% reported having suffered from depression before their pregnancy.

The results of the PPAQ reveal that pregnant women who had not suffered from depression before pregnancy were more physically active (Table 2). Thus, the maximum score obtained by these women in each block was 1043 METS, 105 METS, 739 METS and 287 METS, respectively.

Table 2. PPQA results for the variable previous depression.

		N	Mean	Standard Deviation	Standard Error	95% Confidence Interval for the Mean	
						Lower Limit	Upper Limit
MET Home	No	86	445.12	168.53	18.17	408.98	481.25
	Yes	13	379.45	141.09	39.13	294.19	464.71
	Total	99	436.50	166.04	16.69	403.38	469.61
MET Transport	No	86	35.33	18.22	1.97	31.42	39.23
	Yes	13	34.46	14.98	4.15	25.41	43.51
	Total	99	35.21	17.76	1.79	31.67	38.75
MET Exercise	No	86	155.71	126.41	13.63	128.61	182.81
	Yes	13	141.51	110.02	30.52	75.02	207.99
	Total	99	153.84	123.96	12.46	129.12	178.57
MET Work	No	86	84.12	70.81	7.68	68.84	99.39
	Yes	13	69.19	51.58	14.31	38.02	100.36
	Total	99	82.14	68.54	6.92	68.40	95.88
PPAQ	No	86	719.29	299.23	32.27	655.14	783.45
	Yes	13	624.62	219.25	60.81	492.12	757.11
	Total	99	706.86	290.82	29.23	648.85	764.86

With regard to depression during pregnancy, 87.9% of the women in the sample did not show depression when analysing their responses to the EPDS questionnaire, while 12.1% of the women in the sample showed depression when analysing their responses to the EPDS questionnaire. When correlated with the results of the PPAQ, it was observed that the pregnant women who suffered from depression were the women who obtained the highest activity scores (Table 3).

When the sample was tested for normality (Kolmogorov–Smirnov test) with the intention of further statistical analysis, it was observed that the distribution of the sample is not normal. Therefore, a nonparametric analysis was used to test two different groups. When looking at the differences between the results of first trimester pregnant women and second trimester pregnant women, no significant differences were found in either their physical activity or mood. Then, when no significant differences were found, the level of physical activity of the whole sample was analysed to see if it was having an influence. It was found that 58.6% of the pregnant women engaged in light-intensity physical activity, and 41.4% of the pregnant women were sedentary. To understand the data, a crosstabulation was carried out to study the level of physical activity in relation to whether or not they were depressed during pregnancy, but no significant differences were found (Pearson's chi-square 0.985). When the data on physical activity level were crosstabulated with prepregnancy depression, no significant differences were found (Pearson's chi-square 0.710).

Therefore, there is no correlation between the results of the Edinburgh scale and physical activity that could serve as a diagnostic tool for perinatal depression. However, there is a significant correlation of 0.570** between the score on the Edinburgh scale and having depression during the first and second trimesters of pregnancy in the women in the sample. The correlation between educational level and employment status was 0.321**.

In turn, there was a significant negative correlation between employment status and the Edinburgh scale—0.230*, between employment status and educational level—0.232* and age group with the Edinburgh scale—0.346**.

Table 3. PPQA scores for depression during pregnancy.

		N	Mean	Standard Deviation	Standard Error	95% Confidence Interval for the Mean	
						Lower Limit	Upper Limit
MET Home	No	87	432.79	158.97	17.04	398.91	466.67
	Yes	12	463.34	217.14	62.68	325.38	601.31
	Total	99	436.50	166.04	16.69	403.38	469.61
MET Transport	No	87	34.84	16.88	1.81	31.24	38.44
	Yes	12	37.92	23.96	6.92	22.69	53.14
	Total	99	35.21	17.76	1.79	31.67	38.75
MET Exercise	No	87	147.02	116.52	12.49	122.19	171.86
	Yes	12	203.29	166.45	48.05	97.53	309.05
	Total	99	153.84	123.96	12.46	129.12	178.57
MET Work	No	87	77.27	63.46	6.84	63.66	90.87
	Yes	12	117.02	93.74	27.06	57.45	176.58
	Total	99	82.14	68.54	6.92	68.40	95.88
PPAQ	No	87	691.04	267.82	28.71	633.96	748.12
	Yes	12	821.57	420.02	121.25	554.70	1088.43
	Total	99	706.86	290.82	29.23	648.85	764.86

Finally, a chi-square test was performed to analyse whether there were significant differences between pregnant women who suffered from depression during pregnancy, taking into account whether they had previously developed depression, and the data revealed that there were significant differences (Table 4).

Table 4. Differences between women with depression before and during pregnancy and those who did not.

Chi-square	53.828	56.818
Df [1]	1	1
Asymptotic sig.	0.000	0.000

[1] df = Degree of freedom.

4. Discussion

The research study attempts to discover the possible relationship between physical activity and predisposition to suffer from depression during pregnancy and/or the onset of depression during the postpartum period.

It is known that regular physical activity contributes to good health and reduces the risk of certain concomitant pathologies in pregnancy [3]. In addition, the American College of Obstetrics and Gynecology states that physical activity during pregnancy prevents excessive weight gain during pregnancy, reduces the risk of gestational diabetes, preeclampsia and caesarean delivery. In turn, the British College, the Canadian Society of Obstetrics and Gynaecology and the Spanish Society of Obstetrics and Gynaecology recommend 150 min of moderate physical activity per week throughout pregnancy. Synthesising all this information, the research carried out reveals that the women in the sample put all these physical activity recommendations into practice, as the data show that the average total physical activity carried out was 706.86 METS min/week, with 436.86 METS min/week at home and

436.86 METS min/week at home. Being at home accounted for 436.50 METS, in transport 35.21 METS, as exercise 153.84 METS and at work 82.14 METS. They even put into practice the recommendation proposed by the WHO on physical activity for pregnant women [30], as the pregnant women performed physical activity within the range of 600 to 1500 METS, which corresponds to moderate physical activity, with an average of 706.86 METS.

Studies related to activity in pregnancy show that it is at home that pregnant women have the highest energy expenditure [19,31]. This was confirmed by the research, as the pregnant women in the sample obtained a maximum value of 1043 METS of physical activity at home, regardless of any variable.

Pregnancy is a complex period of time for both the woman and the new life that is being engendered, as the great transformations that occur throughout gestation can lead to the development of fatigue in the pregnant woman, due to the energy requirements demanded by her foetus and the woman's weight gain [32]. Thus, these coexisting factors together with the hormonal changes that occur can interfere with the level of physical activity performed by the mother throughout pregnancy, increasing her level of fatigue [15]. This in turn may alter her emotional response to the problems of everyday life, leading to a variation in her mood [33], which is likely to induce the development of perinatal depression [34]. However, of the 99 women in the sample, only 13.1% of the EPDS questionnaire revealed that they suffered from depression during pregnancy, so, the data show that physical activity prevented the development of this pathology. Furthermore, following the data, they found that women who had never suffered from depression were more active than those who had suffered from depression.

However, if we compare all the results obtained in the research with existing studies on the subject, we can see that the studies confirm that mothers who are more physically active suffer less depression and anxiety than mothers who are less physically active [35,36].

Limitations and Future Prospects

In our study, we found that women who had not been depressed prior to pregnancy were the most active, but at the same time, we found that during pregnancy, they suffer a longer period of depression than those who do not do physical activity. The study documented a correlation between the level of physical activity among pregnant women and their depression status. The weakness of the study is its narrow focus on too few variables. The relationship could be related to other variables that contribute to the existence of the relationship (e.g., health conditions or leadership style in the workplace that contribute to the existence of depression [37]). In a complementary study, we could analyse the reasons why women who do physical activity suffer more depression than those who do not, as subjectively we could think that this is due to different external factors that have not been analysed on this occasion, such as greater difficulty in doing physical activity, extreme bodily changes, etc.

On the other hand, it would be necessary to make a more specific selection of the sample having participants between the three trimesters of pregnancy as well as taking into account as a dependent variable the situation of pregnancy at risk. In addition, if it was intended to analyse whether depression in pregnant women is palliated by the practice of physical activity, it would have been convenient to do a good screening of the sample and compare homogeneous and consistent groups of pregnant women with depression and without depression to observe if the activity physical fitness improves the status in women with depression.

In the future, a longitudinal study should be carried out to provide precise data on each woman. We recommend extending the study with a larger representative sample to avoid sampling bias, as well as using other advanced data analysis techniques, for example, Structural Equation Modelling (SEM) or fsQCA. Especially fsQCA allows working with small samples and overcomes some limitations of the dominant research logic [38].

Lastly, it is recommended that a specialist in sports science, in collaboration with the gynaecologist, prescribes physical activity for pregnant women, since benefits have been found for the health of both the mother and the foetus.

5. Conclusions

In conclusion, the research reveals that regular physical activity is beneficial for the women in the study. In relation to depression, pregnant women without depression are much more active. In addition, having a favourable employment situation or a high level of education is directly related to being more physically active when pregnant. Additionally, the results show that the greatest energy expenditure and the greatest amount of physical activity are carried out by pregnant women at home.

Author Contributions: Conceptualisation, B.Y.-A., S.G.-C. and M.D.-A.; methodology, B.Y.-A., J.S.-I. and I.S.-F.; software, B.Y.-A., I.S.-F. and A.Z.-O.; validation, B.Y.-A., S.G.-C., I.S.-F. and M.D.-A.; formal analysis, B.Y.-A., S.G.-C. and A.Z.-O.; investigation, I.S.-F., S.G.-C., B.Y.-A., J.S.-I., A.Z.-O. and M.D.-A.; resources, S.G.-C. and M.D.-A.; data curation, B.Y.-A. and S.G.-C.; writing—original draft preparation, I.S.-F., S.G.-C., B.Y.-A., J.S.-I., A.Z.-O. and M.D.-A.; writing—review and editing, B.Y.-A., I.S.-F. and M.D.-A.; visualisation, B.Y.-A., S.G.-C., I.S.-F. and M.D.-A.; supervision, S.G.-C. and B.Y.-A.; project administration, S.G.-C. and B.Y.-A. All authors have read and agreed to the published version of the manuscript.

Funding: This research received no external funding.

Institutional Review Board Statement: Ethics Approval: Clinical Research Ethics Committee of the Toledo Hospital Complex. Castilla-La Mancha Public Health Service (SESCAM). REC no. 125 (date of approval: 25 November 2015). Informed Consent Statement: Informed consent was obtained from all subjects involved in the study.

Informed Consent Statement: Informed consent was obtained from all subjects involved in the study.

Data Availability Statement: The data that support the findings of this study are available from the corresponding author upon request.

Conflicts of Interest: The authors declare no conflict of interest.

References

1. Artal, R.; O'toole, M. Guidelines of the American College of Obstetricians and Gynecologists for exercise during pregnancy and the postpartum period. *Br. J. Sports Med.* **2003**, *7*, 6–12. [CrossRef] [PubMed]
2. Casajús, J.A.; Vicente-Rodríguez, G. Ejercicio físico y salud en poblaciones especiales. *Exernet Colección ICD* **2011**, *58*, 169–194.
3. Poudevigne, M.S.; O'Connor, P.J. A review of physical activity patterns in pregnant women and their relationship to psychological health. *Sports Med.* **2006**, *36*, 19–38. [CrossRef]
4. Pescatello, L.S.; Riebe, D.; Thompson, P.D.; (Eds.) *ACSM's Guidelines for Exercise Testing and Prescription*; Lippincott Williams & Wilkins: Philadelphia, PA, USA, 2014.
5. Artal, R. Exercise: The alternative therapeutic intervention for gestational diabetes. *Clin. Obstet. Gynecol.* **2003**, *46*, 479–487. [CrossRef]
6. Clapp, J.F., III; Lopez, B.; Harcar-Sevcik, R. Neonatal behavioral profile of the offspring of women who continued to exercise regularly throughout pregnancy. *Am. J. Obstet. Gynecol.* **1999**, *180*, 91–94. [CrossRef]
7. World Health Organization. Mental Health. Depression: Definition. Available online: http://www.euro.who.int/en/what-we-do/health-topics/noncommunicable-diseases/mental-health/news/news/2012/10/depression-in-europe/depression-definition (accessed on 10 March 2021).
8. Oates, M. Suicide: The leading cause of maternal death. *Br. J. Psychiatry* **2003**, *183*, 279–281. [CrossRef]
9. Yirmiya, K.; Yakirevich-Amir, N.; Preis, H.; Lotan, A.; Atzil, S.; Reuveni, I. Women's Depressive Symptoms during the COVID-19 Pandemic: The Role of Pregnancy. *Int. J. Env. Res. Public Health* **2021**, *18*, 4298. [CrossRef]
10. Ko, J.Y.; Farr, S.L.; Dietz, P.M.; Robbins, C.L. Depression and treatment among U.S. pregnant and non-pregnant women of reproductive age, 2005–2009. *J. Women's Health* **2012**, *28*, 830–835. [CrossRef]
11. Payne, J.L. Depression: Is pregnancy protective? *J. Womens Health* **2012**, *21*, 809–810. [CrossRef] [PubMed]
12. National Institutes of Health. National Institutes of Mental Health. Major Depressive Disorder among Adults. Available online: http://www.nimh.nih.gov/statistics/1mdd_adult.shtml (accessed on 10 January 2021).
13. Nott, P.N.; Franklin, M.; Armitage, C.; Gelder, M.G. Hormonal changes and mood in the puerperium. *Br. J. Psychiatry* **1976**, *128*, 379–383. [CrossRef]

14. Harris, B.; Lovett, L.; Newcombe, R.G.; Read, G.F.; Walker, R.; Riad-Fahmy, D. Maternity blues and major endocrine changes: Cardiff puerperal mood and hormone study II. *BMJ* **1994**, *308*, 949–953. [CrossRef] [PubMed]
15. Bethea, C.L.; Pecins-Thompson, M.; Schutzer, W.E.; Gundlah, C.L.Z.N.; Lu, Z.N. Ovarian steroids and serotonin neural function. *Mol. Neurobiol.* **1998**, *18*, 87–123. [CrossRef] [PubMed]
16. Steiner, M.; Dunn, E.; Born, L. Hormones and mood: From menarche to menopause and beyond. *J. Affect. Disord.* **2003**, *74*, 67–83. [CrossRef]
17. Steiner, M. Postpartum psychiatric disorders. *Can. J. Psychiatry* **1990**, *35*, 89–95. [CrossRef]
18. Reeves, N.; Potempa, K.; Gallo, A. Fatigue in early pregnancy: An exploratory study. *J. Nurse-Midwifery* **1991**, *36*, 303–309. [CrossRef]
19. Costa, D.D.; Rippen, N.; Dritsa, M.; Ring, A. Self-reported leisure-time physical activity during pregnancy and relationship to psychological well-being. *J. Psychosom. Obstet. Gynecol.* **2003**, *24*, 111–119. [CrossRef]
20. Nakamura, A.; van der Waerden, J.; Melchior, M.; Bolze, C.; El-Khoury, F.; Pryor, L. Physical activity during pregnancy and postpartum depression: Systematic review and meta-analysis. *J. Affect. Disord.* **2019**, *246*, 29–41. [CrossRef]
21. Physical Activity and Exercise During Pregnancy and the Postpartum Period: ACOG Committee Opinion, Number 804. *Obstet. Gynecol.* **2020**, *135*, e178–e188. [CrossRef]
22. Poudevigne, M.S.; O'Connor, P.J. Physical activity and mood during pregnancy. *Med. Sci. Sports Exerc.* **2005**, *37*, 1374–1380. [CrossRef]
23. Ng, Q.X.; Venkatanarayanan, N.; Loke, W.; Yeo, W.S.; Lim, D.Y.; Chan, H.W.; Sim, W.S. A meta-analysis of the effectiveness of yoga-based interventions for maternal depression during pregnancy. *Complementary Ther. Clin. Pract.* **2019**, *34*, 8–12. [CrossRef]
24. Montero, I.; León, O.G. A guide for naming research studies in psychology. *Int. J. Clin. Health Psychol.* **2007**, *7*, 847–862.
25. Chasan-Taber, L.; Schmidt, M.D.; Roberts, D.E.; Hosmer, D.; Markenson, G.; Freedson, P.S. Development and validation of a Pregnancy Physical Activity Questionnaire. *Med. Sci. Sports Exerc.* **2004**, *36*, 1750–1760. [CrossRef] [PubMed]
26. Suliga, E.; Sobaś, K.; Król, G. Validation of the Pregnancy Physical Activity Questionnaire (PPAQ). *Med. Stud. Studia Med.* **2017**, *33*, 40–45. [CrossRef]
27. Fernández, M.D.; Sánchez, P.T.; Hermoso, V.M.S. Versiones corta y larga. In *Traducción de la Guía Para el Procesamiento de Datos y Análisis del Cuestionario Internacional de Actividad Física (IPAQ)*; Universidad de Granada; Junta de Andalucía: Granada, Spain, 2005.
28. Cox, J.L.; Holden, J.M.; Sagovsky, R. Detection of postnatal depression. Development of the 10-item Edinburgh Postnatal Depression Scale. *Br. J. Psychiatry J. Ment. Sci.* **1987**, *150*, 782–786. [CrossRef] [PubMed]
29. Rubertsson, C.; Börjesson, K.; Berglund, A.; Josefsson, A.; Sydsjö, G. The Swedish validation of Edinburgh Postnatal Depression Scale (EPDS) during pregnancy. *Nord. J. Psychiatry* **2011**, *65*, 414–418. [CrossRef]
30. World Health Organization. *Recommendations on Antenatal Care for A Positive Pregnancy Experience*; World Health Organization: Geneva, Switzerland, 2016.
31. Goodwin, A.; Astbury, J.; McMeeken, J. Body image and psychological well-being in pregnancy. A comparison of exercisers and non-exercisers. *Aust. N. Z. J. Obstet. Gynaecol.* **2000**, *40*, 442–447. [CrossRef]
32. Dios-Aguado, M.; Agulló-Ortuño, M.T.; Ugarte-Gurrutxaga, M.I.; Yañez-Araque, B.; Molina-Gallego, B.; Gómez-Cantarino, S. Nutritional Health Education in Pregnant Women in a Rural Health Centre: Results in Spanish and Foreign Women. *Healthcare* **2021**, *9*, 1293. [CrossRef]
33. Gómez-Cantarino, S.; García-Valdivieso, I.; Moncunill-Martínez, E.; Yáñez-Araque, B.; Ugarte Gurrutxaga, M.I. Developing a Family-Centered Care Model in the Neonatal Intensive Care Unit (NICU): A New Vision to Manage Healthcare. *Int. J. Environ. Res. Public Health* **2020**, *17*, 7197. [CrossRef]
34. López-Sánchez, I.; Santos-Fonseca, R.S.; Molero-Segrera, M.; Casado-Méndez, P.R.; González-González, A. Associated factors for postpartum depression. *Rev. Arch. Médico Camagüey* **2019**, *23*, 770–779.
35. Koniak-Griffin, D. Aerobic exercise, psychological well-being, and physical discomforts during adolescent pregnancy. *Res. Nurs. Health* **1994**, *17*, 253–263. [CrossRef]
36. Campolong, K.; Jenkins, S.; Clark, M.M.; Borowski, K.; Nelson, N.; Moore, K.M.; Bobo, W.V. The association of exercise during pregnancy with trimester-specific and postpartum quality of life and depressive symptoms in a cohort of healthy pregnant women. *Arch. Women's Ment. Health* **2018**, *21*, 215–224. [CrossRef] [PubMed]
37. Ruiz-Palomino, P.; Yáñez-Araque, B.; Jiménez-Estévez, P.; Gutiérrez-Broncano, S. Can Servant Leadership Prevent Hotel Employee Depression during the COVID-19 Pandemic? A Mediating and Multigroup Analysis. *Technol. Forecast. Soc. Chang.* **2022**, *174*, 121192. [CrossRef] [PubMed]
38. Yáñez-Araque, B.; Gómez-Cantarino, S.; Gutiérrez-Broncano, S.; López-Ruiz, V.-R. Examining the Determinants of Healthcare Workers' Performance: A Configurational Analysis during COVID-19 Times. *Int. J. Environ. Res. Public Health* **2021**, *18*, 5671. [CrossRef] [PubMed]

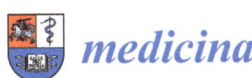

Article

Maternal Periodontal Status as a Factor Influencing Obstetrical Outcomes

Petra Völgyesi [1], Márta Radnai [2], Gábor Németh [1], Krisztina Boda [3], Elena Bernad [4,5,6,*] and Tibor Novák [1]

[1] Department of Obstetrics and Gynecology, Faculty of Medicine, University of Szeged, 6725 109 Szeged, Hungary
[2] Department of Prosthodontics, Faculty of Medicine, University of Szeged, 6725 109 Szeged, Hungary
[3] Department of Medical Physics and Informatics, Faculty of Medicine, University of Szeged, 6725 109 Szeged, Hungary
[4] Department of Obstetrics and Gynecology, Faculty of Medicine, "Victor Babes" University of Medicine and Pharmacy, 300041 Timisoara, Romania
[5] Clinic of Obstetrics and Gynecology, "Pius Brinzeu" County Clinical Emergency Hospital, 300723 Timisoara, Romania
[6] Center for Laparoscopy, Laparoscopic Surgery and In Vitro Fertilization, "Victor Babes" University of Medicine and Pharmacy, 300041 Timisoara, Romania
* Correspondence: bernad.elena@umft.ro

Abstract: *Background and Objectives:* Preterm birth as a complex phenomenon is influenced by numerous endogenic and exogenic factors, although its exact cause often remains obscure. According to epidemiological studies, maternal periodontal diseases, in addition to affecting general health, can also cause adverse pregnancy outcomes. Nonetheless, the existing results in the literature regarding this topic remain controversial. Consequently, our study aimed to determine the connection between poor maternal periodontal status and neonatal birth weight. *Materials and Methods*: A total of 111 primigravida–primiparous pregnant, healthy women underwent a periodontal examination in the second trimester of their pregnancies. Probing depth (PD) and bleeding on probing (BOP) were determined, and based on these diagnostic measurements, the patients were divided into three subgroups according to their dental status: healthy (H, $n = 17$), gingivitis (G, $n = 67$), and periodontitis (P, $n = 27$). *Results:* Considering that poor maternal oral status is an influencing factor for obstetrical outcomes, the presence of PD and BOP (characterized by the sulcus bleeding index, SBI) was evaluated. In the case of P, defined as PD $\geq$ 4 mm in at least one site and BOP $\geq$ 50% of the teeth, a significant correlation between BOP and a low neonatal birth weight at delivery ($p = 0.001$) was found. An analysis of the relationship between SBI and gestational age (GA) at the time of the periodontal examination in the different dental status groups showed a significant correlation between these parameters in the G group ($p = 0.04$). *Conclusions:* Our results suggest that a worse periodontal status during pregnancy may negatively affect obstetrical outcomes, especially the prematurity rate and newborn weight. Therefore, the importance of periodontal screening to prevent these complications is undeniable.

Keywords: preterm birth; gingivitis; periodontitis; neonatal birth weight

1. Introduction

Prematurity is a global health issue that is becoming the leading cause of newborn morbidity and mortality worldwide [1]. According to the latest data from the World Health Organization (WHO), approximately 15 million preterm births (PBs) occur worldwide each year [2]. Over the years, many risk factors have been identified that may be associated with preterm birth and low birth weight, including age, tobacco use, alcohol use, and infections [3]. In 1996, Offenbacher et al. were the first to report a possible correlation between periodontal disease and preterm birth [4], and, since then, an increasing number

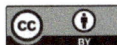

of studies have addressed the relationship between the two conditions [5,6]. Periodontal diseases include gingivitis and periodontitis, mainly caused by inappropriate oral hygiene or dental plaque misalignment [7].

Gingivitis, a milder and reversible pathological condition, manifests itself as inflammation of the gums due to accumulated bacterial plaque. When chronic inflammation extends from superficial to deep tissues, severe damage occurs in the tooth-supporting apparatus, which can lead to periodontitis. Initially, the clinical signs of these periodontal ailments include gingival edema and bleeding, and in the case of insufficient oral hygiene and/or regular dental care, with the deterioration of this condition and the development of periodontal pockets, tooth loss can occur [8]. Interestingly, studies have shown that pregnancy-induced hormonal changes can further aggravate gingival inflammation or the severity of pre-existing periodontal diseases [9,10]. The elevated levels of progesterone and estrogen may increase vascular permeability, making fibrous tissues more vulnerable to bacteria and resulting in adverse gingival changes [11]. With this damaging phenomenon, oral pathogens (e.g., Gram-negative microorganisms) and their bacterial products can easily reach the uterus through the bloodstream, and, at the same time, microbial components and inflammatory mediators derived from periodontal disease can also circulate to the liver, where they can initiate an entire inflammatory cascade. Consequently, prostaglandin production increases, which may cause preterm uterine activity, premature rupture of membranes, cervical insufficiency, and preterm labor [12]. Scientific data have proven that preterm delivery is strongly associated not only with a higher level of gingival prostaglandin E2 but also with increased neonatal immunoglobulin M seropositivity for several oral bacteria.

In recent studies [13], the role and the clinical and microbiological management of the oral microbiota have been described, focusing on the personalization of periodontal clinical practices and a proactive approach.

Primarily, the most reliable diagnostic tools for the identification and classification of periodontal diseases are probing depth (PD) and bleeding on probing (BOP), characterized by the sulcus bleeding index (SBI) [14]. The present study aimed to evaluate the correlation between periodontal status, based on a clinical examination of PD and BOP, and obstetrical outcomes, including neonatal birth weight (BW) and gestational age (GA) at delivery.

2. Materials and Methods

2.1. Study Design

This prospective clinical study was conducted at the University of Szeged, Department of Obstetrics and Gynecology, where, based on the authors' previously published results, a dental unit was installed and where the examination of the selected pregnant patients was carried out. It is important to know that, in Hungary, all pregnancies that finish with deliveries are recorded in the national health system database. Dental examinations are compulsory during pregnancy, and this fact is noted in the Health Booklet, which follows an expectant woman from the start to the end of her pregnancy. A total of 111 healthy, without significant illnesses, primigravida–primiparous pregnant women were involved in this study, which was ethically approved by the Human Investigation Review Board of the Albert Szent-Györgyi Clinical Center, Szeged, Hungary, approval number (123/2019-SZTE). Patients were selected during regular pregnancy-related ultrasound examinations, performed around the gestational ages of 11 and 19 weeks. Multiple gestations or cases with any associated diseases or regular medications were excluded. The study period for the periodontal examinations was between 1 August 2019 and 29 February 2020. Szeged is the county seat of Csongrád-Csanád County, with a population of about 159,000 inhabitants. The Department of Obstetrics and Gynecology, a part of Albert Szent-Györgyi Medical School, is a state-financed unit and the only place where childbirth (about 2500/year) takes place in this city. Only inhabitants of Szeged were selected to take part in this study in order to eliminate problems related to the scheduling of periodontal examinations for pregnant patients from other places. The ultrasound examinations were performed by authorized doctors, based on a previous schedule, with the medical unit conducting about 20 similar examinations/day. This number also includes pregnant women from other cities and villages because the department is the regional tertiary medical unit for the southeastern part of Hungary, serving four counties (Csongrád-Csanád, Békés, Bács-Kiskun, and the southern part of Jász-Nagykun Szolnok), with a total population of about 1.6 million inhabitants. In the study period, there were a total of 2860 ultrasound examinations, of which 1144 were carried out on inhabitants of Szeged. Finally, of this number, 111 primigravida–primipara, healthy women were included in the project and selected for periodontal examinations. The health status of all 111 patients was monitored throughout their pregnancies; all women gave birth at our institution. The patients were fully informed about the aim of this study, and they took part voluntarily after signing a written consent form. A dental unit was installed at the Department of Obstetrics and Gynecology, based on the author's previous studies concerning the association between maternal dental modification and obstetric outcomes, and it was used for the dental examinations. It was equipped with good lighting and the possibility of patient positioning. Gestational age was determined by carrying out sonographic measurements of the embryos in the first trimester.

Periodontal examinations were performed after the ultrasound screening, based on a previous appointment, by an experienced dentist, according to the WHO guidelines. Patients' periodontal status was determined using PD and BOP. A disposable periodontal probe, which had a 0.5 mm diameter tip, was used for these measurements. PD was measured at 6 sites per tooth (the mesiobuccal, midbuccal, distobuccal, mesiolingual, midlingual, and distolingual sites), with the exception of the third molars, while BOP was recorded after 15 s on a Yes/No scale at the same sites as where PD was previously determined. The criteria used in each group were as follows: periodontally healthy patients had a sulcus depth between 1 and 3 mm with non-detectable gingival bleeding; patients with gingivitis had the same PD as healthy individuals, but they also had a BOP $\geq 25\%$; and patients with periodontitis had a PD ≥ 4 mm in at least one site and a BOP $\geq 50\%$ of the teeth. The determination of periodontitis was based on PD and BOP, the two most important periodontal parameters. The selection of these factors was based on our previous clinical studies in this field. PD ≥ 4 mm is regarded as a "critical probing depth", while smaller PD values are considered normal. BOP is a well-accepted sign of periodontal inflammation, and BOP and PD together are significant factors in the staging of periodontal disease [5,6,14]. After the deliveries, GA and neonatal birth weight (BW) were analyzed, and correlations regarding the patient's previous periodontal status were explored. During the examination carried out by the dentist, in all cases, the expectant women were instructed on correct oral hygiene procedures, including toothbrush and dental floss usage. The patients were classified into 3 categories based on the results of the aforementioned measurements: 17 healthy individuals (H), 67 patients with gingivitis (G), and 27 patients with periodontitis (P). The BOP was recorded and determined for each tooth. The percentage of BOP cases was calculated according to the total number of teeth of the patient, and this approach was named the sulcus bleeding index (SBI). For example, if the total number of teeth was 28, and BOP was found in 25 teeth, the SBI was 89.28%.

Delivery was considered at-term if it occurred after the completion of the 37th week. Before this gestational age (24^{+0}–36^{+6} weeks), it was noted as a preterm delivery. A low BW was defined if the newborn weight was under the 5th percentile.

2.2. Statistical Analysis and Graph Editing

The recruited patients were divided into three groups according to their dental status. The samples were characterised as the mean and standard deviation (SD) of the data. The group means were compared by a one-way ANOVA, which can be considered a generalisation of the Student's two-sample t-test for more than two groups. The linear relationship between the examined variables was also examined by the calculation of Pearson's correlation coefficient and the regression line. The significance of the correlation (its p-value) was also given. Statistical analyses were performed using SPSS version 26, and $p < 0.05$ was considered to be statistically significant. Graphs were edited in Microsoft Excel.

3. Results

The recruited patients were divided into three groups, namely, H, G, and P, according to the different dental statuses diagnosed during pregnancy. The low rate of cases with a healthy dental status at the time of the periodontal examination was remarkable, and this can be an important message related to the role of pre-conceptional periodontal care for women who want to have a pregnancy in the near future. All patients enrolled in this study gave birth to their newborns at the Department of Obstetrics and Gynecology, the University of Szeged.

3.1. The Main Gestational Age at Dental Examination, Gestational and Maternal Age at Delivery and Birth Weight at Delivery

The main gestational age at the dental examination, the gestational and maternal ages at delivery, and the birth weight at delivery are presented in Table 1. As shown, the observed difference in the birth weights of the three examined groups was found to be statistically non-significant.

Table 1. Sample characteristics in different dental status groups. Results are shown as means (±SD).

	Healthy (H) $n = 17$	Gingivitis (G) $n = 67$	Periodontitis (P) $n = 27$	ANOVA
Gestational age at dental examination (w)	16.24 ± 3.492	15.00 ± 3.516	14.00 ± 3.150	$p = 0.111$
Gestational age at delivery (w)	38.53 ± 1.772	39.07 ± 1.454	38.67 ± 1.414	$p = 0.253$
Maternal age at delivery (y)	31.25 ± 4.337	30.91 ± 5.197	29.53 ± 6.309	$p = 0.464$
Birth weight (g)	3518.82 ± 548.212	3402.24 ± 541.443	3396.67 ± 611.826	$p = 0.726$

Analysis of invariance: ANOVA.

3.2. Correlation between SBI and BW in Group P

After a further investigation of these data, it was clearly visible that the correlation was the most pronounced and statistically significant in the P group, in which a significantly lower newborn weight was observed with an increase in SBI. This means that a more severe periodontal disease was associated with a lower BW ($r = -0.587$, $p = 0.001$). The data are presented in Figure 1.

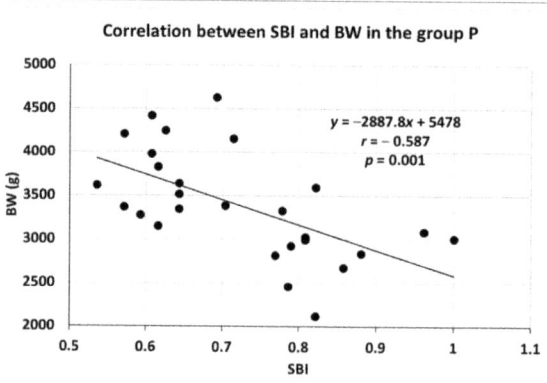

Figure 1. Correlation between SBI and BW in group P. Results are shown as means (±SD). BW = birth weight; SBI = sulcus bleeding index; P = periodontitis; $n = 111$; and $p < 0.05$ was considered statistically significant.

3.3. Correlation between SBI and GA at Dental Examination in Different Dental Status Groups

A detailed analysis showed a significant positive correlation ($r = 0.252$, $p = 0.04$) between SBI and patients' GA at the dental examination in the G group. These detailed data are presented in Figure 2 and Table 2, where the rate of G at the time of the dental examination can be seen. Being a significant linear correlation, Figure 2 gives a more detailed picture of this relationship.

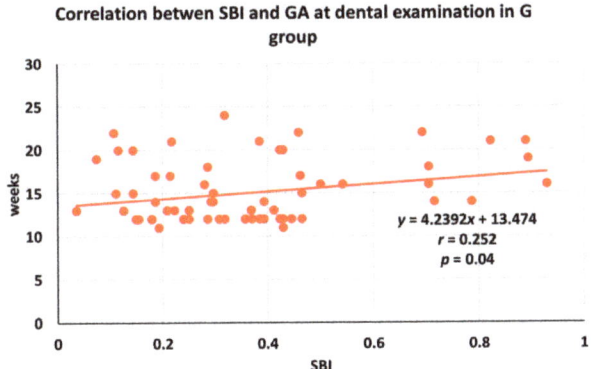

Figure 2. Correlation between SBI and GA at dental examination in the G group. Results are shown as means (±SD). G = gingivitis; GA = gestational age; SBI = sulcus bleeding index; $n = 111$; and $p < 0.05$ was considered statistically significant.

Table 2. Correlation between SBI and GA at periodontal examination in different dental status groups; $p < 0.05$ was considered statistically significant.

Group	N	Correlation Coefficient	p Value
Healthy	17	$r = -0.391$	$p = 0.120$
Gingivitis	67	$r = 0.252$	$p = 0.04$
Periodontitis	27	$r = 0.127$	$p = 0.527$
Total	111	$r = -0.035$	$p = 0.714$

4. Discussion

Dental hygiene is very important during pregnancy. Preventive or diagnostic dental treatment is highly recommended at any time throughout pregnancy, along with a proper oral hygiene routine every day. Although we did not observe a connection between poor dental status and premature delivery (Table 1), our results demonstrate a significant correlation between P and a low BW at delivery ($p = 0.001$), meaning that pregnant women with a higher BOP (and, subsequently, a higher SBI) might have an increased risk of having lower BW newborns. These data are in line with the findings of Sanz et al., who previously revealed the role of hormonal and inflammatory processes in premature birth as a consequence of periodontal disease. Cytokine production and endotoxins released by oral microorganisms evoke the activation of the inflammatory cascade, which may contribute to the initiation of preterm parturition [15]. Preterm birth and a low BW may also carry a risk of predisposition to later neurological and motor impairments, together with malnutrition problems; thus, preventive medical interventions should be performed [16].

Moreover, in line with BW, gestational age at dental examination was also correlated with BOP. Interestingly, G was found to be higher at a significant rate at the time of the dental examinations ($p = 0.04$). In the context of these results, we verified that BOP had a positive correlation with the patient's gestational age at the medical check-ups, drawing our attention to the importance of dental screening. Based on these results, it can be concluded that a worse periodontal status during pregnancy may negatively affect obstetrical outcomes. As a methodological limitation of this study, we note the relatively low number of cases. The most important cause of this was the beginning of the COVID-19 pandemic, which, at that moment, stopped study-related dental examinations. Moreover, this patient number limitation makes it impossible to differentiate between late prematurity (34^{+0}–36^{+6} GW), prematurity (28^{+0}–33^{+6} GW), and extreme prematurity (24^{+0}–27^{+6} GW) and examine their correlations with maternal dental status. Still, regarding these causes, the results of our study have a powerful message, illustrating the importance of oral health during pregnancy.

Similar to our findings, Cho et al. found that pregnant women with dental caries participated in screenings less frequently [17]; however, clinical trials support the fact that preventive dental care can play a major role in the improvement of birth outcomes [18]. Both quantitative and qualitative studies regarding this issue have corroborated that women may have fears of dental examinations during pregnancy [19]. Although a high proportion of pregnant women experience dental problems (e.g., gingival bleeding, dental caries, and tooth mobility), only 30–40% seek medical advice during pregnancy. There may be many factors behind this pattern, but most of the time, it is due to a previous negative experience or a lack of education regarding oral hygiene. Since there is a strong correlation between poor dental status and pregnancy outcomes, raising awareness of oral health is indispensable [20]. Preventive dental and periodontal care, especially before and, if necessary, during pregnancy, is fundamental to maintaining both mothers' and newborns' health, and, for this exact reason, effective collaboration between obstetricians and dentists is essential [21,22]. Oral health promotion and education about proper dental care in pregnancy are indispensable for the prevention of pregnancy-associated complications, such as prematurity and neonatal low BW.

However, Scribante et al. [13] focused on the role of the balance of oral dysbiosis. They stated that using probiotics and paraprobiotics can lead to a statistically significant reduction in oral pathogenic bacterial load.

5. Conclusions

Periodontal diseases, such as gingivitis and periodontitis, mainly occur due to inappropriate oral hygiene. Pregnancy-induced hormonal changes further aggravate pre-existing periodontal diseases and can ultimately lead to adverse pregnancy outcomes. Our results indicate that there is a connection between periodontal status during pregnancy and obstetrical outcomes. We, therefore, believe that periodontal health programs linked to maternity are crucial for the prevention and diagnosis of periodontal diseases in pregnant women. By means of oral health education, a higher proportion of pregnancy and birth-related complications could be prevented.

Based on the obtained results, we can consider that poor maternal oral status is an influencing factor for worse obstetrical outcomes. In particular, the dental modifications associated with hemorrhage of the gingiva and periodontal pockets are involved. These modifications are detectable as early as the first trimester, and they can influence obstetrical outcomes, resulting, for example, in a lower newborn weight.

Author Contributions: Conceptualization, T.N.; methodology, P.V. and M.R.; formal analysis, K.B.; investigation, P.V. and M.R.; resources, G.N.; data curation, T.N. and K.B.; writing—original draft preparation, P.V.; writing—review and editing, T.N.; visualization, K.B. and E.B.; supervision, G.N. All authors have read and agreed to the published version of the manuscript.

Funding: This research received no external funding.

Institutional Review Board Statement: This study was ethically approved by the Human Investigation Review Board of the Albert Szent-Györgyi Clinical Center, Szeged, Hungary, approval number (123/2019-SZTE), approval date was 30/05/2019.

Informed Consent Statement: Informed consent was obtained from all subjects involved in this study.

Data Availability Statement: All data used to support the findings of this study are included within the article.

Conflicts of Interest: The authors declare no conflict of interest.

References

1. Daskalakis, G.; Arabin, B.; Antsaklis, A. CaberoRoura, Preterm Labor: Up to Date. *Biomed. Res. Int.* **2019**, *2019*, 4870938. [CrossRef]
2. Liu, L.; Oza, S.; Hogan, D.; Chu, Y.; Perin, J.; Zhu, J.; Lawn, J.; Cousens, S.; Mathers, C.; Black, R. Global, regional, and national causes of under-5 mortality in 2000–15: An updated systematic analysis with implications for the Sustainable Development Goals. *Lancet* **2016**, *388*, 3027–3035. [CrossRef]
3. Beck, S.; Wojdyla, D.; Say, L.; Betran, A.; Merialdi, M.; Requejo, J.; Rubens, C.; Menon, R.; Van Look, P. The worldwide incidence of preterm birth: A systematic review of maternal mortality and morbidity. *Bull. World Health Organ.* **2010**, *88*, 31–38. [CrossRef]
4. Offenbacher, S.; Katz, V.; Fertik, G.; Collins, J.; Boyd, D.; Maynor, G.; McKaig, R.; Beck, J. Periodontal Infection as a Possible Risk Factor for Preterm Low Birth Weight. *J. Periodontol.* **1996**, *67* (Suppl. S10), 1103–1113. [CrossRef] [PubMed]
5. Novak, T.; Radnai, M.; Gorzo, I.; Urban, E.; Orvos, H.; Eller, J.; Pal, A. Prevention of preterm delivery with periodontal treatment. *Fetal Diagn. Ther.* **2009**, *25*, 230–233. [CrossRef]
6. Novak, T.; Nemeth, G.; Kozinszky, Z.; Urban, E.; Gorzo, I.; Radnai, M. Could Poor Periodontal Status be a Warning Sign for Worse Pregnancy Outcome? *Oral Health Prev. Dent.* **2020**, *18*, 165–170.
7. Kinane, D.; Stathopoulou, P.; Papapanou, P. Periodontal diseases. *Nat. Rev. Dis. Prim.* **2017**, *3*, 17038. [CrossRef] [PubMed]
8. Pihlstrom, B.; Michalowicz, B.; Johnson, N. Periodontal diseases. *Lancet* **2005**, *366*, 1809–1820. [PubMed]
9. Carrillo-de-Albornoz, A.; Figuero, E.; Herrera, D.; Cuesta, P.; Bascones-Martinez, A. Gingival changes during pregnancy: III. Impact of clinical, microbiological, immunological and socio-demographic factors on gingival inflammation. *J. Clin. Periodontol.* **2012**, *39*, 272–283. [CrossRef]
10. Offenbacher, S.; Lin, D.; Strauss, R.; McKaig, R.; Irving, J.; Barros, S.; Moss, K.; Barrow, D.; Hefti, A.; Beck, J.D. Effects of periodontal therapy during pregnancy on periodontal status, biologic parameters, and pregnancy outcomes: A pilot study. *J. Periodontol.* **2006**, *77*, 2011–2024. [CrossRef] [PubMed]
11. Yenen, Z.; Atacag, T. Oral care in pregnancy. *J. Turk. Ger. Gynecol. Assoc.* **2019**, *20*, 264–268. [CrossRef] [PubMed]
12. Takeuchi, N.; Ekuni, D.; Irie, K.; Furuta, M.; Tomofuji, T.; Morita, M.; Watanabe, T. Relationship between periodontal inflammation and fetal growth in pregnant women: A cross-sectional study. *Arch. Gynecol. Obstet.* **2013**, *287*, 951–957. [CrossRef] [PubMed]
13. Scribante, A.; Butera, A.; Alovisi, M. Customized minimally invasive protocols for the clinical and microbiological management of the oral microbiota. *Microorganisms* **2022**, *10*, 675. [CrossRef]
14. Radnai, M.; Pal, A.; Novak, T.; Urban, E.; Eller, J.; Gorzo, I. Benefits of periodontal therapy when preterm birth threatens. *J. Dent. Res.* **2009**, *88*, 280–284. [CrossRef] [PubMed]
15. Sanz, M.; Kornman, K.; Working Group 3 of the Joint EFP/AAP Workshop. Periodontitis and adverse pregnancy outcomes: Consensus report of the Joint EFP/AAP Workshop on Periodontitis and Systemic Diseases. *J. Periodontol.* **2013**, *84* (Suppl. S4), S164–S169. [CrossRef] [PubMed]
16. Ream, M.; Lehwald, L. Neurologic Consequences of Preterm Birth. *Curr. Neurol. Neurosci. Rep.* **2018**, *18*, 48. [CrossRef] [PubMed]
17. Cho, G.; Kim, S.; Lee, H.; Kim, H.; Lee, K.; Han, S.; Oh, M. Association between dental caries and adverse pregnancy outcomes. *Sci. Rep.* **2020**, *10*, 5309. [CrossRef] [PubMed]
18. Hwang, S.; Smith, V.; McCormick, M.; Barfield, W. The association between maternal oral health experiences and risk of preterm birth in 10 states, Pregnancy Risk Assessment Monitoring System, 2004–2006. *Matern. Child Health J.* **2012**, *16*, 1688–1695. [CrossRef]
19. Ressler-Maerlender, J.; Krishna, R.; Robison, V. Oral health during pregnancy: Current research. *J. Women's Health* **2005**, *14*, 880–882. [CrossRef]
20. AlRatroot, S.; Alotaibi, G.; AlBishi, F.; Khan, S.; Nazir, M.A. Dental Anxiety amongst Pregnant Women: Relationship with Dental Attendance and Sociodemographic Factors. *Int. Dent. J.* **2022**, *72*, 179–185. [CrossRef] [PubMed]
21. Terzic, M.; Aimagambetova, G.; Terzic, S.; Radunovic, M.; Bapayeva, G.; Lagana, A. Periodontal Pathogens and Preterm Birth: Current Knowledge and Further Interventions. *Pathogens* **2021**, *10*, 730. [CrossRef] [PubMed]
22. Mainas, G.; Ide, M.; Rizzo, M.; Magan-Fernandez, A.; Mesa, F.; Nibali, L. Managing the Systemic Impact of Periodontitis. *Medicina* **2022**, *58*, 621. [CrossRef] [PubMed]

Disclaimer/Publisher's Note: The statements, opinions and data contained in all publications are solely those of the individual author(s) and contributor(s) and not of MDPI and/or the editor(s). MDPI and/or the editor(s) disclaim responsibility for any injury to people or property resulting from any ideas, methods, instructions or products referred to in the content.

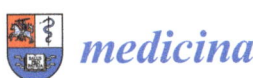

Article

Effect of Lipid-Based Multiple Micronutrients Supplementation in Underweight Primigravida Pre-Eclamptic Women on Maternal and Pregnancy Outcomes: Randomized Clinical Trial

Nabila Sher [1,2], Murad A. Mubaraki [3], Hafsa Zafar [2], Rubina Nazli [2,*], Mashal Zafar [2], Sadia Fatima [2] and Fozia Fozia [4,*]

1. Biochemistry Department, Khyber Girls Medical College, Peshawar 25000, Pakistan
2. Department of Biochemistry, Institute of Basic Medical Science, Khyber Medical University, Peshawar 25000, Pakistan
3. Clinical Laboratory Sciences Department, College of Applied Medical Sciences, King Saud University, Riyadh 11433, Saudi Arabia
4. Department of Biochemistry KMU Institute of Medical Science, Khyber Medical University, Kohat 26000, Pakistan
* Correspondence: rubinanazli44@gmail.com (R.N.); drfoziazeb@yahoo.com (F.F.)

Abstract: *Background and Objectives:* In pre-eclampsia, restricted blood supply due to the lack of trophoblastic cell invasion and spiral artery remodeling is responsible for adverse pregnancies and maternal outcomes, which is added to by maternal undernutrition. This study was designed to observe the effect of multiple nutritional micronutrient supplements on the pregnancy outcomes of underweight pre-eclamptic women. To investigate the effects of lipid-based multiple micr supplementations (LNS-PLW) on pregnancy and maternal outcomes in underweight primigravida pre-eclamptic women. *Materials and Methods:* A total of 60 pre-eclamptic, underweight primigravida women from the antenatal units of tertiary care hospitals in the Khyber Pakhtunkhwa Province, Pakistan, were randomly divided into two groups (Group 1 and Group 2). The participants of both groups were receiving routine treatment for pre-eclampsia: iron (60 mgs) and folic acid (400 ug) IFA daily. Group 2 was given an additional sachet of 75 gm LNS-PLW daily till delivery. The pregnancy outcomes of both groups were recorded. The clinical parameters, hemoglobin, platelet count, and proteinuria were measured at recruitment. *Results:* The percentage of live births in Group 2 was 93% compared to 92% in Group 1. There were more normal vaginal deliveries (NVDs) in Group 2 compared to Group 1 (Group 2, 78% NVD; group 1, 69% NVD). In Group 1, 4% of the participants developed eclampsia. The frequency of cesarean sections was 8/26 (31%) in Group 1 and 6/28 (22%) in Group 2. The number of intrauterine deaths (IUDs) was only 1/28 (4%) in Group 2, while it was 2/26 (8%) in Group 1. The gestational age at delivery significantly improved with LNS-PLW supplementation (Group 2, 38.64 ± 0.78 weeks; Group 1, 36.88 ± 1.55 weeks, p-value 0.006). The Apgar score (Group 2, 9.3; Group 1, 8.4) and the birth weight of the babies improved with maternal supplementation with LNS-PLW (Group 2, 38.64 ± 0.78 weeks: Group 1, 36.88 ± 1.55; p-value 0.003). There was no significant difference in systolic blood pressure, while diastolic blood pressure (Group 2, 89.57 ± 2.08 mmHg; Group 1, 92.17 ± 5.18 mmHg, p-value 0.025) showed significant improvement with LNS-PLW supplementation. The hemoglobin concentration increased with the LNS-PLW supplement consumed in Group 2 (Group 2, 12.15 ± 0.78 g/dL; Group 1, 11.39 ± 0.48 g/dL, p-value < 0.001). However, no significant difference among the platelet counts of the two groups was observed. *Conclusions:* The pregnancy and maternal outcomes of underweight pre-eclamptic women can be improved by the prenatal daily supplementation of LNS-PLW during pregnancy, along with IFA and regular antenatal care and follow-up.

Keywords: pre-eclampsia; lipid-based nutritional supplements; pregnancy outcome; maternal outcome; Khyber Pakhtunkhwa Province of Pakistan

Citation: Sher, N.; Mubaraki, M.A.; Zafar, H.; Nazli, R.; Zafar, M.; Fatima, S.; Fozia, F. Effect of Lipid-Based Multiple Micronutrients Supplementation in Underweight Primigravida Pre-Eclamptic Women on Maternal and Pregnancy Outcomes: Randomized Clinical Trial. *Medicina* 2022, 58, 1772. https://doi.org/10.3390/medicina58121772

Academic Editors: Marius L. Craina and Elena Bernad

Received: 24 October 2022
Accepted: 26 November 2022
Published: 30 November 2022

Publisher's Note: MDPI stays neutral with regard to jurisdictional claims in published maps and institutional affiliations.

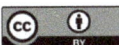

Copyright: © 2022 by the authors. Licensee MDPI, Basel, Switzerland. This article is an open access article distributed under the terms and conditions of the Creative Commons Attribution (CC BY) license (https://creativecommons.org/licenses/by/4.0/).

1. Introduction

Pre-eclampsia is the most common hypertensive disorder in pregnancy. About 3–5% of first pregnancies are complicated by pre-eclampsia globally, with a near 15% recurrence rate in subsequent pregnancies [1]. It is characterized by hypertension, proteinuria, and edema ≥ 20 weeks of gestation in women previously normotensive [2,3]. Pre-eclampsia is a multisystem disorder with a placental origin and creates immediate and long-term fetal and maternal complications. It is documented as one cause of maternal mortality, morbidity, and stillbirths [4–6]. In Pakistan, approximately 19% of maternal mortality is attributed to pre-eclampsia [7], rating only third after postpartum hemorrhage and sepsis [4]. Pre-eclampsia may be subclassified as mild and severe, depending upon the presence of hypertension [1]: mild pre-eclampsia with BP (140–159/90–109 mmHg) and severe pre-eclampsia with BP ($\geq 160/110$ mmHg) [8]. On the bases of gestational age, pre-eclampsia can also be subclassified as being early-onset (≤ 34 weeks) due to fetal disorders, primarily through imperfect placentation. Late-onset (≥ 34 weeks) is due to maternal disorders, lowered maternal thresholds, and excessive physiological placentation [4]. Pre-eclampsia occurs due to abnormal trophoblastic invasion, causing reduced placental perfusion and the replacement of maternal arteriole endothelial cells through an imbalance between the angiogenic and antiangiogenic factors. This, in turn, leads to the damage and dysfunction of the endothelium of maternal arteries, leading to hypertension (due to vasoconstriction), edema due to increased vascular permeability, and proteinuria (due to glomerular damage) [1]. The angiogenic factors are essential for the vessel's health and for new vessel formation and organ development. In pre-eclampsia, the high levels of soluble fms-like tyrosine kinase-1(sFlt-1), soluble Endoglin (sEng), and antiangiogenic factors affect the levels of placental growth factor (PlGF), transforming growth factor β (TGEβ) and vascular endothelial growth factor, respectively [1]. These low levels lead to endothelial dysfunction and the clinical characteristics of pre-eclampsia [6]. The placental growth factor (PlGF) and soluble fms-like tyrosine kinase-1(sFlt-1) are used to differentiate pre-eclampsia from other diseases, like chronic hypertension and kidney diseases [5]. The pathophysiology of pre-eclampsia occurs due to abnormal trophoblastic invasions, causing reduced placental perfusion and the replacement of maternal arteriole endothelial cells through an imbalance between the angiogenic and antiangiogenic factors [5].

Pre-eclampsia is (7.5%) more common among nulliparous women than parous women [7]. A young age, being underweight, and multiple pregnancies are also non-specific risk factors of pre-eclampsia [9]. Moreover, malnutrition, undernutrition, high-fat/fiber diets, and micronutrient deficiency are risk factors for pre-eclampsia [10–12]. The nutritional status of pregnant women plays a vital role in fetal growth and development [13,14]. In low-income countries, maternal undernutrition and anemia are the common causes of maternal mortality and morbidity. Women during pregnancy are at risk of nutritional deficiencies because of the added burden of the metabolism of the fetus and the growing placenta [1]. The deficiency of macro- and micronutrients is common among women of child-bearing age in developing countries [8]. The association between multiple micronutrient deficiencies and the development of pre-eclampsia has also been reported [14,15]. Therefore, undernutrition during pregnancy affects not only the mother's health but also the health of the growing fetus. In order to balance and improve the micronutrient deficiencies and pregnancy outcomes, iron, folic acid, calcium, and multiple micronutrient supplements are used during pregnancy and before conception [4,5]. In order to improve maternal nutrition and pregnancy outcomes, lipid-based multiple micronutrient supplements are given to underweight pregnant and lactating mothers (LNS-PLW) in underdeveloped countries [6,7]. The benefits of lipid-based multiple micronutrient supplementation have been assessed in normotensive undernourished women [6]. The LNS-PLW is a peanut-based product from the World Food Program (WFP) that is packed in a ready-to-use sachet of 75 gm, having an energy of 400 kcal (Table 1). It is provided to childbearing-aged women to improve maternal nutrition and pregnancy outcomes in underdeveloped countries like Pakistan [1,8].

Table 1. Chemical composition of (LNS-PLW).

Nutrient	Value	Nutrient	Value
Carbohydrate	35.4 g	Biotin (Vitamin-B7)	45 mcg
Protein	10.5 g	Folates (Vitamin-B9)	247 mcg
Fat (60%ω-3Fatty Acid, 20%ω-6FA)	24 g	Cobalamine (Vit B12)	2.0 mcg
Retinol (Vitamin-A)	412 mcg	Iron	10 mg
Cholecalciferiol (Vitamin-D)	11.2 mcg	Calcium	400 mg
Phytomenadione (Vitamin-K)	20.2 mcg	Zinc	8.2 mg
Tocoferol acetate (Vit-E)	12 mg	Copper	1.0 mg
Ascorbate (Vitamin C)	45 mg	Selenium	15 mcg
Thiamine (Vitamin-B1)	0.75 mg	Iodine	75 mcg
Riboflavin (Vitamin-B2)	1.57 mg	Magnesium	112 mg
Niacin (Vitamin-B3)	9.75 mg	Phosphorus	337 mg
Pantothenic acid (Vit B5)	3.0 mg	Potassium	675 mg
Pyridoxine (Vitamin-B6)	1.35 mg	Manganese	0.9 mg
Total Energy = 400 kcal			

The World Health Organization has recommended that pre-eclampsia screening should be a part of routine antenatal investigation. Most of the routine antenatal investigations are done for the clinical condition which has already been present like screening for viral disease or ultrasound-based screening for morphological abnormalities of the fetus. There is no predictive screening for diseases that have not yet occurred or developed, for example, pre-eclampsia and eclampsia. The outcomes of such a condition are alarming once it develops; therefore, the early detection and prevention of prophylactic therapy may be beneficial. This would enable the clinician to start timely preventive measures, antenatal care, and prophylactic treatment [16,17]. Pre-eclampsia screening has no real cost or side effect from its implementation; therefore, it must be part of the routine antenatal investigation or examination [18]. There are different screening strategies for pre-eclampsia, ranging from simple maternal history analysis to early screening biomarkers.

The screening approaches, which are in practice nowadays, include a detailed maternal history [18], the measurement of mean arterial blood pressure of the pregnant mother, performing Doppler ultrasounds on uterine arteries [19], the identification of serum cardiometabolic biomarkers [20], the identification of novel markers, like cell-free DNA [21], multiple approaches, etc. [22]. The management of pre-eclampsia is divided into three stages: prevention, early detection, and treatment. Dietary counseling, stopping smoking, the management of pre-existing hepatic and renal diseases, giving low-dose aspirin before 12 weeks of pregnancy, calcium supplementation, antihypertensive drugs, and magnesium sulfate are all prescribed for the prevention of eclampsia. Moreover, during hospitalization due to severe pre-eclampsia (for the termination of the pregnancy), a cesarean section may help in the management of the condition [23].

Pre-eclampsia is more common in primigravida, and it is associated with micronutrient deficiencies. Our country is facing a lack of a proper diet, especially for women of childbearing age, due to poverty. Nutritional deficiency is one of the risk factors of pre-eclampsia. To our knowledge, little evidence is available on the effect of LNS-PLW in pre-eclamptic pregnancy and maternal outcomes in our region. The prevalence of undernutrition at childbearing age is quite high; therefore, the current study was designed and conducted to assess the impact of lipid-based multiple micronutrient supplementation (LNS-PLW) on the maternal and pregnancy outcomes of pre-eclamptic underweight women during their first pregnancy.

2. Methods

After screening, 463 pre-eclamptic women from April 2018-December 2019 (Figure 1) we recruited, considering primigravida pre-eclamptic women whose BMI was less than the requirement for their gestational age retrospectively on their first antenatal visit from their antenatal record file. The BMI is calculated by using a computer pregnancy weight gain calculator. This study was conducted in the tertiary health care facilities of Peshawar (Lady Reading Hospital, Hayatabad Medical Complex) and Swat (Civil Hospital Matta), Khyber Pakhtunkhwa (KP) province of Pakistan. The trial was approved by Khyber Medical University, by the Advanced Study and Research Board, and the Ethical Committee (No: DIR/KMU-AS&RB/EN/000527-18 August 2016) (DIR/KMU = EB/EN/000314 on 27 October 2016). The participants were divided by using a computer randomizer (version 3.0) (Medical University of Graz, Institute for Medical Informatics, Statistics and Documentation Auenbruggerplatz 2/5, A-8036 Graz, Austria) into two groups (Group 1 and Group 2) and informed consent was obtained from them. The participants of both groups received conventional treatment for pre-eclampsia and IFA daily. The Group 2 participants received an additional 75 gm sachet of high-energy LNS-PLW supplement daily till delivery. One participant of Group 2 disliked the taste of LNS-PLW, and another participant lost contact and follow-up, so they dropped out. Two participants in Group 1 refused to continue, and two participants lost contact and dropped out. Therefore, 26 participants from Group 1 and 28 participants from Group 2 completed the follow-up, and we collected their pregnancy and maternal outcomes.

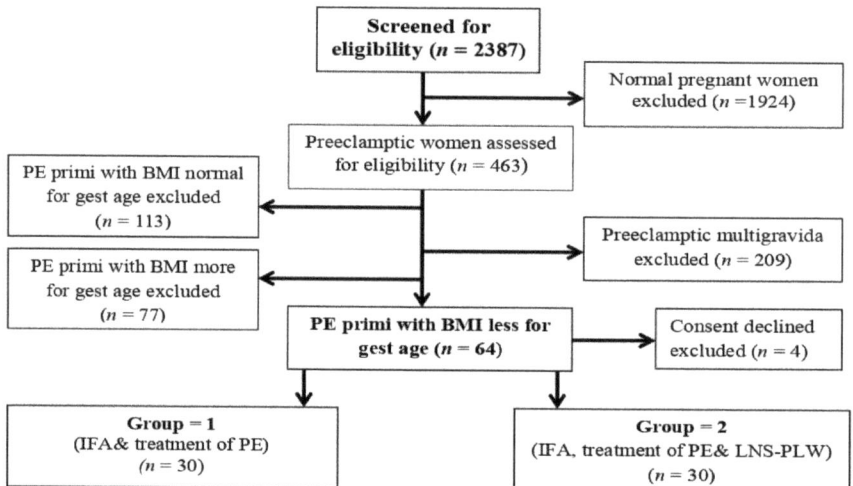

Figure 1. Flow chart showing the enrollment of the participants and intervention allocation. Abbreviations: PE: Preeclampsia, BMI: Basal metabolic index, IFA: Iron folic acid, LNS-PLW: Lipid based nutritional supplements for pregnant and lactating women.

2.1. Data Collection

The socioeconomic data, family, and personal histories were recorded by predesigned questionnaires given to each participant. The age, gestational age, anthropometric measurements (height, weight, BMI), systolic and diastolic blood pressure, and the proteinuria of the participants were measured. About 5 mL of blood was taken from each participant at the time of enrollment and then delivered via an aseptic technique. The hemoglobin and platelet counts were measured by Sysmex XE-2100 hematology analyzer (Sysmex

Corporation, Shisumekkusu Kabushiki-gaisha, Tokyo, Japan). The LNS-PLW was provided weekly and the empty sachets were collected to check their compliance. The leftovers in the sachet were measured. The principal researcher reminded each participant, telephonically, on alternate days to take their medication and LNS-PLW supplement. Their weight was measured by a Beurer digital glass weight scale-GS 200 Allium (Lessingstraße 10 b 89231 Neu-Ulm, Germany), and for their height, a portable stadiometer (Seca Leicester 214) (Hammer Steindamm 9-25. 22089 Hamburg, Germany) was used. The BMI kg/m^2 of the participants was measured. At 10 min intervals, the blood pressure of the patients was measured three times by using a standard mercury sphygmomanometer, and the mean was noted. Proteinuria was measured via the dipstick method. The mode of delivery was also recorded.

2.2. Statistical Analysis

The Shapiro–Wilk test was used for normalizing the data; it was found to be normally distributed. The demographic data were analyzed as descriptive statistics, and the values were presented as mean ± standard deviation. The data of the two groups were compared by student t-testing. For the statistical analyses, we used SPSS software 22 (IBM, Armonk, NY, USA), and $p < 0.05$ was considered significant.

3. Results

The mean age of the participants (Group 1: 22.1 ± 3.3 years; Group 2: 23.3 ± 3.6 years, p-value 0.17) ranged from 15–35 years. Their BMI at the first antenatal visit was calculated retrospectively from their antenatal record (Group 1: 19.6 ± 1.3; Group 2: 19.7 ± 0.9, p-value 0.84). While the BMI kg/m^2 at enrollment was recorded as Group 1: 22.6 ± 1.5 kg/m^2; Group 2, 22.5 ± 1.3 kg/m^2, p-value 0.459. The gestational age (from the first antenatal visit) was calculated retrospectively from participants' antenatal records (Group 1: 19.8 ± 3.5 weeks; Group 2: 20.5 ± 3.1 weeks, p-value 0.45), while the gestational age at enrollment was 30.1 ± 2 weeks for Group 1 and 29.8 ± 2.3 weeks for Group 2 (p-value 0.59). The baseline systolic blood pressure was 146.7 ± 8.9 mmHg for Group 1 and 144.7 ± 6.8 mmHg for Group 2 (p-value 0.63), and the diastolic blood pressure was 95.7 ± 5.2 mmHg for Group 1 and 95.5 ± 4.4 mmHg for Group 2 (p-value 0.89). The proteinuria recorded via the dipstick method at enrollment was as follows: Group 1: 1.8 ± 0.7; Group 2: 1.9 ± 0.7 (p-value 0.34). The baseline hemoglobin concentration was as follows: Group 1: 10.5 ± 0.8 g/dL; Group 2: 10.5 ± 0.9 g/dL (p-value 0.92). The platelets count was as follows: Group 1: 202,166.67 ± 57,770.70/uL; Group 2: 196,200.00 ± 53,832.05/uL (p-value 0.68), taken during recruitment, as shown in Table 2.

The socioeconomic data of the study participants were collected; it was noted that 49% of participants belonged to the low-income group, 28% to the middle-income group, and only 23% belonged to the high-income group. The literacy rate among the participants was also found to be low: 76.66% of women in the control group and 83.33 % in the LNS-PLW group were found to be illiterate.

Maternal Follow-Up at Delivery

The supplements consumed by the two groups during the prenatal periods (IFA by Group 1: 6.8 ± 1.9 weeks; IFA and LNS-PLW by Group 2: 8.8 ± 1.9 weeks; p-value 0.00).

The live birth in Group 2 was 93%, while in Group 1, it was 92%. The number of normal vaginal deliveries in Group 2 was higher: Group 1: 69% NVD; Group 2:78% NVD. In Group 1, 4% of the participants developed eclampsia as shown in Table 3.

The gestational age at delivery was higher in Group 2 (Group 1: 36.9 ± 1.6 weeks; Group 2: 38.6 ± 0.8 weeks, $p = 0.006$).

The blood pressure was calculated after delivery; the systolic BP of both groups was the same (Group 1: 135.7 ± 11.2 mmHg; Group 2: 131.3 ± 4.6 mmHg, p-value 0.07), while the diastolic BP (Group 1: 92.2 ± 5.2 mmHg; Group 2: 89.6 ± 2.1 mmHg, p-value 0.025) showed significant improvement in the LNS-PLW-consuming Group 2 as shown in Table 4.

Table 2. Comparison of baseline parameters of the study groups.

Parameters	Group 1 n = 26 Mean ± SD	Group 2 n = 28 Mean ± SD	p-Value
Age (years)	22.1 ± 3.3	23.3 ± 3.6	0.17
Gest age at first antenatal visit retrospectively (weeks)	20 ± 3.5	20.5 ± 3.1	0.45
BMI Kg/m² at 1st antenatal visit retrospectively	19.6 ± 1.3;	19.7 ± 0.9	0.84
Gestational age at enrollment in weeks	30.1 ± 2	29.8 ± 2.3	0.59
BMI Kg/m² at enrollment	22.6 ± 1.5	22.5 ± 1.3	0.46
Systolic Blood Pressure mmHg	146.7 ± 8.9	144.7 ± 6.8	0.63
Diastolic Blood Pressure mmHg	95.7 ± 5.2	95.5 ± 4.4	0.89
Hb g/dL	10.5 ± 0.8	10.5 ± 0.9	0.92
platelets count/uL	202,166.67 ± 57,770.70	196,200.00 ± 53,832.05	0.68

Table 3. Effect of supplementation on maternal and pregnancy outcomes.

Parameters	Group 1 n = 26	Group 2 n = 28
Live birth	92%	93%
NVD	18 (69%)	22 (78%)
C-section	8 (31%)	6 (22%)
Preterm babies	9 (35%)	-
IUD/stillbirth	2 (8%)	2 (7%)
LBW	16 (61.5%)	8 (28.5%)
Eclampsia	1 (4%)	-

Abbreviations: NVD: normal vaginal delivery; C-section: Caesarean section; IUD: intrauterine death; LBW: low birth weight.

Table 4. Clinical and hematological parameters of study groups at delivery.

Parameters	Group 1 n = 26 Mean ± SD	Group 2 n = 28 Mean ± SD	p-Value
Supplements consume (weeks)	6.8 ± 1.9	8.8 ± 1.9	0.00
Gestational age at delivery	36.9 ± 1.6	38.6 ± 0.8	0.00
Systolic Blood Pressure mmHg	135.7 ± 11.2	131.3 ± 4.6	0.07
Diastolic Blood Pressure mmHg	92.2 ± 5.2	89.6 ± 2.1	0.02
Hemoglobin g/dL	11.4 ± 0.5	12.2 ± 0.8	0.001
BMI(kg/m²) at delivery	27.17 ± 1.39	27.38 ± 0.94	0.570
Birth weight of the baby	2.37 ± 0.21	2.49 ± 0.08	0.003

The blood samples were collected from the women after delivery and during their stay in the hospital in order to compare the hemoglobin concentration. Hemoglobin concentration significantly improved with LNS-PLW supplementation (Group 1: 11.4 ± 0.5 g/dL; Group 2: 12.2 ± 0.8 g/dL, p-value 0.001).

4. Discussion

Pre-eclampsia is a common pregnancy-related complication that occurs in childbearing-age women. It is responsible for poor maternal and fetal outcomes, fetal and maternal mortality, and morbidity [15]. A balance nutritional intake during pregnancy is responsible for the proper functioning of bodily systems [24,25]. Pregnancy is a condition for which appropriate and balanced food intake is needed not only for the mother but also for the growing fetus. Maternal undernutrition and malnutrition increase the risk of pre-eclampsia, gestational hypertension, anemia, premature delivery, fetal and maternal mortality, and morbidity [26,27].

In this study, the hemoglobin concentration significantly increased in Group 2 when compared with Group 1. This may be due to the 10 mg of extra iron in the LNS-PLW supplement with routine IFA (60 mg iron and 400 ug folic acid). In contradiction with findings, a study was conducted in Malawi, in which three groups of women were supplemented from ≤20 weeks of gestation with IFA (containing 60 mg of iron), MMN (containing 20 mg of iron), and LNS (containing 20 mg of iron); at 36 weeks of gestation, the researchers compared the women's hemoglobin levels and reported higher concentrations of hemoglobin in the IFA group [28]. Another study conducted in Bangladesh compared pregnant women (≤20 weeks of gestation) who were receiving either IFA (60 mg of iron and 400 ug of folic acid) or LNS (containing 20 mg of iron). They reported a higher concentration of hemoglobin in the IFA group [29]. Similarly, a study conducted on Ghanaian women reported higher hemoglobin concentrations in women using IFA (containing 60 mg of iron) when compared to those given LNS (containing 20 mg of iron) from ≤20 weeks of gestation [30]. The difference in our study was that, along with IFA (60 mg of iron), we provided an extra 10 mg of iron in the LNS-PLW as well, whereas, in the above studies, the researchers compared three groups of women with different supplements, i.e., IFA, MMN, or LNS individually.

The diastolic blood pressure of the LNS-PLW consumers in the current study decreased significantly at delivery, while no difference was observed for their systolic blood pressure. The LNS-PLW used in the current study was peanut-based, and 80% of its fat content is composed of omega-3 (60%) and omega-6 (20%). Several meta-analyses and trials reported the beneficial effects of ω-3 polyunsaturated fatty acid supplementation on blood pressure control and cardioprotective measures [31]. Moreover, omega-3 may also improve endothelial and vascular functioning and arterioles stiffness [32]. Few other studies conducted on underweight pregnant women showed no difference in systolic and diastolic blood pressure regarding LNS and IFA consumers, presumably due to the subjects being normotensive women [33,34].

Pregnancy outcomes were compared. It was observed that the number of preterm deliveries (<37 weeks) was 35% in Group 1, while all the women on LNS-PLW supplementation delivered after 37 weeks of gestation. The study reported that pre-eclampsia babies are usually preterm [35]. However, a study conducted by Wen et al., 2018, reported that supplementation with folic acid had no effect on babies' gestational age and contradicts our finding [36]. The difference in our observations may be due to the additional intake of the LNS-PLW supplement along with IFA, whereas the study of Wen et al. assessed the effects of folic acid only [36].

The gestational age of our participants at enrollment (in both groups) was found to be below 34 weeks, meaning all were in the early-onset pre-eclampsia class. In the current study, it was observed that the numbers of live births are higher in the LNS-PLW consumers. Moreover, the number of intrauterine deaths (IUDs) is lower in the supplemented group. These findings are in line with another study that reported that supplementation in pre-eclampsia reduces IUD [37]. It was reported that multiple micronutrients (MMNs) supplementations reduced the risk of preterm birth, while LNS supplementation showed no positive effects on the term of pregnancy [13,27]. The number of NVDs was higher in Group 2 compared to Group 1, while 31% of the women in Group 1 had a caesarean section. It is documented that the rate of cesarean section increases with the severity of pre-eclampsia [38], and also micronutrient-deficient women have a greater risk of cesarean delivery [39]. Similarly, Kiattisak et al., 2018, reported that pre-eclamptic women had a higher occurrence of cesarean delivery [35,40]. In contrast to our findings, a study compared the pregnancy outcome of IFA and LNS consumer groups and found no significant difference in pregnancy and fetal outcomes regarding cesarean delivery in rural Bangladesh [41].

The strength of the current study is the participant's compliance and cooperation in maintaining high-quality assurance during supplementation and data collection. Moreover, the low dropout rate was made possible by the main researcher herself collecting the data and following the participants.

This study has some limitations; firstly, the women in both groups were pre-eclamptic, and for comparison, normal pregnant women were not recruited. Secondly, due to time and resource constraints, we analyzed a small number of participants in only three antenatal units.

5. Conclusions

The prenatal use of LNS-PLW daily, along with IFA and regular follow-up, can improve pregnancies and maternal outcomes by increasing the live birth and term of the babies and decreasing maternal complications, like eclampsia and the number of deliveries by cesarean section.

Author Contributions: Conceptualization, N.S., S.F. and R.N.; Data curation, H.Z.; Formal analysis, N.S. and H.Z.; Funding acquisition, F.F.; Investigation, M.Z.; Methodology, N.S., H.Z. and F.F.; Project administration, R.N.; Resources, M.A.M. and M.Z.; Supervision, R.N.; Writing—original draft, N.S. and M.Z.; Writing—review & editing, M.A.M., R.N., S.F. and F.F. All authors have read and agreed to the published version of the manuscript.

Funding: The publication charges for this article are partially borne from Khyber Medical University Publication Fund (No.DIR//ORIC/Ref/22/00004).

Institutional Review Board Statement: The trial was approved by Khyber Medical University, by the Advanced Study and Research Board, and the Ethical Committee (No: DIR/KMU-AS&RB/EN/000527-18 August 2016) (DIR/KMU = EB/EN/000314 on 27 October 2016).

Informed Consent Statement: Informed consent was obtained from all subjects involved in the study.

Data Availability Statement: All data generated or analyzed during this work are included in this published article. Also, all data used to support the findings of this study are available from the corresponding author upon request.

Conflicts of Interest: The authors declare no conflict of interest.

References

1. Brown, M.A.; Magee, L.A.; Kenny, L.C.; Karumanchi, S.A.; McCarthy, F.P.; Saito, S.; Hall, D.R.; Warren, C.E.; Adoyi, G.; Ishaku, S. Hypertensive disorders of pregnancy: ISSHP classification, diagnosis, and management recommendations for international practice. *Hypertension* **2018**, *72*, 24–43. [CrossRef] [PubMed]
2. Pal, B.; Biniwale, P.; Deshpande, H.; Sundari, T.; Govindarajan, M.; Kannan, J.; Mandrupkar, G.; Datar, N.; Pandya, M.; Balamba, P. Diagnosis, management and care of hypertensive disorders of pregnancy (HDP): An Indian Expert Opinion. *Indian J. Obstet. Gynecol. Res.* **2019**, *6*, 122–132. [CrossRef]
3. Baqai, S.M.; Rahim, R.; Ala, H.; Tarar, S.H.; Waqar, F.; Yasmeen, H.; Waheed, A. Society of Obstetricians and Gynaecologists Pakistan (SOGP) Hypertensive Disorders in Pregnancy Guidelines-2022. *Pak. Armed Forces Med. J.* **2022**, *72*, 731–753.
4. Paridaens, H.; Gruson, D. (Eds.) *Pre-Eclampsia: Overview on the Role of Biomarkers in 2016*; Annales de Biologie Clinique: Paris, France, 2017.
5. Hod, T.; Cerdeira, A.S.; Karumanchi, S.A. Molecular mechanisms of preeclampsia. *Cold Spring Harb. Perspect. Med.* **2015**, *5*, a023473. [CrossRef] [PubMed]

6. Massimiani, M.; Lacko, L.A.; Swanson, C.S.B.; Salvi, S.; Argueta, L.B.; Moresi, S.; Ferrazzani, S.; Gelber, S.E.; Baergen, R.N.; Toschi, N.; et al. Increased circulating levels of Epidermal Growth Factor-like Domain 7 in pregnant women affected by preeclampsia. *Transl. Res.* **2019**, *207*, 19–29. [CrossRef]
7. Shah, S. Hypertensive disorders in pregnancy. In *Obstetric and Gynecologic Nephrology*; Springer: Berlin/Heidelberg, Germany, 2020; pp. 11–23.
8. Moori, M.H. A Review of Hypertensive Disorders Management During Pregnancy. *Int. J. Med. Investig.* **2022**, *11*, 27–31.
9. Magee, L.A.; Pels, A.; Helewa, M.; Rey, E.; von Dadelszen, P.; Audibert, F.; Bujold, E.; Côté, A.-M.; Douglas, M.J.; Eastabrook, G. Diagnosis, evaluation, and management of the hypertensive disorders of pregnancy: Executive summary. *J. Obstet. Gynaecol. Can.* **2014**, *36*, 416–438. [CrossRef]
10. Turan, K.; Arslan, A.; Uçkan, K.; Demir, H.; Demir, C. Change of the levels of trace elements and heavy metals in threatened abortion. *J. Chin. Med. Assoc.* **2019**, *82*, 554–557. [CrossRef]
11. Grzeszczak, K.; Kwiatkowski, S.; Kosik-Bogacka, D. The role of Fe, Zn, and Cu in pregnancy. *Biomolecules* **2020**, *10*, 1176. [CrossRef]
12. Habibi, N.; Grieger, J.A.; Bianco-Miotto, T. A review of the potential interaction of selenium and iodine on placental and child health. *Nutrients* **2020**, *12*, 2678. [CrossRef]
13. Mohammad, N.S.; Nazli, R.; Zafar, H.; Fatima, S. Effects of lipid based Multiple Micronutrients Supplement on the birth outcome of underweight pre-eclamptic women: A randomized clinical trial. *Pak. J. Med. Sci.* **2022**, *38*, 219.
14. Lassi, Z.S.; Padhani, Z.A.; Rabbani, A.; Rind, F.; Salam, R.A.; Das, J.K.; Bhutta, Z.A. Impact of dietary interventions during pregnancy on maternal, neonatal, and child outcomes in low-and middle-income countries. *Nutrients* **2020**, *12*, 531. [CrossRef]
15. Nkamba, D.M.; Vangu, R.; Elongi, M.; Magee, L.A.; Wembodinga, G.; Bernard, P.; Ditekemena, J.; Robert, A. Health facility readiness and provider knowledge as correlates of adequate diagnosis and management of pre-eclampsia in Kinshasa, Democratic Republic of Congo. *BMC Health Serv. Res.* **2020**, *20*, 926. [CrossRef]
16. Plasencia, W.; Maiz, N.; Bonino, S.; Kaihura, C.; Nicolaides, K. Uterine artery Doppler at 11 + 0 to 13 + 6 weeks in the prediction of pre-eclampsia. *Ultrasound Obstet. Gynecol.* **2007**, *30*, 742–749. [CrossRef]
17. Groom, K.M.; McCowan, L.M.; Mackay, L.K.; Lee, A.C.; Said, J.M.; Kane, S.C.; Walker, S.P.; van Mens, T.E.; Hannan, N.J.; Tong, S. Enoxaparin for the prevention of preeclampsia and intrauterine growth restriction in women with a history: A randomized trial. *Am. J. Obstet. Gynecol.* **2017**, *216*, 296.e1–296.e14.
18. Lim, K.; Ramus, R. Preeclampsia; practice essentials, overview, pathophysiology. In *Medscape*; medscape medical news, located in the heart of Manhattan, steps from Times Square New York. 2018.
19. Khong, S.L.; Kane, S.C.; Brennecke, S.P.; da Silva Costa, F. First-trimester uterine artery Doppler analysis in the prediction of later pregnancy complications. *Dis. Markers* **2015**, *2015*, 679730. [CrossRef]
20. Zhong, Y.; Zhu, F.; Ding, Y. Serum screening in first trimester to predict pre-eclampsia, small for gestational age and preterm delivery: Systematic review and meta-analysis. *BMC Pregnancy Childbirth* **2015**, *15*, 191. [CrossRef]
21. Bahado-Singh, R.O.; Akolekar, R.; Mandal, R.; Dong, E.; Xia, J.; Kruger, M.; Wishart, D.S.; Nicolaides, K. First-trimester metabolomic detection of late-onset preeclampsia. *Am. J. Obstet. Gynecol.* **2013**, *208*, 58.e1–58.e7. [CrossRef]
22. Russo, M.L.; Blakemore, K.J. (Eds.) A historical and practical review of first trimester aneuploidy screening. In *Seminars in Fetal and Neonatal Medicine*; Elsevier: Amsterdam, The Netherlands, 2014.
23. English, F.A.; Kenny, L.C.; McCarthy, F.P. Risk factors and effective management of preeclampsia. *Integr. Blood Press. Control* **2015**, *8*, 7.
24. Serbesa, M.L.; Iffa, M.T.; Geleto, M. Factors associated with malnutrition among pregnant women and lactating mothers in Miesso Health Center, Ethiopia. *Eur. J. Midwifery* **2019**, *3*, 13. [CrossRef]
25. Chen, X.; Zhao, D.; Mao, X.; Xia, Y.; Baker, P.N.; Zhang, H. Maternal dietary patterns and pregnancy outcome. *Nutrients* **2016**, *8*, 351. [CrossRef] [PubMed]
26. Patel, A.; Prakash, A.A.; Das, P.K.; Gupta, S.; Pusdekar, Y.V.; Hibberd, P.L. Maternal anemia and underweight as determinants of pregnancy outcomes: Cohort study in eastern rural Maharashtra, India. *BMJ Open* **2018**, *8*, e021623. [CrossRef] [PubMed]
27. Tariq, K.; Fatima, S.; Nazli, R.; Habib, S.H.; Shah, M. Supplementation in primi-gravidas and its effect on maternal, birth and infant outcomes: A randomized controlled trial. *Khyber Med. Univ. J.* **2021**, *13*, 187–192. [CrossRef]
28. Jorgensen, J.M.; Ashorn, P.; Ashorn, U.; Baldiviez, L.M.; Gondwe, A.; Maleta, K.; Nkhoma, M.; Dewey, K.G. Effects of lipid-based nutrient supplements or multiple micronutrient supplements compared with iron and folic acid supplements during pregnancy on maternal haemoglobin and iron status. *Matern. Child Nutr.* **2018**, *14*, e12640. [CrossRef] [PubMed]
29. Matias, S.L.; Mridha, M.K.; Young, R.T.; Hussain, S.; Dewey, K.G. Daily maternal lipid-based nutrient supplementation with 20 mg iron, compared with iron and folic acid with 60 mg iron, resulted in lower iron status in late pregnancy but not at 6 months postpartum in either the mothers or their infants in Bangladesh. *J. Nutr.* **2018**, *148*, 1615–1624. [CrossRef]
30. Adu-Afarwuah, S.; Lartey, A.; Okronipa, H.; Ashorn, P.; Zeilani, M.; Baldiviez, L.M.; Oaks, B.M.; Vosti, S.; Dewey, K.G. Impact of small-quantity lipid-based nutrient supplement on hemoglobin, iron status and biomarkers of inflammation in pregnant Ghanaian women. *Matern. Child Nutr.* **2017**, *13*, e12262. [CrossRef]
31. Bonafini, S.; Giontella, A.; Tagetti, A.; Marcon, D.; Montagnana, M.; Benati, M.; Gaudino, R.; Cavarzere, P.; Karber, M.; Rothe, M. Possible role of CYP450 generated omega-3/omega-6 PUFA metabolites in the modulation of blood pressure and vascular function in obese children. *Nutrients* **2018**, *10*, 1689. [CrossRef]

32. Tousoulis, D.; Plastiras, A.; Siasos, G.; Oikonomou, E.; Verveniotis, A.; Kokkou, E.; Maniatis, K.; Gouliopoulos, N.; Miliou, A.; Paraskevopoulos, T. Omega-3 PUFAs improved endothelial function and arterial stiffness with a parallel antiinflammatory effect in adults with metabolic syndrome. *Atherosclerosis* **2014**, *232*, 10–16. [CrossRef]
33. Jahan, K.; Roy, S.; Mihrshahi, S.; Sultana, N.; Khatoon, S.; Roy, H.; Datta, L.R.; Roy, A.; Jahan, S.; Khatun, W. Short-term nutrition education reduces low birthweight and improves pregnancy outcomes among urban poor women in Bangladesh. *Food Nutr. Bull.* **2014**, *35*, 414–421. [CrossRef]
34. Abreu, A.M.; Young, R.R.; Buchanan, A.; Lofgren, I.E.; Okronipa, H.E.; Lartey, A.; Ashorn, P.; Adu-Afarwuah, S.; Dewey, K.G.; Oaks, B.M. Maternal Blood Pressure in Relation to Prenatal Lipid-Based Nutrient Supplementation and Adverse Birth Outcomes in a Ghanaian Cohort: A Randomized Controlled Trial and Cohort Analysis. *J. Nutr.* **2021**, *151*, 1637–1645. [CrossRef]
35. Kongwattanakul, K.; Saksiriwuttho, P.; Chaiyarach, S.; Thepsuthammarat, K. Incidence, characteristics, maternal complications, and perinatal outcomes associated with preeclampsia with severe features and HELLP syndrome. *Int. J. Women's Health* **2018**, *10*, 371. [CrossRef]
36. Wen, S.W.; White, R.R.; Rybak, N.; Gaudet, L.M.; Robson, S.; Hague, W.; Simms-Stewart, D.; Carroli, G.; Smith, G.; Fraser, W.D. Effect of high dose folic acid supplementation in pregnancy on pre-eclampsia (FACT): Double blind, phase III, randomised controlled, international, multicentre trial. *BMJ* **2018**, *362*, k3478. [CrossRef]
37. Ali, A.M.; Alobaid, A.; Malhis, T.N.; Khattab, A.F. Effect of vitamin D3 supplementation in pregnancy on risk of pre-eclampsia—Randomized controlled trial. *Clin. Nutr.* **2019**, *38*, 557–563. [CrossRef]
38. Coppage, K.H.; Polzin, W.J. Severe preeclampsia and delivery outcomes: Is immediate cesarean delivery beneficial? *Am. J. Obstet. Gynecol.* **2002**, *186*, 921–923. [CrossRef]
39. Mosavat, M.; Arabiat, D.; Smyth, A.; Newnham, J.; Whitehead, L. Second-trimester maternal serum vitamin D and pregnancy outcome: The Western Australian Raine cohort study. *Diabetes Res. Clin. Pract.* **2021**, *175*, 108779. [CrossRef]
40. Sanchez, M.P.; Guida, J.P.; Simões, M.; Marangoni-Junior, M.; Cralcev, C.; Santos, J.C.; Dias, T.Z.; Luz, A.G.; Costa, M.L. Can pre-eclampsia explain higher cesarean rates in the different groups of Robson's classification? *Int. J. Gynecol. Obstet.* **2021**, *152*, 339–344. [CrossRef]
41. Mridha, M.K.; Matias, S.L.; Paul, R.R.; Hussain, S.; Sarker, M.; Hossain, M.; Peerson, J.M.; Vosti, S.A.; Dewey, K.G. Prenatal lipid-based nutrient supplements do not affect pregnancy or childbirth complications or cesarean delivery in Bangladesh: A cluster-randomized controlled effectiveness trial. *J. Nutr.* **2017**, *147*, 1776–1784.

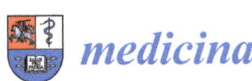

Review

Long QT Syndrome Management during and after Pregnancy

Agne Marcinkeviciene [1,2,3], Diana Rinkuniene [1,2,3,*] and Aras Puodziukynas [1,2,3]

1. Department of Cardiology, Lithuanian University of Health Sciences, LT-44307 Kaunas, Lithuania
2. Department of Cardiology, Hospital of Lithuanian University of Health Sciences Kauno Clinics, LT-50161 Kaunas, Lithuania
3. Kaunas Region Society of Cardiology, LT-44307 Kaunas, Lithuania
* Correspondence: diana.rinkuniene@gmail.com

Abstract: Long QT syndrome (LQTS) is majorly an autosomal dominantly inherited electrical dysfunction, but there are exceptions (Jervell and Lange-Nielsen syndrome is inherited in an autosomal recessive pattern). This disorder prolongs ventricular repolarization and increases the risk of ventricular arrhythmias, syncope, and even sudden cardiac death. The risk of fatal events is reduced during pregnancy, but dramatically increases during the 9 months after delivery, especially in patients with LQT2. In women with LQTS, treatment with β-blockers at appropriate doses is recommended throughout pregnancy and the high-risk postnatal period. In this review, we summarize the management of LQTS during pregnancy and beyond.

Keywords: long QT syndrome; pregnancy; β-blocker

1. Introduction

Concomitant cardiac pathology, including arrhythmogenic channelopathies, can complicate the course of a normal pregnancy and could be related to additional risks for both fetus and mother, including sudden cardiac death (SCD). Long QT syndrome (LQTS) is a cardiac channelopathy, characterized by the prolongation of ventricular repolarization and polymorphic ventricular tachycardia (VT) known as "Torsades de pointes", leading to syncope or SCD. The prevalence of LQTS is approximately 1 in 2000 individuals and can be inherited (approximately 90%) or occur de novo (10%) [1]. LQTS is caused by mutations in several ion-channel genes. The commonest mutations are located in the potassium-channel KCNQ1 (LQT1) and hERG (LQT2) genes, and in the sodium-channel SCN5A (LQT3) gene [2]. These three major genetic subtypes account for approximately 80% of all LQTS cases [3]. There are various subtype-specific triggers for cardiac events in LQTS. Patients with LQT1 experience most of their cardiac incidents as the result of increased adrenergic activity during exercise, especially swimming, or emotional stress. Audible stimulation, such as a ringing telephone or an alarm clock, may provoke LQT2 onset, whereas patients with LQT3 are more likely to have events while resting or sleeping [4]. Women with congenital or acquired LQTS have longer QT intervals and are more likely to develop polymorphic ventricular arrhythmia (VA) or SCD than men [5]. These differences may exist due to alterations of sex hormone levels, dependent on the various menstrual cycle periods, gestation, and the postnatal period, which are related to alterations in QT duration and frequency of cardiac events [6,7].

2. Physiological Changes Induced by Pregnancy

Several gradual physiological developments happen during gestation, such as cardiac remodeling and increased cardiac output. Increased heart pulse in pregnancy results in the shortening of QT intervals, therefore it could be protective in patients with LQTS. Conversely the postnatal period is associated with rapid changes in hemodynamics and increased risk of life-threatening arrhythmias. In women with LQTS, the risk of VT and

SCD is higher in the postpartum period when compared with the relatively low risk during pregnancy [6]. This may be due to the decrease in the heart rate and the prolongation of the QT interval. It has been discussed that altered sleep patterns, physiological stress, and intense auditory stimuli after childbirth may also contribute to adrenergically mediated cardiac events. The risk of SCD in pregnant women with LQTS was evaluated in a retrospective study [7]. It was reported that the first 40 weeks after giving birth are related to an elevated risk of cardiac disturbances (syncope, aborted cardiac arrest (CA), or SCD) compared with the prepregnancy period of 40 weeks. Moreover, the postpartum period increases the risk for first cardiac events in asymptomatic women with LQTS. Seth et al.'s [6] findings indicate that the 9-month period after childbirth is related to a 2.7-fold elevated risk of a cardiac emergency and a 4.1-fold elevated risk of a life-threatening incidents in comparison to the time before the first conception. After the 9-month postpartum period, the risk of cardiac events reverts to the baseline prepregnancy risk. The risk of cardiac events during pregnancy may vary among different LQTS genotypes. Postpartum cardiac events are more commonly reported in patients with the LQT2 mutation than those with the LQT1 or LQT3 genotypes [6,8].

Changes in sex hormone levels may play a role in modulating cardiac repolarization. Estrogen and progesterone are arrhythmogenic sex hormones and their changes during pregnancy and the postpartum period could potentially provoke cardiac events [9]. Rodriguez et al. [10] reported that in patients with a drug-induced LQTS type, the QT interval length varies in different periods of the menses, with a shorter QT interval during the luteal period when progesterone levels are increased, compared to the follicular period with higher estradiol concentrations. This research showed a proarrhythmic effect of estradiol and an antiarrhythmic effect of progesterone, with a reduced susceptibility to sympathetic stimuli. Unfortunately, we could not find any systematic reviews investigating the impact of different sex hormone levels on QT interval duration in women with congenital LQTS. Odening et al. [11] analyzed the prepubertal ovariectomized transgenic LQT2 rabbits, which were treated with estradiol, progesterone, or placebo. The study showed that progesterone significantly reduced potential triggers for polymorphic VT, such as bigeminy and couplets, and completely eliminated the occurrence of polymorphic VT. In addition, it was observed that progesterone prevents against a SCD, suggesting that high progesterone levels during pregnancy are protective. Moreover, the reduction in progesterone levels during the postpartum period is also associated with postpartum arrhythmias and SCD in patients with LQT2 [8]. Contrariwise, estradiol has an effect by steepening the QT/RR ratio, prolonging cardiac refractoriness, and altering the spatial pattern of dispersion of action potential duration, that results in the promotion of polymorphic VA and SCD. Odening et al. [12] published a case report of a female with LQTS in pregnancy and the postnatal period. Although her medical history suggested LQTS type 2, none of the known mutations were found, except for a polymorphism in KCNE1. During pregnancy and while breastfeeding, her QTc interval length continued to be normalized. The electrocardiogram (ECG) showed prolonged QTc duration when the patient was no longer breastfeeding or on hormone-based contraceptives. The alterations of the ECG indicate a hormonal influence on the QTc duration in women with LQTS. Prospective case-control studies are needed to evaluate the arrhythmogenic effect of sex hormones in pregnant women with LQTS.

3. Management of Patients with Long QT Syndrome

Use of β-blockers is the cornerstone of managing congenital LQTS due to its significant reduction in life-threatening arrhythmic risk [13,14]. Their usage significantly reduces a major cardiac event rate during the high-risk postpartum period from 3.7% to 0.8% [6]. According to 2017 American Heart Association (AHA), American College of Cardiology (ACH), and the Heart Rhythm Society (HRS) guidelines on VA and SCD, and the 2018 "European Society of Cardiology (ESC) guidelines" for management of cardiovascular diseases during pregnancy, β-blockers are recommended during and after pregnancy in women with congenital LQTS (recommendation Class I, level of evidence C) [15,16].

Ishibashi et al. [17] in their multicentre study revealed that treatment with β-blockers is essential for the protection of cardiac events during pregnancy and the postnatal period in patients with LQTS. In their study, 136 pregnancies in 76 pregnant women with LQTS were divided into two groups: on β-blocker therapy (β-blockers group) and without β-blocker therapy (non-β-blockers group). During pregnancy and the postnatal period, 14 (11%) cardiac events occurred—all in the non-β-blocker group. Not all β-blockers are the same in the treatment of LQTS. It is shown that the nonselective β-blockers propranolol and nadolol (both are pregnancy risk category C) are significantly more effective than relatively β-1 cardioselective metoprolol (pregnancy risk category C) in preventing cardiac events in symptomatic patients [18]. Furthermore, propranolol has a significantly better QTc shortening effect compared to nadolol and metoprolol, especially in high-risk patients with markedly prolonged QTc. Unfortunately, no randomized clinical trials analyzing the comparative efficacy of different β-blockers for the treatment of LQTS during pregnancy have been conducted [14].

The safety and efficacy of β-blocker use for pregnant women with LQTS and their offspring remains questionable. There is a concern that this treatment may increase the risk of intrauterine grown retardation and malformation in the fetus [17]. In the same study by Ishibashi et al., the frequency of low birthweight infants was significantly higher in the β-blockers group compared with the non-β-blockers group ($p = 0.024$). Although the mean birth weight was within normal range, the birth weight was lower in the β-blockers group than in the non-β-blockers group. This difference between groups may have occurred because the β-blockers group was diagnosed as higher gestational risk, and more than half of the β-blockers group patients had undergone an elective Cesarean delivery before the end of full gestational period. The most used β-blocker in this investigation was propranolol, but events of low birthweight infants did not differ between the different types of β-blockers. Also, there were no significant differences in congenital malformations between the groups.

Huttunen et al. [19] found that LQT1 patients, exposed to maternal β-blocker treatment during pregnancy, were significantly smaller at birth than patients who weren't exposed to β-blocker therapy. However, the study showed a rapid catch-up growth during the first year of life. Marshall et al. [20] observed that β-blocker therapy does not increase the risk of fetal distress and miscarriages, even though these infants weigh lower than infants of mothers with LQTS not receiving this therapy. Based on a meta-analysis [21], the first-trimester β-blocker use in general showed no increased odds of any major (non-organ specific) birth defects. On the other hand, examining organ-specific malformations, a 2-fold increase in the risk of cardiovascular defects and an over 3-fold increase in oral clefts and neural tube defects were observed. These data are difficult to interpret due to small numbers of heterogenous studies, lack of statistical significance and potential biases. In addition, β-blockers are secreted in breast milk, however the risk of adverse effects is low in neonates with normal renal and hepatic functions [22]. Hence, it is safe and recommended to continue β-blockers during pregnancy and the postpartum period, at least 40 weeks after delivery [7], in women with LQTS.

Amiodarone (pregnancy risk category D) is contraindicated, as it promotes additional prolongation of the QT interval, herewith it has been related with fetal growth retardation, premature labor, and hypothyroidism [15]. In select LQT3 patients, mexiletine or ranolazine (pregnancy risk category C) can benefit as an add-on therapy to prevent cardiac events in pregnancy. Mexiletine is a class IB antiarrhythmic agent, a late sodium channel blocker that significantly shortens the QT interval [16]. Ranolazine is an antianginal drug used for the treatment of chronic angina. Chorin et al. [23] reported the first long-term study of this drug for LQT3. Ranolazine has been shown to reduce the QT interval of LQT3 harboring the SCN5A-D1790G mutation. There are many genotypic and phenotypic variants in LQT3 that have differing responses to medications, therefore, patients with LQT3 should have a full biophysical assessment of the individual channel mutants and genotypes [24].

The implantation of an implantable cardioverter-defibrillator (ICD) should be considered prior to the pregnancy in women with high-risk factors for a SCD [25]. Conversely, ICD implantation during pregnancy does not increase the risk of major ICD-related problems, such as lead prolapse, lead dysfunction or lead thrombus, under appropriate management and is recommended if an indication emerges [26,27]. Implantation, for ICD ideally single lead, can be done safely, especially if the fetus is beyond 8 weeks of gestation [25]. Programming of the device should be intended to increase the threshold for shock therapies by prolonging the duration of tachycardia episode detection to prevent shock therapies in self-terminating episodes. Immediate electrical cardioversion is recommended for sustained VT regardless of its impact on hemodynamics [16,25].

4. Risk Evaluation and Delivery Strategy

For all women with an inherited arrhythmia syndrome, such as LQTS, a multidisciplinary team with expertise in pregnancy, cardiac arrhythmias and genetics should carry out risk assessment and provide pre-pregnancy care [15]. The risk evaluation of LQTS is challenging. The most potent factors predicting CA are LQT2 or LQT3 genotypes, previous events, and degree of QT prolongation [13,16]. QT-interval prolonging drugs and safety data should be checked carefully during pregnancy. Pregnant women suffering from hyperemesis should be closely monitored for electrolyte imbalance, such as hypokalemia and hypomagnesemia. Usage of antiemetic medications may also prolong the QT interval. An ECG, heart ultrasound, and an exercise test are recommended before becoming pregnant. Moreover, Holter monitoring may be useful for a channelopathy. All regular prenatal and peripartum examinations and testing, led by obstetrics, remain an important part of care.

Childbirth may be related to changes in volume, electrolyte disturbances, acute pain, adrenaline release, and the urgent use of antiemetics and anesthetics [28]. The above conditions could complicate the course of childbirth and lead to complications. The 2018 ESC guidelines provide the framework of risk stratification, monitoring and treatment during labor and delivery, which has been developed by expert consensus (see Table 1) [15,28]. The induction of labor should be considered at 40 weeks of gestation. Patients with LQTS, who are at moderate to high-risk, should be supervised at a tertiary center by the expert team, including obstetric and cardiac nurses, an anesthesiologist, a cardiologist with the expertise in inherited arrhythmia syndromes, and an expert obstetrician. In high-risk LQTS, Caesarean delivery is recommended, whereas in low-risk or medium-risk LQTS, the mode of delivery is advised by obstetricians. In the absence of obstetric contraindications, vaginal delivery is considered the safest mode of delivery. According to Tanaka et al. [29], each mode of delivery in women with LQTS has a low likelihood of cardiovascular events, but there is a higher Caesarean delivery rate due to non-reassuring fetal status in labor. It is important to mention that most women (92%) used β-blockers in this study, which may have helped to prevent cardiovascular events during labor.

Unfortunately, there are no clinical trials that generalize optimal anesthetic management in pregnant women with LQTS, and thus the findings are derived from case reports. In order to avoid life-threatening arrhythmias in LQTS patients, sympathetic activity should be minimized. It is reported that this goal can be achieved with combined spinal-epidural anesthesia [30]. Spinal anesthesia alone is not administered for LQTS patients, as it leads to sudden hemodynamic changes and increased risk of VA and CA [31]. Conversely, epidural anesthesia is associated with gradual alteration in hemodynamics. However, all possible options during childbirth should be discussed and scheduled in advance. For patients in the high-risk LQTS group, continuous ECG monitoring during labor is recommended. It is important to be prepared for intravenous administration of a β-blocker in moderate to high-risk LQTS patients, and for intravenous administration of selected antiarrhythmic medication, such as lidocaine or mexiletine, in case of an emergency in a high-risk LQTS patient (see Table 2). Esmolol, which is rapidly up-titrated and has a short half-life period, can be used if possible. Commonly available alternatives are intermittent intravenous metoprolol and propranolol [28].

Table 1. Recommended level of care during labor for women with LQTS. Adapted from the 2018 ESC guidelines [15] and Roston et al. [28].

Risk of Arrhythmia with Hemodynamic Impairment during Labor	LQTS Phenotype	Level of Surveillance	Class [a]	Level [b]
Low-risk	• LQTS with no previous events and QTc ≤ 470 ms	1	I	C
Medium-risk	• LQTS with remote events, • LQTS with no previous events and QTc ≥ 470 ms	2	I	C
High-risk	• Any other LQTS with latest incidents *	3	I	C

Descriptions of the planned actions	Level of surveillance		
	1	2	3
Consultation with a cardiologist	+		
Prescribe/terminate the required medication if necessary	+	+	+
Consultation with an expert team at tertiary center		+	+
Method and location of delivery recommended by midwives	+	+	
Labor at thoracic operating theatre (Cesarean delivery advised)			+
Heart rhythm assessment (telemetry, external heart rate monitor)		(+)	+
Intravenous line, administration of β-blocker if necessary		+	+
Arterial line			+
Be prepared to administer selected antiarrhythmic drugs IV			+
Exterior cardioverter-defibrillator on unit		+	+

* Latest incidents are described as arrhythmogenic syncope and/or seizures, CA and/or persistent VA in the last 1 year with adequate medication therapy. CA—cardiac arrest; LQTS—long QT syndrome; ms—milliseconds; QTc—corrected QT interval; IV—intravenous; VA—ventricular arrhythmia. [a] Class of recommendation, [b] level of evidence.

Table 2. Treatment of unstable cardiac rhythm disturbances of LQTS in pregnancy. Adapted from Roston et al. [28].

Therapy for Acute Presentation	Transition to Chronic Therapy
1st line: IV or oral β-blocker	Increase β-blocker ± add mexiletine
2nd line: IV MgSO$_4$, lidocaine, mexiletine	Consider K+ supplement ± LCSD (best delayed until post-partum)
3nd line: transvenous pacing *	Consider for ICD indication **

* Before considering a permanent device, a temporary transvenous pacemaker should be attempted. ** The ICD should only be implanted according to strong recommendations. Echocardiography or other non-radiological technique should be used. IV—intravenous; LCSD—left cardiac sympathetic denervation; ICD—implantable cardioverter-defibrillator.

5. Postpartum Follow Up

So far, there are no general recommendations and approved schemes for how women with LQTS should be supervised after delivery. Different follow up strategies may vary depending on the consensus of the healthcare facility. Women with LQTS should be checked by an experienced cardiologist within the first weeks after delivery and every month for the first 9 months to evaluate efficacy of treatment, ECG, and symptoms [32,33]. Dose adjustment of β-blockers may be needed. Optimal postpartum care remains the same as in routine cases.

6. Conclusions

A pregnancy heart team is necessary to evaluate the risk and monitor women with LQTS carefully throughout the pregnancy and delivery. Changes of estradiol and progesterone levels during pregnancy may play a role in arrhythmogenesis. Additional caution may be required in the 9-month postnatal period, which is associated with an increased risk of cardiac events, especially in patients with LQT2. Consequently, the close cardiac follow up with monitoring of ECG during the postnatal period is essential. Treatment with β-blockers is important to protect women with LQTS from cardiac events during pregnancy and the postnatal period. The benefits of β-blockers are outweighed by the risks to the foetus. Genetic counselling and testing for mutations in LQTS patients provide important prognostic and therapeutic information that can help family members understand the risks. However, a negative genetic result does not rule out the diagnosis of LQTS, as has been confirmed by clinical evaluation. In conclusion, pregnancy planning is mostly safe and not contraindicated in LQTS.

Author Contributions: A.M., D.R. and A.P.; methodology, A.M. and D.R.; writing—original draft preparation, A.M. and D.R.; writing—review and editing, A.M., D.R. and A.P.; visualization, D.R.; supervision, A.P.; funding acquisition, D.R. and A.P. All authors have read and agreed to the published version of the manuscript.

Funding: This research received no external funding.

Institutional Review Board Statement: Ethical review and approval were waived for this study, due to the type of study.

Informed Consent Statement: Not applicable.

Data Availability Statement: Not applicable.

Conflicts of Interest: The authors declare no conflict of interest.

References

1. Schwartz, P.J.; Stramba-Badiale, M.; Crotti, L.; Pedrazzini, M.; Besana, A.; Bosi, G.; Gabbarini, F.; Goulene, K.; Insolia, R.; Mannarino, S.; et al. Prevalence of the congenital long-QT syndrome. *Circulation* **2009**, *120*, 1761–1767. [CrossRef]
2. Wilde, A.A.M.; Bezzina, C.R. Genetics of cardiac arrhythmias. *Heart* **2005**, *91*, 1352–1358. [CrossRef]
3. Bohnen, M.S.; Peng, G.; Robey, S.H.; Terrenoire, C.; Iyer, V.; Sampson, K.J.; Kass, R.S. Molecular pathophysiology of congenital long QT syndrome. *Physiol. Rev.* **2017**, *97*, 89–134. [CrossRef]
4. Schwartz, P.J.; Priori, S.G.; Spazzolini, C.; Moss, A.J.; Vincent, G.M.; Napolitano, C.; Denjoy, I.; Guicheney, P.; Breithardt, G.; Keating, M.T.; et al. Genotype-phenotype correlation in the long-QT syndrome: Gene-specific triggers for life-threatening arrhythmias. *Circulation* **2001**, *103*, 89–95. [CrossRef]
5. Sauer, A.J.; Moss, A.J.; McNitt, S.; Peterson, D.R.; Zareba, W.; Robinson, J.L.; Qi, M.; Goldenberg, I.; Hobbs, J.B.; Ackerman, M.J.; et al. Long QT syndrome in adults. *J. Am. Coll. Cardiol.* **2007**, *49*, 329–337. [CrossRef]
6. Rodriguez, I.; Kilborn, M.J.; Liu, X.K.; Pezzullo, J.C.; Woosley, R.L. Drug-induced QT prolongation in women during the menstrual cycle. *J. Am. Med. Assoc.* **2001**, *285*, 1322–1326. [CrossRef]
7. Seth, R.; Moss, A.J.; McNitt, S.; Zareba, W.; Andrews, M.L.; Qi, M.; Robinson, J.L.; Goldenberg, I.; Ackerman, M.J.; Benhorin, J.; et al. Long QT Syndrome and pregnancy. *J. Am. Coll. Cardiol.* **2007**, *49*, 1092–1098. [CrossRef]
8. Rashba, E.J.; Zareba, W.; Moss, A.J.; Hall, W.J.; Robinson, J.; Locati, E.H.; Schwartz, P.J.; Andrews, M. Influence of pregnancy on the risk for cardiac events in patients with hereditary long QT syndrome. *Circulation* **1998**, *97*, 451–456. [CrossRef]
9. Khositseth, A.; Tester, D.J.; Will, M.L.; Bell, C.M.; Ackerman, M.J. Identification of a common genetic substrate underlying postpartum cardiac events in congenital long QT syndrome. *Heart Rhythm.* **2004**, *1*, 60–64. [CrossRef]
10. Odening, K.E.; Koren, G. How do sex hormones modify arrhythmogenesis in long QT syndrome? Sex hormone effects on arrhythmogenic substrate and triggered activity. *Heart Rhythm.* **2014**, *11*, 2107–2115. [CrossRef]
11. Odening, K.E.; Choi, B.R.; Liu, G.X.; Hartmann, K.; Ziv, O.; Chaves, L.; Schofield, L.; Centracchio, J.; Zehender, M.; Peng, X.; et al. Estradiol promotes sudden cardiac death in transgenic long QT type 2 rabbits while progesterone is protective. *Heart Rhythm.* **2012**, *9*, 823–832. [CrossRef]
12. Odening, K.E.; Koren, G.; Kirk, M. Normalization of QT interval duration in a long QT syndrome patient during pregnancy and the postpartum period due to sex hormone effects on cardiac repolarization. *Hearth Case Rep.* **2016**, *2*, 223–227. [CrossRef]
13. Priori, S.G.; Wilde, A.A.; Horie, M.; Cho, Y.; Behr, E.R.; Berul, C.; Blom, N.; Brugada, J.; Chiang, C.E.; Huikuri, H.; et al. HRS/EHRA/APHRS Expert Consensus Statement on the Diagnosis and Management of Patients with Inherited Primary

Arrhythmia Syndromes: Document endorsed by HRS, EHRA, and APHRS in May 2013 and by ACCF, AHA, PACES, and AEPC in June 2013. *Heart Rhythm.* **2013**, *10*, 1932–1963. [CrossRef]
14. Ackerman, M.J.; Priori, S.G.; Dubin, A.M.; Kowey, P.; Linker, N.J.; Slotwiner, D.; Triedman, J.; Van Hare, G.F.; Gold, M.R. Beta-blocker therapy for long QT syndrome and catecholaminergic polymorphic ventricular tachycardia: Are all beta-blockers equivalent? *Heart Rhythm.* **2017**, *14*, e41–e44. [CrossRef]
15. Regitz-Zagrosek, V.; Roos-Hesselink, J.W.; Bauersachs, J.; Blomström-Lundqvist, C.; Cífková, R.; De Bonis, M.; Iung, B.; Johnson, M.R.; Kintscher, U.; Kranke, P.; et al. 2018 ESC Guidelines for the management of cardiovascular diseases during pregnancy. *Eur. Heart J.* **2018**, *39*, 3165–3241. [CrossRef]
16. Al-Khatib, S.M.; Stevenson, W.G.; Ackerman, M.J.; Bryant, W.J.; Callans, D.J.; Curtis, A.B.; Deal, B.J.; Dickfeld, T.; Field, M.E.; Fonarow, G.C.; et al. 2017 AHA/ACC/HRS guideline for management of patients with ventricular arrhythmias and the prevention of sudden cardiac death. *Circulation* **2018**, *138*, e272–e391.
17. Ishibashi, K.; Aiba, T.; Kamiya, C.; Miyazaki, A.; Sakaguchi, H.; Wada, M.; Nakajima, I.; Miyamoto, K.; Okamura, H.; Noda, T.; et al. Arrhythmia risk and β-blocker therapy in pregnant women with long QT syndrome. *Heart* **2017**, *103*, 1374–1379. [CrossRef]
18. Chockalingam, P.; Crotti, L.; Girardengo, G.; Johnson, J.N.; Harris, K.M.; van der Heijden, J.F.; Hauer, R.N.; Beckmann, B.M.; Spazzolini, C.; Rordorf, R.; et al. Not all beta-blockers are equal in the management of long QT syndrome types 1 and 2: Higher recurrence of events under metoprolol. *J. Am. Coll. Cardiol.* **2012**, *60*, 2092–2099. [CrossRef]
19. Huttunen, H.; Hero, M.; Lääperi, M.; Känsäkoski, J.; Swan, H.; Hirsch, J.A.; Miettinen, P.J.; Raivio, T. The role of KCNQ1 mutations and maternal beta blocker use during pregnancy in the growth of children with long QT syndrome. *Front. Endocrinol.* **2018**, *9*, 194. [CrossRef]
20. Heradien, M.J.; Goosen, A.; Crotti, L.; Durrheim, G.; Corfield, V.; Brink, P.A.; Schwartz, P.J. Does pregnancy increase cardiac risk for LQT1 patients with the KCNQ1-A341V mutation? *J. Am. Coll. Cardiol.* **2006**, *48*, 1410–1415. [CrossRef]
21. Yakoob, M.Y.; Bateman, B.T.; Ho, E.; Hernandez-Diaz, S.; Franklin, J.M.; Goodman, J.E.; Hoban, R.A. The risk of congenital malformations associated with exposure to β-blockers early in pregnancy: A meta-analysis. *Hypertension* **2013**, *62*, 375–381. [CrossRef]
22. Garg, L.; Garg, J.; Krishnamoorthy, P.; Ahnert, A.; Shah, N.; Dusaj, R.S.; Bozorgnia, B. Influence of Pregnancy in Patients with Congenital Long QT Syndrome. *Cardiol. Rev.* **2017**, *25*, 197–201. [CrossRef]
23. Chorin, E.; Hu, D.; Antzelevitch, C.; Hochstadt, A.; Belardinelli, L.; Zeltser, D.; Barajas-Martinez, H.; Rozovski, U.; Rosso, R.; Adler, A.; et al. Ranolazine for congenital long-QT syndrome type III: Experimental and long-term clinical data. *Circ. Arrhythm. Electrophysiol.* **2016**, *9*, e004370. [CrossRef]
24. Lee, M.J.; Monteil, D.C.; Spooner, M.T. Peripartum management of patient with long QT3 after successful implantable cardioverter defibrillator device discharge resulting in device failure: A case report. *Eur. Heart J. Case Rep.* **2021**, *5*, ytab487. [CrossRef]
25. Priori, S.G.; Blomström-Lundqvist, C.; Mazzanti, A.; Blom, N.; Borggrefe, M.; Camm, J.; Elliott, P.M.; Fitzsimons, D.; Hatala, R.; Hindricks, G.; et al. 2015 ESC Guidelines for the management of patients with ventricular arrhythmias and the prevention of sudden cardiac death the Task Force for the Management of Patients with Ventricular Arrhythmias and the Prevention of Sudden Cardiac Death of the European Society of Cardiology (ESC) Endorsed by: Association for European Paediatric and Congenital Cardiology (AEPC). *Eur. Heart J.* **2015**, *36*, 2793–28761.
26. Miyoshi, T.; Kamiya, C.A.; Katsuragi, S.; Ueda, H.; Kobayashi, Y.; Horiuchi, C.; Yamanaka, K.; Neki, R.; Yoshimatsu, J.; Ikeda, T.; et al. Safety and efficacy of implantable cardioverter-defibrillator during pregnancy and after delivery. *Circ. J.* **2013**, *77*, 1166–1170. [CrossRef]
27. Boulé, S.; Ovart, L.; Marquié, C.; Botcherby, E.; Klug, D.; Kouakam, C.; Brigadeau, F.; Guédon-Moreau, L.; Wissocque, L.; Meurice, J.; et al. Pregnancy in women with an implantable cardioverter-defibrillator: Is it safe? *Europace* **2014**, *16*, 1587–1594. [CrossRef]
28. Roston, T.M.; van der Werf, C.; Cheung, C.C.; Grewal, J.; Davies, B.; Wilde, A.A.M.; Krahn, A.D. Caring for the pregnant woman with an inherited arrhythmia syndrome. *Heart Rhythm* **2020**, *17*, 341–348. [CrossRef]
29. Tanaka, H.; Katsuragi, S.; Tanaka, K.; Sawada, M.; Iwanaga, N.; Yoshimatsu, J.; Ikeda, T. Maternal and neonatal outcomes in labor and at delivery when long QT syndrome is present. *J. Matern. Neonatal Med.* **2016**, *29*, 1117–1119. [CrossRef]
30. Hashimoto, E.; Kojima, A.; Kitagawa, H.; Matsuura, H. Anesthetic management of a patient with type 1 long QT syndrome using combined epidural-spinal anesthesia for caesarean section: Perioperative approach based on ion channel function. *J. Cardiothorac. Vasc. Anesth.* **2020**, *34*, 465–469. [CrossRef]
31. Al-Refai, A.; Gunka, V.; Douglas, J. Spinal anesthesia for Cesarean section in a parturient with long QT syndrome. *Can. J. Anaesth.* **2004**, *51*, 993–996. [CrossRef]
32. Taylor, C.; Stambler, B.S. Management of Long QT syndrome in women before, during, and after pregnancy. *US Cardiol. Rev.* **2021**, *15*, e08. [CrossRef]
33. Meregalli, P.G.; Westendorp, I.C.; Tan, H.L.; Elsman, P.; Kok, W.E.; Wilde, A.A. Pregnancy and the risk of torsades de pointes in congenital long-QT syndrome. *Neth. Heart J.* **2008**, *16*, 422–425. [CrossRef]

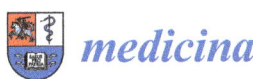

Review

Considering the Effects and Maternofoetal Implications of Vascular Disorders and the Umbilical Cord

Lara Sánchez-Trujillo [1,2,3], Cielo García-Montero [1,2], Oscar Fraile-Martinez [1,2], Luis G. Guijarro [2,4], Coral Bravo [5,6,7], Juan A. De Leon-Luis [5,6,7], Jose V. Saez [8], Julia Bujan [1,2], Melchor Alvarez-Mon [1,2,9], Natalio García-Honduvilla [1,2], Miguel A. Saez [1,2,10,†] and Miguel A. Ortega [1,2,*,†]

1. Department of Medicine and Medical Specialities, Faculty of Medicine and Health Sciences, University of Alcalá, 28801 Alcalá de Henares, Spain
2. Ramón y Cajal Institute of Sanitary Research (IRYCIS), 28034 Madrid, Spain
3. Deparment of Pediatrics, Hospital Universitario Principe de Asturias, 28801 Alcalá de Henares, Spain
4. Department of Systems Biology, Faculty of Medicine and Health Sciences (Networking Research Center on Liver and Digestive Diseases (CIBEREHD), University of Alcalá, 28801 Alcalá de Henares, Spain
5. Department of Public and Maternal and Child Health, School of Medicine, Complutense University of Madrid, 28040 Madrid, Spain
6. Department of Obstetrics and Gynecology, University Hospital Gregorio Marañón, 28009 Madrid, Spain
7. Health Research Institute Gregorio Marañón, 28009 Madrid, Spain
8. Department of Biomedicine and Biotechnology, Faculty of Medicine and Health Sciences, University of Alcalá, 28801 Alcalá de Henares, Spain
9. Immune System Diseases-Rheumatology and Internal Medicine Service, University Hospital Príncipe de Asturias, CIBEREHD, 28806 Alcalá de Henares, Spain
10. Pathological Anatomy Service, Central University Hospital of Defence-UAH Madrid, 28801 Alcala de Henares, Spain
* Correspondence: miguel.angel.ortega92@gmail.com
† These authors contributed equally to this work.

Abstract: The umbilical cord is a critical anatomical structure connecting the placenta with the foetus, fulfilling multiple functions during pregnancy and hence influencing foetal development, programming and survival. Histologically, the umbilical cord is composed of three blood vessels: two arteries and one vein, integrated in a mucous connective tissue (Wharton's jelly) upholstered by a layer of amniotic coating. Vascular alterations in the umbilical cord or damage in this tissue because of other vascular disorders during pregnancy are worryingly related with detrimental maternofoetal consequences. In the present work, we will describe the main vascular alterations presented in the umbilical cord, both in the arteries (Single umbilical artery, hypoplastic umbilical artery or aneurysms in umbilical arteries) and the vein (Vascular thrombosis, aneurysms or varicose veins in the umbilical vein), together with other possible complications (Velamentous insertion, vasa praevia, hypercoiled or hypocoiled cord, angiomyxoma and haematomas). Likewise, the effect of the main obstetric vascular disorders like hypertensive disorders of pregnancy (specially pre-eclampsia) and chronic venous disease on the umbilical cord will also be summarized herein.

Keywords: umbilical cord; vascular malperfusion; pre-eclampsia; chronic venous disease

1. Introduction

The umbilical cord is an anatomical structure composed of two arteries and a vein covered by Wharton's jelly derived from allantois, which in turn is upholstered by a layer of amniotic coating [1]. The umbilical cord connects the foetus and the placenta and ensures adequate nutrition, foetal oxygenation, and proper waste elimination. The integrity of the maternal-foetal circulation is essential for the correct development and survival of the foetus. If foetal oxygenation is compromised, foetal hypoxia can affect essential systems such as the cardiovascular system or the central nervous system. Abnormalities or complications that affect these functions involve foetal and neonatal compromise and increase perinatal morbidity and mortality [2].

Both umbilical arteries arise from the internal iliac arteries and are responsible for returning deoxygenated blood from the foetus to the mother. The two arteries converge in the chorionic arteries of the placenta, and their position in the cord is variable. At the histological level, they are characterized by a small lumen comprising a muscular middle layer and an external circular layer and lacking an internal elastic lamina. There is a variant called the single umbilical artery in which there is only one umbilical artery, which can be the result of aneuploidies or congenital anomalies or simply an incidental finding.

The umbilical vein results from the convergence of the chorionic veins and is responsible for the supply of oxygenated blood to the foetus. It is characterized by a wider lumen, with an internal elastic limiting layer and a lax muscular layer in a circular arrangement. During embryogenesis, a right umbilical vein develops that normally degenerates during embryonic development but can persist as a variant in the form of a supernumerary vessel. The umbilical vein connects with the systemic circulation of the foetus through the ductus venosus, which drains into the inferior vena cava. When the cord is detached after birth, the structures contained in the cord sheath remain at the base. The closed blood vessels remain permeable during the first weeks of life. Finally, the umbilical arteries will be defined at the lateral umbilical ligaments, the umbilical vein at the round ligament, and the ductus venosus at the ligamentum venosus.

Wharton's jelly is derived from mesoblastic cells of the embryonic pedicle and is composed of a hydrophilic extracellular matrix that is rich in water, proteoglycans, and hyaluronic acid. Wharton's jelly provides supportive and protective functions against compression.

The umbilical cord usually inserts in the placenta centrally or eccentrically, which is considered a normal cord insertion. However, there are insertion abnormalities such as marginal insertion, velamentous insertion, or vasa praevia [1].

Velamentous insertion of the umbilical cord consists of the divergence of umbilical vessels, unsupported by the umbilical cord or placental tissue, as they traverse amnion and chorion before reaching the placenta [3]. It is characterized by the presence of membranous umbilical vessels in the region of placental insertion, little Wharton jelly and susceptibility to compression with the danger of hemorrhage and fetal exsanguination. Vasa praevia consists of an anomaly of the umbilical vessels that cross the membranes of the low uterine segment, unsupported by umbilical cord or placental tissue, with a high risk of rupture of the vessels [3].

Ultrasound examination of the umbilical cord can be performed from the eighth gestational week and is key during prenatal follow-up [4]. There is no consensus about umbilical cord examination among the different societies' guidelines. The International Society of Ultrasound in Obstetrics and Gynecology, do not recommend checking specifically for possible umbilical cord abnormalities [5]. However, the American Institute of Ultrasound in Medicine (AIUM) guidelines highlight the importance of umbilical cord ultrasound examination between second and third-ultrasound examinations [4]. At the anatomic level, its foetal and placental insertion, number of vessels, length, diameter, coiling, and vascular anomalies are important [4].

The average thickness of the cord varies and depends on the length of gestation. A cord with a diameter of less than 1 cm is considered thin [6].

The length of the cord is variable between sexes and gestational age; in term gestations, cords shorter than 35 cm are considered short, and those longer than 70 cm are considered long [6].

Coiling corresponds to the winding pattern of the umbilical arteries around the umbilical vein; 1–3 coils per 10 cm of length is considered normal [1]. In most cases, the pattern is to the left and is evaluated by calculating the coiling index (inverse of the distance separating two spiral turns).

Correct foetal growth and development are also determined by correct placental development. Dysregulation of cell differentiation during placental angiogenesis implies an alteration in the primitive foetal circulation, which may indicate abnormal intrauterine growth [7]. The perinatal and neonatal implications of incorrect placental development vary greatly depending on its severity.

Several factors have been linked to changes in foetal blood flow, including the presence of vascular alterations during pregnancy, which in turn encompass anomalies and vascular alterations in the umbilical cord [8].

2. Vascular Alterations of the Umbilical Cord and Its Impact on the Foetus and Newborn

2.1. Arterial Vascular Alterations of the Umbilical Cord

Single umbilical artery (SUA) is a variation of cord anatomy in which only a single umbilical artery is present. The absence of the left umbilical artery is more frequent than the absence of the right artery. SUA occurs in approximately 0.5–5% of spontaneous pregnancies, although it depends on the population studied [9]. It is usually the result of an atresia or secondary atrophy of one of the arteries, but it may also be due to a primary agenesis of an umbilical artery or the persistence of the single allantoic artery that originates the umbilical arteries. It can be properly diagnosed with a color Doppler ultrasound of the paravesical umbilical vessels [3].

There is no clear relationship between SUA and certain foetal or neonatal pathologies, although studies suggest increased risks of preterm delivery, caesarean section, low birth weight, small newborn for gestational age and admission to the NICU [10]. The association of SUA with other chromosomal or anatomical abnormalities may also imply changes in foetal and neonatal development [9,11]. The highest incidence of malformation associated has been found in the urinary sytem, cardiovascular system and digestive system [9] If these malformations are present, a genetic testing should be performed [9] such as amniocentesis for karyotype [11].

A similar anomaly is hypoplastic umbilical artery, in which two umbilical arteries are present but one has a significantly smaller diameter than the other, with an artery-to-artery diameter difference of more than 50 per cent [12], which increases blood flow resistance. It can be explained by an atrophy of an artery in late pregnancy. Its association with other abnormalities also affects foetal and neonatal prognosis [12]. Some abnormalities found included trisomy 18, polyhydramnios, congenital heart disease, and fetal growth restriction [12].

Supernumerary vessels are rare in humans, and it is usually a result of the persistence of the right umbilical vein.

Aneurysms in umbilical arteries have also been described. They are a very rare condition and are identifiable by the turbulent pulsatile flow at the ultrasound level. They usually occur together with SUA [10] and are detected in areas near the placental insertion site that are less protected by Wharton's jelly, usually during the second or third trimester of gestation. They are associated with delayed intrauterine growth, SUA, aneuploidy like trisomy 18, cardiac abnormalities and foetal demise [13]. When aneurysm is detected a detailed ultrasaound examination with fetal echocardiography and karyotype should be considered, as well as early delivery [13].

2.2. Venous Vascular Disorders of the Umbilical Cord and Their Impact on the Foetus and Newborn

Vascular thromboses (umbilical cord thrombi) mainly affect the umbilical vein and have been related to other cord abnormalities such as anomalous venous insertion of the cord, an excess of cord coiling, long cords, narrowed cord and little Wharton jelly [14]. They are related to FGR (Fetal Growth Restriction), foetal demise and hypoxic-ischemic encephalopathy [14], so fetus should be closely monitored and a cesarean section surgery should be recommended even without delay [14,15].

These thromboses can be favoured by aneurysms or varicose veins in the umbilical vein, which are identifiable at the ultrasound level as turbulent nonpulsatile flows in areas of dilation. They are more frequent than umbilical artery aneurysms. Vascular thromboses are diagnosed by visualizing dilations greater than 9 mm in diameter or with a diameter greater than 50% of the unaffected vessel and can be intra- or extra-abdominal [16]. Maternal coagulation disorders, vascular endothelial damage and elevated blood glucose have been proposed as possible determining factors to the formation of thrombosis [14] however, the pathogenesis has not been fully elucidated.

Umbilical vain varix is a focal dilatation of the intrabdominalumbilical vein, which has a varix diameter at least 50% wider than the diameter of the intrahepatic umbilical vein [17]. It appears as a fusiform cystic structure.The presence of umbilical venous varices as the only alteration does not usually have foetal repercussions [18]. However, in some studies, the presence of intra-amniotic varicose veins is also related to an increased risk of intra-amniotic haemorrhage, low birth weight and foetal demise [17,19] so fetal monitoring is highly recommended.

2.3. Other Vascular Disorders

The insertion of the umbilical cord is almost always central or paracentral and coincides with the anchorage of the amnion. Velamentous insertion of the umbilical cord consists of the divergence of umbilical vessels, unsupported by the umbilical cord or placental tissue, as they traverse amnion and chorion before reaching the placenta [3]. It is characterized by the presence of membranous umbilical vessels in the region of placental insertion, little Wharton jelly and susceptibility to compression. Vasa praevia consists in an anomaly of the umbilical vessels that cross the membranes of the low uterine segment, unsupported by umbilical cord or placental tissue, with a hight risk of rupture of the vessels [3]. It occurs in 1% of pregnancies [6] and it is more frequent in twin pregnancies [20]. Membrane rupture can cause vessel rupture with a risk of exsanguination and foetal demise. Flow compression can translate into placental infarcts and limb amputations [21–25]. In addition, the risks of low birth weight and perinatal death are increased [20,26].

Although prenatal diagnosis is difficult, the coiling pattern of the umbilical vessels and its relationships with venous percussion and fetoplacental blood flow have also been studied. A hypercoiled or hypocoiled cord has been associated with increased risks of adverse perinatal events and foetal demise [27].

A hypocoiled or hypercoiled cord has also been associated with increased risks of preterm childbirth, loss of foetal well-being, meconium in amniotic fluid, Apgar > 7, small for gestational age, foetal and cardiac abnormalities, foetal demise and NICU admission [28]. The coil pattern of the umbilical cord also seems to have implications for fetoplacental flow, as cords with segmented patterns and linked patterns may result in chronic foetal vascular obstruction and stillbirth [29].

In addition, the absence of proper cushioning by Wharton jelly in thin cords seems to favour vascular compression, with consequent repercussions for foetal flow and uterine growth [30]. A thin umbilical cord with little Wharton jelly has been associated with small placental size and low birth weight; that is, a thin umbilical cord seems to be related to placental insufficiency, intrauterine growth restriction and low birth weight [31–34].

Regarding the length of the umbilical cord, a short umbilical cord has also been related to a higher incidence of adverse events such as urgent caesarean section or low birth weight [32,34]. A longer cord allows wide foetal movements that can increase the risk of crossed and circular entanglement and true cord knots, which can lead to foetal demise [35].

Angiomyxoma, previously also called haemangioma, is an infrequent tumour that arises from the proliferation of mesenchymal angiogenic cells in close relationship with the umbilical vessels [36]. They are usually incidental ultrasound findings, although they can contribute to the involvement of adjacent vessels, favouring hydrops or cord torsion. They are visualized with solid-cystic, echogenic and vascularized mass lesions, usually located in the area of foetal insertion [37]. In some cases, they have been related to foetal demise due to the risk of compression of vessels, rupture and formation of haematomas that compromise the umbilical flow with the foetus [38].

Haematomas of the cord produced by the extravasation of blood from the umbilical vein to Wharton's jelly have also been described. Although they are infrequent, they can be spontaneous [39] and have a benign course. However, they are usually associated with invasive procedures, infections or morphological abnormalities [40]. They usually have an isoechoic and heterogeneous appearance on ultrasound. This bleeding can be a cause of loss of foetal well-being, intrapartum asphyxia and hypoxic-ischaemic encephalopathy in the newborn [40]. Some studies relate it to oligoamnios in the third trimester, which can increase susceptibility to cord compression [41]. It has also been related to the performance of amniocentesis in the second trimester and an increased risk of prenatal and perinatal death [41].

2.4. Foetal Programming: How Vascular Alterations in the Umbilical Cord Can Impact on the Foetus and Newborn

Vascular alterations of the umbilical cord, among other placental or maternal vascular pathologies such as chorioamnionitis, hypertension or preeclampsia [42–44] can affect foetal oxygenation during pregnancy. Foetal hypoxia results in anaerobic metabolism in which organic acids such as lactate and ketoacids are produced, leading to metabolic or mixed acidosis.

Different environmental or non-environmental stimuli that make up the intrauterine environment can affect gene expression in the umbilical cord and placenta [45]. The epigenetic changes produced by DNA methylation in different tissues can be decisive in the development of the umbilical cord, placenta, and therefore in the fetus and newborn [45]. These changes conform the concept of fetal health programming. During pregnancy, the hypoxia produced by these vascular alterations leads to a state of fetal programming that can affect the health of the newborn and subsequent development during childhood and adulthood [46,47], affecting cardiac, cerebral or renal function [46]. This concept of fetal programming is evolving as the mechanisms that explain it become clearer [46].

Foetal vascular malperfusion is one of the main patterns of placental damage and is the second most frequent cause of cerebral palsy. Involvement of the umbilical cord has been associated with greater foetal vascular malperfusion at the distal villous level [8].

The pH of arterial and venous blood extracted from the cord at the time of birth can be useful to identify newborns at higher risk of an adverse event in the first hours of life [48], although the criteria for performing this measurement are not clearly established. A pH lower than 7 is a criterion of neonatal asphyxia [48], although the extraction of the umbilical vein or artery should be taken into account. Although this is closely related to neonatal morbidity and mortality, the consequences for the foetus and newborn vary [49], and most newborns do not present long-term neurological or behavioural alterations [50–52].

In addition, elevated lactate is a predictor of short-term neonatal morbidity [53] and is associated with increased risks of moderate-severe encephalopathy, cerebral palsy and other cognitive and neurodevelopment alterations [54].

The Apgar Score is used as a quick assessment of the newborn [55] consisting in the assessment of: heart rate, respiratory effort, muscle tone, color and reflex irritability.

Perinatal risk factors can affect the immediate general condition of the newborn [56]. A reduced value in Apgar score could be a predictor of neonatal mortality, especially in very preterm infants [57,58]. However, it is not appropriate to use it alone to identify asphyxia [55]. Also, a high Apgar score could not be sufficient to identify well being newborns as mild metabolic acidosis could be missed [59].

Some studies show a significant and positive correlation between Apgar score and cord pH values [60–62]. This correlation has been proved specially in high-risk pregnancies, where the use of cord pH and Apgar Score could be crucial [56].

3. Umbilical Cord Alterations Related to Non-Hypertensive Maternal Diseases

Many pregnant women suffer endocrine disorders before and during pregnancy. These conditions have been identified as major contributors to stillbirth [63].

Diabetes Mellitus and carbohydrate intolerance are some frequent metabolic diseases during pregnancy that could affect the structure of the umbilical cord. Some studies suggest that even with optimum glycemic control, diabetes mellitus may be a cause of placental alterations and vascular dysfunction [64–66]. Mothers with gestational diabetes mellitus show a down-regulation of vascular endothelial growth factor A (VEGFA), which has a critical role in angiogenesis, producing an abnormal coiling pattern of the umbilical cord [67]. Histopathologic changes have also been described such as a discontinuous endothelial cell of the intima, extravasation of arterial blood to Wharton's jelly, thinner vein wall, and larger lumen [68]. Also, hypo-coiling has been described as one of the main abnormal patterns of coiling in gestational diabetes [69].

Nowadays, obesity has become a frequent condition among pregnant women. Usually is accompanied by other important conditions such as hypertension and diabetes. It is one of the most important preventable causes of stillbirth [70]. A recent study suggests that umbilical cord abnormalities may account for approximately one-fourth of the effect of obesity on the risk of stillbirth at term [71]. Umbilical hyper coiling, velamentous and marginal cord insertion, thrombosis, and long cord have been described in obese women and all these complications are common causes of stillbirth [71]. Moreover, low umbilical cord blood pH has been found in obese pregnant women, proving that obesity can be an independent risk factor for fetal acidosis at birth increasing newborn morbimortality [72].

4. Hypertensive Disorders and Chronic Venous Disease during Pregnancy: Placental and Umbilical Cord Alterations

4.1. Hypertensive Disorders during Pregnancy

Both the placenta and the umbilical cord are vascular structures that can be altered by systemic or local vascular changes, including those produced by hypertensive disorders of pregnancy such as chronic hypertension, pregnancy-induced hypertension, preeclampsia, HELLP syndrome and eclampsia [73].

Pregnancy-induced hypertension has been linked to histopathological changes in umbilical vessels. Specifically, a decrease in the lumen of the umbilical vein has been described, along with thickening of the tunica media, increased elastic fibres and decreased collagen fibres [44]. The haemodynamic alterations resulting from these changes would impact foetal blood flow and the foetus. These vascular histopathological changes produce an increase in resistance to the flow of the uterine artery. Recently, it has been proposed that analysis of flow velocity waveforms using machine learning analysis, could be useful to improve the diagnosis of umbilical cord abnormalities [74].

Preeclampsia is a pregnancy condition in wich new-onset hypertension occurs after 20 weeks of gestation and it is related to severe obstetric complications. If affects 2–8% of pregnancies ant it is associated with complications such as FGR and preterm delivery [43].

Decreases in the venous area and wall thickness of the umbilical cord have been observed in pregnant women with preeclampsia and may impact cardiovascular development in the foetus and newborn [43]. However, other studies have reported increased wall and tunica media thickness and an increase in the wall-luminal ratio [53]; therefore, more studies analysing these structural changes are needed. The utility of Doppler ultrasonography in predicting pre-eclampsia has not been extensively studied [75]. However, some studies show that abnormal Doppler ultrasonography has good overall sensitivity in predicting pre-eclampsia [75]. Some studies have also found relationships of preeclampsia with hypercoiling, marginal and paramarginal insertion, and SUA [73].

4.2. Chronic Venous Disease during Pregnancy: Placental and Umbilical Cord Alterations and Their Impact on the Foetus and the Newborn

Chronic venous disease (CVD) is a vascular disorder characterized by increased venous hypertension and insufficient venous return from the lower limbs [76]. The haemodynamic changes that occur during pregnancy, such as vasodilation, compression of iliac veins and venous stasis, favour its development [77–80]. CVD has been associated with several alterations in placental structure and function [80–82]. However, the foetal and neonatal repercussions remain unclear and require comprehensive investigation.

At the placental level, CVD has been linked to changes at the level of placental angiogenesis [80], including increases in lymphangiogenesis and angiogenesis. However, the impacts of CVD on placental function, the foetus and the newborn are still unclear.

Elevations of the markers VEGF, TGF beta and PEDF have been observed in the placentas of pregnant women with CVD [81]. These changes suggest that CVD affects the proper development and functioning of the circulatory system, which ensures the correct supply of nutrients and oxygen to the foetus.

CVD has been linked to an increase in the production of reactive oxygen species (ROS) in the venous wall and plasma of affected patients. Elevation of oxidized NADPH (NOXs) has been linked to placental pathology [83] and hypertensive disorders of pregnancy, such as preeclampsia [84]. This oxidative stress has also been detected in the umbilical cord and umbilical foetal blood [85]. At the umbilical level, increases in the gene and protein expression of NOX-1, NOX-2, iNOS, HIF-1alpha and MDA have been observed [86].

Oxidative stress has been linked to ultrasound and cardiotocographic alterations [87,88] such as intrauterine growth retardation, foetal growth restriction, or preterm delivery. According to the foetal programming hypothesis, this oxidative stress is thought to affect the subsequent development of neonatal pathology [87].

In addition, decreases in the expression of cadherin, cadherin 17 and cadherin 6 in the placentas of pregnant women with CVD have been described [89]. Some studies suggest that cadherins are involved in changes in placentation [90–92].

Moreover, pregnancy itself is a proinflammatory state [93,94]. The foetus and neonate are also participants in this proinflammatory state [95]. Some studies have shown that gestational CVD favours this proinflammatory state, as indicated by increases in the levels of proinflammatory cytokines (IL-6, IL-12, TNF-α, IL-10, IL-13, IL-2, IL-7, IFN-γ, IL-4, IL-5, IL-21, IL-23, GM-CSF, chemokines (fractalkine), MIP-3α and MIP-1β) in pregnant women with CVD and in the umbilical cord blood of their newborns [76]. At the foetal and neonatal levels, this proinflammatory profile has been related to multiple pathologies, such as preeclampsia, preterm delivery, and the development of bronchial hyperresponsiveness or overweight during the first years of life and therefore forms part of the so-called "foetal programming" [46,47].

5. Conclusions

The umbilical cord is the link between the foetus and mother and is key in the proper functioning of foetal-placental circulation. As showed in Figure 1, there are plenty possible vascular alterations that may affect the umbilical cord and maternofoetal structures. These vascular alterations of the umbilical cord can compromise or modify foetal blood flow. Hence, changes in the umbilical cord can have a variety of perinatal and neonatal level implications depending on clinical severity as showed in Table 1. Alterations at the level of the umbilical cord are closely related to foetal programming and thus impact the health of the newborn at birth and in later childhood. This array of vascular alterations and CVD emphasizes the need for more studies that allow the establishment of ultrasound, anatomical, histological or plasma markers for the early diagnosis of foetal or prenatal pathologies to prevent foetal and neonatal morbidity and mortality.

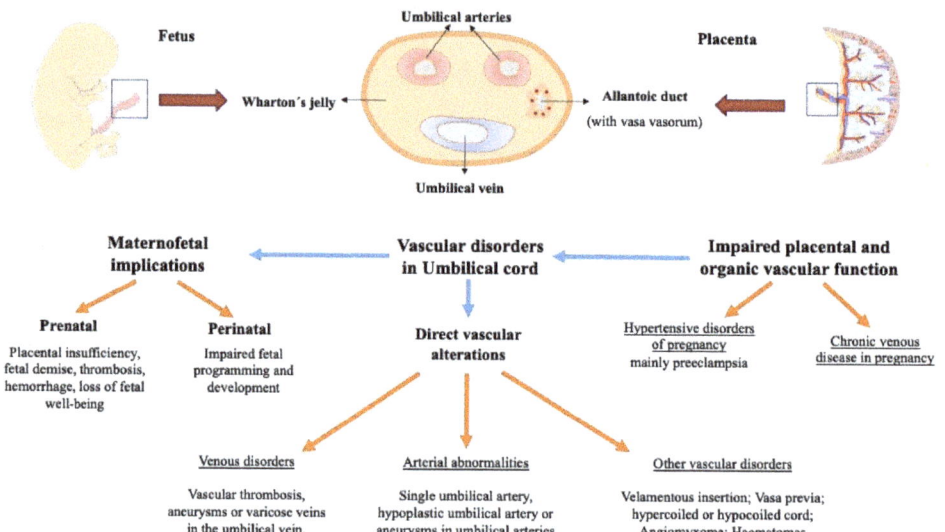

Figure 1. Histological description and vascular alterations observed in the umbilical cord or affecting the umbilical cord, along with the many maternofoetal consequences derived.

Table 1. Main vascular alterations of the umbilical cord and their impact on the foetal well-being and the newborn.

Pathology	Cause and Risk Factors	Vascular Alteration	Impact	References
Single umbilical artery (SUA)	Primary agenesis, atresia, or secondary atrophy. Chromosomal abnormalities.	Variation of the anatomy of the cord in which only a single umbilical artery is present. Absence of the left umbilical artery is more frequent. Occurs in 0.5–5% of spontaneous pregnancies.	There is no clear relationship of this isolated variant with a certain foetal or neonatal pathology, although studies suggest that there could be increased risks of preterm delivery, caesarean section, low birth weight, small for gestational age newborn and admission to the NICU. The association of SUA with other chromosomal or anatomical abnormalities (malformation of the urinary system, cardiovascular system and digestive system) may also imply changes in foetal and neonatal development.	[9–11]
Umbilical artery aneurysm	SUA. Trisomy 18.	Turbulent pulsatile flow at the ultrasound level. Found in areas close to the placental insertion site that are less protected by Wharton's jelly, usually during the second or third trimester of gestation.	They are associated with delayed intrauterine growth, aneuploidy and foetal demise.	[13]

Table 1. *Cont.*

Pathology	Cause and Risk Factors	Vascular Alteration	Impact	References
Pregnancy-induced hypertension	Risk factors: primary hypertension, renal disease, diabetes, multiple gestations.	Decrease in the lumen of the umbilical vein, thickening of the tunica media, increase in elastic fibres and a decrease in collagen fibres.	Influences foetal blood flow and potentially the foetus	[44,74]
Preeclampsia	Unknown cause.	Decreased venous area and wall thickness in the umbilical cords. Other studies show an increased wall thickness, with increases in the thickness of the tunica media and wall-luminal ratio. Some studies also show relationships of preeclampsia with hypercoiling, marginal and paramarginal insertion and SUA.	Associated with FGR (foetal growth restriction) and preterm delivery. Some studies suggest relationship with hyoercoiling, marginal and paramarginal insertion and SUA.	[43,73,75]
Vascular thrombosis: umbilical cord thrombi.	Maternal coagulation disorders, vascular endothelial damage, elevated blood glucose. Risk factors: hypercoiling, long cord, narrowed cord.	They mainly affect the umbilical vein and are related to vellum insertion of the cord and an excess of cord coiling, with long cords and little Wharton jelly.	They are related to FGR and foetal demise.	[14,15]
Varicose veins or umbilical vein aneurysms	No specific causes and risk factors known.	They are more frequent than umbilical artery aneurysms. Turbulent nonpulsatile flows occur in dilation zones. They are diagnosed by visualizing dilations greater than 9 mm in diameter or with a diameter greater than 50% of the unaffected vessel. They can be intra- or extra-abdominal.	They do not usually have foetal repercussions. Some studies have found an increased risk of intra-amniotic haemorrhage, low birth weight or foetal demise.	[17–19]
Velamentous cord insertion and vasa praevia.	No specific causes and risk factors known.	Velamentous insertion of the umbilical cord consists of the divergence of umbilical vessels, unsupported by the umbilical cord or placental tissue, as they traverse amnion and chorion before reaching the placenta with little Wharton jelly and susceptibility to compression. Vasa praevia consists in an anomaly of the umbilical vessels that cross the membranes of the low uterine segment, unsupported by umbilical cord or placental tissue, with a hight risk of rupture of the vessels	The rupture of membranes can cause the rupture of vessels with risk of exsanguination and foetal demise. Flow compression can translate into placental infarcts and limb amputations. In addition, there are increased risks of low birth weight and perinatal death.	[20–26]

Table 1. Cont.

Pathology	Cause and Risk Factors	Vascular Alteration	Impact	References
Hypercoiled umbilical cord	No specific causes and risk factors known.	Modifies fetoplacental flow.	Increased risk of adverse perinatal events and foetal demise, increased risk of preterm delivery, loss of foetal well-being, meconium amniotic fluid, Apgar > 7, small for gestational age, foetal and cardiac abnormalities, foetal demise and admission to the NICU.	[28,29]
Hypocoiled umbilical cord	No specific causes and risk factors known.	Modifies fetoplacental flow.	Increased risk of adverse perinatal events and foetal demise, chronic foetal vascular obstruction, stillbirth, increased risk of preterm delivery, loss of foetal well-being, meconium amniotic fluid, Apgar > 7, small for gestational age, foetal and cardiac abnormalities, foetal demise and admission to the NICU.	[28,29]
Thin umbilical cord	No specific causes and risk factors known.	Favours vascular compression with repercussions for foetal flow and uterine growth.	Small placental size, low birth weight, placental insufficiency, intrauterine growth restriction and low birth weight.	[30,31,33,34]
Long umbilical cord	No specific causes and risk factors known.	Greater than 70 cm.	They allow wide foetal movements with greater risk of crossed and circular entanglement and true cord knots, which increases the risk of foetal demise.	[35]
Short umbilical cord	No specific causes and risk factors known.	Less than 35 cm.	Higher incidence of adverse events such as urgent caesarean section or low birth weight.	[32,34]
Umbilical angiomyxoma or haemangioma	Mostly incidental. Risk factors: Hydrops, cord torsion, foetal demise, rupture, haematomas.	Infrequent tumour that arises from the proliferation of mesenchymal angiogenic cells in a close relationship with the umbilical vessels. Solid cystic mass, echogenic and vascularized lesions, usually located in the area of foetal insertion.	Foetal demise due to the risk of compression of vessels, their rupture and formation of haematomas that compromise the umbilical flow to the foetus.	[36–38]
Umbilical haematoma	Mostly spontaneous. Risk factors: Invasive procedures (amniocentesis), infections, oligoamnios and morphological abnormalities.	Extravasation of blood from the umbilical vein to Wharton's jelly.	Loss of foetal well-being, intrapartum asphyxia and hypoxic-ischaemic encephalopathy in the newborn. Oligoamnios in the third trimester. Increased risks of prenatal and perinatal death.	[39–41]

Table 1. Cont.

Pathology	Cause and Risk Factors	Vascular Alteration	Impact	References
Chronic venous disease	Vsodilation, compression of iliac veins and venous stasis during pregnancy, favour its development.		Increases in the gene and protein expression of NOX-1, NOX-2, iNOS, HIF-1alpha and MDA. This oxidative stress has been linked to ultrasound and cardiotocographic alterations [87,88] such as intrauterine growth retardation, foetal growth restriction, or preterm delivery. Some studies have shown that gestational CVD favours this proinflammatory state, as indicated by increases in the levels of proinflammatory cytokines (IL-6, IL-12, TNF-α, IL-10, IL-13, IL-2, IL-7, IFN-γ, IL-4, IL-5, IL-21, IL-23, GM-CSF, chemokines (fractalkine), MIP-3α and MIP-1β). This proinflammatory profile has been related to multiple pathologies, such as preeclampsia, preterm delivery, and the development of bronchial hyperresponsiveness or overweight during the first years of life and therefore forms part of the so-called "foetal programming	[46,47,76,85,87,88]

Author Contributions: Conceptualization, L.S.-T., M.A.S., M.A.O.; methodology, L.S.-T., M.A.O.; software, L.S.-T., C.G.-M., O.F.-M.; validation, M.A.O.; formal analysis, L.S.-T., M.A.O.; investigation, L.S.-T., C.G.-M., O.F.-M., L.G.G., C.B., J.A.D.L.-L., J.V.S., J.B., M.A.-M., N.G.-H., M.A.S., M.A.O.; resources, M.A.-M., M.A.O.; data curation, L.S.-T., M.A.S., M.A.O.; writing—original draft preparation, L.S.-T., C.G.-M., O.F.-M., L.G.G., C.B., J.A.D.L.-L., J.V.S., J.B., M.A.-M., N.G.-H., M.A.S., M.A.O.; writing—review and editing, L.S.-T., C.G.-M., O.F.-M., L.G.G., C.B., J.A.D.L.-L., J.V.S., J.B., M.A.-M., N.G.-H., M.A.S., M.A.O.; supervision, M.A.O.; project administration, M.A.-M., M.A.O.; funding acquisition, M.A.-M. All authors have read and agreed to the published version of the manuscript.

Funding: This study (FIS-PI21/01244) has been supported by the Instituto de Salud Carlos III (Plan Estatal de I+D+i 2020–2027) and co-financed by the European Regional Development Fund "A Road to Europe" (ERDF) and P2022/BMD-7321 MITIC-CM, Halekulani S.L. and M.J.R.

Institutional Review Board Statement: Not applicable.

Informed Consent Statement: Not applicable.

Data Availability Statement: Not applicable.

Conflicts of Interest: The authors declare no conflict of interest.

References

1. Benirschke, K.; Kaufmann, P.; Baergen, R. *Pathology of the Human Placenta*, 6th ed.; Springer: New York, NY, USA, 2012.
2. Hammad, I.A.; Blue, N.R.; Allshouse, A.A.; Silver, R.M.; Gibbins, K.J.; Page, J.M.; Goldenberg, R.L.; Reddy, U.M.; Saade, G.R.; Dudley, D.J.; et al. Umbilical Cord Abnormalities and Stillbirth. *Obs. Gynecol.* 2020, 135, 644–652. [CrossRef] [PubMed]
3. Bohîlțea, R.E.; Dima, V.; Ducu, I.; Iordache, A.M.; Mihai, B.M.; Munteanu, O.; Grigoriu, C.; Veduță, A.; Pelinescu-Onciul, D.; Vlădăreanu, R. Clinically Relevant Prenatal Ultrasound Diagnosis of Umbilical Cord Pathology. *Diagnostics* 2022, 12, 236. [CrossRef] [PubMed]
4. AIUM-ACR-ACOG-SMFM-SRU Practice Parameter for the Performance of Standard Diagnostic Obstetric Ultrasound Examinations. *J. Ultrasound Med.* 2018, 37, E13–E24. [CrossRef] [PubMed]
5. Salomon, L.J.; Alfirevic, Z.; Berghella, V.; Bilardo, C.M.; Chalouhi, G.E.; Da Silva Costa, F.; Hernandez-Andrade, E.; Malinger, G.; Munoz, H.; Paladini, D.; et al. ISUOG Practice Guidelines (updated): Performance of the routine mid-trimester fetal ultrasound scan. *Ultrasound Obs. Gynecol.* 2022, 59, 840–856. [CrossRef] [PubMed]

6. Krzyżanowski, A.; Kwiatek, M.; Gęca, T.; Stupak, A.; Kwaśniewska, A. Modern Ultrasonography of the Umbilical Cord: Prenatal Diagnosis of Umbilical Cord Abnormalities and Assessement of Fetal Wellbeing. *Med. Sci. Monit.* **2019**, *25*, 3170. [CrossRef]
7. James, J.L.; Boss, A.L.; Sun, C.; Allerkamp, H.H.; Clark, A.R. From stem cells to spiral arteries: A journey through early placental development. *Placenta* **2022**, *125*, 68–77. [CrossRef]
8. Stanek, J. Umbilical cord compromise versus other clinical conditions predisposing to placental fetal vascular malperfusion. *Placenta* **2022**, *127*, 8–11. [CrossRef]
9. Li, T.; Wang, G.; Xie, F.; Yao, J.; Yang, L.; Wang, M.; Wang, J.; Xing, L.; Nie, F. Prenatal diagnosis of single umbilical artery and postpartum outcome. *Eur. J. Obs. Gynecol. Reprod. Biol.* **2020**, *254*, 6–10. [CrossRef]
10. Dagklis, T.; Siargkas, A.; Apostolopoulou, A.; Tsakiridis, I.; Mamopoulos, A.; Athanasiadis, A.; Sotiriadis, A. Adverse perinatal outcomes following the prenatal diagnosis of isolated single umbilical artery in singleton pregnancies: A systematic review and meta-analysis. *J. Perinat. Med.* **2021**, *50*, 244–252. [CrossRef]
11. Prucka, S.; Clemens, M.; Craven, C.; McPherson, E. Single umbilical artery: What does it mean for the fetus? A case-control analysis of pathologically ascertained cases. *Genet. Med.* **2004**, *6*, 54–57. [CrossRef]
12. Petrikovsky, B.; Schneider, E. Prenatal diagnosis and clinical significance of hypoplastic umibilical artery. *Prenat. Diagn.* **1996**, *16*, 938–940. [CrossRef]
13. Vyas, N.M.; Manjeera, L.; Rai, S.; Devdas, S. Prenatal Diagnosis of Umbilical Artery Aneurysm with Good Fetal Outcome and Review of Literature. *J. Clin. Diagn. Res.* **2016**, *10*, QD01. [CrossRef]
14. Zhu, Y.; Beejadhursing, R.; Liu, Y. 10 cases of umbilical cord thrombosis in the third trimester. *Arch. Gynecol. Obs.* **2021**, *304*, 59–64. [CrossRef]
15. Wei, J.; Li, Q.; Zhai, H. Umbilical artery thrombosis diagnosed at different gestational ages and fetal outcomes: A case series. *BMC Pregnancy Childbirth* **2021**, *21*, 788. [CrossRef]
16. Sepulveda, W.; Sebire, N.J.; Harris, R.M.; Nyberg, D.A. The Placenta, Umbilical Cord and Membranes. In *Diagnostic Imaging of Fetal Anomalies*, 2nd ed.; Lippincott Williams & Wilkins: Philadelphia, PA, USA, 2003; pp. 114–115.
17. Lallar, M.; Phadke, S.R. Fetal intra abdominal umbilical vein varix: Case series and review of literature. *Indian J. Radiol. Imaging* **2017**, *27*, 59–61. [CrossRef] [PubMed]
18. Navarro-González, T.; Bravo-Arribas, C.; Pérez-Fernández-Pacheco, R.; Gámez-Alderete, F.; de León-Luis, J. Resultados perinatales luego del diagnóstico ecográfico prenatal de variz de la vena umbilical intraabdominal. *Ginecol. Obs. Mex.* **2013**, *81*, 504–509.
19. Fung, T.Y.; Leung, T.N.; Leung, T.Y.; Lau, T.K. Fetal intra-abdominal umbilical vein varix: What is the clinical significance? *Ultrasound Obstet. Gynecol.* **2005**, *25*, 149–154. [CrossRef]
20. Buchanan-Hughes, A.; Bobrowska, A.; Visintin, C.; Attilakos, G.; Marshall, J. Velamentous cord insertion: Results from a rapid review of incidence, risk factors, adverse outcomes and screening. *Syst. Rev.* **2020**, *9*, 147. [CrossRef]
21. Turnpenny, P.D.; Stahl, S.; Bowers, D.; Bingham, P. Peripheral ischaemia and gangrene presenting at birth. *Eur. J. Pediatr.* **1992**, *151*, 550–554. [CrossRef]
22. Thuring, A.; Maršál, K.; Laurini, R. Placental ischemia and changes in umbilical and uteroplacental arterial and venous hemodynamics. *J. Matern. Fetal Neonatal Med.* **2012**, *25*, 750–755. [CrossRef]
23. McDermott, M.; Gillan, J.E. Chronic reduction in fetal blood flow is associated with placental infarction. *Placenta* **1995**, *16*, 165–170. [CrossRef] [PubMed]
24. Laurini, R.; Laurin, J.; Maršál, K. Placental histology and fetal blood flow in intrauterine growth retardation. *Acta Obs. Gynecol. Scand.* **1994**, *73*, 529–534. [CrossRef] [PubMed]
25. Beken, S.; Sarıyılmaz, K.; Albayrak, E.; Akçay, A.; Korkmaz, A. Extremity Necrosis Due to Intrauterine Arterial Ischemia. *Turk. J. Haematol. Off. J. Turk. Soc. Haematol.* **2021**, *38*, 222–223. [CrossRef]
26. Vahanian, S.A.; Lavery, J.A.; Ananth, C.V.; Vintzileos, A. Placental implantation abnormalities and risk of preterm delivery: A systematic review and metaanalysis. *Am. J. Obs. Gynecol.* **2015**, *213*, S78–S90. [CrossRef] [PubMed]
27. De Laat, M.W.M.; Franx, A.; Bots, M.L.; Visser, G.H.A.; Nikkels, P.G.J. Umbilical coiling index in normal and complicated pregnancies. *Obs. Gynecol.* **2006**, *107*, 1049–1055. [CrossRef]
28. Pergialiotis, V.; Kotrogianni, P.; Koutaki, D.; Christopoulos-Timogiannakis, E.; Papantoniou, N.; Daskalakis, G. Umbilical cord coiling index for the prediction of adverse pregnancy outcomes: A meta-analysis and sequential analysis. *J. Matern. Fetal Neonatal Med.* **2019**, *33*, 4022–4029. [CrossRef]
29. Ernst, L.M.; Minturn, L.; Huang, M.H.; Curry, E.; Su, E.J. Gross patterns of umbilical cord coiling: Correlations with placental histology and stillbirth. *Placenta* **2013**, *34*, 583–588. [CrossRef]
30. Brunelli, R.; de Spirito, M.; Giancotti, A.; Palmieri, V.; Parasassi, T.; di Mascio, D.; Flammini, G.; D'Ambrosio, V.; Monti, M.; Boccaccio, A.; et al. The biomechanics of the umbilical cord Wharton Jelly: Roles in hemodynamic proficiency and resistance to compression. *J. Mech. Behav. Biomed. Mater.* **2019**, *100*, 103377. [CrossRef]
31. Proctor, L.K.; Fitzgerald, B.; Whittle, W.L.; Mokhtari, N.; Lee, E.; MacHin, G.; Kingdom, J.C.P.; Keating, S.J. Umbilical cord diameter percentile curves and their correlation to birth weight and placental pathology. *Placenta* **2013**, *34*, 62–66. [CrossRef]
32. Yamamoto, Y.; Aoki, S.; Oba, M.S.; Seki, K.; Hirahara, F. Relationship Between Short Umbilical Cord Length and Adverse Pregnancy Outcomes. *Fetal Pediatr. Pathol.* **2016**, *35*, 81–87. [CrossRef]

33. Debebe, S.K.; Cahill, L.S.; Kingdom, J.C.; Whitehead, C.L.; Chandran, A.R.; Parks, W.T.; Serghides, L.; Baschat, A.; Macgowan, C.K.; Sled, J.G. Wharton's jelly area and its association with placental morphometry and pathology. *Placenta* **2020**, *94*, 34–38. [CrossRef] [PubMed]
34. Yamamoto, Y.; Aoki, S.; Oba, M.S.; Seki, K.; Hirahara, F. Short umbilical cord length: Reflective of adverse pregnancy outcomes. *Clin. Exp. Obs. Gynecol.* **2017**, *44*, 216–219. [CrossRef]
35. Suzuki, S. Excessively long umbilical cord: A preventive factor of miserable outcomes of pregnancies with true umbilical cord knots. *J. Matern. Fetal Neonatal Med.* **2020**, *33*, 3757–3760. [CrossRef] [PubMed]
36. Kaur, N.; Heerema-McKenney, A.; Kollikonda, S.; Karnati, S. Changing Course of an Umbilical Cord Mass—Chasing the Diagnosis of Angiomyxoma. *Pediatr. Dev. Pathol.* **2022**, *25*, 558–561. [CrossRef] [PubMed]
37. Göksever, H.; Celiloğlu, M.; Küpelioğlu, A. Angiomyxoma: A rare tumor of the umbilical cord. *J. Turk. Ger. Gynecol. Assoc.* **2010**, *11*, 58. [PubMed]
38. Vougiouklakis, T.; Mitselou, A.; Zikopoulos, K.; Dallas, P.; Charalabopoulos, K. Ruptured hemangioma of the umbilical cord and intrauterine fetal death, with review data. *Pathol. Res. Pract.* **2006**, *202*, 537–540. [CrossRef] [PubMed]
39. Khatiwada, P.; Alsabri, M.; Wiredu, S.; Kusum, V.; Kiran, V. Spontaneous Umbilical Cord Hematoma. *Cureus* **2021**, *13*, 185–190. [CrossRef] [PubMed]
40. Gualandri, G.; Rivasi, F.; Santunione, A.L.; Silingardi, E. Spontaneous umbilical cord hematoma: An unusual cause of fetal mortality: A report of 3 cases and review of the literature. *Am. J. Forensic Med. Pathol.* **2008**, *29*, 185–190. [CrossRef]
41. Clermont-Hama, Y.; Thibouw, K.; Devisme, L.; Franquet-Ansart, H.; Stichelbout, M.; Subtil, D. Risk factors for spontaneous hematoma of the umbilical cord: A case-control study. *Placenta* **2020**, *99*, 152–156. [CrossRef]
42. Wright, R.G.; Macindoe, C.; Green, P. Placental Abnormalities Associated with Childbirth. *Acad. Forensic Pathol.* **2019**, *9*, 2–14. [CrossRef]
43. Herzog, E.M.; Eggink, A.J.; Reijnierse, A.; Kerkhof, M.A.M.; de Krijger, R.R.; Roks, A.J.M.; Reiss, I.K.M.; Nigg, A.L.; Eilers, P.H.C.; Steegers, E.A.P.; et al. Impact of early-and late-onset preeclampsia on features of placental and newborn vascular health. *Placenta* **2017**, *49*, 72–79. [CrossRef]
44. Koech, A.; Ndungu, B.; Gichangi, P. Structural Changes in Umbilical Vessels in Pregnancy Induced Hypertension. *Placenta* **2008**, *29*, 210–214. [CrossRef]
45. Green, B.B.; Marsit, C.J. Select Prenatal Environmental Exposures and Subsequent Alterations of Gene-Specific and Repetitive Element DNA Methylation in Fetal Tissues. *Curr. Environ. Health Rep.* **2015**, *2*, 126–136. [CrossRef]
46. Fajersztajn, L.; Veras, M.M. Hypoxia: From Placental Development to Fetal Programming. *Birth Defects Res.* **2017**, *109*, 1377–1385. [CrossRef]
47. Konkel, L. Lasting Impact of an Ephemeral Organ: The Role of the Placenta in Fetal Programming. *Environ. Health Perspect.* **2016**, *124*, A124. [CrossRef]
48. Gilstrap, L.C.; Leveno, K.J.; Burris, J.; Williams, M.L.; Little, B.B. Diagnosis of birth asphyxia on the basis of fetal pH, Apgar score, and newborn cerebral dysfunction. *Am. J. Obs. Gynecol.* **1989**, *161*, 825–830. [CrossRef]
49. Malin, G.L.; Morris, R.K.; Khan, K.S. Strength of association between umbilical cord pH and perinatal and long term outcomes: Systematic review and meta-analysis. *BMJ* **2010**, *340*, 1121. [CrossRef]
50. Andres, R.L.; Saade, G.; Gilstrap, L.C.; Wilkins, I.; Witlin, A.; Zlatnik, F.; Hankins, G.V. Association between umbilical blood gas parameters and neonatal morbidity and death in neonates with pathologic fetal acidemia. *Am. J. Obs. Gynecol.* **1999**, *181*, 867–871. [CrossRef]
51. Knutzen, L.; Svirko, E.; Impey, L. The significance of base deficit in acidemic term neonates. *Am. J. Obs. Gynecol.* **2015**, *213*, e1–e373. [CrossRef]
52. Dain, C.; Roze J christophe Olivier, M.; Bossard, M.; Praud, M.; Flamant, C. Neurodevelopmental outcome at 24 months of healthy infants at birth with an umbilical artery blood pH ≤ 7 and/or hyperlactacidemia ≥ 7 mmol/L. *Birth* **2021**, *48*, 178–185. [CrossRef]
53. Tuuli, M.G.; Stout, M.J.; Shanks, A.; Odibo, A.O.; Macones, G.A.; Cahill, A.G. Umbilical cord arterial lactate compared with pH for predicting neonatal morbidity at term. *Obs. Gynecol.* **2014**, *124*, 756–761. [CrossRef] [PubMed]
54. White, C.R.H.; Doherty, D.A.; Henderson, J.J.; Kohan, R.; Newnham, J.P.; Pennell, C.E. Accurate prediction of hypoxic-ischaemic encephalopathy at delivery: A cohort study. *J. Matern. Fetal Neonatal Med.* **2012**, *25*, 1653–1659. [CrossRef] [PubMed]
55. Watterberg, K.L.; Aucott, S.; Benitz, W.E.; Cummings, J.J.; Eichenwald, E.C.; Goldsmith, J.; Poindexter, B.B.; Puopolo, K.; Stewart, D.L.; Wang, K.S.; et al. The Apgar Score. *Pediatrics* **2015**, *136*, 819–822. [CrossRef]
56. Ahmadpour-Kacho, M.; Asnafi, N.; Javadian, M.; Hajiahmadi, M.; Taleghani, N.H. Correlation between Umbilical Cord pH and Apgar Score in High-Risk Pregnancy. *Iran. J. Pediatr.* **2010**, *20*, 401. [PubMed]
57. Cnattingius, S.; Norman, M.; Granath, F.; Petersson, G.; Stephansson, O.; Frisell, T. Apgar Score Components at 5 Minutes: Risks and Prediction of Neonatal Mortality. *Paediatr. Perinat. Epidemiol.* **2017**, *31*, 328–337. [CrossRef]
58. Mu, Y.; Li, M.; Zhu, J.; Wang, Y.; Xing, A.; Liu, Z.; Xie, Y.; Wang, X.; Liang, J. Apgar score and neonatal mortality in China: An observational study from a national surveillance system. *BMC Pregnancy Childbirth* **2021**, *21*, 47. [CrossRef]
59. Yılmaz, A.; Kaya, N.; Ülkersoy, İ.; Taner, H.E.; Acar, H.C.; Kaymak, D.; Perk, Y.; Vural, M. The Correlation of Cord Arterial Blood Gas Analysis Results and Apgar Scores in Term Infants Without Fetal Distress. *Turk. Arch. Pediatr.* **2022**, *57*, 538–543. [CrossRef]

60. Mlodawska, M.; Mlodawski, J.; Gladys-Jakubczyk, A.; Pazera, G. Relationship between Apgar score and umbilical cord blood acid-base balance in full-term and late preterm newborns born in medium and severe conditions. *Ginekol. Pol.* **2021**, *93*, 57–62. [CrossRef]
61. Omo-Aghoja, L. Maternal and fetal Acid-base chemistry: A major determinant of perinatal outcome. *Ann. Med. Health Sci. Res.* **2014**, *4*, 8. [CrossRef]
62. Kostro, M.; Jacyna, N.; Głuszczak-Idziakowska, E.; Sułek-Kamas, K.; Jakiel, G.; Wilińska, M. Factors affecting the differentiation of the apgar score and the biochemical correlation of fetal well-being—A prospective observational clinical study. *J. Mother Child* **2021**, *22*, 238–246. [CrossRef]
63. Monari, F.; Menichini, D.; Salerno, C.; Donno, V.; Po', G.; Melis, B.; Facchinetti, F. Impact of endocrine disorders on stillbirth: A prospective cohort study. *Gynecol. Endocrinol.* **2022**, *38*, 483–487. [CrossRef]
64. Campbell, I.W.; Duncan, C.; Urquhart, R.; Evans, M. Placental dysfunction and stillbirth in gestational diabetes mellitus. *Br. J. Diabetes Vasc. Dis.* **2009**, *9*, 38–40. [CrossRef]
65. Leach, L.; Taylor, A.; Sciota, F. Vascular dysfunction in the diabetic placenta: Causes and consequences. *J. Anat.* **2009**, *215*, 69. [CrossRef]
66. Pietryga, M.; Brązert, J.; Wender-Ozegowska, E.; Dubiel, M.; Gudmundsson, S. Placental Doppler velocimetry in gestational diabetes mellitus. *J. Perinat. Med.* **2006**, *34*, 108–110. [CrossRef]
67. Najafi, L.; Honardoost, M.; Khajavi, A.; Cheraghi, S.; Kadivar, M.; Khamseh, M.E. The association of umbilical coiling and angiogenesis markers: Impact assessment of gestational diabetes. *Placenta* **2022**, *129*, 70–76. [CrossRef]
68. Tenaw Goshu, B. Histopathologic Impacts of Diabetes Mellitus on Umbilical Cord During Pregnancy. *Pediatr. Health Med.* **2022**, *13*, 37–41. [CrossRef]
69. Najafi, L.; Khamseh, M.E.; Kashanian, M.; Younesi, L.; Abedini, A.; Valojerdi, A.E.; Amoei, Z.; Heiran, E.N.K.; Keshtkar, A.A.; Malek, M. Antenatal umbilical coiling index in gestational diabetes mellitus and non-gestational diabetes pregnancy. *Taiwan J. Obs. Gynecol.* **2018**, *57*, 487–492. [CrossRef]
70. Bodnar, L.M.; Parks, W.T.; Perkins, K.; Pugh, S.J.; Platt, R.W.; Feghali, M.; Florio, K.; Young, O.; Bernstein, S.; Simhan, H.N. Maternal prepregnancy obesity and cause-specific stillbirth. *Am. J. Clin. Nutr.* **2015**, *102*, 858–864. [CrossRef]
71. Åmark, H.; Westgren, M.; Sirotkina, M.; Varli, I.H.; Persson, M.; Papadogiannakis, N. Maternal obesity and stillbirth at term; placental pathology—A case control study. *PLoS ONE* **2021**, *16*, e0250983. [CrossRef]
72. Cardona-Benavides, I.; Mora-González, P.; Pineda, A.; Puertas, A.; Manzanares Galán, S. Maternal obesity and the risk of fetal acidosis at birth. *J. Matern. Fetal Neonatal Med.* **2022**, *35*, 765–769. [CrossRef]
73. Olaya, C.M.; Salcedo-Betancourt, J.; Galvis, S.H.; Ortiz, A.M.; Gutierrezb, S.; Bernal, J.E. Umbilical cord and preeclampsia. *J. Neonatal Perinat. Med.* **2016**, *9*, 49–57. [CrossRef] [PubMed]
74. Naftali, S.; Ashkenazi, Y.N.; Ratnovsky, A. A novel approach based on machine learning analysis of flow velocity waveforms to identify unseen abnormalities of the umbilical cord. *Placenta* **2022**, *127*, 20–28. [CrossRef] [PubMed]
75. Shahid, N.; Masood, M.; Bano, Z.; Naz, U.; Hussain, S.F.; Anwar, A.; Hashmi, A.A. Role of Uterine Artery Doppler Ultrasound in Predicting Pre-Eclampsia in High-Risk Women. *Cureus* **2021**, *13*, e16276. [CrossRef] [PubMed]
76. Ortega, M.A.; Gómez-Lahoz, A.M.; Sánchez-Trujillo, L.; Fraile-Martinez, O.; García-Montero, C.; Guijarro, L.G.; Bravo, C.; De Leon-Luis, J.A.; Saz, J.V.; Bujan, J.; et al. Chronic Venous Disease during Pregnancy Causes a Systematic Increase in Maternal and Fetal Proinflammatory Markers. *Int. J. Mol. Sci.* **2022**, *23*, 8976. [CrossRef] [PubMed]
77. Taylor, J.; Hicks, C.W.; Heller, J.A. The hemodynamic effects of pregnancy on the lower extremity venous system. *J. Vasc. Surg. Venous Lymphat. Disord.* **2018**, *6*, 246–255. [CrossRef]
78. Troiano, N.H. Physiologic and hemodynamic changes during pregnancy. *AACN Adv. Crit. Care* **2018**, *29*, 273–283. [CrossRef]
79. Ortega, M.A.; Fraile-Martínez, O.; García-Montero, C.; Álvarez-Mon, M.A.; Chaowen, C.; Ruiz-Grande, F.; Pekarek, L.; Monserrat, J.; Asúnsolo, A.; García-Honduvilla, N.; et al. Understanding Chronic Venous Disease: A Critical Overview of Its Pathophysiology and Medical Management. *J. Clin. Med.* **2021**, *10*, 3239. [CrossRef]
80. Ortega, M.A.; Saez, M.A.; Fraile-Martínez, O.; Asúnsolo, Á.; Pekarek, L.; Bravo, C.; Coca, S.; Sainz, F.; Mon, M.Á.-; Buján, J.; et al. Increased angiogenesis and lymphangiogenesis in the placental villi of women with chronic venous disease during pregnancy. *Int. J. Mol. Sci.* **2020**, *21*, 2487. [CrossRef]
81. Ortega, M.A.; Saez, M.Á.; Asúnsolo, Á.; Romero, B.; Bravo, C.; Coca, S.; Sainz, F.; Álvarez-Mon, M.; Buján, J.; García-Honduvilla, N. Upregulation of VEGF and PEDF in Placentas of Women with Lower Extremity Venous Insufficiency during Pregnancy and Its Implication in Villous Calcification. *BioMed Res. Int.* **2019**, *2019*, 5320902. [CrossRef]
82. Ortega, M.A.; Fraile-Martínez, O.; García-Montero, C.; Sáez, M.A.; Álvarez-Mon, M.A.; Torres-Carranza, D.; Álvarez-Mon, M.; Bujan, J.; García-Honduvilla, N.; Bravo, C.; et al. The Pivotal Role of the Placenta in Normal and Pathological Pregnancies: A Focus on Preeclampsia, Fetal Growth Restriction, and Maternal Chronic Venous Disease. *Cells* **2022**, *11*, 568. [CrossRef]
83. Schoots, M.H.; Gordijn, S.J.; Scherjon, S.A.; van Goor, H.; Hillebrands, J.L. Oxidative stress in placental pathology. *Placenta* **2018**, *69*, 153–161. [CrossRef] [PubMed]
84. Bedard, K.; Krause, K.H. The NOX family of ROS-generating NADPH oxidases: Physiology and pathophysiology. *Physiol. Rev.* **2007**, *87*, 245–313. [CrossRef] [PubMed]
85. Perrone, S.; Laschi, E.; Buonocore, G. Biomarkers of oxidative stress in the fetus and in the newborn. *Free Radic. Biol. Med.* **2019**, *142*, 23–31. [CrossRef] [PubMed]

86. Ortega, M.A.; Romero, B.; Asúnsolo, Á.; Martínez-Vivero, C.; Sainz, F.; Bravo, C.; de León-Luis, J.; Álvarez-Mon, M.; Buján, J.; García-Honduvilla, N. Pregnancy-associated venous insufficiency course with placental and systemic oxidative stress. *J. Cell. Mol. Med.* **2020**, *24*, 4157–4170. [CrossRef] [PubMed]
87. Perrone, S.; Laschi, E.; Buonocore, G. Oxidative stress biomarkers in the perinatal period: Diagnostic and prognostic value. *Semin. Fetal Neonatal Med.* **2020**, *25*, 101087. [CrossRef] [PubMed]
88. Draganovic, D.; Lucic, N.; Jojic, D.; Milicevic, S. Correlation of oxidative stress markers with ultrasound and cardiotocography parameters with hypertension induced pregnancy. *Acta Inf. Med.* **2017**, *25*, 19–23. [CrossRef]
89. Ortega, M.A.; Chaowen, C.; Fraile-Martinez, O.; García-Montero, C.; Saez, M.A.; Cruza, I.; Pereda-Cerquella, C.; Alvarez-Mon, M.A.; Guijarro, L.G.; Fatych, Y.; et al. Chronic Venous Disease in Pregnant Women Causes an Increase in ILK in the Placental Villi Associated with a Decrease in E-Cadherin. *J. Pers. Med.* **2022**, *12*, 277. [CrossRef]
90. Incebiyik, A.; Kocarslan, S.; Camuzcuoglu, A.; Hilali, N.G.; Incebiyik, H.; Camuzcuoglu, H. Trophoblastic E-cadherin and TGF-beta expression in placenta percreta and normal pregnancies. *J. Matern. Fetal Neonatal Med.* **2016**, *29*, 126–129. [CrossRef]
91. Duzyj, C.M.; Buhimschi, I.A.; Motawea, H.; Laky, C.A.; Cozzini, G.; Zhao, G.; Funai, E.F.; Buhimschi, C.S. The invasive phenotype of placenta accreta extravillous trophoblasts associates with loss of E-cadherin. *Placenta* **2015**, *36*, 645–651. [CrossRef]
92. Li, H.W.; Cheung, A.N.Y.; Tsao, S.W.; Cheung, A.L.M.; Wai-Sum, O. Expression of e-cadherin and beta-catenin in trophoblastic tissue in normal and pathological pregnancies. *Int. J. Gynecol. Pathol.* **2003**, *22*, 63–70. [CrossRef]
93. Raghupathy, R.; Kalinka, J. Cytokine imbalance in pregnancy complications and its modulation. *Front. Biosci.* **2008**, *13*, 985–994. [CrossRef]
94. Velez, D.R.; Fortunato, S.J.; Morgan, N.; Edwards, T.L.; Lombardi, S.J.; Williams, S.M.; Menon, R. Patterns of cytokine profiles differ with pregnancy outcome and ethnicity. *Hum. Reprod.* **2008**, *23*, 1902–1909. [CrossRef]
95. Agarwal, S.; Karmaus, W.; Davis, S.; Gangur, V. Immune markers in breast milk and fetal and maternal body fluids: A systematic review of perinatal concentrations. *J. Hum. Lact.* **2011**, *27*, 171–186. [CrossRef]

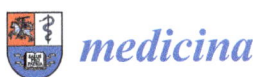

Review

Infective Endocarditis during Pregnancy—Keep It Safe and Simple!

Viviana Aursulesei Onofrei [1,2,†], Cristina Andreea Adam [1,3,*], Dragos Traian Marius Marcu [1,4,†], Radu Crisan Dabija [1,4,†], Alexandr Ceasovschih [1,2], Mihai Constantin [1,2], Elena-Daniela Grigorescu [1], Antoneta Dacia Petroaie [1] and Florin Mitu [1,3,5,6]

1. Department of Medical Specialties I, II, III and Preventive Medicine and Interdisciplinary, "Grigore T. Popa" University of Medicine and Pharmacy, University Street No. 16, 700115 Iasi, Romania
2. "St. Spiridon" Clinical Emergency Hospital, Independence Boulevard No. 1, 700111 Iasi, Romania
3. Cardiovascular Rehabilitation Clinic, Clinical Rehabilitation Hospital, Pantelimon Halipa Street No. 14, 700661 Iasi, Romania
4. Clinical Hospital of Pneumophthisiology Iași, Doctor Iosif Cihac Street No. 30, 700115 Iasi, Romania
5. Academy of Medical Sciences, Ion C. Brătianu Boulevard No. 1, 030167 Bucharest, Romania
6. Academy of Romanian Scientists, Professor Dr. Doc. Dimitrie Mangeron Boulevard No. 433, 700050 Iasi, Romania
* Correspondence: adam.cristina93@gmail.com
† This author has the same contribution as the first author.

Abstract: The diagnosis of infective endocarditis (IE) during pregnancy is accompanied by a poor prognosis for both mother and fetus in the absence of prompt management by multidisciplinary teams. We searched the electronic databases of PubMed, MEDLINE and EMBASE for clinical studies addressing the management of infective endocarditis during pregnancy, with the aim of realizing a literature review ranging from risk factors to diagnostic investigations to optimal therapeutic management for mother and fetus alike. The presence of previous cardiovascular pathologies such as rheumatic heart disease, congenital heart disease, prosthetic valves, hemodialysis, intravenous catheters or immunosuppression are the main risk factors predisposing patients to IE during pregnancy. The identification of modern risk factors such as intracardiac devices and intravenous drug administration as well as genetic diagnostic methods such as cell-free deoxyribonucleic acid (DNA) next-generation sequencing require that these cases be addressed in multidisciplinary teams. Guiding treatment to eradicate infection and protect the fetus simultaneously creates challenges for cardiologists and gynecologists alike.

Keywords: infective endocarditis; pregnancy; cardiovascular maternal risk; multidisciplinary approach; heart team

1. Infective Endocarditis during Pregnancy—An Introduction to a Complex Issue

Cardiovascular disease is responsible for complications in 1–4% of pregnancies and 25% of maternal deaths [1]. Infective endocarditis (IE) is a rare condition during pregnancy, with an extremely rare incidence rate of less than 0.01% [2]. From 1893 when the first case of IE was reported by William Bart Osler to the present day, advances in diagnostic methods and the development of new therapeutic molecules have allowed for prompt diagnosis as well as the possibility of quickly administering a targeted antibiotic regimen to reduce the risk of morbidity and mortality for both mother and fetus. The use of multiple imaging assessment methods affords the possibility of surgical intervention during the acute infectious process as well as the development of therapeutic guidelines with clear indications for the use of antibiotics in pregnancy which have laid the foundation for the clear management of this pathology, but with multiple challenges remaining for both mother and fetus [3,4].

IE is an infection of the endocardium and predominantly affects the anatomical structures on the left side of the heart [5]. The emergence of bacterial agents resistant to standard antibiotic therapy, the increasing identification of "modern" risk factors such as intracardiac devices and intravenous drug administration and the increasing prevalence of nosocomial infections are current challenges with multiple implications for pregnant women with IE, both medically, socially and economically [6,7].

The prognosis of patients with IE depends on the age at which pregnancy is achieved, as it is known that young age is associated with a high risk of obstetric complications. Epidemiological data in the literature highlights the high mortality rate of these pathologies, both for the mother (22%) and the fetus (15%) in the absence of prompt management from multidisciplinary teams [8].

Cardiovascular risk assessment is important to perform at every pregnancy, especially in patients with a history of heart disease prior to pregnancy. The guidelines of the European Society of Cardiology [9] for the assessment of cardiovascular disease recommend the application of the World Health Organization (WHO) classification of maternal cardiovascular risk assessment, with prognostic and therapeutic implications alike. A large proportion of clinical cases reported in the literature present as complications or cause of death the occurrence of heart failure or an acute embolic cardiovascular event [10].

This article aims to review the latest information from the literature on the complex management of IE during pregnancy starting from modern risk factors, plus genetic and molecular diagnostic methods, to potential therapeutic targets contributing to a multidisciplinary and integrative approach to these cases.

2. Materials and Methods

We searched the electronic databases of PubMed, MEDLINE and EMBASE for clinical studies addressing the management of infective endocarditis during pregnancy, with the aim of conducting a review of recent literature on this topic, from pathophysiological mechanisms to risk factors, signs and symptoms, as well as therapeutic management, maternal and fetal outcome and future research directions.

We used the following words or phrases for searching: "infective endocarditis" or "pregnancy", plus one of the following (in various associations): "cardiovascular risk", "cardiovascular mortality", "cardiovascular prognosis", "cardiovascular risk factors", "fetal risk", "fetal outcome". Observational studies, including prospective or retrospective cohort studies, RCTs, meta-analyses, guidelines and case reports related to our topic were included. All selected articles were then reviewed individually to select additional relevant publications from the reference section. Two independent reviewers selected studies by analyzing the title and abstract.

3. From Pathophysiology to Multidisciplinary Assessment

There are few cases reported in the literature of IE in pregnant women, which increases the importance for the academic world to understand the underlying mechanisms, the risk factors involved, the discovery of incriminating microorganisms and optimal therapeutic management, with maximum benefits for both fetus and mother.

3.1. Hemodynamic and Immunologic Adaptations during Pregnancy

The main physiological changes occur in the first weeks of pregnancy when some of the pregnant patients will exhibit clinical manifestations suggestive for various cardiovascular pathologies which were subclinical until that moment [11]. During pregnancy, a number of hemodynamic changes occur at the cardiovascular level predominantly affecting the hemodynamic status [12,13].

Heart rate increases on average by up to 25%, steady throughout pregnancy until the third trimester [14–16]. Starting from the 25th week of pregnancy, there is an increase in plasma volume on the one hand and on the other hand a 30% reduction in red blood cells which leads to dilution anemia [17,18].

The cardiac output increases as the pregnancy progresses, reaching in the third trimester 45% higher than baseline. Some patients may experience increases in cardiac output both at onset through increased stroke volume and in progression through vena cava compression [19].

Changes in blood pressure values should be carefully monitored during pregnancy to assess the hemodynamic impact on both mother and fetus [20,21]. Vascular resistance occurring in the first trimester of pregnancy will lead to a decrease in blood pressure values, especially for the systolic component where values can be up to 15 mmHg lower [11,22,23]. In a patient with right heart IE, the increased blood volume and hemodynamic changes described above create an increased pressure environment that can easily lead to pulmonary embolism. Systemic embolisms can occur in a similar way in pregnant patients with left heart IE [24].

During pregnancy a number of immunological adaptations occur to adapt to the fetus which increase the risk of infections [25,26]. During pregnancy, there are oscillations in immune status, with data in the literature showing a global suppression [27]. Different stages of pregnancy are associated with a distinct maternal immunological profile. Thus, if in the first trimester studies have shown the existence of a significant inflammatory substrate, the second trimester is characterized by a reduced inflammatory status creating a predisposition for the occurrence of infections [28]. If we corroborate these data with the presence of the risk factors mentioned above, we get a picture of a complex pathology, which requires a rapid and efficient multidisciplinary approach.

3.2. Demographics and Risk Factors

Demographic Data

The risk of developing IE for women with congenital heart disease is lower than that of men due to better dental and hand hygiene as well as lower rates of smoking and intravenous drug use [29–31]. Increased life expectancy and the rise in healthcare-associated infections have led to an increased incidence of IE among women, while in men studies have reported a decrease in incidents with age [32]. Gender also influences the mortality rate, with women having a higher risk than men [33]. An increased susceptibility to infections secondary to the relative immunosuppression associated with pregnancy exacerbates the negative impact of IE on both mother and fetus, both during pregnancy and in the first weeks postpartum [34].

Kebed et al. [35] conducted a systematic review based on an analysis of 72 clinical trials including 90 patients with peripartum IE. 98% of patients had native valve infections, with the most common cardiac structure involved being the mitral valve. In the antibiotic era, IE is no longer a disease of underdeveloped countries. Similar epidemiological phenomena have been reported in high income countries due to rising living standards and prophylactic antibiotic administration [36,37].

Risk Factors

The risk factors responsible for the development of IE in pregnant women are similar to those of the general population, the three main etiologies being intravenous drug administration, congenital heart disease and rheumatic heart disease [38,39]. 0.5% of patients with congenital heart disease develop IE during pregnancy [9].

In the past, the most common causes of IE in young people were rheumatic heart disease or congenital heart disease. Advances in technology have led to changes in the panel of predisposing factors over time, with age, frailty or the presence of comorbidities increasingly being blamed instead of prosthetic valves, hemodialysis, intravenous catheters or immunosuppression [40,41] (Figure 1).

Over 75% of patients who develop IE secondary to intravenous drug administration have endocardial damage, most commonly secondary to septic embolization at injection sites [42]. Tricuspid valve involvement is objectified in most cases, whereas pulmonary valve lesions are much rarer [43,44]. Isolated pulmonary valve IE is a rare entity, with few such cases reported in the literature, especially in pregnant women. Risk factors include pulmonary valve abnormalities, intravenous drugs or the presence of right heart catheters [45].

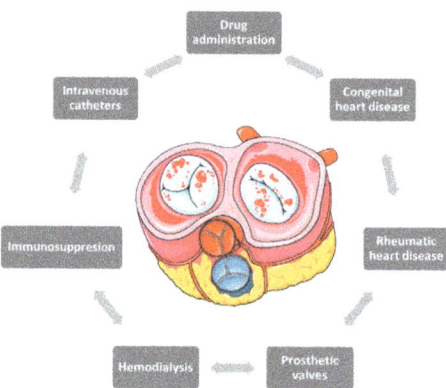

Figure 1. Risk factors involved in the onset of infective endocarditis in pregnancy.

There are few cases in the literature of IE involving devices used to close atrial septal defects in pregnant patients one year after the procedure. In a case series published by Amedro et al. [46], none of the 22 patients with atrial septal defects closed with minimally invasive surgery developed IE at more than one year. This clinical finding has a pathophysiological basis in the observation that bacterial insemination occurs before neo-endothelialization of implanted devices, most commonly in the first 3 months [47].

Pregnant women may associate a partially immunocompromised status that increases their risk of developing IE in the context of the presence of comorbidities with prognostic implications on the course of pregnancy or fetal viability. This justifies the continuation of antibiotic therapy beyond the 6-month period indicated by current clinical guidelines [48,49]. The susceptibility of pregnant women to certain infectious diseases or the modulation of their severity is closely related to the placental immune response and its tropism for certain pathogens [49,50]. These rare cases present diagnostic and treatment challenges, due to the lack of accurate therapeutic recommendations. Most pregnant women have been excluded from clinical trials that have investigated the indications for percutaneous closure of atrial septal defects or patent foramen ovale [51–53].

Bicuspid aortic valve is the most common congenital disease, affecting 1–2% of the general population. The occurrence of IE in these patients involves the presence of a susceptible endothelium which allows for the aggregation of platelets and fibrin at this level, with the consequent formation of thrombi which represent a favorable site for the proliferation of microorganisms [54].

In the literature, there are extremely few clinical cases reported of patients with mitral valve IE requiring simultaneous valve replacement and assisted cesarean delivery. One of the main concerns in these situations is the safety of the fetus which may be jeopardized by the need for a cardiopulmonary bypass [55]. The highest risks have been reported in fetuses with a gestational age of 26 weeks and a reported survival rate of less than 28% [56].

Etiological Agents

Streptococci and staphylococci are the main etiological determinants of IE [57]. Staphylococci are the most common pathogens, with *Staphylococcus aureus* being an increasingly isolated pathogen that has a negative prognostic role [58–60]. IE can coexist with other infections, usually caused by the same pathogen. The etiological agents of left heart IE are predominantly streptococci, with staphylococci more commonly associated with right heart involvement [61]. These cases are extremely rare in pregnancy, with very few such clinical scenarios reported in the literature. One such example is a *Streptococcus oralis* infection that caused IE and meningitis simultaneously [62]. *Streptococcus oralis* causes meningitis in patients undergoing spinal anesthesia or certain dental procedures, and is rarely associated with neonatal meningitis or maternal sepsis [63].

Bacillus cereus is a rare pathogen responsible for the occurrence of IE in the general population, with less than 20 such clinical cases reported to date. It occurs most commonly in drug users or those with implanted cardiac devices. Shah et al. [64] isolated *Bacillus cereus* in the tricuspid valve of a 25-week pregnant patient, this being the first case of *Bacillus cereus* infection in a pregnant woman. Khafaga et al. [58] reported for the first time *Staphylococcus lugdunensis* as an etiologic agent of IE in a pregnant woman. *Staphylococcus lugdunensis* is a coagulase-negative, skin commensal staphylococcus that colonizes the perineum [65,66].

Most cases of pregnant IE reported in the literature have a bacterial infection as a microbiological substrate, with rare cases of fungi underlying this potentially fatal complication for both mother and fetus [67,68]. IE with fungal pathogens such as *Zygomycetes* are frequently nosocomial, secondary to prolonged antibiotic therapy or intravenous catheterization [69,70]. Such a clinical situation was encountered in a pregnant woman previously diagnosed with positive serology for hepatitis B [67].

3.3. Diagnosis and Management

The diagnostic and therapeutic management of these cases must be prompt, taking into account the maternal impact of the associated morbidity and mortality as well as the high risk of fetal death [29,35,71]. The management of IE in pregnant women must be carried out in multidisciplinary teams that individualize the therapeutic plan and identify the optimal time for surgery (in selected situations) and pregnancy termination [72]. Literature data show a reduction of in-hospital ($p < 0.001$) and one-year mortality for pregnant patients treated with multidisciplinary teams [73–75]. The development of such models of good practice for the benefit of patients is an ongoing concern of clinicians and researchers in the field alike, with the well-being of the mother and the fetus at the center [75,76].

Clinical Picture

The clinical picture of pregnant patients with IE may be the classic one with fever, vascular murmurs, petechiae and clinical signs associated with anemia and embolization [2], or may be partially masked by other symptoms associated with pregnancy. Special attention should be paid to fever in pregnancy, as it is a symptom frequently associated with various causes such as chorioamnionitis, pneumonia, various viral infections and pyelonephritis [77].

Diagnostic Methods

The diagnostic algorithm of pregnant patients with IE is similar to that of the pathology in the general population. Identification of the infectious agent is achieved by bacterial cultures which remain the standard test for pregnancy IE. In patients with negative cultures, direct serological testing is performed. The guidelines of the European Society of Cardiology recommend the collection of three blood cultures from different venipuncture sites, taken at an interval of at least one hour between the first and the last [31,78]. Alternatively, molecular testing (e.g., PCR testing for *Tropheryma whipplei*) or histopathological testing using resected valves can be used. The modified Duke criteria help establish the diagnosis of IE based on clinical, echocardiographic or microbiological findings [79,80].

Cell-free deoxyribonucleic acid (DNA) next-generation sequencing is a useful diagnostic tool, superior to the methods presented above because of the longer time interval in which it can identify the pathogen compared to standard blood cultures [81–83]. Circulating cell-free DNA was first discovered in 1948 by Mandel et al. [84,85]. Blood contains small amounts of it, predominantly from bacteria, and is a veritable reservoir of genetic material from all the body's cells [86,87]. There are different types of cell-free DNA, the most common being circulating tumor DNA, cell-free mitochondrial DNA, cell-free fetal DNA and donor-derived cell-free DNA [88]. Recent studies have appreciated cell-free DNA as a potential clinical biomarker associated with endothelial dysfunction [89].

Cell-free DNA sequencing provides a rapid, non-invasive diagnosis, representing the only diagnostic resource in some cases of IE in which the infectious agent could not be identified by conventional microbiological identification methods [90]. In addition to diagnosis, this method can also be used for monitoring infectious pathologies or for early identification of recurrences, but further studies are needed on the decay of it in blood after treatment [91]. Decay kinetics after treatment have not been extensively reviewed in the literature to date, with few reports in the literature. Solanky et al. [91] presented the case of a 53-year-old patient diagnosed with IE involving *Bartonella quintana* at the level of the biological aortic prosthesis and periodically monitored decay kinetics after parenteral antibiotic therapy and valve resection. The group of investigators observed that after 4 weeks of parenteral antibiotic therapy, the cell-free DNA sequencing signal decreased by approximately 80%. Following excision of the aortic bioprosthesis, the decrease in cell-free DNA sequencing occurred in two phases, a rapid one in the first 24 h and a slow one occurring up to 48 h after surgery, which justifies its use as a method of monitoring the response to antibiotic therapy.

Cell-free DNA sequencing and other state-of-the-art molecular methods are showing their usefulness in the etiological diagnosis of IE, especially in those with negative bacterial cultures [92,93]. A representative example is metagenomic next-generation sequencing, which according to clinical studies published to date has a higher sensitivity than classical diagnostic methods [94,95]. Duan et al. [96] analyzed a group of 109 patients, both with and without different infectious pathologies, and demonstrated that although the sensitivity of the method is superior, no statistically significant differences were reported in specificity compared to cultures ($p = 0.41$). Comparing the infectious and non-infectious groups of patients, the investigators demonstrated that the duration of hospitalization and the 28-day death rate in the first group were statistically significant and superior. Advanced statistical techniques identified age as a determinant parameter in obtaining positive metagenomic next-generation sequencing analysis results.

Microbial cell-free DNA has a sensitivity of 89.3% and a specificity of 74.3% compared to blood cultures, with each additional day that positive results are reported associated with a 2.89-fold increased risk of metastatic infection ($p = 0.0011$) [97]. A recently published systematic review included a total of 13 clinical trials using this genetic diagnostic method in IE. Until August 2022, metagenomic next-generation sequencing has been used to identify gram positive cocci (8.9% of cases), coagulase-negative staphylococci (17.6% of cases), streptococci (37.5% of cases) and *Enterococcus faecalis* (6.6% of cases) [92]. This method not only enjoys advantages such as reduced processing time, the provision of real-time information and ease of obtaining a blood sample, but also a number of disadvantages such as the high cost of the molecular extraction technique and the lack of guidelines to give this method the status of an alternative technique to conventional diagnostic methods due to the lack of large clinical studies on large groups of patients confirming the data existing so far from limited reports (Figure 2) [98].

Cell-Free DNA has also been identified in pregnant patients in the maternal circulation. In 1997, a group of investigators identified Y-specific DNA fragments in the serum and plasma of pregnant patients, representing approximately 3.4–6.2% of the plasma [99]. This discovery led over time to the use of this genetic material for prenatal aneuploidy screening. Particularly for pregnant women, the significant correlations are between the vegetation length and the serum matrix metalloproteinase-9 level and the occurrence of embolic events. Based on this observation, Thruny et al. [100] demonstrated that 64% of patients with new embolic events had vegetations greater than 10 mm in size and a serum matrix metalloproteinase-9 titer greater than 167 ng/mL [101].

Multimodal Imaging Assessment

The imaging assessment of a pregnant woman with IE should focus on reducing the risk of fetal irradiation. The most commonly used methods of assessment and diagnosis are transthoracic echocardiography and nuclear magnetic resonance [77,102,103]. Echocardiographic identification of vegetations requires transesophageal echocardiography as soon as possible in patients at high risk of complications [78] (Figure 3). The CAPREG II study evaluated pregnant patients with various cardiovascular pathologies to identify predictors associated with a high risk of maternal complications such as mechanical prosthesis, high-risk associated aortic disease, pulmonary hypertension and chronic coronary syndrome [104]. Echocardiography also identifies a number of negative prognostic factors such as the presence of systolic dysfunction, the presence of a subaortic gradient of more than 30 mmHg or a pulmonary artery systolic pressure value of more than 50 mmHg in the absence of obstruction in the right ventricular outflow tract [105]. In addition to transthoracic echocardiography, transesophageal echocardiography is an additional imaging investigation required for patients with IE and mechanical valve prosthesis [106].

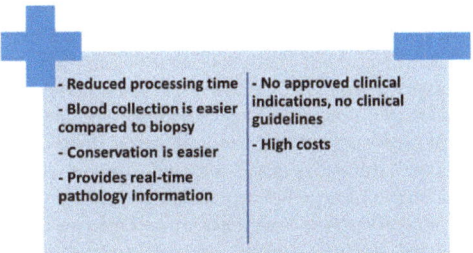

Figure 2. Advantages and disadvantages of using cell-free DNA sequencing in patients with IE.

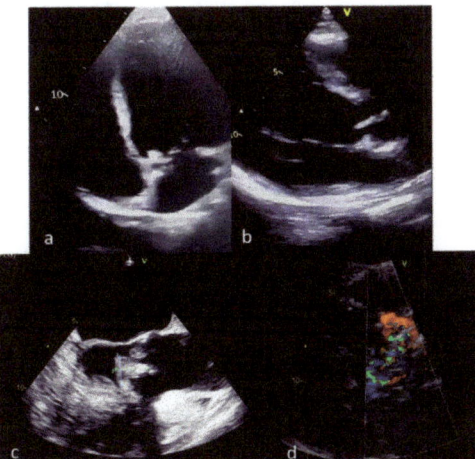

Figure 3. Echocardiographic findings in pregnant patients with IE (**a**,**b**): transthoracic echocardiography, aortic valve vegetations; (**c**): transesophageal echocardiography; (**d**): transthoracic echocardiography, aortic regurgitation secondary to aortic valve vegetation).

The persistence of the vegetation after the appearance of clinical signs of systemic embolization, plus the presence of a vegetation at the level of the anterior mitral valve of more than 10 mm, as well as the increase in the size of the vegetation at the end of the antimicrobial treatment, are echocardiographic arguments suggesting the need for surgery [107]. In terms of valve damage, a systematic review published by Kebed et al. [61] on 90 patients with peripartum IE highlights predominantly mitral valve damage in 30% of cases and then tricuspid valve damage in 25.6% of cases. The presence of IE involving the aortic valve was reported in a small number of cases (17.8%), with the percentage being half for the pulmonary valve (7.8%). The investigators of the same study highlighted concomitant damage to several valves in 12% of patients.

Valve dysfunction suggested by acute aortic or mitral regurgitation with associated signs of ventricular dysfunction or acute heart failure unresponsive to treatment along with valve perforation or rupture complete the list of indications for surgical treatment [78]. The greatest risk of embolization is for vegetations larger than 10 mm located in the anterior mitral valve [108,109]. Valvular perforations, valvular or perivalvular destructions, as well as myocardial abscesses, are echocardiographic features frequently encountered in patients with aortic bicuspid disease [110]. Lack of echocardiographic signs does not exclude IE, requiring a comprehensive, multidisciplinary interpretation of the clinical and paraclinical picture [7].

Therapeutic Management

Antibiotic administration must follow several principles in pregnant woman with IE and must be prompt, prolonged, personalized and combined [111]. Drug treatment of IE in pregnancy follows the principles of that given to the general population, but special attention must be paid to the fetotoxic effects of certain antibiotics [29]. Antibiotics are divided into several categories according to the safety associated with administration during pregnancy. Penicillin, ampicillin, amoxypenicillin, cephalosporins and erythromycin have no toxic effects on the fetus and can be administered to pregnant patients with IE in all trimesters according to clinical guidelines. Aminoglycosides, quinolones and tetracycline are recommended to be used in severe cases with a reserved prognosis for the mother, taking into account the associated risks. The same careful discernment is required for vancomycin, imipenem, rifampicin and teicoplanin, whose effects on the fetus cannot be excluded [9].

In pregnancy, it is recommended to delay surgery until the infection is eradicated. In high-risk situations for both mother and fetus, it is recommended to initiate antibiotic treatment for a short period of time prior to surgery despite the associated risk of pulmonary embolism [112]. Surgeries performed at a low gestational age are accompanied by low maternal risk, but fetal complications are frequently reported [113]. It is not recommended to perform surgery under 24 weeks of pregnancy, but to postpone it until 28 weeks of gestation due to the high risk of fetal death associated with insufficient growth [114]. Intravenous systems used with extracorporeal circulation for the removal of vegetation can be used as an alternative in the case of high-risk pregnancies [115].

In this population, special attention should be paid to metabolism in relation to the metabolism of administered medication, especially anesthetics [113]. From an obstetrical point of view, it is recommended to monitor the uteroplacental perfusion to maintain a mean arterial value above 70 mmHg in order to maximize its vascularity [116,117]. Pregnancy imposes a number of restrictions on the medications that can be administered, with current European guidelines recommending avoidance of renin-angiotensin-aldosterone system inhibitors and aldosterone antagonists [9,118,119]. Restrictions are also placed on inhaled anesthetics, propofol and ketamine, which stimulate neuronal apoptosis and thus negatively modulate the neuronal development of the fetus [120–122].

Intravenous tocolytics and antiepileptic medication are recommended during surgery to prevent the onset of labor [123]. Continuous monitoring of the fetus with cardiotocography is also recommended [2].

3.4. Complications and Prognostic Aspects of IE in Pregnant Women

The presence of IE in a pregnant patient, regardless of etiology, is accompanied by a high risk of short- and medium-term mortality due to multiple associated complications. Fetal viability may also be compromised in the absence of prompt management [124]. More than half of patients with IE deliver before term, at an average gestational age of 32 weeks [125]. The small number of cases presented in the literature provides little data on neonatal prognosis [126].

The most common complications that occur are congestive heart failure, perivalvular extension and systemic embolization (up to 50%) [127]. Literature data states that 50–60% of pregnant patients with IE develop some form of heart failure [128]. A recent clinical study published by Pillai et al. shows a correlation between the risk of occurrence of maternal complications (especially acute pulmonary oedema or congestive heart failure) and the risk class associated with pregnancy according to the WHO classification [124]. A recent analysis of 382 pregnant patients with IE reports cerebrovascular thrombosis ($p < 0.001$) and gastrointestinal ($p = 0.007$) and obstetric clots ($p < 0.001$) as the main postpartum complications, with negative socio-economic and medical impact [34]. Moreover, the percentage of patients where cesarean delivery was performed was higher compared to a cohort of pregnant women without an IE (56.1% vs. 2.2%) [34]. Humbert et al. [129] developed an algorithm to predict patients at high risk of cerebral embolism in which six variables were included: age, diabetes mellitus, atrial fibrillation, embolism prior to antibiotics, vegetation length and *Staphylococcus aureus* as etiologic agent. The greatest risk of embolization is in the first week after diagnosis [6,130]. Depending on the associated comorbidities, systemic embolization can occur in up to 50% of cases [65].

Mycotic aneurysms are another common complication in patients with IE, most commonly affecting the cerebral arteries in the intracranial segments [131,132]. Other complications rarely seen in pregnant patients with IE are splenic infarction and pulmonary embolism, the latter secondary to right heart IE [133,134]. Coronary embolization is a rare complication in pregnant women with IE and may be the etiological cause of silent myocardial infarction [55].

Complications in fetus are also varied and are accompanied by increased morbidity and mortality. IE during pregnancy increases the risk of stillbirth (odds ratio 2.96) or preterm birth (odds ratio 3.61) at an average gestational age of 32 weeks [34]. Premature birth is associated with a variety of fetal complications, the most common being low birth weight, low APGAR scores at birth, respiratory distress syndrome and intraventricular hemorrhage [73,135,136]. Clinical data show that about half of all newborns require prolonged hospitalization in the intensive care unit [73].

The appearance of pseudoaneurysms, fistulas and abscesses are other complications reported so far [137]. Surgical treatment becomes necessary if drug therapy is ineffective. Fetal viability also guides the need to induce labor before or during cardiac surgery [9]. Indications for surgery in pregnancy-associated IE are heart failure secondary to acute valvular regurgitation, large vegetations, sepsis or embolization [138].

The management of these cases is extremely complex, in which multidisciplinary teams must choose the best therapeutic strategy for mother and fetus alike [73]. Based on literature data, three types of clinical scenarios have been synthesized, with varying implications depending on the clinical and paraclinical data of the pregnant woman. The performance of cardiac surgery and continuation of pregnancy depends on several prognostic factors, the most important being the negative impact of cardiopulmonary bypass on the fetus and adverse effects associated with medication, especially vasoactive agents such as warfarin [55]. Vaginal or cesarean delivery followed by surgery is the second clinical scenario, which may induce worsening of heart failure in patients with hemodynamic instability. Another treatment option is to perform simultaneous caesarean section and cardiac surgery, paying special attention to the increased bleeding risk secondary to heparinization associated with cardiovascular bypass.

Cardiac surgery is also associated with a high risk for the fetus. Clinical guidelines recommend postponing cardiac surgery as much as possible until 6 weeks postpartum, and if not possible then to perform cardiac surgery in the second trimester between 13–28 weeks of pregnancy [139,140]. In some cases, the fetus may have transient or spontaneous bradycardia, which may subside at the end of surgery. As an alternative to fetal heart rate monitoring, uterine activity can be monitored. Early surgical treatment reduces the risk of embolization compared to conventional drug management by up to 25% ($p = 0.02$) [141]. Pre-pregnancy valve damage negatively influences the prognosis of pregnant women after surgery [142].

Cardiopulmonary bypass (CPB) is the biggest challenge of surgery, with literature data recommending caesarean birth prior to surgery to minimize the risk of death, which can be as high as 15% [143]. Cardiopulmonary bypass was first used in 1959 in a 6-week pregnant woman who underwent surgery to close an atrial septal defect [144]. CPB performed immediately postpartum carries a high risk of uterine bleeding, but the literature confirms that it can be performed relatively safely during pregnancy [58,145]. The main effects of cardiovascular bypass on the fetus are related to a number of factors such as timing of heparinization, infusion fluid temperature, infusion rate and associated pressure and temperature of the pregnant woman. Fetal death most commonly occurs during the cooling and rewarming periods of the bypass [39]. Maintaining the activated clotting time for more than 300 s prevents blood clots in the CPB circuit.

In the case of fetuses with a low gestational age, it is recommended to adjust cardiopulmonary bypass parameters by increasing infusion rates, maintaining normothermia and pulsatile flow and continuous monitoring of fetal heart rate [146]. The viability of the placenta is dependent on both maternal and fetal factors. Utero-placental hypoperfusion leads to bradycardia and fetal hypoxia [147]. Approximately one hour after interruption of a cardiopulmonary bypass, the fetus progressively develops respiratory acidosis secondary to increased placental vascular resistance through activation of eicosanoid products. This increase in fetal vascular resistance is poorly tolerated by the immature fetal myocardium [148–150].

Prematurity and stillbirth occur most frequently in urgent cases, accompanied by high surgical risk, multiple maternal co-morbidities or low gestational age [145]. Perioperatively, administration of progesterone prevents uterine contractions and magnesium sulphate and atosiban contribute to fetal protection and maintenance of viability [140]. It is recommended as much as possible to reduce the CBP time, increase the infusion rate and continue antibiotic therapy for up to 6 weeks after surgery [151].

Prevention of massive postpartum hemorrhage events is achieved in some situations by uterine balloon tamponade, ligation of branches of the uterine artery and concomitant administration of intravenous oxytocin [151].

IE is associated with a higher risk of death for both mother and fetus. Cardiac surgery during pregnancy is associated with a high maternal mortality rate of up to 7%, regardless of the gestational age of the fetus or the practice of caesarean section before [139]. Fetal survival is superior in the case of caesarean birth prior to surgery [139]. The highest risk of death is reported in fetuses under 26 weeks gestational age [56]. Death rates vary according to the location of the lesions, being about 40% for the aortic valve, 22% for the mitral valve and 10% for the tricuspid valve [152]. There is a direct proportional relationship between maternal and fetal mortality in relation to cardiac surgery. Thus, if the risk of maternal death is minimal in the second trimester (4.6%), and doubles in the third trimester (8.8%), the risk of fetal death decreases with increasing gestational age, reaching 29% in the third trimester compared to 45% in the first weeks of pregnancy. Cesarean birth before valve replacement is accompanied by the lowest risk for the fetus (6.7%), while for the mother no significant differences were reported compared to the existing statistical data for the 3rd trimester (8.8% vs. 8.3%) [139].

4. Impact of COVID-19 on the Etiopathogenic Mechanisms of IE

The COVID-19 pandemic was the biggest medical, economic and human challenge of the last decade [153,154]. Since the first infections and until now, multiple clinical studies have been conducted on the impact of this virus on patients with cardiovascular disease or who are apparently healthy. These results involving both diagnostic and therapeutic roles have ensured the dynamics of therapeutic strategies. A number of specific physiological conditions, such as pregnancy, were also investigated.

Epidemiological studies have shown that SARS-COV2 infection per se has been associated with a high risk of complications in pregnant patients (regardless of gestational stage), with these complications including high risk of pre-eclampsia, premature birth and gestational diabetes [155,156]. Pregnant women are more susceptible to significant complications, with a high risk of death secondary to a viral infection due to physiological changes in the respiratory and immune systems during pregnancy and the puerperal period [157].

The link between COVID-19 and IE has been investigated in several clinical trials and two potential, independent mechanisms have been proposed [158]. Based on an animal model, Liesenborghs et al. [159] emphasize the idea that endothelial injury predisposes patients to IE secondary to *S. aureus* insemination. The same group of investigators point to a second potential mechanism, focusing on the inflammatory process in heart valves that stimulates bacterial adhesion by increasing the expression of certain structures. Rajan et al. [160] analyzed the effects of COVID-19 on pregnant women with rheumatic heart disease and observed a high risk in both groups, with no statistical significance, however, in terms of both maternal and fetal risk. The proposed mechanisms require further clinical studies to confirm or disprove the connection between the two pathologies.

5. Future Directions

The management of IE during pregnancy is extremely challenging in terms of the complications that can arise for both mother and fetus, as well as the limitations of medication [161]. Changing the mode of antibiotic therapy administration from intravenous to oral (with the use of two different antibiotics with different mechanisms of action) in patients with left heart IE is non-inferior according to the results of the Partial Oral Treatment of Endocarditis trial [162,163]. Overuse of antibiotics has led to the emergence of resistance in many bacterial strains, which requires clinical research to find new molecules that can be administered to pregnant women with IE [164]. One such example is daptomycin which is recommended for patients with right-sided *Staphylococcus aureus* IE, unresponsive to conventional treatment [165,166]. There are not enough clinical trials to date to allow or prohibit its use in pregnancy [167].

Clinical data on the use of ultrasound contrast agents during pregnancy are conflicting, but current recommendations are still directed towards avoiding its use as much as possible [168]. Sonobactericide non-invasively removes IE biofilm using ultrasound-activated lipid-coated microbubbles [169,170]. Recent in vitro clinical studies have demonstrated the efficacy of microbubbles against IE-associated biofilm caused by *Staphylococcus aureus* by 84% degradation [171]. In a similar study, Kouijzer et al. [172] demonstrated that vancomycin-decorated microbubbles are able to bind to the cell walls of gram-positive bacteria. However, the promising results presented above require further clinical research specifically targeting pregnant patients with IE.

Recently, the first non-antibiotic antimicrobial direct lytic agent was tested by Fowler et al. [173] in a cohort of patients with both right- and left-sided IE determined by *Staphylococcus aureus*. The investigators demonstrated that this potential therapeutic target induced a rapid bacteriolytic effect by eradicating the biofilm to which the synergistic effect associated with antibiotic therapy was added [174]. This direction of research is a promising one, with multiple therapeutic and prognostic implications among IE patients.

6. Conclusions

IE in pregnancy is an ongoing challenge both diagnostically and therapeutically because of the poor prognosis (for both mother and fetus) in the absence of prompt and comprehensive management. The approach to these cases must be multidisciplinary in order to decrease the risk of maternal and fetal morbidity and mortality. The development of new diagnostic methods based on molecular genetics (such as cell-free DNA) offers future prospects for the early identification of rare microbial agents encountered in everyday practice. Facilitating the opportunity for surgical intervention, decreasing maternal mortality and choosing the optimal antibiotic therapy are some of the benefits of considering cases of pregnant IE in multidisciplinary teams.

Author Contributions: All authors contributed equally to this work. V.A.O., C.A.A. and D.T.M.M. wrote the paper; R.C.D. and M.C. helped revise the language; A.C., E.-D.G. and A.D.P. undertook review editing; V.A.O. and F.M. revised the final script. All authors have read and agreed to the published version of the manuscript.

Funding: This research received no external funding.

Institutional Review Board Statement: Not applicable.

Informed Consent Statement: Not applicable.

Data Availability Statement: Not applicable.

Acknowledgments: Figure 1 was partly generated using Servier Medical Art, provided by Servier, licensed under a Creative Commons Attribution 3.0 unported license, https://creativecommons.org/licenses/by/3.0/ (accessed on 10 February 2023). The images in Figure 3 belong to the personal collection of Aursulesei Onofrei.

Conflicts of Interest: The authors declare no conflict of interest.

References

1. Petersen, E.E. Racial/Ethnic Disparities in Pregnancy-Related Deaths—United States, 2007–2016. *Morb. Mortal. Wkly. Rep.* **2019**, *68*, 762. [CrossRef] [PubMed]
2. Yuan, S.-M. Infective Endocarditis during Pregnancy. *J. Coll. Physicians Surg. Pak.* **2014**, *25*, 6.
3. Grinberg, M.; Solimene, M.C. Historical Aspects of Infective Endocarditis. *Rev. Assoc. Médica Bras.* **2011**, *57*, 228–233. [CrossRef] [PubMed]
4. Kamani, C.H.; Allenbach, G.; Jreige, M.; Pavon, A.G.; Meyer, M.; Testart, N.; Firsova, M.; Fernandes Vieira, V.; Boughdad, S.; Nicod Lalonde, M.; et al. Diagnostic Performance of 18F-FDG PET/CT in Native Valve Endocarditis: Systematic Review and Bivariate Meta-Analysis. *Diagnostics* **2020**, *10*, 754. [CrossRef]
5. Frontera, J.A.; Gradon, J.D. Right-Side Endocarditis in Injection Drug Users: Review of Proposed Mechanisms of Pathogenesis. *Clin. Infect. Dis.* **2000**, *30*, 374–379. [CrossRef]
6. Prendergast, B.D. The Changing Face of Infective Endocarditis. *Heart* **2006**, *92*, 879–885. [CrossRef]
7. Habib, G.; Hoen, B.; Tornos, P.; Thuny, F.; Prendergast, B.; Vilacosta, I.; Moreillon, P.; de Jesus Antunes, M.; Thilen, U.; Lekakis, J.; et al. Guidelines on the Prevention, Diagnosis, and Treatment of Infective Endocarditis (New Version 2009): The Task Force on the Prevention, Diagnosis, and Treatment of Infective Endocarditis of the European Society of Cardiology (ESC). Endorsed by the European Society of Clinical Microbiology and Infectious Diseases (ESCMID) and the International Society of Chemotherapy (ISC) for Infection and Cancer. *Eur. Heart J.* **2009**, *30*, 2369–2413. [CrossRef]
8. Bigi, M.A.B.; Mollazadeh, R. Fatal Outcome of Infective Endocarditis in a Pregnant Marfan Woman. *Internet J. Cardiol.* **2007**, *4*. [CrossRef]
9. Regitz-Zagrosek, V.; Roos-Hesselink, J.W.; Bauersachs, J.; Blomström-Lundqvist, C.; Cífková, R.; De Bonis, M.; Iung, B.; Johnson, M.R.; Kintscher, U.; Kranke, P.; et al. 2018 ESC Guidelines for the Management of Cardiovascular Diseases during Pregnancy: The Task Force for the Management of Cardiovascular Diseases during Pregnancy of the European Society of Cardiology (ESC). *Eur. Heart J.* **2018**, *39*, 3165–3241. [CrossRef]
10. Montoya, M.E.; Karnath, B.M.; Ahmad, M. Endocarditis during Pregnancy. *South. Med. J.* **2003**, *96*, 1156–1157. [CrossRef]
11. Morton, A. Physiological Changes and Cardiovascular Investigations in Pregnancy. *Heart Lung Circ.* **2021**, *30*, e6–e15. [CrossRef]
12. Taranikanti, M. Physiological Changes in Cardiovascular System during Normal Pregnancy: A Review. *Indian J. Cardiovasc. Dis. Women WINCARS* **2018**, *03*, 062–067. [CrossRef]
13. Loerup, L.; Pullon, R.M.; Birks, J.; Fleming, S.; Mackillop, L.H.; Gerry, S.; Watkinson, P.J. Trends of Blood Pressure and Heart Rate in Normal Pregnancies: A Systematic Review and Meta-Analysis. *BMC Med.* **2019**, *17*, 167. [CrossRef]
14. Visentin, S.; Palermo, C.; Camerin, M.; Daliento, L.; Muraru, D.; Cosmi, E.; Badano, L.P. Echocardiographic Techniques of Deformation Imaging in the Evaluation of Maternal Cardiovascular System in Patients with Complicated Pregnancies. *BioMed Res. Int.* **2017**, *2017*, 4139635. [CrossRef]
15. Coad, F.; Frise, C. Tachycardia in Pregnancy: When to Worry? *Clin. Med.* **2021**, *21*, e434–e437. [CrossRef]
16. Sarhaddi, F.; Azimi, I.; Axelin, A.; Niela-Vilen, H.; Liljeberg, P.; Rahmani, A.M. Trends in Heart Rate and Heart Rate Variability During Pregnancy and the 3-Month Postpartum Period: Continuous Monitoring in a Free-Living Context. *JMIR mHealth uHealth* **2022**, *10*, e33458. [CrossRef]
17. Litmanovich, D.E.; Tack, D.; Lee, K.S.; Shahrzad, M.; Bankier, A.A. Cardiothoracic Imaging in the Pregnant Patient. *J. Thorac. Imaging* **2014**, *29*, 38–49. [CrossRef]
18. Datta, S.; Kodali, B.S.; Segal, S. Maternal Physiological Changes During Pregnancy, Labor, and the Postpartum Period. In *Obstetric Anesthesia Handbook*; Springer: New York, NY, USA, 2010; pp. 1–14, ISBN 978-0-387-88601-5.
19. Adeyeye, V.O.; Balogun, M.O.; Adebayo, R.A.; Makinde, O.N.; Akinwusi, P.O.; Ajayi, E.A.; Ogunyemi, S.A.; Akintomide, A.O.; Ajayi, E.O.; Adeyeye, A.G.; et al. Echocardiographic Assessment of Cardiac Changes during Normal Pregnancy among Nigerians. *Clin. Med. Insights Cardiol.* **2016**, *10*, 157–162. [CrossRef]
20. Abe, M.; Arima, H.; Yoshida, Y.; Fukami, A.; Sakima, A.; Metoki, H.; Tada, K.; Mito, A.; Morimoto, S.; Shibata, H.; et al. Optimal Blood Pressure Target to Prevent Severe Hypertension in Pregnancy: A Systematic Review and Meta-Analysis. *Hypertens. Res.* **2022**, *45*, 887–899. [CrossRef]
21. Mustafa, R.; Ahmed, S.; Gupta, A.; Venuto, R.C. A Comprehensive Review of Hypertension in Pregnancy. *J. Pregnancy* **2012**, *2012*, 105918. [CrossRef]
22. James, S.L.; Abate, D.; Abate, K.H.; Abay, S.M.; Abbafati, C.; Abbasi, N.; Abbastabar, H.; Abd-Allah, F.; Abdela, J.; Abdelalim, A.; et al. Global, Regional, and National Incidence, Prevalence, and Years Lived with Disability for 354 Diseases and Injuries

for 195 Countries and Territories, 1990–2017: A Systematic Analysis for the Global Burden of Disease Study 2017. *Lancet* **2018**, *392*, 1789–1858. [CrossRef] [PubMed]
23. Garovic, V.D.; Dechend, R.; Easterling, T.; Karumanchi, S.A.; McMurtry Baird, S.; Magee, L.A.; Rana, S.; Vermunt, J.V.; August, P. Hypertension in Pregnancy: Diagnosis, Blood Pressure Goals, and Pharmacotherapy: A Scientific Statement from the American Heart Association. *Hypertension* **2022**, *79*, e21–e41. [CrossRef] [PubMed]
24. Wang, J.; Wang, A.; Cui, Y.; Wang, C.; Zhang, J. Diagnosis and Treatment of Infective Endocarditis in Pregnancy: A Case Report. *J. Cardiothorac. Surg.* **2020**, *15*, 109. [CrossRef] [PubMed]
25. Kourtis, A.P.; Read, J.S.; Jamieson, D.J. Pregnancy and Infection. *N. Engl. J. Med.* **2014**, *370*, 2211–2218. [CrossRef]
26. Abu-Raya, B.; Michalski, C.; Sadarangani, M.; Lavoie, P.M. Maternal Immunological Adaptation During Normal Pregnancy. *Front. Immunol.* **2020**, *11*, 2627. [CrossRef]
27. Mor, G.; Aldo, P.; Alvero, A.B. The Unique Immunological and Microbial Aspects of Pregnancy. *Nat. Rev. Immunol.* **2017**, *17*, 469–482. [CrossRef]
28. Kumar, M.; Saadaoui, M.; Al Khodor, S. Infections and Pregnancy: Effects on Maternal and Child Health. *Front. Cell. Infect. Microbiol.* **2022**, *12*, 690. [CrossRef]
29. D'Alto, M.; Budts, W.; Diller, G.P.; Mulder, B.; Egidy Assenza, G.; Oreto, L.; Ciliberti, P.; Bassareo, P.P.; Gatzoulis, M.A.; Dimopoulos, K. Does Gender Affect the Prognosis and Risk of Complications in Patients with Congenital Heart Disease in the Modern Era? *Int. J. Cardiol.* **2019**, *290*, 156–161. [CrossRef]
30. Tutarel, O.; Alonso-Gonzalez, R.; Montanaro, C.; Schiff, R.; Uribarri, A.; Kempny, A.; Grübler, M.R.; Uebing, A.; Swan, L.; Diller, G.-P.; et al. Infective Endocarditis in Adults with Congenital Heart Disease Remains a Lethal Disease. *Heart* **2018**, *104*, 161–165. [CrossRef]
31. Habib, G.; Lancellotti, P.; Antunes, M.J.; Bongiorni, M.G.; Casalta, J.-P.; Del Zotti, F.; Dulgheru, R.; El Khoury, G.; Erba, P.A.; Iung, B.; et al. 2015 ESC Guidelines for the Management of Infective Endocarditis: The Task Force for the Management of Infective Endocarditis of the European Society of Cardiology (ESC). Endorsed by: European Association for Cardio-Thoracic Surgery (EACTS), the European Association of Nuclear Medicine (EANM). *Eur. Heart J.* **2015**, *36*, 3075–3128. [CrossRef]
32. Correa de Sa, D.D.; Tleyjeh, I.M.; Anavekar, N.S.; Schultz, J.C.; Thomas, J.M.; Lahr, B.D.; Bachuwar, A.; Pazdernik, M.; Steckelberg, J.M.; Wilson, W.R.; et al. Epidemiological Trends of Infective Endocarditis: A Population-Based Study in Olmsted County, Minnesota. *Mayo Clin. Proc.* **2010**, *85*, 422–426. [CrossRef]
33. Chen, H.; Zhan, Y.; Zhang, K.; Gao, Y.; Chen, L.; Zhan, J.; Chen, Z.; Zeng, Z. The Global, Regional, and National Burden and Trends of Infective Endocarditis From 1990 to 2019: Results From the Global Burden of Disease Study 2019. *Front. Med.* **2022**, *9*, 774224. [CrossRef]
34. Dagher, M.M.; Eichenberger, E.M.; Addae-Konadu, K.L.; Dotters-Katz, S.K.; Kohler, C.L.; Fowler, V.G., Jr.; Federspiel, J.J. Maternal and Fetal Outcomes Associated With Infective Endocarditis in Pregnancy. *Clin. Infect. Dis.* **2021**, *73*, 1571–1579. [CrossRef]
35. Kebed, K.Y.; Bishu, K.; Al Adham, R.I.; Baddour, L.M.; Connolly, H.M.; Sohail, M.R.; Steckelberg, J.M.; Wilson, W.R.; Murad, M.H.; Anavekar, N.S. Pregnancy and Postpartum Infective Endocarditis: A Systematic Review. *Mayo Clin. Proc.* **2014**, *89*, 1143–1153. [CrossRef]
36. Nappi, F.; Martuscelli, G.; Bellomo, F.; Avtaar Singh, S.S.; Moon, M.R. Infective Endocarditis in High-Income Countries. *Metabolites* **2022**, *12*, 682. [CrossRef]
37. Nappi, F.; Spadaccio, C.; Mihos, C. Infective Endocarditis in the 21st Century. *Ann. Transl. Med.* **2020**, *8*, 1620. [CrossRef]
38. Adesomo, A.; Gonzalez-Brown, V.; Rood, K.M. Infective Endocarditis as a Complication of Intravenous Drug Use in Pregnancy: A Retrospective Case Series and Literature Review. *Am. J. Perinatol. Rep.* **2020**, *10*, e288–e293. [CrossRef]
39. Patel, C.; Akhtar, H.; Gupta, S.; Harky, A. Pregnancy and Cardiac Interventions: What Are the Optimal Management Options? *J. Card. Surg.* **2020**, *35*, 1589–1596. [CrossRef]
40. Slipczuk, L.; Codolosa, J.N.; Davila, C.D.; Romero-Corral, A.; Yun, J.; Pressman, G.S.; Figueredo, V.M. Infective Endocarditis Epidemiology over Five Decades: A Systematic Review. *PLoS ONE* **2013**, *8*, e82665. [CrossRef]
41. Murdoch, D.R.; Corey, G.R.; Hoen, B.; Miró, J.M.; Fowler, V.G.; Bayer, A.S.; Karchmer, A.W.; Olaison, L.; Pappas, P.A.; Moreillon, P.; et al. Clinical Presentation, Etiology, and Outcome of Infective Endocarditis in the 21st Century: The International Collaboration on Endocarditis-Prospective Cohort Study. *Arch. Intern. Med.* **2009**, *169*, 463–473. [CrossRef]
42. Basak, S.; Solomonsz, F.A.; Anumba, D.O.C. Infective Endocarditis Affecting the Pulmonary Valves in Pregnant Intravenous Drug Users. *J. Obstet. Gynaecol.* **2011**, *31*, 78–80. [CrossRef] [PubMed]
43. Johnstone, R.; Khalil, N.; Shojaei, E.; Puka, K.; Bondy, L.; Koivu, S.; Silverman, M. Different Drugs, Different Sides: Injection Use of Opioids Alone, and Not Stimulants Alone, Predisposes to Right-Sided Endocarditis. *Open Heart* **2022**, *9*, e001930. [CrossRef] [PubMed]
44. Pang, P.Y.K.; Yang, L.W.Y.; Zhu, L.; Chua, Y.L. Isolated Tricuspid Valve Replacement for Infective Endocarditis. *Cardiol. Res.* **2022**, *13*, 110–117. [CrossRef] [PubMed]
45. Dayan, V.; Gutierrez, F.; Cura, L.; Soca, G.; Lorenzo, A. Two Cases of Pulmonary Homograft Replacement for Isolated Pulmonary Valve Endocarditis. *Ann. Thorac. Surg.* **2009**, *87*, 1954–1956. [CrossRef] [PubMed]
46. Amedro, P.; Soulatges, C.; Fraisse, A. Infective Endocarditis after Device Closure of Atrial Septal Defects: Case Report and Review of the Literature. *Catheter. Cardiovasc. Interv.* **2017**, *89*, 324–334. [CrossRef]

47. Lock, J.E.; Rome, J.J.; Davis, R.; Van Praagh, S.; Perry, S.B.; Van Praagh, R.; Keane, J.F. Transcatheter Closure of Atrial Septal Defects. Experimental Studies. *Circulation* **1989**, *79*, 1091–1099. [CrossRef]
48. Sharma, N.; Weena, U.; Medamana, J.; Mann, N.; Strachan, P.; Chikwe, J.; Kort, S. Atrial Septal Defect Closure Device–Related Infective Endocarditis in a 20-Week Pregnant Woman. *JACC Case Rep.* **2021**, *3*, 300–303. [CrossRef]
49. Mor, G.; Cardenas, I. The Immune System in Pregnancy: A Unique Complexity. *Am. J. Reprod. Immunol.* **2010**, *63*, 425–433. [CrossRef]
50. Sharma, S.; Rodrigues, P.R.S.; Zaher, S.; Davies, L.C.; Ghazal, P. Immune-metabolic adaptations in pregnancy: A potential stepping-stone to sepsis. *EBioMedicine* **2022**, *86*, 104337. [CrossRef]
51. Fraisse, A.; Latchman, M.; Sharma, S.-R.; Bayburt, S.; Amedro, P.; di Salvo, G.; Baruteau, A.E. Atrial Septal Defect Closure: Indications and Contra-Indications. *J. Thorac. Dis.* **2018**, *10*, S2874–S2881. [CrossRef]
52. Majunke, N.; Bialkowski, J.; Wilson, N.; Szkutnik, M.; Kusa, J.; Baranowski, A.; Heinisch, C.; Ostermayer, S.; Wunderlich, N.; Sievert, H. Closure of Atrial Septal Defect with the Amplatzer Septal Occluder in Adults. *Am. J. Cardiol.* **2009**, *103*, 550–554. [CrossRef]
53. Osteraas, N.D.; Vargas, A.; Cherian, L.; Song, S. Role of PFO Closure in Ischemic Stroke Prevention. *Curr. Treat. Options Cardiovasc. Med.* **2019**, *21*, 63. [CrossRef]
54. He, S.; Huynh, C.A.; Deng, Y.; Markan, S.; Nguyen, A. Bicuspid Aortic Valve in Pregnancy Complicated by Aortic Valve Vegetation, Aortic Root Abscess, and Aortic Insufficiency. *Cureus* **2021**, *13*, e20209. [CrossRef]
55. Maruichi-Kawakami, S.; Nagao, K.; Kanazawa, T.; Inada, T. Infective Endocarditis in Pregnancy Requiring Simultaneous Emergent Caesarean Section and Mitral Valve Replacement: A Case Report. *Eur. Heart J. Case Rep.* **2021**, *5*, ytab461. [CrossRef]
56. Kong, X.; Xu, F.; Wu, R.; Wu, H.; Ju, R.; Zhao, X.; Tong, X.; Lv, H.; Ding, Y.; Liu, F.; et al. Neonatal Mortality and Morbidity among Infants between 24 to 31 Complete Weeks: A Multicenter Survey in China from 2013 to 2014. *BMC Pediatr.* **2016**, *16*, 174. [CrossRef]
57. Lapinsky, S.E. Obstetric Infections. *Crit. Care Clin.* **2013**, *29*, 509–520. [CrossRef]
58. Khafaga, M.; Kresoja, K.-P.; Urlesberger, B.; Knez, I.; Klaritsch, P.; Lumenta, D.B.; Krause, R.; von Lewinski, D. *Staphylococcus Lugdunensis* Endocarditis in a 35-Year-Old Woman in Her 24th Week of Pregnancy. *Case Rep. Obstet. Gynecol.* **2016**, *2016*, e7030382. [CrossRef]
59. Selton-Suty, C.; Célard, M.; Le Moing, V.; Doco-Lecompte, T.; Chirouze, C.; Iung, B.; Strady, C.; Revest, M.; Vandenesch, F.; Bouvet, A.; et al. Preeminence of *Staphylococcus aureus* in Infective Endocarditis: A 1-Year Population-Based Survey. *Clin. Infect. Dis.* **2012**, *54*, 1230–1239. [CrossRef]
60. Hoen, B.; Duval, X. Infective Endocarditis. *N. Engl. J. Med.* **2013**, *368*, 1425–1433. [CrossRef]
61. Perez-Viloria, M.E.; Lopez, K.; Malik, F.; Lopez, O.; Yatham, P.; Malik, R.; Rosen, G. A Rare Case of Pulmonic and Aortic Valve Infective Endocarditis: A Case Report. *Cureus* **2022**, *14*, e31820. [CrossRef]
62. Wydall, S.; Durrant, F.; Scott, J.; Cheesman, K. Streptococcus Oralis Endocarditis Leading to Central Nervous System Infection in Pregnancy. *Anaesth. Rep.* **2021**, *9*, e12133. [CrossRef] [PubMed]
63. Poi, B.N.; Pasupulety Venkata, N.K.; Auckland, C.R.; Paul, S.P. Neonatal Meningitis and Maternal Sepsis Caused by Streptococcus Oralis. *J. Neonatal-Perinat. Med.* **2018**, *11*, 331–334. [CrossRef] [PubMed]
64. Shah, M.; Patnaik, S.; Wongrakpanich, S.; Alhamshari, Y.; Alnabelsi, T. Infective Endocarditis Due to Bacillus Cereus in a Pregnant Female: A Case Report and Literature Review. *IDCases* **2015**, *2*, 120–123. [CrossRef]
65. Connolly, C.; O'Donoghue, K.; Doran, H.; McCarthy, F.P. Infective Endocarditis in Pregnancy: Case Report and Review of the Literature. *Obstet. Med.* **2015**, *8*, 102–104. [CrossRef] [PubMed]
66. Liu, P.-Y.; Huang, Y.-F.; Tang, C.-W.; Chen, Y.-Y.; Hsieh, K.-S.; Ger, L.-P.; Chen, Y.-S.; Liu, Y.-C. Staphylococcus Lugdunensis Infective Endocarditis: A Literature Review and Analysis of Risk Factors. *J. Microbiol. Immunol. Infect.* **2010**, *43*, 478–484. [CrossRef] [PubMed]
67. Vaideeswar, P.; Shah, R. Zygomycotic Infective Endocarditis in Pregnancy. *Cardiovasc. Pathol.* **2017**, *28*, 28–30. [CrossRef]
68. Cinteza, E.; Nicolescu, A.; Ciomartan, T.; Gavriliu, L.-C.; Voicu, C.; Carabas, A.; Popescu, M.; Margarint, I. Disseminated Cunninghamella Spp. Endocarditis in a Beta-Thalassemia Patient after Asymptomatic COVID-19 Infection. *Diagnostics* **2022**, *12*, 657. [CrossRef]
69. Giamarellou, H. Nosocomial Cardiac Infections. *J. Hosp. Infect.* **2002**, *50*, 91–105. [CrossRef]
70. Arulkumaran, N.; Singer, M. Puerperal Sepsis. *Best Pract. Res. Clin. Obstet. Gynaecol.* **2013**, *27*, 893–902. [CrossRef]
71. Francis, K.; Viscount, D. An Unusual Case of Infectious Endocarditis in Pregnancy. *J. Obstet. Gynecol. Neonatal Nurs.* **2013**, *42*, S98–S99. [CrossRef]
72. Chu, L.; Zhang, J.; Li, Y.N.; Meng, X.; Liu, Y.Y. Clinical treatment of infective endocarditis with vegetations in pregnant women and the outcomes of gestation. *Zhonghua Fu Chan Ke Za Zhi* **2016**, *51*, 331–338.
73. Shapero, K.S.; Nauriyal, V.; Megli, C.; Berlacher, K.; El-Dalati, S. Management of Infective Endocarditis in Pregnancy by a Multidisciplinary Team: A Case Series. *Ther. Adv. Infect. Dis.* **2022**, *9*, 20499361221080644. [CrossRef]
74. Botelho-Nevers, E.; Thuny, F.; Casalta, J.P.; Richet, H.; Gouriet, F.; Collart, F.; Riberi, A.; Habib, G.; Raoult, D. Dramatic Reduction in Infective Endocarditis-Related Mortality with a Management-Based Approach. *Arch. Intern. Med.* **2009**, *169*, 1290–1298. [CrossRef]

75. El-Dalati, S.; Cronin, D.; Riddell, J.; Shea, M.; Weinberg, R.L.; Washer, L.; Stoneman, E.; Perry, D.A.; Bradley, S.; Burke, J.; et al. The Clinical Impact of Implementation of a Multidisciplinary Endocarditis Team. *Ann. Thorac. Surg.* **2022**, *113*, 118–124. [CrossRef]
76. Davierwala, P.M.; Marin-Cuartas, M.; Misfeld, M.; Borger, M.A. The Value of an "Endocarditis Team". *Ann. Cardiothorac. Surg.* **2019**, *8*, 621–629. [CrossRef]
77. Botea, R.; Porterie, J.; Marcheix, B.; Breleur, F.-O.; Lavie-Badie, Y. Infective Endocarditis in a Third Trimester Pregnant Woman. *JACC Case Rep.* **2020**, *2*, 521–525. [CrossRef]
78. Baddour, L.M.; Wilson, W.R.; Bayer, A.S.; Fowler, V.G.; Tleyjeh, I.M.; Rybak, M.J.; Barsic, B.; Lockhart, P.B.; Gewitz, M.H.; Levison, M.E.; et al. Infective Endocarditis in Adults: Diagnosis, Antimicrobial Therapy, and Management of Complications: A Scientific Statement for Healthcare Professionals From the American Heart Association. *Circulation* **2015**, *132*, 1435–1486. [CrossRef]
79. Liesman, R.M.; Pritt, B.S.; Maleszewski, J.J.; Patel, R. Laboratory Diagnosis of Infective Endocarditis. *J. Clin. Microbiol.* **2017**, *55*, 2599–2608. [CrossRef]
80. Li, J.S.; Sexton, D.J.; Mick, N.; Nettles, R.; Fowler, V.G.; Ryan, T.; Bashore, T.; Corey, G.R. Proposed Modifications to the Duke Criteria for the Diagnosis of Infective Endocarditis. *Clin. Infect. Dis.* **2000**, *30*, 633–638. [CrossRef]
81. Eichenberger, E.M.; Degner, N.; Scott, E.R.; Ruffin, F.; Franzone, J.; Sharma-Kuinkel, B.; Shah, P.; Hong, D.; Dalai, S.C.; Blair, L.; et al. Microbial Cell-Free DNA Identifies the Causative Pathogen in Infective Endocarditis and Remains Detectable Longer Than Conventional Blood Culture in Patients with Prior Antibiotic Therapy. *Clin. Infect. Dis.* **2023**, *76*, e1492–e1500. [CrossRef]
82. Cai, S.; Yang, Y.; Pan, J.; Miao, Q.; Jin, W.; Ma, Y.; Zhou, C.; Gao, X.; Wang, C.; Hu, B. The Clinical Value of Valve Metagenomic Next-Generation Sequencing When Applied to the Etiological Diagnosis of Infective Endocarditis. *Ann. Transl. Med.* **2021**, *9*, 1490. [CrossRef] [PubMed]
83. Shishido, A.A.; Noe, M.; Saharia, K.; Luethy, P. Clinical Impact of a Metagenomic Microbial Plasma Cell-Free DNA next-Generation Sequencing Assay on Treatment Decisions: A Single-Center Retrospective Study. *BMC Infect. Dis.* **2022**, *22*, 372. [CrossRef] [PubMed]
84. Pietrzak, B.; Kawacka, I.; Olejnik-Schmidt, A.; Schmidt, M. Circulating Microbial Cell-Free DNA in Health and Disease. *Int. J. Mol. Sci.* **2023**, *24*, 3051. [CrossRef] [PubMed]
85. Mandel, P. Les Acides Nucleiques Du Plasma Sanguin Chez 1 Homme. *C. R. Seances Soc. Biol. Fil.* **1948**, *142*, 241–243. [PubMed]
86. Bronkhorst, A.J.; Ungerer, V.; Oberhofer, A.; Gabriel, S.; Polatoglou, E.; Randeu, H.; Uhlig, C.; Pfister, H.; Mayer, Z.; Holdenrieder, S. New Perspectives on the Importance of Cell-Free DNA Biology. *Diagnostics* **2022**, *12*, 2147. [CrossRef]
87. Ranucci, R. Cell-Free DNA: Applications in Different Diseases. *Methods Mol. Biol.* **2019**, *1909*, 3–12. [CrossRef]
88. Martignano, F. Cell-Free DNA: An Overview of Sample Types and Isolation Procedures. In *Cell-Free DNA as Diagnostic Markers*; Methods in Molecular Biology; Casadio, V., Salvi, S., Eds.; Springer: New York, NY, USA, 2019; Volume 1909, pp. 13–27, ISBN 978-1-4939-8972-0.
89. De Miranda, F.S.; Barauna, V.G.; dos Santos, L.; Costa, G.; Vassallo, P.F.; Campos, L.C.G. Properties and Application of Cell-Free DNA as a Clinical Biomarker. *Int. J. Mol. Sci.* **2021**, *22*, 9110. [CrossRef]
90. Camargo, J.F.; Ahmed, A.A.; Lindner, M.S.; Morris, M.I.; Anjan, S.; Anderson, A.D.; Prado, C.E.; Dalai, S.C.; Martinez, O.V.; Komanduri, K.V. Next-Generation Sequencing of Microbial Cell-Free DNA for Rapid Noninvasive Diagnosis of Infectious Diseases in Immunocompromised Hosts. *F1000Research* **2020**, *8*, 1194. [CrossRef]
91. Solanky, D.; Ahmed, A.A.; Fierer, J.; Golts, E.; Jones, M.; Mehta, S.R. Utility of Plasma Microbial Cell-Free DNA Decay Kinetics After Aortic Valve Replacement for Bartonella Endocarditis: Case Report. *Front. Trop. Dis.* **2022**, *3*, 842100. [CrossRef]
92. Haddad, S.F.; DeSimone, D.C.; Chesdachai, S.; Gerberi, D.J.; Baddour, L.M. Utility of Metagenomic Next-Generation Sequencing in Infective Endocarditis: A Systematic Review. *Antibiotics* **2022**, *11*, 1798. [CrossRef]
93. Bragg, L.; Tyson, G.W. Metagenomics Using Next-Generation Sequencing. *Methods Mol. Biol.* **2014**, *1096*, 183–201. [CrossRef]
94. Metagenomic Next Generation Sequencing: How Does It Work and Is It Coming to Your Clinical Microbiology Lab? Available online: https://asm.org:443/Articles/2019/November/Metagenomic-Next-Generation-Sequencing-How-Does-It (accessed on 24 April 2023).
95. Wu, D.; Wang, W.; Xun, Q.; Wang, H.; Liu, J.; Zhong, Z.; Ouyang, C.; Yang, Q. Metagenomic Next-Generation Sequencing Indicates More Precise Pathogens in Patients with Pulmonary Infection: A Retrospective Study. *Front. Cell. Infect. Microbiol.* **2022**, *12*, 1500. [CrossRef]
96. Duan, H.; Li, X.; Mei, A.; Li, P.; Liu, Y.; Li, X.; Li, W.; Wang, C.; Xie, S. The Diagnostic Value of Metagenomic Next-generation Sequencing in Infectious Diseases. *BMC Infect. Dis.* **2021**, *21*, 62. [CrossRef]
97. Eichenberger, E.M.; de Vries, C.R.; Ruffin, F.; Sharma-Kuinkel, B.; Park, L.; Hong, D.; Scott, E.R.; Blair, L.; Degner, N.; Hollemon, D.H.; et al. Microbial Cell-Free DNA Identifies Etiology of Bloodstream Infections, Persists Longer Than Conventional Blood Cultures, and Its Duration of Detection Is Associated With Metastatic Infection in Patients With *Staphylococcus aureus* and Gram-Negative Bacteremia. *Clin. Infect. Dis.* **2022**, *74*, 2020–2027. [CrossRef]
98. Luke, J.; Oxnard, G.; Paweletz, C.; Camidge, R.; Heymach, J.; Solit, D.; Johnson, B. Realizing the Potential of Plasma Genotyping in an Age of Genotype-Directed Therapies. *J. Natl. Cancer Inst.* **2014**, *106*, dju214. [CrossRef]
99. Grace, M.R.; Hardisty, E.; Dotters-Katz, S.K.; Vora, N.L.; Kuller, J.A. Cell-Free DNA Screening: Complexities and Challenges of Clinical Implementation. *Obstet. Gynecol. Surv.* **2016**, *71*, 477–487. [CrossRef]

100. Thuny, F.; Habib, G.; Dolley, Y.L.; Canault, M.; Casalta, J.-P.; Verdier, M.; Avierinos, J.-F.; Raoult, D.; Mege, J.-L.; Morange, P.-E.; et al. Circulating Matrix Metalloproteinases in Infective Endocarditis: A Possible Marker of the Embolic Risk. *PLoS ONE* **2011**, *6*, e18830. [CrossRef]
101. Thuny, F.; Disalvo, G.; Belliard, O.; Avierinos, J.-F.; Pergola, V.; Rosenberg, V.; Casalta, J.-P.; Gouvernet, J.; Derumeaux, G.; Iarussi, D.; et al. Risk of Embolism and Death in Infective Endocarditis: Prognostic Value of Echocardiography: A Prospective Multicenter Study. *Circulation* **2005**, *112*, 69–75. [CrossRef]
102. Lupu, S.; Pop, M.; Mitre, A. Loeffler Endocarditis Causing Heart Failure with Preserved Ejection Fraction (HFpEF): Characteristic Images and Diagnostic Pathway. *Diagnostics* **2022**, *12*, 2157. [CrossRef]
103. Todde, G.; Gargiulo, P.; Canciello, G.; Borrelli, F.; Pilato, E.; Esposito, G.; Losi, M.A. Rapid Evolution of an Aortic Endocarditis. *Diagnostics* **2022**, *12*, 327. [CrossRef]
104. Silversides, C.K.; Grewal, J.; Mason, J.; Sermer, M.; Kiess, M.; Rychel, V.; Wald, R.M.; Colman, J.M.; Siu, S.C. Pregnancy Outcomes in Women With Heart Disease: The CARPREG II Study. *J. Am. Coll. Cardiol.* **2018**, *71*, 2419–2430. [CrossRef] [PubMed]
105. Hennessey, K.C.; Ali, T.S.; Choi, E.; Ortengren, A.R.; Hickerson, L.C.; Lee, J.M.; Taub, C.C. Association between Abnormal Echocardiography and Adverse Obstetric Outcomes in Low-Risk Pregnant Women. *J. Cardiovasc. Dev. Dis.* **2022**, *9*, 394. [CrossRef] [PubMed]
106. Holcman, K.; Rubiś, P.; Ząbek, A.; Boczar, K.; Podolec, P.; Kostkiewicz, M. Advances in Molecular Imaging in Infective Endocarditis. *Vaccines* **2023**, *11*, 420. [CrossRef] [PubMed]
107. Baddour, L.M.; Epstein, A.E.; Erickson, C.C.; Knight, B.P.; Levison, M.E.; Lockhart, P.B.; Masoudi, F.A.; Okum, E.J.; Wilson, W.R.; Beerman, L.B.; et al. Update on Cardiovascular Implantable Electronic Device Infections and Their Management: A Scientific Statement From the American Heart Association. *Circulation* **2010**, *121*, 458–477. [CrossRef]
108. Steckelberg, J.M. Emboli in Infective Endocarditis: The Prognostic Value of Echocardiography. *Ann. Intern. Med.* **1991**, *114*, 635. [CrossRef]
109. Bhatia, P.; Dwivedi, D.; Gautam, A.R.; Singh, S. Implications of Active Infective Endocarditis with Pregnancy and Its Management. *J. Obstet. Anaesth. Crit. Care* **2021**, *11*, 128. [CrossRef]
110. Park, M.-Y.; Jeon, H.-K.; Shim, B.-J.; Kim, H.-N.; Lee, H.-Y.; Kang, J.-H.; Kim, J.-J.; Koh, Y.-S.; Shin, W.-S.; Lee, J.-M. Complete Atrioventricular Block Due to Infective Endocarditis of Bicuspid Aortic Valve. *J. Cardiovasc. Ultrasound* **2011**, *19*, 140–143. [CrossRef]
111. Yu, B.; Zhao, Y.Y.; Zhang, Z.; Wang, Y.Q. Infective endocarditis in pregnancy: A case report. *Beijing Da Xue Xue Bao* **2022**, *54*, 578–580. [CrossRef]
112. Vizzardi, E.; De Cicco, G.; Zanini, G.; D'Aloia, A.; Faggiano, P.; Lo Russo, R.; Chiari, E.; Dei Cas, L. Infectious Endocarditis during Pregnancy, Problems in the Decision-Making Process: A Case Report. *Cases J.* **2009**, *2*, 6537. [CrossRef]
113. Tamura, T.; Yokota, S. Mitral Valve Repair in Infective Endocarditis during Pregnancy. *Ann. Card. Anaesth.* **2018**, *21*, 189–191.
114. Mahli, A.; Izdes, S.; Coskun, D. Cardiac Operations during Pregnancy: Review of Factors Influencing Fetal Outcome. *Ann. Thorac. Surg.* **2000**, *69*, 1622–1626. [CrossRef]
115. Ayzenbart, V.; Fuentes, H.; Fuentes, F.; Aziz, S.; Joseph, M. AngioVac use in endocarditis during pregnancy: A novel approach for recurrent debulking of tricuspid infective vegetations in a 27-year-old woman in her 22nd and 26th weeks of pregnancy. *Chest* **2021**, *160*, A786. [CrossRef]
116. Strickland, R.A.; Oliver, W.C.; Chantigian, R.C.; Ney, J.A.; Danielson, G.K. Anesthesia, Cardiopulmonary Bypass, and the Pregnant Patient. *Mayo Clin. Proc.* **1991**, *66*, 411–429. [CrossRef]
117. Velauthar, L.; Plana, M.N.; Kalidindi, M.; Zamora, J.; Thilaganathan, B.; Illanes, S.E.; Khan, K.S.; Aquilina, J.; Thangaratinam, S. First-Trimester Uterine Artery Doppler and Adverse Pregnancy Outcome: A Meta-Analysis Involving 55,974 Women. *Ultrasound Obstet. Gynecol.* **2014**, *43*, 500–507. [CrossRef]
118. Alwan, S.; Polifka, J.E.; Friedman, J.M. Angiotensin II Receptor Antagonist Treatment during Pregnancy. *Birt. Defects Res. A. Clin. Mol. Teratol.* **2005**, *73*, 123–130. [CrossRef]
119. Cooper, W.O.; Hernandez-Diaz, S.; Arbogast, P.G.; Dudley, J.A.; Dyer, S.; Gideon, P.S.; Hall, K.; Ray, W.A. Major Congenital Malformations after First-Trimester Exposure to ACE Inhibitors. *N. Engl. J. Med.* **2006**, *354*, 2443–2451. [CrossRef]
120. Dolovich, L.R.; Addis, A.; Vaillancourt, J.M.; Power, J.D.; Koren, G.; Einarson, T.R. Benzodiazepine Use in Pregnancy and Major Malformations or Oral Cleft: Meta-Analysis of Cohort and Case-Control Studies. *BMJ* **1998**, *317*, 839–843. [CrossRef]
121. Olsen, E.A.; Brambrink, A.M. Anesthetic Neurotoxicity in the Newborn and Infant. *Curr. Opin. Anaesthesiol.* **2013**, *26*, 535–542. [CrossRef]
122. Davidson, A.J. Anesthesia and Neurotoxicity to the Developing Brain: The Clinical Relevance. *Paediatr. Anaesth.* **2011**, *21*, 716–721. [CrossRef]
123. Marcoux, J.; Rosin, M.; Mycyk, T. CPB-Assisted Aortic Valve Replacement in a Pregnant 27-Year-Old with Endocarditis. *Perfusion* **2009**, *24*, 361–364. [CrossRef]
124. Pillai, S.K.; Monisha, S. A Study on Foetomaternal Outcome of Pregnancies Complicated by Cardiac Diseases. *J. Fam. Med. Prim. Care* **2022**, *11*, 4655–4660. [CrossRef] [PubMed]
125. Barth, W.H., Jr. Cardiac surgery in pregnancy. *Clin. Obstet. Gynecol.* **2009**, *52*, 630–646. [CrossRef] [PubMed]
126. Kastelein, A.W.; Oldenburger, N.Y.; van Pampus, M.G.; Janszen, E.W.M. Severe Endocarditis and Open-Heart Surgery during Pregnancy. *BMJ Case Rep.* **2016**, *2016*, bcr2016217510. [CrossRef] [PubMed]

127. Task Force on the Management of Cardiovascular Diseases During Pregnancy of the European Society of Cardiology. Expert consensus document on management of cardiovascular diseases during pregnancy. *Eur. Heart. J.* **2003**, *24*, 761–781. [CrossRef]
128. Krcmery, V.; Gogová, M.; Ondrusová, A.; Buckova, E.; Doczeova, A.; Mrazova, M.; Hricak, V.; Fischer, V.; Marks, P.; Slovak Endocarditis Study Group. Etiology and Risk Factors of 339 Cases of Infective Endocarditis: Report from a 10-Year National Prospective Survey in the Slovak Republic. *J. Chemother.* **2003**, *15*, 579–583. [CrossRef]
129. Hubert, S.; Thuny, F.; Resseguier, N.; Giorgi, R.; Tribouilloy, C.; Le, D.Y.; Casalta, J.-P.; Riberi, A.; Chevalier, F.; Rusinaru, D.; et al. Prediction of Symptomatic Embolism in Infective Endocarditis. *J. Am. Coll. Cardiol.* **2013**, *62*, 1384–1392. [CrossRef]
130. Tackett, M.S.; Ahmed, T.; El-Dalati, S.A.; Ahmed, T. Paradoxical embolisation to the brain in right-sided infective endocarditis and patent foramen ovale in a pregnant woman. *BMJ Case Rep* **2023**, *16*, e254403. [CrossRef]
131. Kuo, I.; Long, T.; Nguyen, N.; Chaudry, B.; Karp, M.; Sanossian, N. Ruptured Intracranial Mycotic Aneurysm in Infective Endocarditis: A Natural History. *Case Rep. Med.* **2010**, *2010*, 168408. [CrossRef]
132. Aziz, F.; Perwaiz, S.; Penupolu, S.; Doddi, S.; Gongireddy, S. Intracranial Hemorrhage in Infective Endocarditis: A Case Report. *J. Thorac. Dis.* **2011**, *3*, 134–137.
133. Wojda, T.R.; Cornejo, K.; Lin, A.; Cipriano, A.; Nanda, S.; Amortegui, J.D.; Wojda, B.T.; Stawicki, S.P. Septic Embolism: A Potentially Devastating Complication of Infective Endocarditis. In *Contemporary Challenges in Endocarditis*; Firstenberg, M.S., Ed.; InTech: London, UK, 2016; ISBN 978-953-51-2769-7.
134. Mamoun, C.; Houda, F. Infarctus splénique révélant une endocardite infectieuse chez une femme enceinte: À propos d'un cas et brève revue de littérature. *Pan Afr. Med. J.* **2018**, *30*. [CrossRef]
135. Klebermass-Schrehof, K.; Czaba, C.; Olischar, M.; Fuiko, R.; Waldhoer, T.; Rona, Z.; Pollak, A.; Weninger, M. Impact of Low-Grade Intraventricular Hemorrhage on Long-Term Neurodevelopmental Outcome in Preterm Infants. *Childs Nerv. Syst.* **2012**, *28*, 2085–2092. [CrossRef]
136. Bourke, J.; Wong, K.; Srinivasjois, R.; Pereira, G.; Shepherd, C.C.J.; White, S.W.; Stanley, F.; Leonard, H. Predicting Long-Term Survival Without Major Disability for Infants Born Preterm. *J. Pediatr.* **2019**, *215*, 90–97.e1. [CrossRef]
137. Chambers, C.E.; Clark, S.L. Cardiac Surgery during Pregnancy. *Clin. Obstet. Gynecol.* **1994**, *37*, 316–323. [CrossRef]
138. Campuzano, K.; Roqué, H.; Bolnick, A.; Leo, M.V.; Campbell, W.A. Bacterial Endocarditis Complicating Pregnancy: Case Report and Systematic Review of the Literature. *Arch. Gynecol. Obstet.* **2003**, *268*, 251–255. [CrossRef]
139. Van Steenbergen, G.J.; Tsang, Q.H.Y.; van der Heijden, O.W.H.; Vart, P.; Rodwell, L.; Roos-Hesselink, J.W.; van Kimmenade, R.R.J.; Li, W.W.L.; Verhagen, A.F.T.M. Timing of Cardiac Surgery during Pregnancy: A Patient-Level Meta-Analysis. *Eur. Heart J.* **2022**, *43*, 2801–2811. [CrossRef]
140. You, Y.; Liu, S.; Wu, Z.; Chen, D.; Wang, G.; Chen, G.; Pan, Y.; Zheng, X. Cardiac Surgery under Cardiopulmonary Bypass in Pregnancy: Report of Four Cases. *J. Cardiothorac. Surg.* **2021**, *16*, 268. [CrossRef]
141. Kang, D.-H.; Kim, Y.-J.; Kim, S.-H.; Sun, B.J.; Kim, D.-H.; Yun, S.-C.; Song, J.-M.; Choo, S.J.; Chung, C.-H.; Song, J.-K.; et al. Early Surgery versus Conventional Treatment for Infective Endocarditis. *N. Engl. J. Med.* **2012**, *366*, 2466–2473. [CrossRef]
142. Olmos, C.; Vilacosta, I.; Fernández, C.; Sarriá, C.; López, J.; Del Trigo, M.; Ferrera, C.; Vivas, D.; Maroto, L.; Hernández, M.; et al. Comparison of Clinical Features of Left-Sided Infective Endocarditis Involving Previously Normal Versus Previously Abnormal Valves. *Am. J. Cardiol.* **2014**, *114*, 278–283. [CrossRef]
143. Ward, H.; Hickman, R.C. Bacterial endocarditis in pregnancy. *Aust. N. Z. J. Obstet. Gynaecol.* **1971**, *11*, 189–191. [CrossRef]
144. Dubourg, G.; Broustet, P.; Bricaud, H.; Fontan, F.; Trarieux, M.; Fontanille, P. Complete correction of a triad of Fallot, in extracorporeal circulation, in a pregnant woman. *Arch. Mal. Coeur Vaiss.* **1959**, *52*, 1389–1391.
145. John, A.S.; Gurley, F.; Schaff, H.V.; Warnes, C.A.; Phillips, S.D.; Arendt, K.W.; Abel, M.D.; Rose, C.H.; Connolly, H.M. Cardiopulmonary Bypass During Pregnancy. *Ann. Thorac. Surg.* **2011**, *91*, 1191–1196. [CrossRef] [PubMed]
146. Shook, L.L.; Barth, W.H.J. Cardiac Surgery during Pregnancy. *Clin. Obstet. Gynecol.* **2020**, *63*, 429. [CrossRef] [PubMed]
147. Kapoor, M.C. Cardiopulmonary Bypass in Pregnancy. *Ann. Card. Anaesth.* **2014**, *17*, 33–39. [CrossRef] [PubMed]
148. Hawkins, J.A.; Paape, K.L.; Adkins, T.P.; Shaddy, R.E.; Gay, W.A. Extracorporeal Circulation in the Fetal Lamb. Effects of Hypothermia and Perfusion Rate. *J. Cardiovasc. Surg.* **1991**, *32*, 295–300.
149. Lamb, M.P.; Ross, K.; Johnstone, A.M.; Manners, J.M. Fetal Heart Monitoring during Open Heart Surgery. Two Case Reports. *Br. J. Obstet. Gynaecol.* **1981**, *88*, 669–674. [CrossRef]
150. Parry, A.J.; Westaby, S. Cardiopulmonary Bypass during Pregnancy. *Ann. Thorac. Surg.* **1996**, *61*, 1865–1869. [CrossRef]
151. Shore-Lesserson, L.; Baker, R.A.; Ferraris, V.A.; Greilich, P.E.; Fitzgerald, D.; Roman, P.; Hammon, J.W. The Society of Thoracic Surgeons, The Society of Cardiovascular Anesthesiologists, and The American Society of ExtraCorporeal Technology: Clinical Practice Guidelines*—Anticoagulation During Cardiopulmonary Bypass. *Ann. Thorac. Surg.* **2018**, *105*, 650–662. [CrossRef]
152. Abbassi-Ghanavati, M.; Greer, L.G.; Cunningham, F.G. Pregnancy and Laboratory Studies: A Reference Table for Clinicians. *Obstet. Gynecol.* **2009**, *114*, 1326–1331. [CrossRef]
153. Ahmad, M.S.; Shaik, R.A.; Ahmad, R.K.; Yusuf, M.; Khan, M.; Almutairi, A.B.; Alghuyaythat, W.K.Z.; Almutairi, S.B. "LONG COVID": An Insight. *Eur. Rev. Med. Pharmacol. Sci.* **2021**, *25*, 5561–5577. [CrossRef]
154. Figliozzi, S.; Masci, P.G.; Ahmadi, N.; Tondi, L.; Koutli, E.; Aimo, A.; Stamatelopoulos, K.; Dimopoulos, M.; Caforio, A.L.P.; Georgiopoulos, G. Predictors of Adverse Prognosis in COVID-19: A Systematic Review and Meta-analysis. *Eur. J. Clin. Invest.* **2020**, *50*, e13362. [CrossRef]

155. Gajbhiye, R.K.; Sawant, M.S.; Kuppusamy, P.; Surve, S.; Pasi, A.; Prusty, R.K.; Mahale, S.D.; Modi, D.N. Differential Impact of COVID-19 in Pregnant Women from High-Income Countries and Low- to Middle-Income Countries: A Systematic Review and Meta-Analysis. *Int. J. Gynaecol. Obstet.* **2021**, *155*, 48–56. [CrossRef]
156. Wei, S.Q.; Bilodeau-Bertrand, M.; Liu, S.; Auger, N. The Impact of COVID-19 on Pregnancy Outcomes: A Systematic Review and Meta-Analysis. *CMAJ Can. Med. Assoc. J.* **2021**, *193*, E540–E548. [CrossRef]
157. Vale, A.J.M.; Fernandes, A.C.L.; Guzen, F.P.; Pinheiro, F.I.; de Azevedo, E.P.; Cobucci, R.N. Susceptibility to COVID-19 in Pregnancy, Labor, and Postpartum Period: Immune System, Vertical Transmission, and Breastfeeding. *Front. Glob. Womens Health* **2021**, *2*, 602572. [CrossRef]
158. Roshdy, A.; Zaher, S.; Fayed, H.; Coghlan, J.G. COVID-19 and the Heart: A Systematic Review of Cardiac Autopsies. *Front. Cardiovasc. Med.* **2020**, *7*, 626975. [CrossRef]
159. Liesenborghs, L.; Meyers, S.; Lox, M.; Criel, M.; Claes, J.; Peetermans, M.; Trenson, S.; Vande Velde, G.; Vanden Berghe, P.; Baatsen, P.; et al. *Staphylococcus aureus* Endocarditis: Distinct Mechanisms of Bacterial Adhesion to Damaged and Inflamed Heart Valves. *Eur. Heart J.* **2019**, *40*, 3248–3259. [CrossRef]
160. Rajan, M.; Sachan, S.; Abhinay, A.; Verma, B. Maternal and Fetal Outcomes of COVID-19 Infection in Pregnant Women with Chronic Rheumatic Heart Disease in a South Asian Population: A Case Series. *J. Obstet. Gynaecol. Res.* **2022**, *48*, 1480–1483. [CrossRef]
161. Rezar, R.; Lichtenauer, M.; Haar, M.; Hödl, G.; Kern, J.M.; Zhou, Z.; Wuppinger, T.; Kraus, J.; Strohmer, B.; Hoppe, U.C.; et al. Infective Endocarditis—A Review of Current Therapy and Future Challenges. *Hellenic J. Cardiol.* **2021**, *62*, 190–200. [CrossRef]
162. Bundgaard, H.; Ihlemann, N.; Gill, S.U.; Bruun, N.E.; Elming, H.; Madsen, T.; Jensen, K.T.; Fursted, K.; Christensen, J.J.; Schultz, M.; et al. Long-Term Outcomes of Partial Oral Treatment of Endocarditis. *N. Engl. J. Med.* **2019**, *380*, 1373–1374. [CrossRef]
163. Iversen, K.; Ihlemann, N.; Gill, S.U.; Madsen, T.; Elming, H.; Jensen, K.T.; Bruun, N.E.; Høfsten, D.E.; Fursted, K.; Christensen, J.J.; et al. Partial Oral versus Intravenous Antibiotic Treatment of Endocarditis. *N. Engl. J. Med.* **2019**, *380*, 415–424. [CrossRef]
164. Bloem, A.; Bax, H.I.; Yusuf, E.; Verkaik, N.J. New-Generation Antibiotics for Treatment of Gram-Positive Infections: A Review with Focus on Endocarditis and Osteomyelitis. *J. Clin. Med.* **2021**, *10*, 1743. [CrossRef]
165. Guleri, A.; Utili, R.; Dohmen, P.; Petrosillo, N.; Piper, C.; Pathan, R.; Hamed, K. Daptomycin for the Treatment of Infective Endocarditis: Results from European Cubicin® Outcomes Registry and Experience (EU-CORE). *Infect. Dis. Ther.* **2015**, *4*, 283–296. [CrossRef] [PubMed]
166. Peiffer-Smadja, N.; Abbara, S.; Rizk, N.; Pogliaghi, M.; Rondinaud, E.; Tesmoingt, C.; Massias, L.; Lucet, J.C.; Alkhoder, S.; Armand-Lefèvre, L.; et al. High-Dose Daptomycin in Patients with Infective Endocarditis or Sternal Wound Infections. *Clin. Microbiol. Infect.* **2018**, *24*, 1106–1108. [CrossRef] [PubMed]
167. Daptomycin Use During Pregnancy. Available online: https://www.drugs.com/pregnancy/daptomycin.html (accessed on 12 February 2023).
168. Perelli, F.; Turrini, I.; Giorgi, M.G.; Renda, I.; Vidiri, A.; Straface, G.; Scatena, E.; D'Indinosante, M.; Marchi, L.; Giusti, M.; et al. Contrast Agents during Pregnancy: Pros and Cons When Really Needed. *Int. J. Environ. Res. Public. Health* **2022**, *19*, 16699. [CrossRef] [PubMed]
169. Kouijzer, J.J.P.; Noordermeer, D.J.; van Leeuwen, W.J.; Verkaik, N.J.; Lattwein, K.R. Native Valve, Prosthetic Valve, and Cardiac Device-Related Infective Endocarditis: A Review and Update on Current Innovative Diagnostic and Therapeutic Strategies. *Front. Cell Dev. Biol.* **2022**, *10*, 995508. [CrossRef]
170. Lattwein, K.R.; Shekhar, H.; Kouijzer, J.J.P.; van Wamel, W.J.B.; Holland, C.K.; Kooiman, K. Sonobactericide: An Emerging Treatment Strategy for Bacterial Infections. *Ultrasound Med. Biol.* **2020**, *46*, 193–215. [CrossRef]
171. Lattwein, K.R.; Beekers, I.; Kouijzer, J.J.P.; Leon-Grooters, M.; Langeveld, S.A.G.; van Rooij, T.; van der Steen, A.F.W.; de Jong, N.; van Wamel, W.J.B.; Kooiman, K. Dispersing and Sonoporating Biofilm-Associated Bacteria with Sonobactericide. *Pharmaceutics* **2022**, *14*, 1164. [CrossRef]
172. Kouijzer, J.J.P.; Lattwein, K.R.; Beekers, I.; Langeveld, S.A.G.; Leon-Grooters, M.; Strub, J.-M.; Oliva, E.; Mislin, G.L.A.; de Jong, N.; van der Steen, A.F.W.; et al. Vancomycin-Decorated Microbubbles as a Theranostic Agent for *Staphylococcus aureus* Biofilms. *Int. J. Pharm.* **2021**, *609*, 121154. [CrossRef]
173. Fowler, V.G.; Das, A.F.; Lipka-Diamond, J.; Schuch, R.; Pomerantz, R.; Jáuregui-Peredo, L.; Bressler, A.; Evans, D.; Moran, G.J.; Rupp, M.E.; et al. Exebacase for Patients with *Staphylococcus aureus* Bloodstream Infection and Endocarditis. *J. Clin. InvestIG.* **2020**, *130*, 3750–3760. [CrossRef]
174. Ye, J.; Chen, X. Current Promising Strategies against Antibiotic-Resistant Bacterial Infections. *Antibiotics* **2022**, *12*, 67. [CrossRef]

Disclaimer/Publisher's Note: The statements, opinions and data contained in all publications are solely those of the individual author(s) and contributor(s) and not of MDPI and/or the editor(s). MDPI and/or the editor(s) disclaim responsibility for any injury to people or property resulting from any ideas, methods, instructions or products referred to in the content.

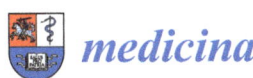

Article

The Impact of SARS-CoV-2 Infection on Premature Birth—Our Experience as COVID Center

Tina-Ioana Bobei [1,2], Bashar Haj Hamoud [3], Romina-Marina Sima [2,4,*], Gabriel-Petre Gorecki [2,5], Mircea-Octavian Poenaru [2,4], Octavian-Gabriel Olaru [2,4] and Liana Ples [2,4]

1. Department PhD, IOSUD, "Carol Davila" University of Medicine and Pharmacy, 020021 Bucharest, Romania; tina-ioana.bobei@drd.umfcd.ro
2. "Bucur" Maternity, Saint John Hospital, 012361 Bucharest, Romania; gabriel.gorecki@doc.utm.ro (G.-P.G.); mircea.poenaru@umfcd.ro (M.-O.P.); octavian_olaru@umfcd.ro (O.-G.O.); liana.ples@umfcd.ro (L.P.)
3. Department for Gynaecology, Obstetrics and Reproductive Medicine, Saarland University Hospital, Kirrberger Straße 100, Building 9, 66421 Homburg, Germany; bashar.hajhamoud@uks.eu
4. Department of Obstetrics and Gynecology, Carol Davila University of Medicine and Pharmacy, 050474 Bucharest, Romania
5. Faculty of Medicine, Titu Maiorescu University, 040441 Bucharest, Romania
* Correspondence: romina.sima@umfcd.ro

Abstract: Information about the impact of SARS-CoV-2 infection on pregnant women is still limited and raises challenges, even as publications are increasing rapidly. The aim of the present study was to determine the impact of SARS-CoV-2 infection on preterm birth pregnancies. We performed a prospective, observational study in a COVID-only hospital, which included 34 pregnant women with SARS-CoV-2 infection and preterm birth compared with a control group of 48 healthy women with preterm birth. The rate of cesarean delivery was 82% in the study group versus 6% for the control group. We observed a strong correlation between premature birth and the presence of COVID-19 symptoms (cough $p = 0.029$, fever $p = 0.001$, and chills $p = 0.001$). The risk for premature birth is correlated to a lower value of oxygen saturation ($p = 0.001$) and extensive radiologic pulmonary lesions ($p = 0.025$). The COVID-19 pregnant women with preterm delivery were older, and experienced an exacerbation of severe respiratory symptoms, decreased saturation of oxygen, increased inflammatory markers, severe pulmonary lesions and decreased lymphocytes.

Keywords: COVID-19; pregnant women; gestation age; preterm birth; birth rate; SARS-CoV-2

1. Introduction

Coronavirus disease-2019 (COVID-19) was declared a pandemic on 11th March 2020 [1]. For pregnant women, the mortality rate in cases of SARS-CoV-2 infection was reported at around 25% in the early studies [2]. These studies found no evidence that indicates an increased susceptibility in pregnant women. However, more recent studies suggest a role of this virus in mortality and morbidity due to cardiorespiratory and immune system involvement, which may determine an abnormal response to SARS-CoV-2 infection in pregnancy [3–5].

Information about SARS-CoV-2 infection in pregnant women, the fetus, and the neonatal prognosis is still limited even if the number of published articles is increasing. There are studies that describe the prevalence of maternal and neonatal SARS-CoV-2 outcomes [1,2] and suggest a possible increased risk of preterm delivery in cases of pregnant women with COVID-19 [3]. The aim of the present study was to evaluate the impact of SARS-CoV-2 infection on preterm birth among COVID-positive pregnant women.

2. Methods

We conducted a prospective cohort observational study (based on STROBE Statement) which included pregnant women with SARS-CoV-2 infection and preterm delivery. Patients delivered at "Saint John" Hospital, "Bucur" Maternity, a tertiary COVID-only health facility. Since 19 March 2020, "Bucur" Maternity was destinated by the Romanian Ministry of Health as the Department of Obstetrics and Gynecology responsible only for obstetrical and gynecological SARS-CoV-2 infection pathology associated.

The center where the study was conducted had an operating permit from the Bucharest Public Health Directorate for only 17 places in the obstetrics and gynecology ward and six places in the intensive care unit exclusive for COVID-19 patients. In this situation, only pregnant SARS-CoV-2-positive patients were admitted and cared for and we acted as a tertiary referral center for the whole south part of Romania (more than half of the Romanian population which is about 19 million persons).

Therefore, among the whole cohort of patients with SARS-CoV-2 infection, we selected women with preterm delivery from March 2020 to June 2021, which constituted the study group. The study obtained the approval of the ethical committee. Patients were included after signing their informed consent. We compared the study group with SARS-CoV-2 infection and preterm birth (COVID-19) with a historical control group of healthy women with preterm birth (non-COVID-19) who were hospitalized between March 2018 and March 2020 in the same department. The study was non-randomized. The control group was selected using the DRG (Diagnosis-Related-Group) code O.60 for preterm delivery.

The inclusion criteria were: singleton pregnancy, spontaneous pregnancy, gestational age between 24 and 36 weeks, RT-PCR (Real Time-Polymerase Chain Reaction) test positive for SARS-CoV-2, live fetus (ultrasound fetal viability), and adult women (range: 18–47).

The exclusion criteria were: age under 18 years, ART (Assisted Reproduction Techniques), pregnancy-associated pathologies, stillbirth, multiple pregnancies, previous premature birth, cervical incompetence, presence of pessary or cerclage, and the refusal of different investigations or treatment.

The analyzed parameters were: maternal age, obstetrical history of abortion, parity, rupture of membranes, gestational age at birth, days of ongoing COVID infection, birth type, COVID-19 symptoms, maternal and newborn evolution, CRP (C-Reactive Protein) level, leucocyte and lymphocyte values, and thoracic X-ray. All variables were obtained from the patient's observation file.

Statistical analysis was performed using Statistical Package for Social Sciences SPSS Statistic software, version 23 (Armonk, New York, NY, USA). (SPSS). Frequencies and descriptive data as well as correlations were recorded. A p-value < 0.05 was considered statistically significant. Pearson correlation was used for bivariate variables.

3. Results

In the period of study, 377 pregnancies with COVID 19 were admitted and 238 births (204 at term and 34 preterm births) occurred in our tertiary center. The overall rate of premature births was 14.28%; this rate was 8.2% during the previous non-COVID period in our clinic.

Our study included 34 pregnant patients with SARS-CoV-2 infection and preterm delivery compared with 48 patients from the control group.

Within the control group, we had eight cases of extremely preterm birth (<28 weeks gestational age, seven cases of moderately preterm birth (28 weeks to 31 weeks gestational age), and 33 cases of late preterm birth (32 weeks to 36 weeks+ 6 days gestational age), whereas within the SARS-CoV-2 group, there were three cases of extremely preterm births, four cases of moderate preterm, and 27 cases of late preterm births. The compared control and study group characteristics are illustrated in Table 1.

The obstetrical characteristics of the studied groups were similar. There was a higher percentage of pregnant women over 41 years old with COVID-19 who gave birth prematurely compared with healthy women. Within the COVID-19 group, we observed a lower percentage of extremely preterm births and higher percentages of moderate to late preterm births compared with the control. The major and significant difference among the two studied groups was the highest rate of cesarean section performed in COVID-19 patients for preterm delivery. The rate of cesarean delivery was increased in the COVID-19 period due to clinical indications, severe maternal clinical conditions and fetal distress (Table 2), which also justifies the increased rate of induced preterm births.

Table 1. Clinical characteristics of the patients.

MATERNAL CHARACTERISTICS	COVID-19 PATIENTS (%)	NON-COVID-19 PATIENTS (%)	p VALUE
MATERNAL AGE (YEARS)			
18–30	41	52.1	<0.001
31–40	46.2	43.8	<0.001
≥41	12.5	4.2	<0.001
GESTATIONAL AGE (WEEKS)			
<28	7.7	16.7	<0.01
28–31	12.8	14.6	<0.01
32–36	79.5	68.8	<0.01
BIRTH TYPE			
VAGINAL	18	94	<0.001
CESAREAN SECTION	82	6	<0.001
SPONTANOUS PRETERM BIRTHS	24	84	0.024
INDUCED BIRTH PRETERM BIRTHS	76	16	0.012

Table 2. Cesarean section indications.

Cesarean Indications (Percentage)	COVID-19 Patients (n = 34)	Non-COVID-19 Patients (n = 48)
Previous C-section	4.7	67
Exacerbation of symptoms	33.5	-
Labor dystocia	37.2	-
Fetal distress	24.6	33

We observed that the rate of cesarean section in the COVID-19 group of preterm labor was increased (82%) in this period and that two of the most frequent indications were the symptoms exacerbation, such as severe acute respiratory distress (33.5%) and fetal distress (24.6%), in comparison with only 6% in the non-COVID-19 group with previous C-section and fetal distress as indications.

The mean gestational age for COVID-19 diagnosis was 33.8 ± 8.2 weeks, with 7.4% of women being diagnosed in the first trimester, 9.7% in the second trimester, and 82.9% in the third trimester of pregnancy. Patients were asymptomatic in 63.2% of cases. The most common symptoms were cough (23%), followed by shortness of breath (21.6%), and fever (12.2%). Overall, 82% had cesarean section and 18% had a vaginal birth.

The distribution of the group according to the interval since the positive result of the RT-PCR test is illustrated in Table 3, from which we can observe that the highest proportion of premature births is represented by patients in the first four days of disease.

Regarding the biological markers, we found an inversed correlation between the value of CRP (C-Reactive Protein) and gestational age at birth (p = 0.001) or leucocyte count (p = 0.001). So, the risk of premature birth increases with the augmented value of inflammatory markers (Table 4). The lymphocyte count was indirectly correlated with the COVID-19 symptoms and the necessity of delivery. Patients with lower number of lymphocytes had more severe COVID-19 symptoms and more often underwent induced preterm delivery (p = 0.001).

In the group of pregnant women with SARS-CoV-2 infection, a strong correlation was established between premature birth and the presence of COVID-19 symptoms (cough p = 0.029, fever p = 0.001, and chills p = 0.001). The risk for premature birth is correlated with the decreased value for oxygen saturation (p = 0.001) and extensive radiologic pulmonary lesions (p = 0.025); the chest X-ray were taken with all standard protective measures for the patient. So, the risk for premature birth increased with moderate and severe infection with SARS-CoV-2 in the present study.

Table 3. COVID-19-related characteristics in the study group.

COVID-19 Characteristics	Days	Percentage (%)
Days of infection	1–4 days	59
	5–9 days	32
	10–14 days	9
Symptoms	asymptomatic	53
	mild	25.7
	moderate	11
	severe	10.3
Maternal outcome	curred	58.82
	improved	20.59
	transfer	20.59
Newborn outcome	good	41.2
	improved	50
	transfer	2.9
	dead	5.9

Table 4. CRP level.

CRP Level (Values Interval/mg/dL-Percentage)	COVID-19 Patients ($n = 34$)	Non-COVID-19 Patients ($n = 48$)
<0.5	7.8	52.1
0.5–49	73.4	43.7
50–99	13.6	2.1
>100	5.2	2.1

We also identified a strong correlation between severe maternal symptoms such as respiratory distress and newborns' outcome ($p = 0.001$). Women with severe respiratory distress delivered newborns who required neonatal intensive care. In the study group, the rate of perinatal death was about 5.9%, mainly related to prematurity. Gestational age at diagnosis, birth weight, and maternal ventilatory support were the main risk factors associated with adverse fetal outcomes.

The severity of symptomatology was correlated with cesarean birth rate ($p = 0.034$). Patients who experienced an exacerbation of severe respiratory symptoms delivered mostly by cesarean section. A total of 20.59% of patients had an unfavorable outcome, with mechanical ventilation and intubation before or after delivery and the transfer in intensive care units that could provide a higher degree of support.

4. Discussions

Pregnant women have a higher susceptibility to respiratory pathogens due to the adaptive anatomical and physiological changes in the respiratory system that occur during pregnancy, and these viral infections can induce pregnancy complications [3,6].

The purpose of this study was to determine the impact of SARS-CoV-2 infection on preterm birth, and we demonstrated that the rate of cesarean delivery was higher in the COVID-19 period due to severe maternal clinical conditions and fetal distress in comparison with the non-COVID-19 group. A strong correlation was observed between severe maternal symptoms such as respiratory distress and poor newborns' outcome ($p = 0.001$).

Oltean et al.'s review suggests elevated rates of ICU admission, C-sections, preeclampsia, placenta praevia, gestational diabetes, placental abruption, preterm birth, and elevated levels of CRP in women with COVID-19 in comparison to pregnant women without SARS-CoV-2 [7]. In our study, we identified that an increased CRP level is a risk factor for preterm birth.

Women with severe symptoms are more susceptible to adverse outcomes such as premature birth, even if pregnancy itself does not appear to aggravate the course of clinical characteristics or symptomatology of COVID-19 pneumonia [3,8]. Our study revealed the same pattern.

Increased levels of inflammatory markers are a risk factor that associated with other immunologically mediated processes are thought to play a role in the preterm birth syndrome [9].

According to Silva et al., the inflammatory status can promote conditions such as pre-eclampsia, intrauterine growth restriction, or premature birth [10]. Based on our clinical research, the gestational age decreased with the increased levels of inflammatory markers, so the inflammatory status may be the promotor factor for preterm delivery also in SARS-CoV-2-associated pregnancies.

We found a decreased rate of extremely preterm births in the COVID-19 group and an increased rate of moderate to late preterm births within the control group. In a Danish review, the rate of extremely premature birth also decreased during the COVID-19 lockdown [11].

As DiMascio et al. found, the main determinants of adverse perinatal outcomes in fetuses from mothers with COVID-19 infection are maternal ventilatory support, early gestational age at infection, and low birth weight [12]. We identified a strong correlation between severe maternal symptoms such as respiratory distress and newborns' outcome. The results of our study showed that in pregnancies with COVID-19, the rate of perinatal death was also increased, mainly related to prematurity. Gestational age at diagnosis, birth weight, and maternal ventilatory support were the factors associated with adverse fetal outcomes.

Since the onset of the COVID-19 epidemic, pregnant women with suspected or confirmed SARS-CoV-2 infections have undergone cesarean delivery in the absence of other obstetric indications in order to reduce the risk of intrapartum transmission, as some authors showed [13]. According to Bellos's meta-analysis, from currently available case series, a higher than expected number of preterm deliveries and cesarean sections are found in SARS-CoV-2 pregnancies [14]. Several studies have established that the incidence of premature and cesarean births increased during the pandemic period. There are cohort studies describing a limitation of risk in patients with severe forms of the disease, possibly with associated comorbidities. The main factors that may increase the risk of preterm labor, premature rupture of membranes, preterm birth, and abnormal fetal heart rate are fever and hypoxemia, but preterm births also occur in pregnant women with mild to moderate forms of the disease. Changes in prenatal care and increased stress during the pandemic may also increase the incidence of preterm births. One of the limitations of multiple studies is that spontaneous preterm birth is not differentiated from iatrogenic preterm birth. It appears that most cases of COVID-19 in the third trimester are delivered by planned cesarean section for the management of severe maternal illness, which may be partly explained by the obstetric decision to deliver due to the severity of the maternal infection (bilateral pneumonia with respiratory failure and shock) [14].

As can be seen in our results, the rate of preterm births and cesarean sections are increased due to severe maternal clinical conditions, and fetal distress compared to non-COVID patients. Unless fetal extraction is required to improve maternal oxygenation, SARS-CoV-2 infection is not an indication for delivery. There are several studies describing a direct association between preterm birth and COVID-19 infection [15,16]. From the onset of the pandemic, the majority of pregnant women confirmed with SARS-CoV-2 infection have given birth by cesarean section, with no other obstetrical indication [17].

Other poor outcomes in pregnant women with COVID-19, such as pre-eclampsia, preterm birth, and delivery by emergency cesarean section, are responsible in a cohort study for a high rate of fetal deaths [18]. In our study, there is a strong correlation between the type of delivery and COVID-19 symptoms. All symptomatic pregnant women delivered by cesarean section. In Allotey's analysis, an increased rate of preterm birth was observed in the COVID-19 pandemic compared to the worldwide reference rate. The same finding was observed in our study as well. The vaginal preterm birth rate was relatively low (5–6%), which is comparable to the general population [19,20] as the rate in the present.

The placental characteristics of pregnant women confirmed with SARS-CoV-2 infection were associated with perinatal outcomes, and it was determined that placental patterns indicate no clear evidence of transplacental transmission of SARS-CoV-2 or significant impact on perinatal outcomes in both mild and severe cases [21]. Multiple studies have reported no evidence of SARS-CoV-2 presence in the placenta, amniotic fluid, or cord blood [15,22]. Since there is no proof of vertical transmission, COVID-19 is not an indication for cesarean section in order to prevent transmission during expulsion [15,23]. In our study, no newborn was confirmed with SARS-CoV-2 infection by RT-PCR testing at 24 h and 48 h after birth within.

Similar to the results of Papanou's meta-analysis, the present study finds that the rate of preterm births increased during the pandemic due to iatrogenic involvement [24]. At the time when our study started, the vaccination of pregnant women against SARS-CoV-2 was not yet approved. As a consequence, no pregnant women were vaccinated and we could not determine what impact it would have had in reducing the risk of maternal, birth, and neonatal outcomes. According to Heather S. Lipkind et al., COVID-19 vaccination during pregnancy was not related to preterm birth or low gestational age at birth overall, compared with unvaccinated pregnant women [25]. The available data suggest that vaccination during pregnancy is associated with antibodies against SARS-CoV-2 transmission to the fetus, but the level of protection of the newborn provided by transplacental and breast milk antibodies is unclear [26].

The limitations of our study were: the reduced number of patient, the study was performed during the first period of the pandemic and there were no evidence about the vaccine anti SARS-CoV-2 on pregnant women. Meanwhile, the number of patient treated in our COVID exclusive center provided the largest cohort of the pregnancies infected with SARS-CoV-2 in our country and can be considered also the main strength.

The impact of the SARS-CoV-2 pandemic on obstetrical population and neonates is a subject of intense debate with the unpredictable outcome and frequent changes in pathogenicity and contagiosity of the virus variants. Considering morbidity and mortality of the prematurity SARS-CoV2 impact on premature birth is a matter of intense debate.

5. Conclusions

The present study investigates the main characteristics of COVID-19-associated preterm deliveries in a tertiary center providing exclusive care for those patients and having the highest level of experience in Romania. The pregnant women with COVID-19 with preterm delivery were older women, who experienced an exacerbation of severe respiratory symptoms, decreased saturation of oxygen, increased inflammatory markers, extensive pulmonary lesions and decreased lymphocytes. The preterm delivery was mainly induced and by cesarean section and the newborns required intensive care more often than the ones delivered by healthy mothers.

Author Contributions: Conceptualization: T.-I.B. and L.P.; original draft preparation: T.-I.B. and M.-O.P.; critical review and editing: B.H.H., O.-G.O. and G.-P.G.; supervision: R.-M.S. and L.P. All authors have read and agreed to the published version of the manuscript.

Funding: This research received no external funding.

Institutional Review Board Statement: The study was conducted according to the guidelines of the Declaration of Helsinki, and approved by the Ethics Committee of "Sf. Ioan" Emergency Hospital, Bucharest, Romania (no 30386/16 December 2021).

Informed Consent Statement: Informed consent was obtained from all subjects involved in the study.

Conflicts of Interest: The authors declare that the research was conducted in the absence of any commercial or financial relationships that could be construed as a potential conflict of interest.

References

1. World Health Organization. WHO Director-General's Opening Remarks at the Media Briefing on COVID-19. Available online: https://www.who.int/dg/speeches/detail/who-director-general-s-opening-remarks-at-the-media-briefing-on-covid-19%2D%2D-11-march-2020 (accessed on 14 January 2022).
2. Wong, S.F.; Chow, K.M.; Leung, T.N.; Ng, W.F.; Ng, T.K.; Shek, C.C.; Ng, P.C.; Lam, P.W.; Ho, L.C.; To, W.W.; et al. Pregnancy and perinatal outcomes of women with severe acute respiratory syndrome. *Am. J. Obstet. Gynecol.* **2004**, *191*, 292–297. [CrossRef] [PubMed]
3. Wastnedge, E.A.; Reynolds, R.M.; Van Boeckel, S.R.; Stock, S.J.; Denison, F.C.; Maybin, J.A.; Critchley, H.O. Pregnancy and COVID-19. *Physiol. Rev.* **2021**, *101*, 303–318. [CrossRef] [PubMed]
4. Qiao, J. What are the risks of COVID-19 infection in pregnant women? *Lancet* **2020**, *395*, 760–762. [CrossRef]
5. Albuquerque, L.P.; Monte, A.V.L.; Araújo, R.M.S. Implications of COVID-19 for pregnant patients. *Rev. Eletrônica Acervo Saúde* **2020**, *12*, e4632.
6. Schwartz, D.A.; Graham, A.L. Potential maternal and infant outcomes from (Wuhan) coronavirus 2019-nCoV infecting pregnant women: Lessons from SARS, MERS, and other human coronavirus infections. *Viruses* **2020**, *12*, 194. [CrossRef] [PubMed]
7. Oltean, I.; Tran, J.; Lawrence, S.; Ruschkowski, B.A.; Zeng, N.; Bardwell, C.; Nasr, Y.; de Nanassy, J.; El Demellawy, D. Impact of SARS-CoV-2 on the clinical outcomes and placental pathology of pregnant women and their infants: A systematic review. *Heliyon* **2021**, *7*, 06393. [CrossRef] [PubMed]
8. Liu, D.; Li, L.; Wu, X.; Zheng, D.; Wang, J.; Yang, L.; Zheng, C. Pregnancy and Perinatal Outcomes of Women With Coronavirus Disease (COVID-19) Pneumonia: A Preliminary Analysis. *Am. J. Roentgenol.* **2020**, *215*, 127–132. [CrossRef] [PubMed]
9. Goldenberg, R.L.; Culhane, J.F.; Iams, J.D.; Romero, R. Epidemiology and causes of preterm birth. *Lancet* **2008**, *371*, 75–84. [CrossRef]
10. De Souza Silva, G.A.; da Silva, S.P.; da Costa, M.; da Silva, A.R.; de Vasconcelos Alves, R.R.; Ângelo Mendes Tenório, F.; da Silva Melo, A.R.; de Freitas, A.C.; Lagos de Melo, C.M. SARS-CoV, MERS-CoV and SARS-CoV-2 infections in pregnancy and fetal development. *J. Gynecol. Obstet. Hum. Reprod.* **2020**, *49*, 101846. [CrossRef] [PubMed]
11. Hedermann, G.; Hedley, P.L.; Bækvad-Hansen, M.; Hjalgrim, H.; Rostgaard, K.; Poorisrisak, P.; Breindahl, M.; Melbye, M.; Hougaard, D.M.; Christiansen, M.; et al. Danish premature birth rates during the COVID-19 lockdown. *Arch. Dis. Child. Fetal Neonatal Ed.* **2021**, *106*, 93–95. [CrossRef]
12. Di Mascio, D.; Sen, C.; Saccone, G.; Galindo, A.; Grünebaum, A.; Yoshimatsu, J.; Stanojevic, M.; Kurjak, A.; Chervenak, F.; Suárez, M.J.R.; et al. Risk factors associated with adverse fetal outcomes in pregnancies affected by Coronavirus disease 2019 (COVID-19): A secondary analysis of the WAPM study on COVID-19. *J. Périnat. Med.* **2020**, *48*, 950–958. [CrossRef] [PubMed]
13. Chen, H.; Guo, J.; Wang, C.; Luo, F.; Yu, X.; Zhang, W.; Li, J.; Zhao, D.; Xu, D.; Gong, Q.; et al. Clinical characteristics and intrauterine vertical transmission potential of COVID-19 infection in nine pregnant women: A retrospective review of medical records. *Lancet* **2020**, *395*, 809–815. [CrossRef]
14. Bellos, I.; Pandita, A.; Panza, R. Maternal and perinatal outcomes in pregnant women infected by SARS-CoV-2: A meta-analysis. *Eur. J. Obstet. Gynecol. Reprod. Biol.* **2020**, *256*, 194–204. [CrossRef] [PubMed]
15. Wang, X.; Zhou, Z.; Zhang, J.; Zhu, F.; Tang, Y.; Shen, X. A Case of 2019 Novel Coronavirus in a Pregnant Woman with Preterm Delivery. *Clin. Infect. Dis.* **2020**, *71*, 844–846. [CrossRef] [PubMed]
16. Mullins, E.; Evans, D.; Viner, R.M.; O'Brien, P.; Morris, E. Coronavirus in pregnancy and delivery: Rapid review. *Ultrasound Obs. Gynecol.* **2020**, *55*, 586–592. [CrossRef] [PubMed]
17. Wei, S.; Bilodeau-Bertrand, M.; Liu, S.; Auger, N. The impact of COVID-19 on pregnancy outcomes: A systematic review and meta-analysis. *CMAJ.* **2021**, *193*, 540–548. [CrossRef]
18. Gurol-Urganci, I.; Jardine, J.E.; Carroll, F.; Draycott, T.; Dunn, G.; Fremeaux, A.; Harris, T.; Hawdon, J.; Morris, E.; Muller, P.; et al. Maternal and perinatal outcomes of pregnant women with SARS-CoV-2 infection at the time of birth in England: National cohort study. *Am. J. Obstet. Gynecol.* **2021**, *225*, 522.e1–522.e11. [CrossRef]
19. Allotey, J.; Stallings, E.; Bonet, M.; Yap, M.; Chatterjee, S.; Kew, T.; Debenham, L.; Llavall, A.C.; Dixit, A.; Zhou, D.; et al. Clinical manifestations, risk factors, and maternal and perinatal outcomes of coronavirus disease 2019 in pregnancy: Living systematic review and meta-analysis. *BMJ* **2020**, *370*, m3320. [CrossRef]
20. Turan, O.; Hakim, A.; Dashraath, P.; Jeslyn, W.J.L.; Wright, A.; Kadir, R.A. Clinical characteristics, prognostic factors, and maternal and neonatal outcomes of SARS-CoV-2 infection among hospitalized pregnant women: A systematic review. *Int. J. Gynecol. Obstet.* **2020**, *151*, 7–16. [CrossRef]
21. Giordano, G.; Petrolini, C.; Corradini, E.; Campanini, N.; Esposito, S.; Perrone, S. COVID-19 in pregnancy: Placental pathological patterns and effect on perinatal outcome in five cases. *Diagn. Pathol.* **2021**, *16*, 88. [CrossRef]
22. Li, Y.; Zhao, R.; Zheng, S.; Chen, X.; Wang, J.; Sheng, X.; Zhou, J.; Cai, H.; Fang, Q.; Yu, F.; et al. Lack of Vertical Transmission of Severe Acute Respiratory Syndrome Coronavirus 2, China. *Emerg. Infect. Dis.* **2020**, *26*, 1335–1336. [CrossRef] [PubMed]
23. Zhu, H.; Wang, L.; Fang, C.; Peng, S.; Zhang, L.; Chang, G.; Xia, S.; Zhou, W. Clinical analysis of 10 neonates born to mothers with 2019-nCoV pneumonia. *Transl. Pediatr.* **2020**, *9*, 51–60. [CrossRef] [PubMed]
24. Papapanou, M.; Papaioannou, M.; Petta, A.; Routsi, E.; Farmaki, M.; Vlahos, N.; Siristatidis, C. Maternal and Neonatal Characteristics and Outcomes of COVID-19 in Pregnancy: An Overview of Systematic Reviews. *Int. J. Environ. Res. Public Health* **2021**, *18*, 596. [CrossRef] [PubMed]

25. Lipkind, H.S.; Vazquez-Benitez, G.; DeSilva, M.; Vesco, K.K.; Ackerman-Banks, C.; Zhu, J.; Boyce, T.G.; Daley, M.F.; Fuller, C.C.; Getahun, D.; et al. Receipt of COVID-19 Vaccine During Pregnancy and Preterm or Small-for-Gestational-Age at Birth—Eight Integrated Health Care Organizations, United States, December 15, 2020–July 22, 2021. *MMWR Morb. Mortal. Wkly. Rep.* **2022**, *71*, 26–30. [CrossRef] [PubMed]
26. Jamieson, D.J.; Rasmussen, S.A. An update on COVID-19 and pregnancy. *Am. J. Obstet. Gynecol.* **2022**, *226*, 177–186. [CrossRef] [PubMed]

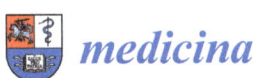

Article

Unraveling the Efficacy of Therapeutic Interventions for Short Cervix: Insights from a Retrospective Study for Improved Clinical Management

Alina-Madalina Luca [1], Elena Bernad [2,*], Dragos Nemescu [1,*], Cristian Vaduva [3,†], Anamaria Harabor [4,†], Ana-Maria Adam [4], Valeriu Harabor [4], Aurel Nechita [4], Cristina Strobescu [5,†], Raluca Mogos [1,†], Alexandru Carauleanu [1], Ingrid-Andrada Vasilache [1] and Demetra Socolov [1]

1. Department of Obstetrics and Gynecology, 'Grigore T. Popa' University of Medicine and Pharmacy, 700115 Iasi, Romania
2. Department of Obstetrics and Gynecology, Faculty of Medicine, "Victor Babes" University of Medicine and Pharmacy, 300041 Timisoara, Romania
3. Department of Mother and Child Medicine, Faculty of Medicine, University of Medicine and Pharmacy, 200349 Craiova, Romania
4. Clinical and Surgical Department, Faculty of Medicine and Pharmacy, 'Dunarea de Jos' University, 800216 Galati, Romania; adam.anamaria89@gmail.com (A.-M.A.)
5. Department of Vascular Surgery, University of Medicine and Pharmacy "Grigore T. Popa", 700111 Iasi, Romania
* Correspondence: bernad.elena@umft.ro (E.B.); dnemescu@yahoo.com (D.N.)
† These authors contributed equally to this work.

Abstract: *Background and Objectives*: Preterm birth (PTB) is associated with important neonatal mortality and morbidity. The aim of this study was to retrospectively evaluate the average treatment effects on the treated and the efficacy of various therapeutic interventions for PTB in a cohort of patients with singleton pregnancies and short cervical lengths. *Materials and Methods*: This observational retrospective study included 1146 singleton pregnancies at risk of PTB that were segregated into the following groups: intravaginal progesterone (group 1), Arabin pessary (group 2), McDonald cerclage (group 3), intravaginal progesterone and Arabin pessary (group 4), and intravaginal progesterone and cerclage (group 5). Their treatment effects were evaluated and compared. *Results*: All evaluated therapeutic interventions significantly reduced the occurrence of late and early preterm births. The risk of late and early PTB was lowered for those pregnant patients who received progesterone and pessaries or progesterone and cerclage in comparison with those who received only progesterone. The extremely PTB risk of occurrence was significantly lowered only by the administration of progesterone in association with cervical cerclage in comparison with progesterone monotherapy. *Conclusions*: The combined therapeutic interventions had the highest efficacy in preventing preterm birth. An individualized evaluation is needed to establish the best therapeutic approach in particular cases.

Keywords: preterm birth; progesterone; cervical cerclage; pessary

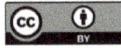

1. Introduction

Preterm birth (PTB), defined as any birth before 37 complete weeks of gestation, is an important public health problem responsible for approximately 2.5 million neonatal deaths per year worldwide [1]. Gestational age sub-groups (such as extremely preterm, very preterm, moderate preterm, and late preterm), the occurrence of preterm birth (spontaneous versus medically induced), and pathophysiological background are examples of common classification criteria of categorization systems [2]. PTB may occur naturally, as a result of spontaneous preterm labor and/or preterm pre-labor membrane rupture, or under the direction of a healthcare professional by cesarean delivery or labor induction.

The complications of PTB include acute respiratory distress syndrome (ARDS), necrotizing enterocolitis (NE), sepsis, intraventricular hemorrhage (IVH), hypoxic–ischemic encephalopathy (HIE), seizures, and cerebral palsy, as well as feeding difficulties and visual or hearing impairment [3–6]. Follow-ups of these patients reveal a higher prevalence of neurodevelopmental problems, along with social-emotional and learning difficulties [7,8].

A plethora of risk factors for the prediction of preterm birth have been proposed [9–12], but only a few of them have remained consistent throughout the literature. Maternal characteristics are the most studied, and it was proven that ethnicity, extremes of maternal age, low maternal education, smoking, illicit drug consumption, personal history of preterm birth, short cervical length (less than 2.5 cm), and maternal comorbidities (vaginal or systemic infections, autoimmune disorders, thrombophilia, etc.) were significantly associated with the occurrence of PTB [13–16]. Moreover, some hormonal and vitamin imbalances have been proposed as risk factors for pregnancy complications, such as PTB [17]. Thus, correcting these imbalances will result in improving the overall health status of these patients [18,19].

Preterm birth has also been linked to placental, uterine, or fetal abnormalities such as placental abruption, placenta previa, polyhydramnios, uterine malformations, uterine fibromas, and fetal structural or chromosomal defects [20–23]. There is a lack of agreement over whether prior uterine surgery (curettage, hysteroscopy, myomectomy, and multiple previous cesarean surgeries) increases the risk of preterm birth or not, and although systematic reviews have found only modest associations, they were unable to account for all possible confounders [24–27].

Various treatment strategies for PTB have been proposed, including vaginal progesterone, pessaries, and cerclage, with or without the association of tocolysis. For a woman with a short cervix and a history of spontaneous preterm delivery, the National Institute for Health and Care Excellence's (NICE) preterm birth guidelines suggest giving the option of vaginal progesterone or cervical cerclage [28]. NICE also advises women with low cervical lengths (25 m) or histories of spontaneous preterm birth to take into account vaginal progesterone [28]. Vaginal progesterone has recently been the subject of large, negative, randomized controlled trials [10,11], which have raised questions regarding its efficacy [29,30].

On the other hand, Care et al. evaluated, in a systematic review and meta-analysis, 61 trials that compared the efficacy of various interventions for the prevention of preterm birth in singleton pregnancies, and the authors concluded that vaginal progesterone was associated with fewer women with preterm births <34 weeks (odds ratio (OR): 0.50, 95% confidence interval (CI): 0.34–0.70), along with Shirodkar cerclage (effect size (ES): 0.06, 95% CI: 0.00–0.84), and vaginal pessary (ES: 0.65, 95% CI: 0.39 to 1.08) [31]. Still, there is a great heterogeneity regarding the recommendations of various therapeutic strategies, and the PTB prevention protocols differ between healthcare institutions. Moreover, current data from observational studies were determined after the evaluation of small cohorts of patients over short timeframes, thus providing low-quality evidence.

In 2022, Pacagnella et al. published a multicenter, open-label, randomized controlled trial that evaluated the efficacy of the cervical pessary in addition to vaginal progesterone for the prevention of preterm birth in women with shortened cervixes, and the authors concluded that the combination therapy did not decrease rates of neonatal morbidity or mortality [32]. On the other hand, they showed that the combination progesterone–pessary had significantly lower rates of overall preterm births compared to monotherapy.

There are various formulations of progesterone that can be administered orally, intravaginally, or intramuscularly. A recent randomized clinical trial of 150 pregnant patients at risk of preterm birth, who had received oral Dydrogesterone (30 mg/day), 17α-hydroxyprogesterone caproate (17α-OHPC, 250 mg intramuscular, weekly), or nothing, showed that progesterone caproate obtained superior results in prolonging the latency period until birth and improving neonatal outcomes in comparison with oral progesterone and placebo [33].

Very few observational studies have evaluated the treatment effects of various strategies used in monotherapy or combined therapies. Therefore, the aim of this study was to retrospectively evaluate the average treatment effects and efficacies of various therapeutic interventions for preterm birth in a cohort of patients with singleton pregnancies and short cervical lengths.

2. Materials and Methods

This observational retrospective study included 1146 singleton pregnancies with asymptomatic short cervixes that were evaluated at the tertiary maternity hospital 'Cuza-Voda', Iasi, Romania, between January 2017 and December 2021. Ethical approval for this study was obtained from the Institutional Ethics Committees of 'Cuza-Voda' Maternity Hospital (No. 2052/16.02.2021) and the University of Medicine and Pharmacy 'Grigore T. Popa' (No. 101/08.07.2021). Informed consent was waived for this study, but all participants included in the study signed a consent form for the use of anonymized clinical data in further studies. All methods were carried out in accordance with relevant guidelines and regulations.

Inclusion criteria comprised singleton pregnancies with certain first-trimester dating, maternal age ≥ 18 years old, and short cervical lengths (less than 2.5 cm) that presented at our institution between 18 and 22 weeks of gestation for fetal morphological evaluation. The exclusion criteria referred to twin pregnancies, structural or chromosomal fetal abnormalities, patients with preterm labor, premature rupture of membranes, or vaginal infections, patients with clinical emergencies who could not receive one of the proposed therapeutic approaches, stillbirth, and incomplete medical records.

The risk of preterm birth was considered in the presence of short cervical length (less than 2.5 cm) measured by transvaginal ultrasound using an E8 scanner with a 5–15 MHz transvaginal probe (GE Medical Systems, Milwaukee, WI, USA), as recommended by ISUOG [34].

Each physician chose the therapeutic approach for these pregnant patients based on local protocols and international guidelines [35–38], while taking into account the patient's preference and compliance with a specific treatment. Intravaginal progesterone was administered to asymptomatic patients with or without a personal history of PTB and short cervical length (less than 25 mm). The Arabin pessary was chosen for a patient with or without a personal history of PTB if the vaginal ultrasound indicated signs of cervical incompetence (cervical shortening and funneling). Cervical cerclage was recommended for a patient with a personal history of PTB and short cervical length or in the presence of major clinical modifications of the cervix (cervical effacement or dilation), with or without a protrusion of the amniotic sac, even in the absence of a personal history of PTB. Intravaginal progesterone was added to cervical cerclage or Arabin pessary at the physician's discretion, especially when the cervical length was less than 15 mm.

The patients were segregated into the following groups depending on the employed therapeutic approach: intravaginal progesterone (200 mg/day)—group 1 (n = 562 patients), Arabin pessary—group 2 (n = 286 patients), McDonald cerclage—group 3 (n = 128 patients), intravaginal progesterone and Arabin pessary—group 4 (n = 101 patients), and intravaginal progesterone and cerclage—group 5 (n = 69 patients).

The evaluated outcomes were represented by preterm birth between 32 and 36 + 6 weeks of gestation (late preterm), 28 and 31 + 6 weeks of gestation (early preterm), and at less than 28 weeks of gestation (extremely preterm). From the patient's medical records, we also retrieved demographic data, a personal history of preterm birth, thrombosis, or ischemic placental disease, and comorbidities (thrombophilia, autoimmune disorders, etc.), as well as neonatal outcomes, such as birth through cesarean delivery, Apgar scores at 1 and 5 min, neonatal intensive care unit admission (NICU), the presence of IVH, cerebral palsy, ARDS, necrotizing enterocolitis, the need for mechanical ventilation, and neonatal death.

Pearson's chi-squared test was used to determine whether there is a statistically significant difference between the expected frequencies and the observed frequencies in one or more categories of clinical characteristics. For continuous variables, results were given as mean and standard deviation (SD), and between-group differences were assessed using ANOVA. For the multivariate analysis of treatment groups, we used multinomial logistic regression, adjusted for maternal age, smoking status, and the presence of comorbidities. For binary outcomes, relative risk (RR) and 95% CI values were calculated. We also calculated average treatment effects on the treated (ATT) using regression adjustment and compared the logarithmic odds ratios (logORs) of various therapeutic interventions for the evaluated outcomes. A p-value less than 0.05 was considered statistically significant. The statistical analyses were performed using STATA SE (version 17, 2022; StataCorp LLC, College Station, TX, USA).

3. Results

This observational retrospective study included 1146 pregnant patients with singleton pregnancies, segregated into five groups: intravaginal progesterone—group 1 (n = 562 patients), Arabin pessary—group 2 (n = 286 patients), McDonald cerclage—group 3 (n = 128 patients), intravaginal progesterone and Arabin pessary—group 4 (n = 101 patients), and intravaginal progesterone and cerclage—group 5 (n = 69 patients).

The clinical characteristics of the evaluated groups and the results from the univariate analysis are presented in Table 1. Pregnant patients who underwent cervical cerclage had the highest rates of preterm births in their personal history (39.06%), followed by patients who received intravaginal progesterone and Arabin pessaries (30.69%) and intravaginal progesterone and cerclage (26.08%). We found a statistically significant difference regarding this aspect between groups (p < 0.001).

Table 1. Univariate analysis of the clinical characteristics of the patients included in our study.

Patient's Data	Group 1 (n = 562 Patients)	Group 2 (n = 286 Patients)	Group 3 (n = 128 Patients)	Group 4 (n = 101 Patients)	Group 5 (n = 69 Patients)	p-Value
Maternal age, years (mean and standard deviation)	29.46 ± 6.59	30.34 ± 6.54	29.98 ± 6.60	29.83 ± 6.85	30.67 ± 6.19	0.31
Medium (n/%)	Rural = 291 (51.9%) Urban = 270 (48.1%)	Rural = 138 (48.1%) Urban = 149 (51.9%)	Rural = 68 (53.1%) Urban = 60 (46.9%)	Rural = 52 (51.5%) Urban = 49 (48.5%)	Rural = 42 (60.9%) Urban = 39.1 (47%)	0.41
Smoking (n/%)	Yes = 13 (2.3%)	Yes = 10 (3.49%)	Yes = 7 (5.5%)	Yes = 5 (5.0%)	Yes = 4 (5.8%)	0.19
Personal history of preterm birth (n/%)	Yes = 34 (6.04%)	Yes = 47 (16.43%)	Yes = 50 (39.06%)	Yes = 31 (30.69%)	Yes = 18 (26.08%)	<0.001
Personal history of thrombosis (n/%)	Yes = 2 (0.35%)	Yes = 1 (0.34%)	Yes = 0 (0%)	Yes = 0 (0%)	Yes = 0 (0%)	0.47
Diabetes (n/%)	Yes = 6 (1.1%)	Yes = 2 (0.7%)	Yes = 1 (0.8%)	Yes = 1 (1%)	Yes = 0 (0%)	0.91
Thrombophilia (n/%)	Yes = 5 (0.88%)	Yes = 2 (0.69%)	Yes = 1 (0.8%)	Yes = 0 (0%)	Yes = 0 (0%)	0.98
Personal history of autoimmune disorders (n/%)	Yes = 18 (3.2%)	Yes = 14 (4.89%)	Yes = 8 (6.25%)	Yes = 5 (4.95%)	Yes = 0 (0%)	0.33
Personal history of ischemic placental disease (n/%)	Yes = 7 (1.24%)	Yes = 4 (1.39%)	Yes = 2 (1.56%)	Yes = 1 (1%)	Yes = 0 (0%)	0.98
Cervical length, mm (mean and standard deviation)	22.1 ± 2.16	20.25 ± 2.21	19.75 ± 1.70	18.75 ± 3.59	16.5 ± 3.87	0.14

We evaluated the average treatment effects of various therapeutic interventions, and we described them considering the main outcomes. The average treatment effects on the treated (ATT) analysis (Table 2) revealed that all therapeutic interventions significantly reduced the occurrence of late and early preterm births. Progesterone in combination with cervical cerclage had the highest impact on the occurrence of both late (ATT = −0.28; 95%CI: −0.48–0.08; p = 0.006) and early (ATT = −0.21; 95%CI: −0.35–0.37; p = 0.009) PTB. On the other hand, only progesterone intravaginally administered significantly reduced the occurrence of extremely preterm birth (ATT = −0.07; 95%CI: −0.13–0.10; p < 0.001).

Table 2. Average treatment effects on the treated of the evaluated therapeutic interventions for preterm birth.

Treatment	Late Preterm Birth				Early Preterm Birth				Extremely Preterm Birth			
	ATT	95%CI Lower Bound	95%CI Upper Bound	p-Value	ATT	95%CI Lower Bound	95%CI Upper Bound	p-Value	ATT	95%CI Lower Bound	95%CI Upper Bound	p-Value
Progesterone	−0.14	−0.19	−0.09	<0.001	−0.07	−0.13	0.11	<0.001	−0.07	−0.13	0.10	<0.001
Pessary	−0.16	−0.28	−0.05	<0.001	−0.10	−0.17	0.21	0.03	−0.01	−0.13	0.13	0.09
Cerclage	−0.14	−0.31	−0.01	0.01	−0.08	−0.19	0.23	0.02	−0.04	−0.13	0.17	0.255
Progesterone and pessary	−0.18	−0.35	−0.01	0.03	−0.07	−0.21	0.16	0.01	0.16	−0.03	0.35	0.09
Progesterone and cerclage	−0.28	−0.48	−0.08	0.006	−0.21	−0.35	0.37	0.009	0.09	−0.09	0.29	0.306

Table legend: ATT—average treatment effect on the treated; CI—confidence interval.

Graphical representations of the comparisons between evaluated therapeutic interventions for the reduction of various types of preterm birth are presented in Figures 1–3. The highest performance in the reduction of late PTB was achieved by the combination of progesterone and cerclage (logOR: −5.34; 95% CI: −6.34−−4.34), followed by progesterone and pessary (logOR: −4.79; 95% CI: −5.58−−4.00). The lowest performance, in this case, was achieved by the administration of progesterone in monotherapy (logOR: −2.02; 95% CI: −2.29−−1.74).

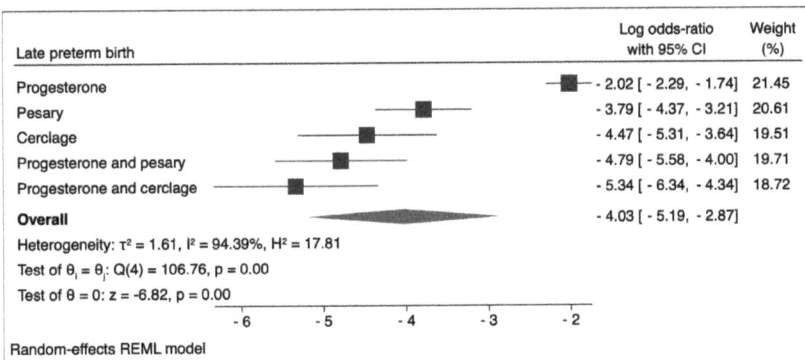

Figure 1. Comparison between therapeutic interventions for the reduction of late preterm birth.

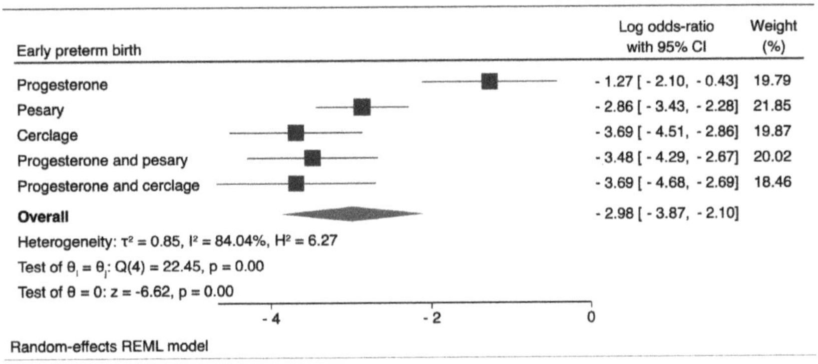

Figure 2. Comparison between therapeutic interventions for the reduction of early preterm birth.

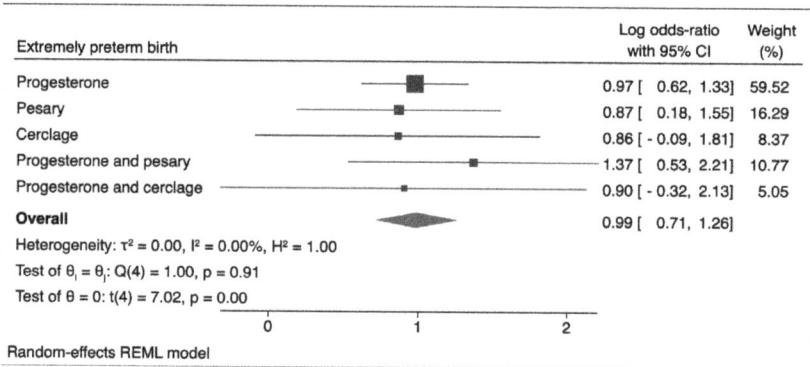

Figure 3. Comparison between therapeutic interventions for the reduction of extremely preterm birth.

When evaluating the reduction of early preterm birth through therapeutic interventions, our results indicated that both cervical cerclage (logOR: −3.69; 95% CI: −4.51−−2.86) and the combination of progesterone and cerclage (logOR: −3.69; 95% CI: −4.68−−2.69) achieved similar performances, closely followed by the combination of progesterone and pessary (logOR: −3.48; 95%CI: −4.29−−2.67).

In the case of extremely preterm birth, the results indicated a non-significant influence of the evaluated therapeutic interventions over the pregnancy's course and a tendency for these interventions to be associated with increased odds of PTB.

In our cohort of patients, the risk of occurrence of late preterm birth was significantly higher for pregnant patients who received progesterone in comparison with those who received Arabin pessaries (RR: 3.13; 95% CI: 2.42–4.04; $p < 0.001$) or cervical cerclage (RR: 2.73; 95% CI: 1.93–3.86; $p < 0.001$) (Table 3). On the other hand, the risk was significantly lower for patients who received progesterone and pessaries (RR: 0.36; 95% CI: 0.24–0.54; $p < 0.001$) or progesterone and cerclage (RR: 0.30; 95% CI: 0.18–0.52; $p < 0.001$) in comparison with those who received only progesterone, translating into a risk reduction of 64% for the first treatment option and 70% for the second treatment option.

Table 3. Calculated relative risks for various therapeutic interventions in relationship with the evaluated outcomes.

Therapeutic Intervention	Late Preterm Birth		Early Preterm Birth		Extremely Preterm Birth	
	RR and 95% CI	p-Value	RR and 95% CI	p-Value	RR and 95% CI	p-Value
Progesterone vs. pessary	3.13 (2.42–4.04)	<0.001	3.73 (2.37–5.88)	<0.001	4.81 (2.49–9.26)	<0.001
Progesterone vs cerclage	2.73 (1.93–3.86)	<0.001	3.57 (1.87–6.83)	<0.001	4.16 (1.71–10.12)	0.001
Cerclage vs. pessary	0.87 (0.57–1.32)	0.52	1.04 (0.49–2.20)	0.11	1.15 (0.40–3.28)	0.78
Progesterone + pessary vs progesterone alone	0.36 (0.24–0.54)	<0.001	0.44 (0.24–0.78)	0.005	0.59 (0.28–1.23)	0.15
Progesterone + pessary vs. cerclage	0.79 (0.47–1.32)	0.37	1.58 (0.69–3.61)	0.27	2.45 (0.82–7.35)	0.10
Progesterone + pessary vs. pessary	1.14 (0.72–1.82)	0.55	1.65 (0.82–3.28)	0.15	2.83 (1.13–7.11)	0.05
Progesterone + cerclage vs. progesterone alone	0.30 (0.18–0.52)	<0.001	0.49 (0.26–0.91)	0.02	0.27 (0.08–0.84)	0.02
Progesterone + cerclage vs. pessary	0.96 (0.53–1.73)	0.91	1.84 (0.88–3.81)	0.10	1.31 (0.37–4.60)	0.66

Table 3. Cont.

Therapeutic Intervention	Late Preterm Birth		Early Preterm Birth		Extremely Preterm Birth	
	RR and 95% CI	p-Value	RR and 95% CI	p-Value	RR and 95% CI	p-Value
Progesterone + cerclage vs. cerclage	0.84 (0.45–1.58)	0.60	1.76 (0.74–4.17)	0.19	1.13 (0.28–4.56)	0.85
Progesterone + pessary vs. progesterone +cerclage	1.18 (0.61–2.29)	0.61	0.89 (0.39–2.01)	0.79	1.61 (0.43–5.92)	0.47

Table legend: RR—relative risk; CI—confidence interval; vs.—versus.

The risk of occurrence of early preterm birth was similarly increased in patients who received progesterone in comparison with those who received Arabin pessaries (RR: 3.73; 95% CI: 2.37–5.88; $p < 0.001$) or cervical cerclage (RR: 3.57; 95% CI: 1.87–6.83; $p < 0.001$). The risk was also lowered for those patients who received progesterone and pessaries (RR: 0.44; 95% CI: 0.24–0.78; $p = 0.005$) or progesterone and cerclage (RR: 0.49; 95% CI: 0.26–0.91; $p \leq 0.02$) in comparison with those who received only progesterone, translating into a risk reduction of 56% for the first treatment option and 51% for the second treatment option.

The same pattern of increased risk of extremely preterm birth was observed for patients who received progesterone in comparison with those who received Arabin pessaries (RR: 4.81; 95% CI: 2.49–9.26; $p < 0.001$) or cervical cerclage (RR: 4.16; 95% CI: 1.71–10.12; $p = 0.001$). However, the risk of occurrence was significantly lowered only by the administration of progesterone in association with cervical cerclage in comparison with progesterone monotherapy (RR: 0.27; 95% CI: 0.08–0.84; $p = 0.02$).

Finally, we evaluated and compared neonatal outcomes using multinomial logistic regression (Table 4). Our analysis revealed that late preterm neonates were born significantly more frequently through cesarean section ($p < 0.001$), required significantly more invasive ventilation ($p < 0.001$), and developed ARDS after birth ($p < 0.001$). Moreover, the Apgar scores at 1 and 5 min of less than seven were significantly prevalent in this group.

Table 4. Pregnancy and neonatal outcomes in preterm deliveries.

Outcome	Late Preterm Birth		Early Preterm Birth		Extremely Preterm Birth	
	aOR and 95% CI	p-Value	aOR and 95% CI	p-Value	aOR and 95% CI	p-Value
Cesarean delivery	2.11 (0.35–5.41)	<0.001	0.95 (0.70–1.29)	0.78	0.88 (0.49–1.57)	0.68
Apgar score at 1 min < 7	1.82 (1.42–2.31)	<0.001	1.79 (0.68–4.41)	0.007	1.83 (0.19–4.51)	0.008
Apgar score at 5 min < 7	1.21 (0.45–3.58)	<0.001	2.65 (1.55–4.55)	<0.001	1.28 (0.45–3.44)	0.03
NICU admission	0.96 (0.67–1.38)	0.84	1.26 (0.17–4.21)	<0.001	0.72 (0.18–2.87)	<0.001
Necrotizing enterocolitis	0.44 (0.16–1.85)	0.79	1.04 (0.55–2.65)	<0.001	1.97 (0.49–3.35)	<0.001
Invasive ventilation	1.39 (0.54–3.09)	<0.001	1.42 (0.73–2.10)	<0.001	1.47 (0.25–2.75)	<0.001
ARDS	1.56 (0.37–3.32)	<0.001	1.38 (0.38–2.44)	<0.001	2.32 (0.92–3.37)	<0.001
Cerebral palsy	0.96 (0.08–4.83)	0.67	0.20 (−0.30–0.72)	0.42	1.99 (0.26–4.04)	0.035
Visual or hearing impairment	0.48 (0.02–2.52)	0.43	0.90 (−0.86–2.68)	0.31	1.67 (0.08–4.68)	0.003
Intraventricular hemorrhage	0.56 (0.37–1.32)	0.06	0.38 (−0.38–1.14)	0.32	2.32 (0.92–3.37)	<0.001
Neonatal death	0.68 (0.36–1.82)	0.79	1.04 (−0.55–2.65)	<0.001	1.97 (0.49–3.35)	<0.001

Table legend: aOR—adjusted OR; CI—confidence interval; NICU—neonatal intensive care unit; ARDS—acute respiratory distress syndrome.

Early preterm neonates were admitted to the NICU significantly more frequently ($p < 0.001$), were diagnosed more frequently with necrotizing enterocolitis and ARDS ($p < 0.001$), and required more invasive ventilation ($p < 0.001$). In addition, they were more prone to receive an Apgar score of less than seven at 1 ($p = 0.007$) and 5 min ($p < 0.001$) and had higher rates of neonatal death ($p < 0.001$).

Extremely preterm neonates were the most fragile group, having significantly higher rates of NICU admission ($p < 0.001$), necrotizing enterocolitis ($p < 0.001$), intraventricular hemorrhage ($p < 0.001$), cerebral palsy ($p = 0.035$), visual or hearing impairment ($p = 0.003$), neonatal deaths ($p < 0.001$), ARDS ($p < 0.001$), and invasive ventilation ($p < 0.001$), as well as lower Apgar scores at 1 ($p = 0.008$) and 5 min ($p = 0.03$).

4. Discussion

This retrospective study evaluated the effectiveness of various therapeutic interventions for preterm birth and compared their treatment effects, considering preterm delivery as an outcome in three gestational age categories. The average treatment effects on the treated indicated that all therapeutic interventions significantly reduced the occurrence of late and early preterm birth, with the highest impact achieved using the combination of progesterone with cervical cerclage. On the other hand, only progesterone intravaginally administered significantly reduced the occurrence of extremely preterm birth.

Similar results were obtained when we compared the occurrence of various types of preterm birth depending on the therapeutic interventions employed. The highest performance for the reduction in late PTB was achieved using the combination of progesterone and cerclage, followed by progesterone and pessary. The lowest performance, in this case, was achieved by the administration of progesterone in monotherapy.

When evaluating the reduction in early preterm birth using therapeutic interventions, our results indicated that both cervical cerclage and the combination of progesterone and cerclage achieved similar performances, closely followed by the combination of progesterone and pessary. On the other hand, in the case of extremely preterm birth, the results indicated a non-significant influence of the evaluated therapeutic interventions over the pregnancy's course and a tendency for these interventions to be associated with increased odds of PTB.

These results can be explained by the fact that extremely preterm labor is more difficult to manage and that therapeutic interventions such as cervical cerclage are often performed in emergencies. A meta-analysis of 12 observational studies, which evaluated the effectiveness of emergency cerclage versus expectant management on maternal and perinatal outcomes, indicated that cerclage was superior to expectant management for the reduction in preterm delivery rates before 28 and 32 weeks of gestation, but these results were based on low-quality evidence [39]. Nevertheless, the intraoperative rupture of membranes is a risk associated with emergency cerclage that ranges from 4% to 9%, and this procedure's apparently positive effects appear to be greatly reduced in the presence of chorioamnionitis [40–42].

In our cohort of patients, the risk of the occurrence of late preterm birth was significantly higher for pregnant patients who received progesterone in comparison with those who received Arabin pessaries or cervical cerclage. On the other hand, the risk was significantly lower for patients who received progesterone and pessaries or progesterone and cerclage in comparison with those who received only progesterone. Our results are in line with previously published data.

A Cochrane systematic review that evaluated the efficacy of cervical pessaries for preventing preterm birth in comparison with other therapeutic interventions in women with singleton pregnancies at risk of preterm delivery indicated that the cervical pessary reduced the risk of delivery before 34 weeks (RR: 0.72; 95%CI: 0.52–1.02) or before 37 weeks (RR: 0.89; 95%CI: 0.73–1.09) in comparison with vaginal progesterone administration [43].

Another Cochrane systematic review that evaluated the effect of cervical cerclage versus other therapeutic interventions in patients at risk of premature delivery concluded that there is not enough quality evidence to determine whether cerclage is more or less effective than progesterone administration, either vaginally or intramuscularly, for the prevention of PTB [44]. On the contrary, a recent indirect comparison meta-analysis concluded that both vaginal progesterone and cervical cerclage are equally effective in preventing PTB [45].

Our results indicated that the risk of early PTB was also lowered for those pregnant patients who received progesterone and pessaries or progesterone and cerclage in comparison with those who received only progesterone, translating into a risk reduction of 56% for the first treatment option, and 51% for the second treatment option. Our results were confirmed by a randomized controlled trial that evaluated the outcomes of combined therapy (cervical cerclage with progesterone) in comparison with progesterone monotherapy and that outlined pregnancy prolongation for preterm labor at 24–28 weeks in the case of combined intervention [46]. Moreover, another recent randomized controlled trial concluded that the cervical pessary was not non-inferior to vaginal progesterone for preventing spontaneous birth before 34 weeks of gestation in pregnant women with short cervixes [47].

The extremely PTB risk of occurrence was significantly lowered only by the administration of progesterone in association with cervical cerclage in comparison with progesterone monotherapy. Similar results were obtained in a retrospective cohort study by Enakpene et al., that revealed a higher performance of the combination therapy (cerclage and progesterone) in preventing extremely preterm birth (<28 weeks of gestation) in comparison with progesterone monotherapy (RR: 0.23; 95%CI: 0.10−0.54, $p = 0.001$) [48].

Our study also outlined significant personal histories of preterm birth for pregnant patients who received cervical cerclage, intravaginal progesterone and Arabin pessary, or intravaginal progesterone and cerclage, in accordance with the published data [49]. Regarding neonatal outcomes, both late and early preterm neonates were significantly associated with adverse outcomes, such as acute respiratory distress syndrome, the need for mechanical ventilation, or low Apgar scores. Extremely preterm neonates were significantly more fragile, with higher rates of neonatal deaths, intraventricular hemorrhage, cerebral palsy, and visual or hearing impairment in addition to the previously mentioned adverse neonatal outcomes, which are commonly encountered after preterm deliveries as stated in the literature [50–52].

The limitations of this study are represented by its retrospective approach, unicentric design, and small sample size. On the other hand, this study has the advantage of following pregnancy outcomes in a 4-year timeframe for patients with singleton pregnancies at risk of PTB who received therapeutic interventions in monotherapy or combined therapies.

Further prospective multicentric randomized controlled trials should be conducted in order to comparatively evaluate the performance of combined therapeutic interventions such as cerclage and progesterone versus progesterone monotherapy for the prevention of PTB.

5. Conclusions

All evaluated therapeutic interventions significantly reduced the occurrence of late and early preterm births. The highest performance in the reduction of late PTB was achieved by the combination of progesterone and cerclage, followed by progesterone and pessary. Both cervical cerclage and the combination of progesterone and cerclage achieved similar performances regarding the rates of early PTB, closely followed by the combination of progesterone and pessaries.

The risk of late and early PTB was lowered for those pregnant patients who received progesterone and pessaries or progesterone and cerclage in comparison with those who received only progesterone. The extremely PTB risk of occurrence was significantly lowered only with the administration of progesterone in association with cervical cerclage in comparison with progesterone monotherapy.

Further prospective studies will be needed in order to elucidate the performance of combined therapies for the prevention of PTB. In addition, an individualized assessment of pregnant patients, with the identification of maternal or sonographic risk factors for preterm birth, will allow prompt administration of treatment tailored to their risk profile.

Author Contributions: Conceptualization, A.-M.L., E.B., D.N. and D.S.; methodology, C.V., A.H., C.S. and R.M.; software, I.-A.V. and A.C.; validation, A.-M.A., V.H., A.N., I.-A.V. and A.C.; formal analysis, A.-M.L., E.B., D.N. and D.S.; investigation, C.V., A.H., C.S. and R.M.; resources, A.-M.A., V.H., A.N., I.-A.V. and A.C.; data curation, A.-M.A., V.H., A.N., I.-A.V. and A.C; writing—original draft preparation A.-M.L., E.B., D.N., D.S., C.V., A.H., C.S. and R.M.; writing—review and editing, A.-M.L., E.B., D.N., D.S., C.V., A.H., C.S. and R.M.; visualization, I.-A.V. and A.C.; supervision, D.S.; project administration, D.S. All authors have read and agreed to the published version of the manuscript.

Funding: This research received no external funding.

Institutional Review Board Statement: The study was conducted in accordance with the Declaration of Helsinki and approved by the Institutional Ethics Committees of 'Cuza-Voda' Maternity Hospital (No. 2052/16.02.2021) and the University of Medicine and Pharmacy 'Grigore T. Popa' (No. 101/08.07.2021).

Informed Consent Statement: Patient consent was waived by the Institutional Ethics Committees because of the retrospective design of the current study.

Data Availability Statement: The data presented in this study are available upon request from the corresponding author. The data are not publicly available because of local policies.

Conflicts of Interest: The authors declare no conflict of interest.

References

1. Rosa-Mangeret, F.; Benski, A.-C.; Golaz, A.; Zala, P.Z.; Kyokan, M.; Wagner, N.; Muhe, L.M.; Pfister, R.E. 2.5 Million Annual Deaths—Are Neonates in Low- and Middle-Income Countries Too Small to Be Seen? A Bottom-Up Overview on Neonatal Morbi-Mortality. *Trop. Med. Infect. Dis.* **2022**, *7*, 64. [CrossRef]
2. Kramer, M.S.; Papageorghiou, A.; Culhane, J.; Bhutta, Z.; Goldenberg, R.L.; Gravett, M.; Iams, J.D.; Conde-Agudelo, A.; Waller, S.; Barros, F.; et al. Challenges in defining and classifying the preterm birth syndrome. *Am. J. Obstet. Gynecol.* **2012**, *206*, 108–112. [CrossRef] [PubMed]
3. Delnord, M.; Zeitlin, J. Epidemiology of late preterm and early term births—An international perspective. *Semin. Fetal Neonatal Med.* **2019**, *24*, 3–10. [CrossRef] [PubMed]
4. De Luca, D. Respiratory distress syndrome in preterm neonates in the era of precision medicine: A modern critical care-based approach. *Pediatr. Neonatol.* **2021**, *62*, S3–S9. [CrossRef] [PubMed]
5. Duchon, J.; Barbian, M.E.; Denning, P.W. Necrotizing Enterocolitis. *Clin. Perinatol.* **2021**, *48*, 229–250. [CrossRef] [PubMed]
6. Ophelders, D.R.M.G.; Gussenhoven, R.; Klein, L.; Jellema, R.K.; Westerlaken, R.J.; Hütten, M.C.; Vermeulen, J.; Wassink, G.; Gunn, A.J.; Wolfs, T.G. Preterm brain injury, antenatal triggers, and therapeutics: Timing is key. *Cells* **2020**, *9*, 1871. [CrossRef]
7. Luu, T.M.; Rehman Mian, M.O.; Nuyt, A.M. Long-Term Impact of Preterm Birth: Neurodevelopmental and Physical Health Outcomes. *Clin. Perinatol.* **2017**, *44*, 305–314. [CrossRef]
8. Carmo, A.L.S.D.; Fredo, F.W.; Bruck, I.; de Lima, J.D.R.M.; Janke, R.N.R.G.H.; Fogaça, T.d.G.M.; Glaser, J.A.; Riechi, T.I.J.d.S.; Antoniuk, S.A. Neurological, cognitive and learning evaluation of students who were born preterm. *Rev. Paul. Pediatr.* **2021**, *40*, e2020252. [CrossRef]
9. Hoffman, M.K. Prediction and Prevention of Spontaneous Preterm Birth: ACOG Practice Bulletin, Number 234. *Obstet. Gynecol.* **2021**, *138*, 945–946. [CrossRef]
10. Filip, C.; Socolov, D.G.; Albu, E.; Filip, R.; Serban, R.; Popa, R.F. Serological Parameters and Vascular Investigation for a Better Assessment in DVT during Pregnancy—A Systematic Review. *Medicina* **2021**, *57*, 160. [CrossRef]
11. Albu, D.F.; Albu, C.C.; Gogănău, A.M.; Albu, Ş.D.; Mogoantă, L.; Edu, A.; Ditescu, D.; Vaduva, C.C. Borderline Brenner tumors associated with ovarian cyst—Case presentation. *Rom. J. Morphol. Embryol.* **2016**, *57*, 893–898. [PubMed]
12. Săndulescu, M.S.; Văduva, C.-C.; Siminel, M.A.; Dijmărescu, A.L.; Vrabie, S.C.; Camen, I.V.; Tache, D.E.; Neamțu, S.D.; Nagy, R.D.; Carp-Velişcu, A.; et al. Impact of COVID-19 on fertility and assisted reproductive technology (ART): A systematic review. *Rom. J. Morphol. Embryol.* **2022**, *63*, 503–510. [CrossRef] [PubMed]
13. Vicoveanu, P.; Vasilache, I.A.; Scripcariu, I.S.; Nemescu, D.; Carauleanu, A.; Vicoveanu, D.; Covali, A.R.; Filip, C.; Socolov, D. Use of a Feed-Forward Back Propagation Network for the Prediction of Small for Gestational Age Newborns in a Cohort of Pregnant Patients with Thrombophilia. *Diagnostics* **2022**, *12*, 1009. [CrossRef]
14. Vicoveanu, P.; Vasilache, I.-A.; Nemescu, D.; Carauleanu, A.; Scripcariu, I.-S.; Rudisteanu, D.; Burlui, A.; Rezus, E.; Socolov, D. Predictors Associated with Adverse Pregnancy Outcomes in a Cohort of Women with Systematic Lupus Erythematosus from Romania—An Observational Study (Stage 2). *J. Clin. Med.* **2022**, *11*, 1964. [CrossRef]

15. Cobo, T.; Kacerovsky, M.; Jacobsson, B. Risk factors for spontaneous preterm delivery. *Int. J. Gynecol. Obstet.* **2020**, *150*, 17–23. [CrossRef]
16. Liu, B.; Xu, G.; Sun, Y.; Du, Y.; Gao, R.; Snetselaar, L.G.; Santillan, M.K.; Bao, W. Association between maternal pre-pregnancy obesity and preterm birth according to maternal age and race or ethnicity: A population-based study. *Lancet Diabetes Endocrinol.* **2019**, *7*, 707–714. [CrossRef]
17. Fanni, D.; Gerosa, C.; Nurchi, V.M.; Manchia, M.; Saba, L.; Coghe, F.; Crisponi, G.; Gibo, Y.; Van Eyken, P.; Fanos, V.; et al. The Role of Magnesium in Pregnancy and in Fetal Programming of Adult Diseases. *Biol. Trace Element Res.* **2021**, *199*, 3647–3657. [CrossRef]
18. Bezerra Espinola, M.S.; Laganà, A.S.; Bilotta, G.; Gullo, G.; Aragona, C.; Unfer, V. D-chiro-inositol Induces Ovulation in Non-Polycystic Ovary Syndrome (PCOS), Non-Insulin-Resistant Young Women, Likely by Modulating Aromatase Expression: A Report of 2 Cases. *Am. J. Case Rep.* **2021**, *22*, e932722. [CrossRef]
19. Gullo, G.; Carlomagno, G.; Unfer, V.; D'Anna, R. Myo-inositol: From induction of ovulation to menopausal disorder management. *Minerva Ginecol.* **2015**, *67*, 485–486.
20. Vahanian, S.A.; Lavery, J.A.; Ananth, C.V.; Vintzileos, A. Placental implantation abnormalities and risk of preterm delivery: A systematic review and metaanalysis. *Am. J. Obstet. Gynecol.* **2015**, *213*, S78–S90. [CrossRef]
21. Berger, V.; Moghadassi, M.; Gosnell, K.; Sparks, T.; Velez, J.G.; Norton, M. The Risk of Preterm Birth in Pregnancies with Fetal Anomalies [11Q]. *Obstet. Gynecol.* **2017**, *129*, 176S. [CrossRef]
22. Herkert, D.; Wheeler, S.M.; Weaver, K.; Grace, M.; Dotters-Katz, S. The risk for recurrent preterm birth after prior preterm birth complicated by major fetal anomaly. *J. Matern. Neonatal Med.* **2022**, *35*, 8147–8149. [CrossRef] [PubMed]
23. Bernad, S.I.B.E.; Barbat, T.; Barbu, D.; Albulescu, V. Assessment of the placental blood flow in the normally developing and growth-restricted fetus. In *Proceedings of 22nd European Congress of Perinatal Medicine, Granada, Spain, 26–20 May 2010*; Monduzzi Editore SPA: Bologna, Italy, 2010; pp. 127–130.
24. Noventa, M.; Spagnol, G.; Marchetti, M.; Saccardi, C.; Bonaldo, G.; Laganà, A.S.; Cavallin, F.; Andrisani, A.; Ambrosini, G.; Vitale, S.G.; et al. Uterine Septum with or without Hysteroscopic Metroplasty: Impact on Fertility and Obstetrical Outcomes—A Systematic Review and Meta-Analysis of Observational Research. *J. Clin. Med.* **2022**, *11*, 3290. [CrossRef] [PubMed]
25. Lemmers, M.; Verschoor, M.; Hooker, A.; Opmeer, B.; Limpens, J.; Huirne, J.; Ankum, W.; Mol, B. Dilatation and curettage increases the risk of subsequent preterm birth: A systematic review and meta-analysis. *Hum. Reprod.* **2016**, *31*, 34–45. [CrossRef] [PubMed]
26. Rault, E.; Delorme, P.; Goffinet, F.; Girault, A. Impact of history of myomectomy on preterm birth risk in women with a leiomyomatous uterus: A propensity score analysis. *BMC Pregnancy Childbirth* **2020**, *20*, 720. [CrossRef]
27. Gedikbasi, A.; Akyol, A.; Bingol, B.; Cakmak, D.; Sargin, M.A.; Uncu, R.; Ceylan, Y. Multiple Repeated Cesarean Deliveries: Operative Complications in the Fourth and Fifth Surgeries in Urgent and Elective Cases. *Taiwan. J. Obstet. Gynecol.* **2010**, *49*, 425–431. [CrossRef]
28. NICE. NIoHaCE. Preterm Labour and Birth (NICE Guideline 25). Available online: https://www.ncbi.nlm.nih.gov/books/NBK553008/ (accessed on 16 March 2023).
29. Norman, J.E.; Marlow, N.; McConnachie, A.; Petrou, S.; Sebire, N.J.; Lavender, T.; Whyte, S.; Norrie, J.; Messow, C.-M.; Shennan, A.; et al. Vaginal progesterone prophylaxis for preterm birth (the OPPTIMUM study): A multicentre, randomised, double-blind trial. *Lancet* **2016**, *387*, 2106–2116. [CrossRef]
30. Crowther, C.A.; Ashwood, P.; McPhee, A.J.; Flenady, V.; Tran, T.; Dodd, J.M.; Robinson, J.S. For the PROGRESS Study Group Vaginal progesterone pessaries for pregnant women with a previous preterm birth to prevent neonatal respiratory distress syndrome (the PROGRESS Study): A multicentre, randomised, placebo-controlled trial. *PLoS Med.* **2017**, *14*, e1002390. [CrossRef]
31. Care, A.; Nevitt, S.J.; Medley, N.; Donegan, S.; Good, L.; Hampson, L.; Smith, C.T. Interventions to prevent spontaneous preterm birth in women with singleton pregnancy who are at high risk: Systematic review and network meta-analysis. *BMJ* **2022**, *376*, e064547. [CrossRef]
32. Pacagnella, R.C.; Silva, T.V.; Cecatti, J.G.; Passini, R., Jr.; Fanton, T.F.; Borovac-Pinheiro, A.; Pereira, C.M.; Fernandes, K.; Franca, M.S.; Li, W.; et al. Pessary Plus Progesterone to Prevent Preterm Birth in Women With Short Cervixes: A Randomized Controlled Trial. *Obstet. Gynecol.* **2022**, *139*, 41–51. [CrossRef]
33. Alizadeh, F.; Mahmoudinia, M.; Mirteimoori, M.; Pourali, L.; Niroumand, S. Comparison of oral Dydrogesterone and 17-α hydroxyprogesterone caprate in the prevention of preterm birth. *BMC Pregnancy Childbirth* **2022**, *22*, 167. [CrossRef] [PubMed]
34. Kagan, K.O.; Sonek, J. How to measure cervical length. *Ultrasound Obstet. Gynecol.* **2015**, *45*, 358–362. [CrossRef] [PubMed]
35. American College of Obstetricians and Gynecologists' Committee on Practice Bulletins—Obstetrics. Prediction and Prevention of Spontaneous Preterm Birth: ACOG Practice Bulletin Summary, Number 234. *Obstet. Gynecol.* **2021**, *138*, 320–323. [CrossRef] [PubMed]
36. Sentilhes, L.; Sénat, M.-V.; Ancel, P.-Y.; Azria, E.; Benoist, G.; Blanc, J.; Brabant, G.; Bretelle, F.; Brun, S.; Doret, M.; et al. Prevention of spontaneous preterm birth: Guidelines for clinical practice from the French College of Gynaecologists and Obstetricians (CNGOF). *Eur. J. Obstet. Gynecol. Reprod. Biol.* **2017**, *210*, 217–224. [CrossRef] [PubMed]
37. Berger, R.; Abele, H.; Bahlmann, F.; Bedei, I.; Doubek, K.; Felderhoff-Müser, U. Prevention and Therapy of Preterm Birth. Guideline of the DGGG, OEGGG and SGGG (S2k Level, AWMF Registry Number 015/025, February 2019)—Part 2 with Recommendations on the Tertiary Prevention of Preterm Birth and the Management of Preterm Premature Rupture of Membranes. *Geburtshilfe Frauenheilkd* **2019**, *79*, 813–833.

38. Berger, R.; Abele, H.; Bahlmann, F.; Bedei, I.; Doubek, K.; Felderhoff-Müser, U. Prevention and Therapy of Preterm Birth. Guideline of the DGGG, OEGGG and SGGG (S2k Level, AWMF Registry Number 015/025, February 2019)—Part 1 with Recommendations on the Epidemiology, Etiology, Prediction, Primary and Secondary Prevention of Preterm Birth. *Geburtshilfe Frauenheilkd* **2019**, *79*, 800–812. [CrossRef]
39. Chatzakis, C.; Efthymiou, A.; Sotiriadis, A.; Makrydimas, G. Emergency cerclage in singleton pregnancies with painless cervical dilatation: A meta-analysis. *Acta Obstet. Gynecol. Scand.* **2020**, *99*, 1444–1457. [CrossRef]
40. Mönckeberg, M.; Valdés, R.; Kusanovic, J.P.; Schepeler, M.; Nien, J.K.; Pertossi, E.; Silva, P.; Silva, K.; Venegas, P.; Guajardo, U.; et al. Patients with acute cervical insufficiency without intra-amniotic infection/inflammation treated with cerclage have a good prognosis. *J. Périnat. Med.* **2019**, *47*, 500–509. [CrossRef]
41. Stupin, J.H.; David, M.; Siedentopf, J.-P.; Dudenhausen, J.W. Emergency cerclage versus bed rest for amniotic sac prolapse before 27 gestational weeks. *Eur. J. Obstet. Gynecol. Reprod. Biol.* **2008**, *139*, 32–37. [CrossRef]
42. Ito, A.; Maseki, Y.; Ikeda, S.; Tezuka, A.; Kuribayashi, M.; Furuhashi, M. Factors associated with delivery at or after 28 weeks gestation in women with bulging fetal membranes before 26 weeks gestation. *J. Matern. Neonatal Med.* **2017**, *30*, 2046–2050. [CrossRef]
43. Abdel-Aleem, H.; Shaaban, O.M.; Abdel-Aleem, A.M.; Mohamed, A.A. Cervical pessary for preventing preterm birth in singleton pregnancies. *Cochrane Database Syst. Rev.* **2022**, *2022*, Cd014508.
44. Alfirevic, Z.; Stampalija, T.; Medley, N. Cervical stitch (cerclage) for preventing preterm birth in singleton pregnancy. *Cochrane Database Syst. Rev.* **2017**, *6*, Cd008991. [CrossRef]
45. Conde-Agudelo, A.; Romero, R.; Da Fonseca, E.; O'brien, J.M.; Cetingoz, E.; Creasy, G.W.; Hassan, S.S.; Erez, O.; Pacora, P.; Nicolaides, K.H. Vaginal progesterone is as effective as cervical cerclage to prevent preterm birth in women with a singleton gestation, previous spontaneous preterm birth, and a short cervix: Updated indirect comparison meta-analysis. *Am. J. Obstet. Gynecol.* **2018**, *219*, 10–25. [CrossRef] [PubMed]
46. Ragab, A.; Mesbah, Y. To do or not to do emergency cervical cerclage (a rescue stitch) at 24–28 weeks gestation in addition to progesterone for patients coming early in labor? A prospective randomized trial for efficacy and safety. *Arch. Gynecol. Obstet.* **2015**, *292*, 1255–1260. [CrossRef] [PubMed]
47. Cruz-Melguizo, S.; San-Frutos, L.; Martínez-Payo, C.; Ruiz-Antorán, B.; Adiego-Burgos, B.; Campillos-Maza, J.M.; Garcia-Gonzalez, C.; Martinez-Guisasola, M.; Perez-Carbajo, E.; Teulon-Gonzalez, M.; et al. Cervical Pessary Compared with Vaginal Progesterone for Preventing Early Preterm Birth: A Randomized Controlled Trial. *Obstet. Gynecol.* **2018**, *132*, 907–915. [CrossRef] [PubMed]
48. Enakpene, C.A.; DiGiovanni, L.; Jones, T.N.; Marshalla, M.; Mastrogiannis, D.; Della Torre, M. Cervical cerclage for singleton pregnant patients on vaginal progesterone with progressive cervical shortening. *Am. J. Obstet. Gynecol.* **2018**, *219*, 397.e1–397.e10. [CrossRef] [PubMed]
49. Goldenberg, R.L.; Culhane, J.F.; Iams, J.D.; Romero, R. Epidemiology and causes of preterm birth. *Lancet* **2008**, *371*, 75–84. [CrossRef]
50. Vogel, J.P.; Chawanpaiboon, S.; Moller, A.-B.; Watananirun, K.; Bonet, M.; Lumbiganon, P. The global epidemiology of preterm birth. *Best Pract. Res. Clin. Obstet. Gynaecol.* **2018**, *52*, 3–12. [CrossRef]
51. da Fonseca, E.B.; Damião, R.; Moreira, D.A. Preterm birth prevention. *Best Pract. Res. Clin. Obstet. Gynaecol.* **2020**, *69*, 40–49. [CrossRef]
52. Petre Izabella, C.M.; Bernad, E.; DOrneanu, F.; Citu, I.; Citu, C.; Stelea, L.; Iacob, D.; Boglut, A.; Moleriu, R.M. Procalcitonin—Neonatal Sepsis Biomarker. In Proceedings of the 13th Conference of the Romanian-German Society of Obstetrics and Gynecology, Timisoara, Romania, 14–16 September 2017; pp. 232–236.

Disclaimer/Publisher's Note: The statements, opinions and data contained in all publications are solely those of the individual author(s) and contributor(s) and not of MDPI and/or the editor(s). MDPI and/or the editor(s) disclaim responsibility for any injury to people or property resulting from any ideas, methods, instructions or products referred to in the content.

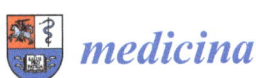

Article

Assessment of the Particularities of Thrombophilia in the Management of Pregnant Women in the Western Part of Romania

Miruna Samfireag [1,2], Cristina Potre [3,*], Ovidiu Potre [3], Lavinia-Cristina Moleriu [4], Izabella Petre [5], Ema Borsi [3], Teodora Hoinoiu [1,2], Marius Preda [6], Tudor-Alexandru Popoiu [4] and Andrei Anghel [7]

1. Department of Internal Medicine, Discipline of Clinical Practical Skills, "Victor Babes" University of Medicine and Pharmacy, No. 2 Eftimie Murgu Square, 300041 Timisoara, Romania; samfireag.miruna@umft.ro (M.S.); tstoichitoiu@umft.ro (T.H.)
2. Advanced Cardiology and Hemostaseology Research Center, "Victor Babes" University of Medicine and Pharmacy, No. 2 Eftimie Murgu Square, 300041 Timisoara, Romania
3. Department of Internal Medicine, Discipline of Hematology, "Victor Babes" University of Medicine and Pharmacy, No. 2 Eftimie Murgu Square, 300041 Timisoara, Romania; potre.ovidiu@umft.ro (O.P.); borsi.ema@umft.ro (E.B.)
4. Department III of Functional Sciences, Discipline of Medical Informatics and Biostatistics, "Victor Babes" University of Medicine and Pharmacy, No. 2 Eftimie Murgu Square, 300041 Timisoara, Romania; moleriu.lavinia@umft.ro (L.-C.M.); tudor.popoiu@student.umft.ro (T.-A.P.)
5. Department XII of Obstetrics and Gynaecology, Discipline III of Obstetrics and Gynaecology, "Victor Babes" University of Medicine and Pharmacy, No. 2 Eftimie Murgu Square, 300041 Timisoara, Romania; petre.izabella@umft.ro
6. Department IX of Surgery I, Discipline II of Surgical Semiology, "Victor Babes" University of Medicine and Pharmacy, No. 2 Eftimie Murgu Square, 300041 Timisoara, Romania; marius.preda@umft.ro
7. Department of Biochemistry and Pharmacology, Discipline of Biochemistry, "Victor Babes" University of Medicine and Pharmacy, No. 2 Eftimie Murgu Square, 300041 Timisoara, Romania; biochim@umft.ro
* Correspondence: potre.cristina@umft.ro

Abstract: *Background and objectives*: Thrombophilia in pregnant women is a condition whose incidence is constantly increasing worldwide, and, under these conditions, the development of preventive procedures is becoming essential. In this study, we aimed to evaluate thrombophilia in pregnant women in the western part of Romania and to establish anthropometric characteristics, socioeconomic features, and genetic and risk factors. *Material and Methods*: 178 pregnant women were divided into three study groups, according to the type of thrombophilia, aiming to carry out the genetic profile and the acquired one. Anthropometric measures and biological tests were performed. *Results*: The mixed type of thrombophilia predominates. The particularities of pregnant women diagnosed with thrombophilia are higher age, living in an urban environment, with normal BMI, approximately 36 weeks of gestational period, and having at least one miscarriage. Regarding the most frequent thrombophilic genetic markers, we obtained the MTFHR gene mutation C677T and A1298C, followed by the PAI-1 4G/5G gene mutation. Smoking represents an aggravating factor in the evolution of this pathology, manifested through the increase of D-dimers and the decrease in antithrombin values, simultaneously with the increase in therapeutic need. *Conclusions*: The predominance of MTHFR and PAI-1 4G/5G gene polymorphism is a particularity of pregnant women with thrombophilia from the western part of Romania. Smoking is confirmed as an important risk factor in spontaneous abortion.

Keywords: thrombophilia; pregnant women; miscarriage

1. Introduction

Thrombophilias can be categorized as either acquired or inherited [1]. Mixed thrombophilia is a condition that can result from both hereditary and nongenetic sources. The risk of venous thromboembolism (VTE) is associated with thrombophilia—a condition that ultimately results in thrombosis, particularly in women who are pregnant [2]. Although expensive, testing for thrombophilia entails a comprehensive range of coagulation and genetic tests, and interpretations call for clinical expertise [3]. Strong evidence linking unfavorable pregnancy outcomes with thrombophilia in pregnancy is limited. The most common factor in maternal thromboembolism is inherited thrombophilia. This is also linked to a higher risk of some unfavorable pregnancy outcomes, such as fetal loss in the second and third trimesters, abruptions, severe intrauterine growth restriction, and early-onset, severe preeclampsia [4,5]. The hemostatic system changes during pregnancy to become hypercoagulable, which raises the risk of thrombosis throughout pregnancy and reaches its peak at term [5]. One of the risk factors among reproductive diseases is represented by hereditary thrombophilia [1].

While acquired forms of thrombophilia are linked with both venous and arterial events, inherited forms are mostly linked with a tendency to VTE. Antiphospholipid antibodies (aPL) are what define antiphospholipid syndrome (APS) as an acquired form of thrombophilia, which is clinically indicated by arterial or venous thrombosis. The diagnosis is based on the Sydney criteria, which include one clinical criterion (pregnancy morbidity or serious or venous thrombosis) and one laboratory criterion (detection of abnormally high levels of high levels of IgM/IgG anticardiolipin antibodies, of anti-beta 2 glycoprotein-I antibodies, or of lupus anticoagulant). This is also linked to obstetric difficulties [1]. There are two categories of inheritable thrombophilic states, classified by Pinjala et al., namely, major or common inherited thrombophilias [6]. However, factor V Leiden and the prothrombin gene mutation G20210A are the most frequent causes of hereditary thrombophilia. Protein C and S and antithrombin abnormalities are less frequent but they represent the most severe triggers [6]. In addition, there is a connection between heritable thrombophilias and homozygosity for the methylene tetrahydrofolate reductase (MTHFR), which causes hyperhomocysteinemia, and poor pregnancy outcomes [5]. In addition to genetic thrombophilia, acquired hemostasis disorders can also result in hypercoagulable diseases. Due to increased procoagulant factors and decreased anticoagulants, as well as other alterations of the hemostasis, acquired states might maintain a prothrombotic situation [7]. Hyperhomocysteinemia, antiphospholipid antibody syndrome, increased levels of procoagulant factors, and decreased levels of anticoagulants are the main acquired diseases associated with thrombophilia [7]. A pregnant woman diagnosed with thrombophilia should be assessed for most risk factors, often referred to as triggers for first or recurrent thrombosis, while determining the best prophylaxis [7]. One identified pathogenic factor causing severe pregnancy problems is thrombophilia. Procoagulant factors that have undergone modifications—mutant genes with a high prevalence that raise the risk of developing thrombosis—have been researched [1,8,9]: MTHFR homozygous or heterozygous mutation in the C677T and A1298C positions, FVL gene homozygous or heterozygous mutation in the G1691A position, prothrombin gene homozygous or heterozygous mutation in the G20210A position, or the polymorphism of PAI-1 [1]. The hemostasis undergoes major alterations throughout a normal pregnancy, which favors procoagulants. On the other hand, during pregnancy, anticoagulant levels may slightly rise (in the case of tissue factor pathway inhibitor, or TFPI, the principal coagulation initiator), remain stable (in the case of antithrombin and protein C), or certainly decrease (protein S) [4]. A pregnancy's favorable outcome is correlated with good placental development [10]. Women who have a prior history of pregnancy difficulties, notably recurrent loss or a prior stillbirth, are treated with a thromboprophylactic dose of low-molecular-weight heparin (LMWH). The use of aspirin and LMWH increases the chance of live births [5]; the follow-up is adjusted based on the side effects that may occur in each patient.

Either laboratory proof of a thrombophilic deficiency or discoveries of thrombotic alterations in placental histology specimens from the affected pregnancy serve as the foundation for this statement [5]. The use of medicine must begin early in pregnancy (preferably at six weeks gestation) before the main trophoblast invasion is complete to reap the full benefits of these treatment approaches [5]. Preterm birth, which affects

5–13% of deliveries in affluent nations, is a significant contributor to infant morbidity and mortality. Though the role of thrombophilia as a risk factor is unknown, genetic thrombophilia has the potential to induce preterm delivery [11]. Prematurity, whose causes are still unknown, is a public health issue due to its multifactorial nature, but also because of associated factors such as social class, demographics, biological, genetic, reproductive, environmental, behavioral, and psychosocial conditions. The accessibility to the quality of healthcare services [12] can also lead to premature birth. Newborns delivered before 37 weeks of pregnancy are considered preterm. Based on gestational age, preterm birth is divided into the following subcategories: extremely early (less than 28 weeks), very early (28 to 32 weeks), and moderate to late preterm (32 to 37 weeks) [13]. Premature newborns have more pronounced hemostatic system differences than term infants, although their hemostatic system development is hastened [14]. It is debatable as to how to treat expectant women who have thrombophilia. There is a wealth of research on the possible connection between thrombophilia and several obstetric problems. Placenta-mediated problems, miscarriages, and fetal losses are the most common obstetric complications that thrombophilia has been linked to [15].

This study aims to comprehensively evaluate thrombophilia in pregnant women in the western part of Romania, taking into account anthropometric characteristics—such as age, body mass index, gestational period, the weight of the newborns, socioeconomic, and risk factors and the genetic markers involved in thrombophilia.

2. Materials and Methods

We started our case-control study with 450 patients grouped into three samples: patients with inherited thrombophilia, acquired thrombophilia, and mixed (inherited and acquired) thrombophilia, with 150 individuals in each group. After applying the inclusion and exclusion criteria, we were left with 178 patients: based on the type of thrombophilia, we had 28.65% (51 patients) with inherited thrombophilia, 28.65% (51 patients) with acquired thrombophilia, and 42.7% (76 patients) with mixed (inherited and acquired) thrombophilia.

The thrombophilia-specific investigation panel aims to carry out the genetic profile and the acquired one: methylenetetrahydrofolate reductase (MTHFR) gene mutation, prothrombin (factor II) gene mutation, factor V Leiden gene mutation, plasminogen activator inhibitor gene mutation-1 (PAI-1), factor XIII gene mutation, glycoprotein IIb/IIIa gene mutation, fibrinogen gene mutation, the angiotensin converting enzyme gene mutation (ACE_insertion_deletion), the angiotensinogen gene mutation (AGT mutation M235T), the serine/threonine kinase gene mutation (ATR-1 Mutation A1166C), respectively, the Cystathionine Beta-Synthase gene mutation (CBS 844ins68), the evaluation of the status of antithrombin, lupus anticoagulant, anticardiolipin, and antiphospholipid antibodies, homocysteine, protein C, protein S, and of D dimers. Genetic testing for thrombophilia mutations entails the analysis of genes using various techniques such as DNA microarrays and real-time polymerase chain reactions.

The database was gathered using the Microsoft Excel software. For the statistical analysis we used two different software: JASPv16.4 and Microsoft Excel. After applying a descriptive analysis to our database, we applied the Shapiro–Wilk test to see the data distribution and decide upon the type of tests that would be used. The Mann–Whitney U-test was used to see if we had significant differences between the two different groups. The Kruskal–Wallis test was used when we analyzed medical tests between our three groups, and the Friedman test was applied to see the D-dimers' value evolution during pregnancy. At the end of the study, we ran a regression analysis and calculated the correlation coefficients. The significance level was set at $\alpha = 0.05$ for the whole study. The noninvasive, case–control study was conducted on a cohort of 450 pregnant women, diagnosed with thrombophilia, in the western part of Romania, evaluated in routine clinical practice between 2018 and 2020. Because of the pandemic situation, in the last year of our study period (2020), the number of patients who sought proper care decreased significantly.

The cohort was divided into three groups, depending on the type of thrombophilia. In the first group, 150 patients diagnosed with hereditary thrombophilia were enrolled. The second group of 150 patients was diagnosed with acquired thrombophilia. Finally, the third group consisted of 150 patients diagnosed with mixed thrombophilia. The study population included Caucasian women, with singleton pregnancy at the time of enrolment, with available results for inherited, acquired, and mixed thrombophilia, and with positive obstetrical history (recurrent pregnancy losses); the exclusion criteria were nonpregnant women, subjects with twin pregnancies, and pregnant women that had incomplete results for the thrombophilia screen. The use of the database was possible with the agreement of the Bioethics Commission of Victor Babes University of Medicine and Pharmacy, No. 2 Eftimie Murgu Square, Timisoara, Romania (51/28.09.2018); the informed consent was obtained from all subjects involved in the study. The study was conducted following the ethical principles set out in the Helsinki Declaration.

3. Results

In Table 1, the impact of age, the body mass index (BMI), the gestational period (GP), and the newborns' weight are presented. It may be observed that the differences appear in the GP and the weight of the newborns (see Figures 1 and 2). If we study the number of pregnancies and miscarriages, we observe that higher values are detected in the case of inherited thrombophilia (see Figure 3). Regarding the environmental setting, 79.78% of our patients were from an urban environment having a median age higher than those living in rural areas (32 years old vs. 28 years old), an outcome that is expected for a Western type of society [16]. A 2019 study on 818 pregnant women [17] determined that the mean age of the enrolled pregnant woman diagnosed with thrombophilia who used LWMH during pregnancy was 33.9 years old, with an SD ± 4.9 years. Similar to these findings, our patients have approximately the same age range (group 1—33 years old, with an IQR ± 5 years, group 2—30 years old, with an IQR ± 7 years, and group 3—30.5 years old, with an IQR ± 7 years). The risk of maternal and fetal difficulties during pregnancy, such as stillbirth, small-for-gestational-age births, preterm birth, preeclampsia, and maternal death, increases in women as age enhances, presenting as hazard gain as age increases [18]. Smoking is one of the most important risk factors for worse pregnancy outcomes [19], and it affected all three groups of our study by aggravating some biological changes such as an increase in D-dimers levels during the last trimester of pregnancy and a decline in antithrombin levels; we also obtained that pregnant smokers needed higher doses of anticoagulant, approximatively over 20%. We tested the D-dimers evolution during pregnancy for all the studied groups and we registered a significant increase in our values in all scenarios, regardless of the type of thrombophilia that our patients had.

According to the objectives of the study, to highlight the particularities of thrombophilia in the western part of Romania, the characteristic profile of the patient with thrombophilia regarding the anthropometric parameters provides an average age of the patients of 32.8 years in the first group, 31 years in the second group, and 31.3 years in group 3, an average BMI value of 22.9 in the first group, 22.2 in the second group, and 22.9 in the third group, and an average gestational period of 37.3 weeks in the first group, 35.8 weeks in the second group, and 35.4 weeks in the third group. In terms of the average weight of the newborn, we observe a value of 2842.2 g in the first group, 2724.5 g in the second group, and 2634.5 g in the third group. To properly provide therapies for preterm labor and premature infants, accurate gestational dates during pregnancy are necessary; we also investigated this aspect, and we obtained that the gestational period (GP) and the newborns' weights show discrepancies.

Table 1. Descriptive analysis upon anthropometric characteristics (IQR—interquartile range).

Variables	Age (Years)			BMI (G (kg)/h² (m²))			GP (Weeks)			Newborn Weight (g)		
	1	2	3	1	2	3	1	2	3	1	2	3
Valid	51	51	76	51	51	76	51	51	76	51	51	76
Missing	0	0	0	0	0	0	0	0	0	0	0	0
Mean	32.8	31	31.3	22.9	22.2	22.9	37.3	35.8	35.4	2842.2	2724.5	2634.5
Median	33	30	30.5	20.8	19.8	20.8	38	37	36	3100	2700	2780
Minimum	21	23	23	15.9	17.2	15.9	30	30	30	1240	1300	1240
Maximum	45	49	49	34.9	34.9	34.9	40	40	42	3770	3740	3880
IQR	5	7	7	6.8	3.8	5.8	1	6	6	660	1000	935

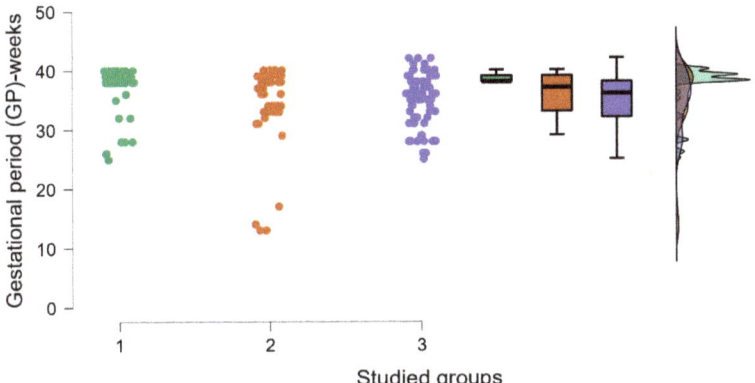

Figure 1. The gestational period is presented in three studied groups, using raincloud plots (in this type of graphical representation, we can see a complete data distribution, by density and by box plots). In group 1, the GP was significantly higher ($p = 0.032 < 0.05$, p value obtained from Kruskal–Wallis test; groups 1 and 2 contain 51 patients each, group 3 contains 76 patients).

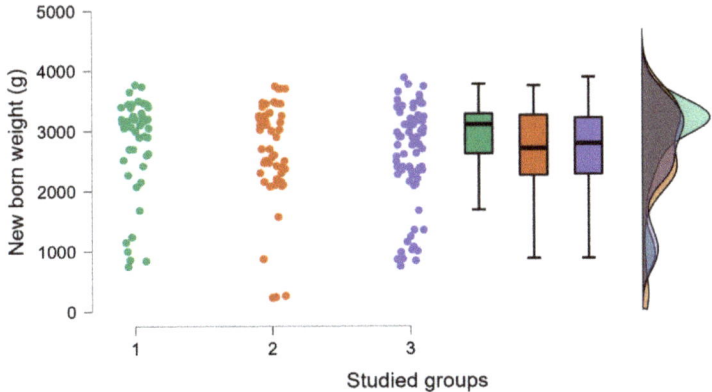

Figure 2. The newborn weight is presented in three studied groups, using raincloud plots; there were no statistically significant differences between the studied groups ($p > 0.05$, p value obtained from Kruskal–Wallis test; groups 1 and 2 contain 51 patients each, group 3 contains 76 patients).

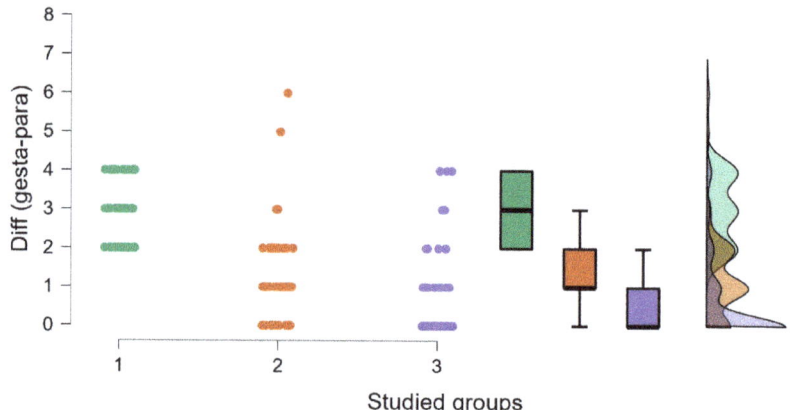

Figure 3. The differences between the number of pregnancies and miscarriages in all studied groups, using raincloud plots. A significant decrease was observed ($p < 0.001$, p value obtained from Kruskal–Wallis test; groups 1 and 2 contain 51 patients each, group 3 contains 76 patients).

To monitor the treatment response during pregnancy, we ran some specific medical tests such as D-dimers (ng/mL) and the levels of antiXa (anti Xa levels UI/mL) in all three pregnancy trimesters; the results are presented in Table 2. To establish the acquired form of thrombophilia, we ran the tests presented in Table 3.

Table 2. The quarterly evolution of the parameters studied for therapeutical orientation (95% confidence interval (median ± 1.5 IQR); IQR—interquartile range).

Medical Tests	95% Confidence Interval		
	Group 1 (n = 51)	Group 2 (n = 51)	Group 3 (n = 76)
D-dimers ng/mL—Trim1	(102.87; 790.87)	(116.3; 672.3)	(121.82; 889.82)
D-dimers ng/mL—Trim2	(1108.3; 1719.7)	(1106.8; 1778.3)	(1105.5; 1715.3)
D-dimers ng/mL—Trim3	(1688.8; 2400.5)	(1690.5; 2409.9)	(1637.1; 2408.2)
anti Xa levels UI/mL—Trim1	(0.24; 0.52)	(0.13; 0.77)	(0.10; 0.79)
anti Xa levels UI/mL—Trim2	(0.26; 0.44)	(0.22; 0.44)	(0.21; 0.43)
anti Xa levels UI/mL—Trim3	(0.35; 0.48)	(0.34; 0.47)	(0.29; 0.47)

The analysis of the genetic markers is presented in Table 4. In terms of the genetic markers involved, the highest frequency is represented by the MTFHR gene mutation C677T and A1298C, followed by the PAI-1 4G/5G gene mutation and the factor XIII gene mutation. In our research, the MTHFR_C677T mutation was homozygous in 11.76% of the cases from group 1 and heterozygous in 52.95% of the cases from the same group. The MTHFR_A1298C mutation was heterozygous in 35.29% of group 1 and 46.05% of group 3. We found the homozygote form of PAI-1 4G/5G in 31.37% of our patients diagnosed with hereditary thrombophilia, and in 22.37% diagnosed with the mixed type. Likewise, the women from our study diagnosed with mixed thrombophilia tested positive in 3.95% of the cases for the homozygote form of ACE_insertion_deletion mutation (angiotensin converting enzyme gene), which was demonstrated to increase miscarriage risk in European women [20,21]. We obtained that 10.53% of the women diagnosed with mixed thrombophilia in our analysis tested positive for the heterozygous form of this mutation. However, early pregnancy loss is linked to homozygosity for the FXIII 34Leu polymorphism [22], which was the case in 13.72% of our patients (diagnosed with inherited thrombophilia, the factor XIII G1002T mutation (Val34Leu) was in the homozygote form).

Table 3. The analysis of the parameters involved in tests performed to establish existence of the acquired form of thrombophilia (95% confidence interval (median ± 1.5 IQR); IQR—interquartile range).

Medical Tests	95% Confidence Interval		
	Group 1 (n = 51)	Group 2 (n = 51)	Group 3 (n = 76)
Lupus Anticoagulant (ratio)	(1.03; 36.35)	(0.97; 33.09)	(0.05; 44.77)
Anti Cardiolipin antibodies IgG (U/mL)	(0.25; 2.49)	(0.16; 2.2)	(0.14; 1.9)
Anti Cardiolipin antibodies IgM (U/mL)	(0.02; 1.5)	(0.05; 1.21)	(0.01; 1.29)
Protein C (%)	(6.92; 131.48)	(1.28; 120.88)	(20.6; 132.2)
Protein S (%)	(4.3; 106.3)	(0.7; 98.3)	(3.9; 115.5)
Antithrombin (%)	(15.77; 122.57)	(3.99; 104.15)	(24.23; 123.83)
Homocysteine (micromole/L)	(0.16; 8.56)	(0.13; 9.73)	(0.1; 10.5)

The most frequent form of thrombophilia found in our study was the mixed one (42.7%). None of the patients was diagnosed with APS. Regarding the genetic factors involved in thrombophilia, it is important to start monitoring an early pregnancy of a woman diagnosed with this pathology to know when to start the proper treatment. Nevertheless, a 2002 study presented that mothers who have the factor V G1691A or factor II A (20210) mutation are far more likely to give birth to babies who are underweight at birth [23]. All women with a known personal history of preeclampsia, recurrent miscarriages, fetal growth restriction, first-trimester abortion, mid-trimester abortion, placental abruption, or intrauterine mortality should undergo a clinical and paraclinical examination for thrombophilia [7,24,25]. We applied the Mann–Whitney U-test to see if there were statistically significant differences in the age of our patients based on their environment, and we obtained significant differences ($p < 0.001$) in all three groups (see Table 5, Appendix A); the age of the patients who were from an urban environment is significantly higher compared with the patients from a rural area. This can be explained by the fact that patients from urban areas tend to form families later than those from rural areas. To quantify the impact of thrombophilia type in miscarriages, we applied a Kruskal–Wallis test, and we obtained significant differences ($p < 0.001$). The highest chance of a miscarriage was registered in the case of inherited thrombophilia (see Figure 4). We applied the Friedman test to see the D-dimers evolution in the pregnancy trimesters for all the studied groups. We obtained in all scenarios a significant increase ($p < 0.001$) in our values, regardless of the type of thrombophilia that our patients had. All the results are plotted in Figure 5.

Table 4. Analysis of the genetic markers of thrombophilia in the three studied groups.

Mutation	Group 1 (n = 51)		Group 2 (n = 51)		Group 3 (n = 76)	
	Present	Absent	Present	Absent	Present	Absent
MTHFR_C677T	11.76% homozygote 52.95% heterozygote	35.29%	0%	100%	13.16% homozygote 56.58% heterozygote	30.26%
MTHFR_A1298C	7.84% homozygote 35.29% heterozygote	56.86%	0%	100%	6.58% homozygote 46.05% heterozygote	47.37%
Factor V Leiden	9.2% heterozygote	90.2%	0%	100%	11.84% heterozygote	88.16%
Prothrombin gene G20210A (Factor II)	1.96% heterozygote	98.04%	0%	100%	10.53% heterozygote	89.47%
Glycoprotein IIb/IIIa T1565C	13.72% heterozygote	86.28%	0%	100%	10.53% heterozygote	89.47%
PAI_1_4G/4G	0%	100%	0%	100%	9.21% homozygote	90.79%
PAI_1_4G_5G	31.37% homozygote 39.22% heterozygote	29.41%	0%	100%	22.37% homozygote 35.53% heterozygote	42.11%
PAI_1_5G_5G	0%	100%	0%	100%	6.58% homozygote 1.32% heterozygote	92.11%
FactorV_R2	1.96% heterozygote	98.04%	0%	100%	17.11% heterozygote	82.89%
B_Fibrinogen G455A	7.84% heterozygote	92.16%	0%	100%	3.95% homozygote 7.89% heterozygote	88.16%
ACE_insertion_deletion (angiotensin converting enzyme gene)	0%	100%	0%	100%	3.95% homozygote 10.53% heterozygote	85.53%
AGT mutationM235T (the angiotensinogen gene)	0%	100%	0%	100%	2.63% homozygote 11.84% heterozygote	85.53%
FactorV 4070_AgtG	0%	100%	0%	100%	2.63% homozygote	97.37%
factor XIII G1002T mutation (Val34Leu)	13.72% homozygote 23.53% heterozygote	62.75%	0%	100%	2.63% homozygote 40.79% heterozygote	56.58%
ATR-1 Mutation A1166C (serine/threonine kinase gene)	0%	100%	0%	100%	1.32% homozygote 7.89% heterozygote	90.79%
CBS 844ins68 (the Cystathionine Beta-Synthase gene)	0%	100%	0%	100%	2.63% homozygote	97.37%

Table 5. Comparative analysis of thrombophilia-specific parameters (groups 1 and 2 contain 51 patients each, group 3 contains 76 patients).

Variables in Study	Type of Test	Obtained p Value	Conclusion
Differences in age based on the patient's environment	Mann–Whitney U-test	$p < 0.001$—group 1 $p < 0.001$—group 2 $p < 0.001$—group 3	The age is higher for the patients who are living in urban areas
LMWH dose (mL) for smokers and nonsmokers	Mann–Whitney U-test	$p = 0.048$—group 1 $p = 0.046$—group 2 $p = 0.038$—group 3	Smokers have higher values for LMWH doses in all groups
D-dimers values in the third trimester of pregnancy for smokers and nonsmokers	Mann–Whitney U-test	$p = 0.019$—group 1 $p = 0.023$—group 2 $p = 0.013$—group 3	Smokers have higher values of D-dimers in all groups

Table 5. Cont.

Variables in Study	Type of Test	Obtained p Value	Conclusion
Antithrombin values in the third trimester of pregnancy for smokers and nonsmokers	Mann–Whitney U-test	$p = 0.009$—group 1 $p = 0.003$—group 2 $p = 0.007$—group 3	Smokers have lower values of antithrombin in all groups
Thrombophilia type—the impact in miscarriages	Kruskal–Wallis test	$p < 0.001$	The highest chance for a miscarriage is in the case of inherited thrombophilia
The antithrombin values within the three groups	Kruskal–Wallis test	$p = 0.045$	The lowest values are in the second group—acquired thrombophilia
The D-dimers evolution during the pregnancy trimesters for all three groups	Friedman test	$p < 0.001$—group 1 $p < 0.001$—group 2 $p < 0.001$—group 3	The D-dimers values are increasing significantly in all three groups

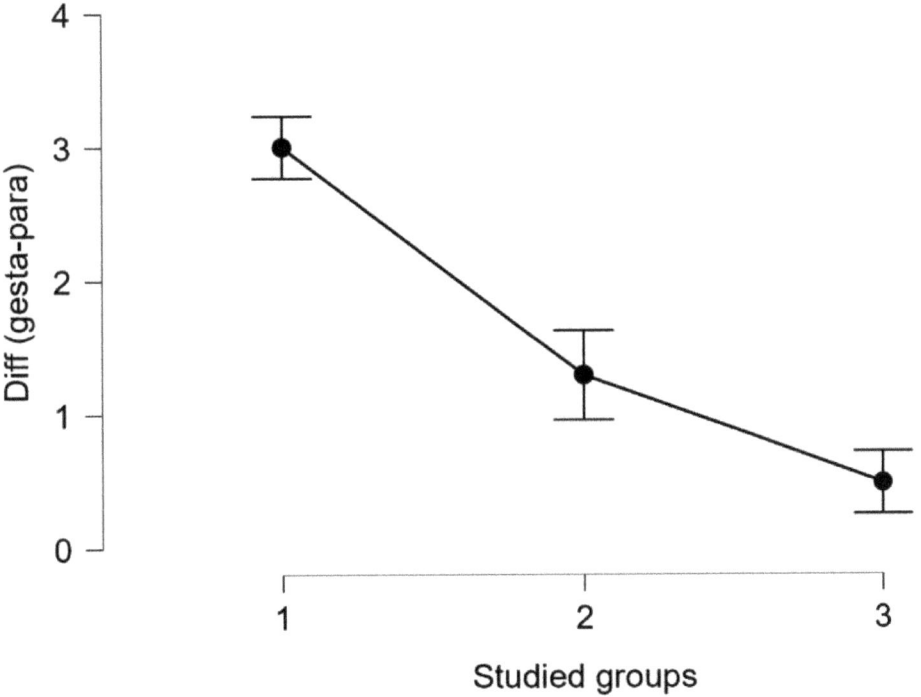

Figure 4. The miscarriage risk, compared between our groups. A significant decrease can be observed within the studied groups, and the lowest rate was reported in group 3 ($p < 0.001$, p value obtained from Kruskal–Wallis's test; groups 1 and 2 contain 51 patients each, group 3 contains 76 patients).

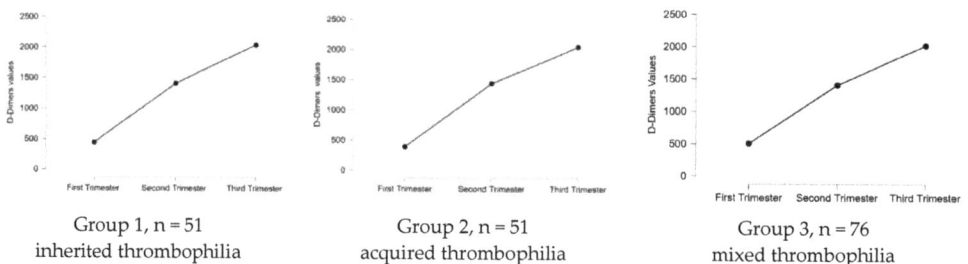

Figure 5. The D-dimers evolution during pregnancy, based on the type of thrombophilia (groups 1, 2, and 3—$p < 0.001$, p value obtained from the Friedman test).

4. Discussion

In our research, our results show that women diagnosed with thrombophilia are more likely to suffer pregnancy losses. Studying thrombophilic conditions will help us develop preventative strategies. This could be a new area of study for Romania's western region addressing women who have experienced previous miscarriages and could undergo a national screening protocol. A wide variety of coagulation and genetic tests are required to be performed, and their interpretations necessitate clinical knowledge. Therefore, women ought to, at the very least, undergo genetic testing.

Analysis of the miscarriage risk shows that women who had a history of losses before the current pregnancy were more likely to develop recurrent pregnancy loss (RPL) in the absence of appropriate treatment, confirming similar observations of other groups [26].

A meta-analysis of 81 case–control studies conducted in 2021 summarized that the risk of RPL may be greatly increased by the FVL mutation [27]; if the death was a stillbirth, FVL and fetal loss were significantly linked [28]. We found the heterozygote form of this mutation in 9.2% of our patients diagnosed with hereditary thrombophilia, and in 11.84% diagnosed with the mixed type.

Considered to be a crucial regulator of the fibrinolytic system is PAI-1. Therefore, any deviation from normal in this gene may impact hemostasis. Increased fibrin formation is linked to the PA1-1 4G/5G and may disrupt placenta circulation and implantation, potentially leading to pregnancy loss [20]. Pregnancy complications tested positive for the prothrombin G20210A mutation in 57.9% of patients [29] with an additional increased risk of early pregnancy loss and preterm placental abruption linked to the heterozygous GA variation [29,30].

According to research carried out in 2018 [22], women who experienced several miscarriages had a considerable increase in factor XIII V34L mutations.

Hyperhomocysteinemia is primarily caused by MTHFR gene polymorphism [31]. Dai et al. hypothesized that excessive homocysteine levels and the MTHFR 677CT and 1298AC genotypes together enhanced the aberrant lipid metabolism in RPL patients [31], so this may be a further direction of research for the western part of Romania regarding women with a history of miscarriages. We prescribed thrombolytics, namely Aspirin, to women with antithrombin, protein C, or protein S deficiency, following recommendations of a certain study in which aspirin enhances implantation and placentation and has vasodilatory effects through boosting prostacyclin production, according to multiple earlier studies [32]. Aspirin may help endothelial dysfunction and appears to have a direct impact on platelets [33].

Smoking is a risk factor manifested in all three groups by the aggravation of some characteristic biological changes, such as the increase in D-dimers values in the last trimester of pregnancy and the decrease in antithrombin values. We applied the Mann–Whitney U-test to the thrombophilia-specific medical tests to see if smoking habit can influence the parameter of thrombophilia-specific medical tests. We evaluated in groups a part of it as well as the whole sample and we obtained significant results ($p < 0.05$) in the case of LMWH dose (ml) in all three groups (group 1, $p = 0.048$; group 2, $p = 0.046$; group 3, $p = 0.038$); the values of smoker patients are significantly higher. We have significant results ($p < 0.05$) in the case of D-dimers ng/mL in the third trimester of pregnancy in all three groups (group 1, $p = 0.019$; group 2, $p = 0.023$; group 3, $p = 0.013$); the smoker patients had higher values. Finally, significant results ($p < 0.05$) were obtained in the case of antithrombin values in all our groups (group 1, $p = 0.009$; group 2, $p = 0.003$; group 3, $p = 0.007$); the smoker patients in this case had significantly lower values. When we analysed the antithrombin values within our groups, we obtained significant differences ($p = 0.045 < 0.05$), the lowest values being registered in the second group—acquired thrombophilia; in groups 1 and 3 we observed almost the same mean values.

Combining preventive dosages of LMWH and aspirin starting before the second trimester of pregnancy has been shown to minimize the incidence of miscarriage in women with genetic thrombophilia [34,35]. LMWH dose adjustments during pregnancy by antifactor Xa activity levels were typical in this retrospective observational cohort analysis of gravidas maintained on LMWH for prophylaxis or treatment of VTE. More frequent monitoring of antifactor Xa levels is recommended in pregnant patients for which a specified target of antifactor Xa is aimed for [36,37].

Various studies [5,38,39] have suggested that certain thrombophilic variants are linked to miscarriages. All of these matched the findings of our study.

5. Conclusions

From the point of view of the thrombophilia profile performed in the western part of Romania, the mixed type of thrombophilia predominates. The particularities of pregnant women diagnosed with thrombophilia are higher age, living in an urban environment, normal BMI, approximately 36 weeks of gestational period, and having at least one miscarriage. Regarding the most frequent thrombophilic genetic markers, we obtained the MTFHR gene mutation C677T and A1298C, followed by the PAI-1 4G/5G gene mutation. Another important aspect was the impact of the smoking habit in thrombophilic pregnant women: smoking represents an aggravating factor in the evolution of this pathology, manifested through the increase of D-dimers and the decrease in antithrombin values, simultaneously with the increase in therapeutic need.

Author Contributions: Conceptualization, M.S. and A.A.; data curation, M.S., C.P., I.P. and A.A.; formal analysis, L.-C.M.; investigation, O.P., I.P. and E.B.; methodology, T.H. and M.P.; project administration, M.S. and A.A.; resources, E.B., T.H. and M.P.; software, L.-C.M. and T.-A.P.; supervision, A.A.; validation, M.S., T.-A.P. and A.A.; visualization, C.P., O.P., E.B., T.H. and M.P.; writing—original draft, M.S., C.P., L.-C.M., I.P. and A.A.; writing—review and editing, C.P., O.P. and T.-A.P. All authors have read and agreed to the published version of the manuscript.

Funding: This research received no external funding.

Institutional Review Board Statement: The study was conducted in accordance with the Declaration of Helsinki and approved by the Bioethics Commission of Victor Babes University of Medicine and Pharmacy, No. 2 Eftimie Murgu Square, Timisoara, Romania (51/28.09.2018).

Informed Consent Statement: Written informed consent was obtained from all subjects involved in the study.

Data Availability Statement: The use of the database was possible with the agreement of the Bioethics Commission.

Conflicts of Interest: The authors declare no conflict of interest.

Appendix A

A raincloud plot was used in order to obtain a complete picture of data dynamics (when we had to analyze the difference between two samples (e.g., environment, smoker), the p value was obtained from the Mann–Whitney U-test; when we had to analyze the differences between the studied groups, we applied the Kruskal–Wallis test).

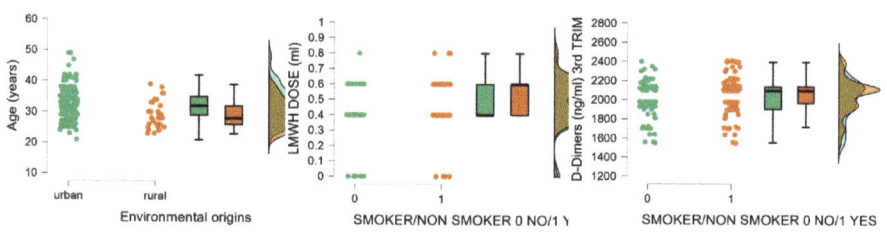

Differences in age based on the patient's environment, a significant decrease was observed in the age of patients coming from a rural environment ($p < 0.01$).

LMWH dose (mL) for smokers and nonsmokers—a significantly higher value of LMWH was registered in smoking patients ($p = 0.048$).

D-dimers values in the third trimester of pregnancy for smokers and nonsmokers; a significantly higher value was registered in smoking patients ($p = 0.013$).

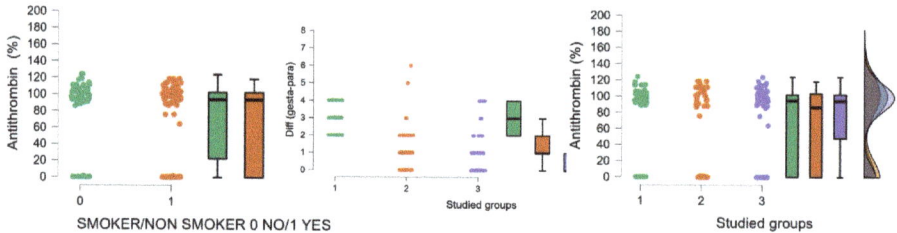

Antithrombin values in the third trimester of pregnancy (smokers and nonsmokers). A significant decrease was observed in smoking patients ($p = 0.007$).

Thrombophilia type—the impact in miscarriages—a significant decrease was observed in the third group ($p < 0.001$).

The antithrombin values within the three groups. A significantly lower antithrombin value was registered in the second group ($p = 0.045$).

References

1. Samfireag, M.; Potre, C.; Potre, O.; Tudor, R.; Hoinoiu, T.; Anghel, A. Approach to Thrombophilia in Pregnancy—A Narrative Review. *Medicina* **2022**, *58*, 692. [CrossRef] [PubMed]
2. Bates, S.M.; Middeldorp, S.; Rodger, M.; James, A.H.; Greer, I. Guidance for the treatment and prevention of obstetric-associated venous thromboembolism. *J. Thromb. Thrombolysis* **2016**, *41*, 92–128. [CrossRef] [PubMed]
3. MacCallum, P.; Bowles, L.; Keeling, D. Diagnosis and management of heritable thrombophilias. *BMJ* **2014**, *349*, g4387. [CrossRef] [PubMed]
4. Lockwood, C.J. High-Risk Pregnancy Series: An Expert's View Inherited Thrombophilias in Pregnant Patients: Detection and Treatment Paradigm. *Obstet. Gynecol.* **2002**, *99*, 333–341. [PubMed]
5. Simcox, L.E.; Ormesher, L.; Tower, C.; Greer, I.A. Thrombophilia and pregnancy complications. *Int. J. Mol. Sci.* **2015**, *16*, 28418–28428. [CrossRef]
6. Pinjala, R.K.; Reddy, L.R.C.; Nihar, R.P.; Praveen, G.V.A.; Sandeep, M. Thrombophilia-How Far and How Much to Investigate? *Indian J. Surg.* **2012**, *74*, 157–162. [CrossRef]
7. Campello, E.; Spiezia, L.; Adamo, A.; Simioni, P. Thrombophilia, risk factors and prevention. In *Expert Review of Hematology*; Taylor and Francis Ltd.: Thames, UK, 2019; Volume 12, pp. 147–158.
8. Younis, J.S.; Samueloff, A. Gestational vascular complications. *Best Pract. Res. Clin. Haematol.* **2003**, *16*, 135–151. [CrossRef]
9. Szecsi, P.B.; Jørgensen, M.; Klajnbard, A.; Andersen, M.R.; Colov, N.P.; Stender, S. Haemostatic reference intervals in pregnancy. *Thromb. Haemost.* **2010**, *103*, 718–727.
10. Dossenbach-Glaninger, A.; van Trotsenburg, M.; Oberkanins, C.; Atamaniuk, J. Risk for early pregnancy loss by factor XIII Val34Leu: The impact of fibrinogen concentration. *J. Clin. Lab. Anal.* **2013**, *27*, 444–449. [CrossRef]
11. Hiltunen, L.M.; Laivuori, H.; Rautanen, A.; Kaaja, R.; Kere, J.; Krusius, T.; Rasi, V.; Paunio, M. Factor V Leiden as a risk factor for preterm birth-a population-based nested case-control study. *J. Thromb. Haemost.* **2011**, *9*, 71–78. [CrossRef]
12. Defilipo, É.C.; Chagas, P.S.; Drumond, C.D.M.; Ribeiro, L.C. Factors associated with premature birth: A case-control study. *Rev. Paul. Pediatr.* **2022**, *40*, e2020486. [CrossRef]

13. Perin, J.; Mulick, A.; Yeung, D.; Villavicencio, F.; Lopez, G.; Strong, K.L.; Prieto-Merino, D.; Cousens, S.; E Black, R.; Liu, L. Global, regional, and national causes of under-5 mortality in 2000-19: An updated systematic analysis with implications for the Sustainable Development Goals. *Lancet Child Adolesc. Health* **2022**, *6*, 106–115. [CrossRef] [PubMed]
14. Haley, K.M. Neonatal Venous Thromboembolism. *Front. Pediatr.* **2017**, *5*, 136. [CrossRef] [PubMed]
15. Clavijo, M.M.; Mahuad, C.V.; de Los Angeles Vicente Reparaz, M.; Aizpurua, M.F.; Ventura, A.; Casali, C.E. Risk factors and role of low molecular weight heparin in obstetric complications among women with inherited thrombophilia-a cohort study. *Hematol. Transfus. Cell Ther.* **2019**, *41*, 303–309. [CrossRef]
16. Lisonkova, S.; Sheps, S.B.; Janssen, P.A.; Lee, S.K.; Dahlgren, L.; Macnab, Y.C. Birth Outcomes Among Older Mothers in Rural Versus Urban Areas: A Residence-Based Approach. *J. Rural. Health* **2010**, *27*, 211–219. [CrossRef] [PubMed]
17. Papadakis, E.; Pouliakis, A.; Aktypi, A.; Christoforidou, A.; Kotsi, P.; Anagnostou, G.; Foifa, A.; Grouzi, E. Low molecular weight heparins use in pregnancy: A practice survey from Greece and a review of the literature. *Thromb. J.* **2019**, *17*, 23. [CrossRef] [PubMed]
18. Heazell, A.E.P.; Newman, L.; Lean, S.C.; Jones, R.L. Pregnancy outcome in mothers over the age of 35. *Curr. Opin. Obstet. Gynecol.* **2018**, *30*, 337–343. [CrossRef]
19. Larsen, T.B.; Sørensen, H.T.; Gislum, M.; Johnsen, S.P. Maternal smoking, obesity, and risk of venous thromboembolism during pregnancy and the puerperium: A population-based nested case-control study. *Thromb. Res.* **2007**, *120*, 505–509. [CrossRef]
20. Shaala, I.Y.; Moneim, D.A.A.; Elwafa, R.A.H.A.; Hosny, T.A.; Ammar, E.T. Detection of plasminogen activator inhibitor-1 (-675 4G/5G) gene polymorphism in women with recurrent abortion. *Hematol. Transfus. Int. J.* **2019**, *19*, 7.
21. Buchholz, T.; Lohse, P.; Rogenhofer, N.; Kosian, E.; Pihusch, R.; Thaler, C.J. Polymorphisms in the ACE and PAI-1 genes are associated with recurrent spontaneous miscarriages. *Hum. Reprod.* **2003**, *18*, 2473–2477. [CrossRef]
22. Bigdeli, R.; Younesi, M.R.; Panahnejad, E.; Asgary, V.; Heidarzadeh, S.; Mazaheri, H.; Aligoudarzi, S.L. Association between thrombophilia gene polymorphisms and recurrent pregnancy loss risk in the Iranian population. *Syst. Biol. Reprod. Med.* **2018**, *64*, 274–282. [CrossRef] [PubMed]
23. Grandone, E.; Margaglione, M.; Colaizzo, D.; Pavone, G.; Paladini, D.; Martinelli, P.; Di Minno, G. Lower birth-weight in neonates of mothers carrying factor V G1691A and factor II A(20210) mutations. *Haematologica* **2002**, *87*, 177–181. [PubMed]
24. Colucci, G.; Tsakiris, D.A. Thrombophilia screening revisited: An issue of personalized medicine. *J. Thromb. Thrombolysis* **2020**, *49*, 618–629. [CrossRef] [PubMed]
25. Ahangari, N.; Doosti, M.; Mousavifar, N.; Attaran, M.; Shahrokhzadeh, S.; Memarpour, S.; Karimiani, E.G. Hereditary thrombophilia genetic variants in recurrent pregnancy loss. *Arch. Gynecol. Obstet.* **2019**, *300*, 777–782. [CrossRef]
26. Bhave, A.A. Coagulopathies in Pregnancy: What an Obstetrician Ought to Know! *J. Obstet. Gynaecol. India* **2019**, *69*, 479–482. [CrossRef]
27. Liu, X.; Chen, Y.; Ye, C.; Xing, D.; Wu, R.; Li, F.; Chen, L.; Wang, T. Hereditary thrombophilia and recurrent pregnancy loss: A systematic review and meta-analysis. *Hum. Reprod.* **2021**, *36*, 1213–1229. [CrossRef]
28. Abu-Asab, N.S.; Ayesh, S.K.; Ateeq, R.O.; Nassar, S.M.; El-Sharif, W.A. Association of inherited thrombophilia with recurrent pregnancy loss in palestinian women. *Obstet. Gynecol. Int.* **2011**, *2011*, 689684. [CrossRef]
29. Nikolaeva, M.G.; Momot, A.P.; Zainulina, M.S.; Yasafova, N.N.; Taranenko, I.A. Pregnancy complications in G20210A mutation carriers associated with high prothrombin activity. *Thromb. J.* **2021**, *19*, 41. [CrossRef]
30. Momot, A.P.; Nikolaeva, M.G.; Yasafova, N.N.; Zainulina, M.S.; Momot, K.A.; Taranenko, I.A. Clinical and laboratory manifestations of the prothrombin gene mutation in women of reproductive age. *J. Blood Med.* **2019**, *10*, 255–263. [CrossRef]
31. Dai, C.; Fei, Y.; Li, J.; Shi, Y.; Yang, X. Novel Review of Homocysteine and Pregnancy Complications. *BioMed Res. Int.* **2021**, *2021*, 6652231. [CrossRef]
32. Croles, F.N.; Nasserinejad, K.; Duvekot, J.J.; Kruip, M.J.; Meijer, K.; Leebeek, F.W. Pregnancy, thrombophilia, and the risk of a first venous thrombosis: Systematic review and bayesian meta-analysis. *BMJ* **2017**, *359*, j4452. [CrossRef] [PubMed]
33. Mayer-Pickel, K.; Kolovetsiou-Kreiner, V.; Stern, C.; Münzker, J.; Eberhard, K.; Trajanoski, S.; Lakovschek, I.-C.; Ulrich, D.; Csapo, B.; Lang, U.; et al. Effect of Low-Dose Aspirin on Soluble FMS-Like Tyrosine Kinase 1/Placental Growth Factor (sFlt-1/PlGF Ratio) in Pregnancies at High Risk for the Development of Preeclampsia. *J. Clin. Med.* **2019**, *8*, 1429. [CrossRef] [PubMed]
34. De Vries, J.I.P.; van Pampus, M.G.; Hague, W.M.; Bezemer, P.D.; Joosten, J.H.; FRUIT Investigators. Low-molecular-weight heparin added to aspirin in the prevention of recurrent early-onset pre-eclampsia in women with inheritable thrombophilia: The FRUIT-RCT. *J. Thromb. Haemost.* **2012**, *10*, 64–72. [CrossRef] [PubMed]
35. Bates, S.M.; Rajasekhar, A.; Middeldorp, S.; McLintock, C.; Rodger, M.; James, A.H.; Vazquez, S.R.; Greer, I.A.; Riva, J.J.; Bhatt, M.; et al. American Society of Hematology 2018 guidelines for management of venous thromboembolism: Venous thromboembolism in the context of pregnancy. *Blood Adv.* **2018**, *2*, 3317–3359. [CrossRef] [PubMed]
36. Shapiro, N.L.; Kominiarek, M.A.; Nutescu, E.A.; Chevalier, A.; Hibbard, J.U. Dosing and monitoring of low-molecular-weight heparin in high-risk pregnancy: Single-center experience. *Pharmacotherapy* **2011**, *31*, 678–685. [CrossRef]
37. Lebaudy, C.; Hulot, J.-S.; Amoura, Z.; Costedoat-Chalumeau, N.; Serreau, R.; Ankri, A.; Conard, J.; Cornet, A.; Dommergues, M.; Piette, J.; et al. Changes in enoxaparin pharmacokinetics during pregnancy and implications for antithrombotic therapeutic strategy. *Clin. Pharmacol. Ther.* **2008**, *84*, 370–377. [CrossRef]

38. Dobbenga-Rhodes, Y. Shedding Light on Inherited Thrombophilias: The Impact on Pregnancy. *J. Perinat. Neonatal Nurs.* **2016**, *30*, 36–44. [CrossRef]
39. Fogerty, A.E.; Connors, J.M. Management of inherited thrombophilia in pregnancy. *Curr. Opin. Endocrinol. Diabetes* **2009**, *16*, 464–469. [CrossRef]

Disclaimer/Publisher's Note: The statements, opinions and data contained in all publications are solely those of the individual author(s) and contributor(s) and not of MDPI and/or the editor(s). MDPI and/or the editor(s) disclaim responsibility for any injury to people or property resulting from any ideas, methods, instructions or products referred to in the content.

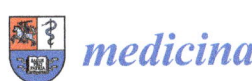

Review

Approach to Thrombophilia in Pregnancy—A Narrative Review

Miruna Samfireag [1,2], Cristina Potre [3,*], Ovidiu Potre [3], Raluca Tudor [4], Teodora Hoinoiu [1,2] and Andrei Anghel [5]

[1] Department of Internal Medicine, Discipline of Clinical Practical Skills, "Victor Babes" University of Medicine and Pharmacy, No. 2 Eftimie Murgu Square, 300041 Timisoara, Romania; samfireag.miruna@umft.ro (M.S.); tstoichitoiu@umft.ro (T.H.)
[2] Advanced Cardiology and Hemostaseology Research Center, "Victor Babes" University of Medicine and Pharmacy, No. 2 Eftimie Murgu Square, 300041 Timisoara, Romania
[3] Department of Internal Medicine, Discipline of Hematology, "Victor Babes" University of Medicine and Pharmacy, No. 2 Eftimie Murgu Square, 300041 Timisoara, Romania; potre.ovidiu@umft.ro
[4] Department of Neurosciences, Discipline of Neurology, "Victor Babes" University of Medicine and Pharmacy, No. 2 Eftimie Murgu Square, 300041 Timisoara, Romania; tudor.raluca@umft.ro
[5] Department of Biochemistry and Pharmacology, Discipline of Biochemistry, "Victor Babes" University of Medicine and Pharmacy, No. 2 Eftimie Murgu Square, 300041 Timisoara, Romania; biochim@umft.ro
* Correspondence: potre.cristina@umft.ro

Abstract: Thrombophilia is a genetic predisposition to hypercoagulable states caused by acquired haemostasis conditions; pregnancy causes the haemostatic system to become hypercoagulable, which grows throughout the pregnancy and peaks around delivery. Genetic testing for thrombophilic gene mutations is evaluated using different methodologies of real-time polymerase chain reaction and DNA microarrays of specific genes. Adapting the general care of the pregnant woman to the particularities caused by thrombophilia is an important component, so screening is preferred to assess the degree of genetic damage that manifests itself as a risk of thrombosis. The major goal of this narrative review was to quantitatively evaluate the literature data on the specific care of pregnant women with thrombophilia that are at risk of developing unplanned miscarriages.

Keywords: thrombophilia; pregnancy; genetic testing; screening; narrative review

1. Introduction

Thrombophilia [1,2] is defined as a predisposition for thrombosis, occurred as a result to a genetic defect (hereditary); it may be diagnosed postnatally (acquired). Thrombosis develops secondary to the alteration of one or more components of the haemostasis, which includes coagulation factors, plasmatic proteins, blood flow, vascular surfaces and cellular elements that finally lead to a hypercoagulable state. This results in arterial or venous thrombosis. A reasonable approach of a patient with thrombosis starts with the attempt to characterize the hypercoagulable condition as hereditary or acquired. Pregnancy modifies the haemostatic system into a hypercoagulable condition, which is absolute around delivery. Recurrent pregnancy loss (RPL) is described as two or more unplanned miscarriages, which involves about 5% of women of reproductive age [3]. Novel studies indicate that thrombophilia is one of the causes that leads to RPL [2,3]. Hereditary states develop due to the presence of some mutations that change a gene that codifies a plasmatic protein involved in the anticoagulant mechanism [4].

Hereditary thrombophilia represents one of the risk factors among reproductive disorders. Thrombophilia expresses an important trend that finally leads to thrombosis [5]. The coagulation system may deviate to a thrombotic condition, which may be characterized as a thromboembolic pathology. This deviation is generated due to various factors, mainly because of the coagulation factors and their synergy, but likewise, because of their connection with blood components and other cells [5]. The possibility of getting diagnosed with thrombosis enhances with age, as a result of various factors, pregnancy being one of them. Venous thromboembolism (VTE) is known as a pathology expressed by multiple factors, being the ultimate clinical clue of genetic or acquired ones. A patient that may develop thrombosis should be tested for thrombophilia, so a woman with a known prothrombotic condition has to be evaluated as such [6]. Bates et al. confirmed in one of their latest studies that 1.2 in every 1000 deliveries are complicated by VTE. The necessity to consider both foetal and mother well-being makes diagnosis, prevention, and treatment of pregnancy associated VTE particularly problematic. Current guidelines [6] deal with these difficult challenges. Thrombophilia testing is frequently requested in clinical practice by asymptomatic persons with a family history of VTE. The presence of thrombophilia is not predicted by having a family history of VTE, but women who plan to become pregnant may benefit from thrombophilia testing [7].

2. Aetiology of Thrombophilia

The phrase "thrombophilia" was first mentioned in 1937, when Nygaard and Brown characterized unexpected occlusion of large arteries, sometimes with associated VTE, but the familial habit of thromboembolic pathology was largely analysed by Jordan and Nandorff in 1956 [5]. The research of hereditary thrombophilia began by studying families with a known history of VTE [5]. Back in the 1900s, hereditary thrombophilia was considered to be a rare genetic disorder. Specific tests for hereditary thrombophilia developed throughout time [5]. The chance of a thrombotic episode to occur increases in the presence of several risk factors like aging, immobilization, prolonged orthostatism, obesity, diet, smoking, elevated oestrogen levels, birth control intakes (increases the chances of a VTE up to three times), and last but not least, pregnancy and the postpartum period [4,5]. The relation made among VTE and inherited thrombophilia was proved after performing case–control studies (Figure 1) [5]. It was estimated that 50% of the thrombotic episodes may happen all of a sudden, 30% are related to pregnancy and 20% are linked with surgery [5].

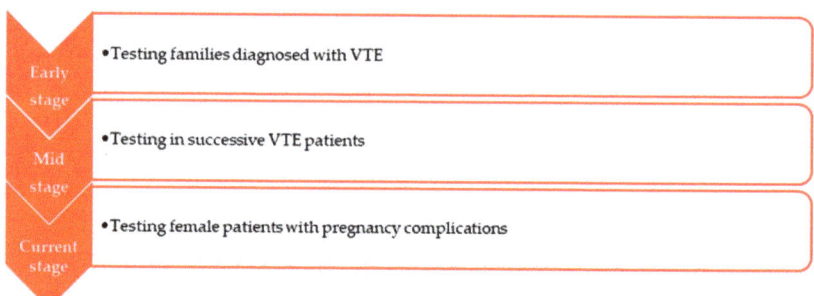

Figure 1. Progression of hereditary thrombophilia testing (information taken from [5]).

Friederich et al. confirmed in their research that if a venous thromboembolic episode happens during pregnancy or within three months of childbirth, it is pregnancy related [8]. The incidence of VTE in pregnancy increases up to five times, with a rate of 0.76-1.72 out of 1000 pregnancies, but most thrombotic events occur mostly in the puerperal period [9].

When assessing the optimal prophylaxis, a patient diagnosed with thrombophilia should be evaluated for the majority of risk factors, known as triggers for first or recurrent thrombosis. Along these lines, when concluding the thrombotic profile of the patients, genetic risk factors should be considered as well as acquired ones, considering that obesity, trauma, acute medical conditions, surgery or malignancies are defined by increased levels of procoagulant factors. In contrast, pregnancy is associated with decreased anticoagulant factors levels [1].

Knowledge about the aetiology of VTE is improving as time goes by, but screening for hereditary thrombophilia is most of the times not convenient, even though it should be noted that pregnant females have an undoubtedly elevated risk of developing VTE, especially if they have affirmative family antecedents for VTE [5].

Particularities of the Hemostatic System in Pregnancy

The chances of bleeding and thromboembolic events are elevated during pregnancy. The utero-placental entity is unique, and its most significant function is to maintain contact between the maternal and foetal circulations, which is a necessity for foetal survival, so the circulation must be developed and sustained [10].

In humans, foetal haemoglobin (HbF) represents almost 2% of the total haemoglobin (Hb) in adults [10]. It is assumed that the physiological function of HbF enables the transition of oxygen from maternal to foetal blood. The interchange of gases such as oxygen and carbon dioxide as well as nutrients must be allowed at the boundary between the maternal and foetal circulations, so, since bleeding and thrombotic activities may impair this critical feature, the rehabilitation of the utero-placental circulation requires multiple systems [10,11]. Coagulopathies in pregnancy, such as deep venous thrombosis (DVT) and repeated pregnancy losses (RPL), may contribute to obstetric emergencies, but these events might be obviated if women would be carefully observed for warning signs that could suggest the need for testing to detect these undesired incidents [12]. Coagulopathies could be predicted by basic laboratory studies, such as a global coagulation panel like complete blood count (CBC), prothrombin time (PT), partial thromboplastin time (PTT) and plasma fibrinogen. The placenta is a highly advanced pregnancy organ that facilitates natural foetal growth and development [13]. Changes in the growth and function of placentas' have dramatic implications on the foetus and its capacity to deal with the intrauterine habitat. In the existence of genetic thrombophilic mutations, considering the number of studies supporting or not the link between hereditary thrombophilia and pregnancy complications, it is impossible to determine the precise risk figures for serious adverse effects [11]. Pregnancy is a prothrombotic condition, and prothrombotic events are obvious as gestation advances. The development of sufficient placental circulation is needed for a healthy pregnancy, and hereditary thrombophilia can be a risk factor for placenta-mediated pregnancy adverse effects [12]. Gestation induces a 2 to 3-fold rise in fibrinogen concentrations, as well as a 20% to 1000% raise in factors VII, VIII, IX, X, and XII, all of which peak at delivery [14]. During normal pregnancy, blood coagulation factor XIII, XII, X, VIII, von Willebrand factor, ristocetin cofactor, factor VII, and fibrinogen increase dramatically, and the most pronounced improvements are observed in the third trimester [10]. These modifications guard against potentially lethal haemorrhage during pregnancy and through the third stage of gestation, but they also raise the likelihood of maternal thromboembolism [10]. In 1000 patients, the incidence VTE is estimated to be between 0.5 and 2.2. It is five times higher among pregnant women, with the highest risk of thrombosis registered between week 6 and 12 after childbirth [15]. The increased levels of oestrogen and progesterone during gestation lead to a hypercoagulable condition, resulting in an upregulation of the clotting factors and a reduction in the levels of anticoagulants [15].

Inherited thrombophilia is assumed to be present in up to 50% of venous thrombotic events that occur during gestation and puerperium, and is well-known that thrombosis during pregnancy, as well as underlying thrombophilia, may have severe consequences for both the mother and the foetus [15,16]. Biological hypercoagulability is a term used to explain variations in blood coagulation and fibrinolysis which have a thrombotic aspect during gestation, and increased fibrin turnover is a result of hypercoagulation. This is demonstrated by increased concentrations of D-Dimers (D-D), the most susceptible marker of secondary fibrinolytic activation [17].

3. Classification of Thrombophilias

Thrombophilia is divided in two main groups—inherited and acquired.

3.1. Hereditary Thrombophilia

The inheritable thrombophilic states [18] may be subdivided in two parts: common, respectively, major inherited thrombophilias [1]. Additionally, they may be classified into two categories: in the first one, inhibitors of coagulation are decreased—deficiency of coagulation inhibitor factor such as antithrombin III (AT III), protein C and protein S deficiency; in the second category, coagulation factors are elevated—activated Protein C resistance (APC), Factor V Leiden, prothrombin gene mutation, increased levels of VIII, IX, XI factors, and dysfibrinogenemias. The first category is more predisposed to thrombosis than the second one, which is more likely to be associated with the first event of thrombosis [18].

Therefore, regarding inherited thrombophilia, the most common causes are the prothrombin gene mutation G20210A and factor Leiden, concluding up to 70% of the diagnosed inherited forms of thrombophilia. The less common but most severe triggers are the defects of protein C and S and of antithrombin III [1,4,5,18].

3.2. Acquired Thrombophilia

Besides inherited thrombophilia, hypercoagulable conditions may also be generated by acquired pathologies of the haemostasis. Acquired states can sustain a prothrombotic condition due to increased procoagulant factors and decreased anticoagulants besides other modifications of the haemostasis [1]. The major acquired pathologies linked to thrombophilia are the following: hyperhomocysteinemia, antiphospholipid antibody syndrome (APS), elevated levels of procoagulant factors and reduced levels of anticoagulants. Normally, these levels are balanced naturally, but they can be modified due to acquired factors or because of aging [1,4]. APS is an immune mediated disorder, defined by obstetrical or thrombotic circumstances [1]. An obstetrical APS is represented by preeclampsia (PE), recurrent miscarriages, foetal growth restriction (FGR), first trimester abortion (FTA), mid-trimester abortion (MTA), placental abruption (PA) or intrauterine death [1,3], yet a thrombotic APS is defined by venous or arterial thrombosis [1]. Antiphospholipids antibodies [aPL] (primarily anticardiolipin) are responsible for setting the APS, together with the detection of lupus anticoagulant [1,3]. The diagnosis of this immune mediated disorder is confirmed if at least one of the clinical manifestations specified earlier is proven and if aPL are described in more than two occasions.

Regarding the risk for thrombosis, it may be subdivided into high risk, moderate and low risk thrombophilia; high risk thrombophilia includes antithrombin III, protein C and protein S deficiency, moderate risk thrombophilia consists of factor V Leiden, prothrombin gene mutation and factor VIII, and last but not least, low risk thrombophilia covers for factor IX, factor XI and hyperhomocysteinemia [19].

3.3. Grading the Risk

3.3.1. High Risk Thrombophilia

Antithrombin III Deficiency (AT III)

AT III is one of the essential plasmatic inhibitors for the activated coagulation factors, immediate aim being for sure thrombin [20]. Deficiency of AT III is established to be a risk factor for venous thrombosis, considering that acquired deficiencies are more common, but it may be fixed by administrating the proper anticoagulation regimen [20]. When heterozygous mutations are detected in the AT gene, this may be followed by AT defects, which are defined by decreased inhibition of factor Xa [1]. Measuring the level of AT III should be performed before administrating the anticoagulation with heparins or with low molecular weight heparins. It is established to increase the risk of thrombosis up to 50%.

Protein C and S Deficiencies

Protein C and S deficiencies, rare pathologies are described by a reduction in the activity of protein C, respectively S, [21,22]; protein C deficiency was identified by Mammen et al. in 1960, yet Stenflo et al. named it the way we know it today. It is known to increase the risk of thrombosis up to 20%, unlike protein S, which increases this risk up to 10%. Thus, hereditary deficiency of both protein C and S leads to an elevated thrombin production and predilection to thrombosis [1].

3.3.2. Moderate Risk Thrombophilia
Activated Protein C Resistance and Factor V Leiden

Activated Protein C Resistance was described for the first time in the early 1990s by Dahlback and Hildebrand [18]; they discovered an error regarding the anticoagulant response while activating protein C (APC). APC resistance was demonstrated to be inherited and linked with hereditary thrombophilia [23]. Factor V Leiden, a hereditary defect of haemostasis, and also a low risk factor for thrombosis, linked with the possibility of developing first and recurrent venous thromboembolism, was included in various screening programs. It is also associated with thrombosis, particularly in women known with other risks factors, such as pregnancy, older age, oral contraceptive intakes, hyperhomocysteinemia, and deficiencies of protein C and protein S [18,24].

Prothrombin Gene Mutation (Factor II)

Prothrombin, or factor II, precursor of the thrombin [25], was first mentioned in 1996 by Poort et al. [18]; prothrombin G20210A mutation is known for the changing of the guanine nucleotide (G) with the adenine nucleotide (A) in the 20210 position, and it affects up to 6% of the population, increasing eventually the risk of thrombosis. Even though its heterozygous posture is known as a low risk factor for developing associated VTE complications, this risk is increased during pregnancy [25]. Nevertheless, both oral contraceptives intakes and pregnancy eventually develop an increased prothrombin activity [25].

Factor VIII

Patients with records of VTE have presented elevated levels of factors VIII, IX and XI [18], although it is uncertain how increased levels of coagulation factors interfere with the risk of thrombosis, but once the level of factor VIII increases, so does the risk of thrombosis (up to 10%).

3.3.3. Low Risk Thrombophilia
Hyperhomocysteinemia

The demethylation of methionine forms the amino-acid-homocysteine [1]. Homocysteine is a commonly developing amino-acid [26]. Increased levels of homocysteine, called hyperhomocysteinemia may result from all sorts of hereditary factors or from a diet poor in folic acid and B vitamins. Elevated levels in pregnancy may end up with recurrent pregnancy loss, but the presence of methylenetetrahydrofolate reductase gene (MTHFR) in the absence of elevated levels of homocysteine is not linked with a significant risk of thrombosis [1].

4. Thrombophilias and Complications in Pregnancy

Pregnancy is a state described as carrying a foetus within the female body that usually ends through miscarriage or delivery [27]. Hereditary and acquired thrombophilias are responsible for more than 50% of the thrombotic events diagnosed during pregnancy and the postnatal period [28]. Along with birth and the postnatal period, haemostatic problems may occur, which involve important complications regarding morbidity and mortality for the mother and foetus as well [29]. Because pregnancy and the postnatal period are well known risk factors for thrombosis, it is established that pregnant women may develop venous thromboembolism in 50% of the cases. On the other hand, any pregnant woman deals with physiological adjustments during pregnancy that end up interfering with biochemical parameters. These adjustments lead to a hypercoagulable condition, so the risk of venous thromboembolism affects 1 in 1600 births [30].

Haemostasis is a vital equilibrium that includes the natural anticoagulation system, fibrinolysis and procoagulants [31]. Normal pregnancy is linked with significant changes in the haemostasis [31], so the procoagulants outcome end up being predominant. Serious pregnancy complications—preeclampsia (PE), recurrent miscarriages, fetal growth restriction (FGR), first trimester abortion (FTA), mid-trimester abortion (MTA), placental abruption (PA) or intrauterine death [3,32]—increase both maternal and foetal morbidity and mortality [28]. Adequate uterine blood flow and normal placental evolution contribute to a typical pregnancy outcome, which is related with significant changes in the coagulation and anticoagulation process, and there is noticed an important boost towards the coagulation factors—fibrinogen, prothrombin, VII, VII, X and XII [28].

On the other hand, in pregnancy, anticoagulant levels might increase lightly (tissue factor pathway inhibitor -TF- the primary initiator of coagulation) [33]; they may also remain stable (antithrombin III and protein C) or they may diminish unquestionably (protein S).

Thrombophilia is known as a pathogenic factor for serious pregnancy complications. Modifications of the procoagulants factors—mutant genes with great prevalence able to increase the risk in developing thrombosis have been studied [28,30]: homozygous or heterozygous mutation in the methylenetetrahydrofolate reductase gene (MTHFR) in the C677T and A1298C positions, the homozygous or heterozygous mutation of the factor V Leiden (FVL) gene in the G1691A position, homozygous or heterozygous mutation of the prothrombin gene in the G20210A position (factor II) or the polymorphism of plasminogen activator inhibitor-1 (PAI-1) 4G/4G mutations [28,30,34].

A favourable result of a pregnancy is related to normal placental formation [34]. Coagulation factor XIII has an important impact regarding its formation, since it is implied in cross-linking fibrin and it is known to be affecting the fibrinolysis. For factor XIII, a frequent polymorphism is connected with an early cross-link and a diminished perceptivity to fibrinolysis. Therefore, factor XIII Val34Leu polymorphism may destroy fibrinolysis, and might increase the general risk for RPL [34]. An equivalence between thrombosis, pregnancy complications and thrombophilia persists to be studied [30].

4.1. Screening Options

Screening for thrombophilia does not interfere with the proper management practiced in pregnancy, recurrent pregnancy losses or infertility issues. A study conducted by Ashraf in 2019 highlighted findings from 1995 to 2017 regarding the importance of genetic thrombophilia testing, in patients that were susceptible of having hypercoagulable conditions [35]. Thrombophilia screening is questionable [36]. Nowadays, laboratories performing various sets of tests regarding the diagnosis of thrombophilia are developing quickly [37]. Screening for hereditary thrombophilia was first mentioned in 1965, when a family was diagnosed with a deficiency of the serine protease inhibitor antithrombin. Later, a few irregularities have been linked with hereditary thrombophilia, and a vast set of tests have been implemented by laboratories in order to identify patients with these irregularities. Testing for hereditary thrombophilia implies a wide variety of coagulation and genetic tests [38], although testing is costly, and interpretations require clinical competence. Specific tests for thrombophilia should not be performed during a thrombotic episode, because the results may be influenced by a few factors, and yet the existence of inherited thrombophilia does not interfere with the primary management of VTE. Screening for thrombophilia involves an ample set of tests, that may include the following parameters: prothrombin G20210A, factor V Leiden (FVL), factor V HR2, factor XIII V34L, plasminogen activator inhibitor-1 4G/5G (PAI-1), methylene tetrahydrofolate reductase (MTHFR) C677T, MTHFR A1298C, β-fibrinogen-455 G>A, apolipoprotein E (Apo E), angiotensin-converting enzyme I/D, apolipoprotein B R3500Q [39]; measurements of protein C, protein S, antithrombin III are also performed, as well as analysis of homocysteine levels [38], and last but not least, tests to distinguish values of lupus anticoagulant, anticardiolipin antibodies and anti-beta 2 glicoprotein-I antibodies in order to confirm or infirm the presence of antiphospolipid syndrome (APS) [37,40]. It is essential to be aware of the drugs taken at the time of testing—for instance, while administrating low molecular weight heparin (LMWH), antithrombin levels may decrease [38]. It is well known that screening for acquired conditions of thrombophilia should be taken into consideration in all situations of thrombosis, although testing for hereditary conditions is improbable to be always useful [41].

Therefore, when should specific tests be performed and who should be tested? In most of the cases, where VTE is suspected and where trigger factors are obvious. Determining proper conditions in order to initiate screening may be useful for the patient as soon as a suitable treatment is prescribed.

Thrombophilic states should be studied in order to be able to take precautionary measures such as: improved prophylaxis in case of pregnancy, avoidance of combined oral contraceptive pill intake (OCP) or of hormonal therapy [41]. Inherited thrombophilia may be associated with VTE in pregnancy, and it may lead to complications such as recurrent pregnancy loss. Based on consensus expert opinion, a manuscript published in 2016 by the Anticoagulation Forum provides practical clinical guidelines on the prevention and specific treatment of obstetric-associated VTE [42].

Screening for thrombophilia in pregnancy is tempting and is widely used, because it raises the occasion of prescribing antiplatelet drugs and anticoagulant therapy in order to reduce the risks of thrombotic events. Thrombophilia, a disorder that finally leads to thrombosis, is linked with an important risk of VTE, especially in women who are prescribed OCP, hormonal therapy or who are pregnant. A few analysis performed over the years have tried to set up the cost effectiveness of testing for thrombophilia. In a study conducted by Wu et al. [43], it was established that performing routine screening for thrombophilia in women before pregnancy it is not profitable, economically speaking [41]. This cost effectiveness study was carried out through UK National Health Services, in order to establish the cost effectiveness of common and selective screening, regarding personal or/and a family history of VTE in comparison with no testing for thrombophilia. The unfavourable complications were linked with screening and no screening in the assumed groups, so four screening theories were tested, as follows: screening 10.000 women in each theory—prior OCP intake, at week 6 of pregnancy, prior prescribing hormonal therapy and last but not least, prior surgeries [43]. The women from the pregnancy group, who were tested positive for thrombophilia, in order to prevent RPL and VTE, would be prescribed prophylaxis drugs. In the common testing, all the patients would be screened; still, in the selective testing, only the patients known with a previous VTE or a family history of thrombosis would be screened. Therefore, in an assumed model of 10,000 patients, where the routine testing has not been performed, unfavourable complications would be encountered in 7 women on OCP, 2921 pregnant ones, 104 patients prescribed hormonal therapy and 1265 women subject to surgeries [43]. Regardless, thrombophilia screening still remains questionable [36].

4.2. Clinical Evaluation

A clinical evaluation for thrombophilia should be performed for all of the patients who had experienced an episode of VTE [44], or for women with a known personal history of preeclampsia, recurrent miscarriages, foetal growth restriction, first trimester abortion, mid-trimester abortion, placental abruption or intrauterine deaths [1,3]. The evaluation starts with an accurate family and personal history for thrombosis, past clinical antecedents, associated pathologies and interpretation of the existing risk factors. An entire physical examination is recommended, paying increased concentration to skin, lymphatic, peripheral arterial and venous, cardiorespiratory, abdominal, urinary and neurological system.

VTE may be separated in idiopathic–unprovoked and secondary-provoked. Provoked VTE is characterized by transitory–reversible, minor and major risk factors or by irreversible–persistent ones; thrombophilic conditions should be evaluated in order to improve prophylaxis in case of the existence of the following risk factors—non-provoking ones—age, sex, combined oral contraceptive pill intake (OCP) or of hormonal therapy, and of provoking ones—pregnancy, long-distance-travel, trauma, surgery, immobilization or cancer [42,44]. Distinction between forms of VTE influences the treatment judgment.

One in 1000 pregnancies is known with associated VTE, and the risk of thrombosis is higher in the postpartum period [45,46]. The majority of the symptoms that may claim deep venous thrombosis (DVT) like dyspnea, tachycardia, groin discomfort, unilateral leg pain and swelling are known as physiological transformations in pregnancy, and eventually most of the women presenting these changes will not develop DVT, but the risk of pregnancy-associated-VTE is increased up to ten times in this category, unlike the non-pregnant same age control-lot [45]. Women with a history of recurrent miscarriages are investigated for thrombophilia in order to set the proper pregnancy-management [45].

4.3. Methodology and Patient Management

Inherited thrombophilias are associated with early pregnancy loss, taking into account an important risk of VTE. This state continues to be a valuable cause of maternal morbidity and mortality [47]. Pregnancy is known to have a five-fold increase in developing VTE, this risk being multiplied up to twenty times during the postpartum period [48]. Due to probable maternal and foetal complications, a proper therapeutic strategy during pregnancy is quite demanding. Various therapeutic methods have been taken into consideration regarding the management of pregnant women diagnosed with hereditary thrombophilia, such as: anticoagulants, antiplatelets drugs and vitamins [6,42,49]. When choosing an ideal treatment for a pregnant woman with inherited thrombophilia, additional risks must be deliberated, regarding its efficacy and safety. Evidence and guidance are followed in order to establish clinical decisions regarding duration of thrombolytics and anticoagulation in pregnant women diagnosed with hereditary thrombophilia. The novel guidelines of American Society of Hematology for the management of venous thromboembolism in the context of pregnancy are improved from the ones followed in 2012 and in 2016 [6,42,50].

4.3.1. Anticoagulants during Pregnancy

When inherited thrombophilia is confirmed, antepartum prophylaxis should be initiated immediately, since the risk of VTE seems to develop early in pregnancy [49]. The administration of anticoagulants during pregnancy is challenging, due to possible associated complications [47]. Likely side effects of maternal anticoagulant treatment may include teratogenicity, bleeding, and recurrent pregnancy loss [47]. The anticoagulants of choice are low-molecular-weight heparin (LMWH) and unfractionated heparin (UFH), owing the ability of not crossing the placenta, being safe for the foetus [47]. Vitamin K antagonists, warfarin for instance, crosses the placenta, being disclosed as potential causer for the enumerated complications—for example, it may lead to the hypoplasia of the nasal bone, if it is administrated between weeks 6 and 12 of pregnancy, or it may cause anomalies of the central nervous system in any trimester [47]. In a study conducted in vitro in 2002 [49,51], there was no trace of transplacental transfer of fondaparinux, which is a synthetic pentasaccharide, an antithrombotic agent that selectively inhibit coagulation factor Xa. Even though it has been described being a safe agent, it may cause foetal teratogenicity, so its usage is mainly restrictive. LMWH known for their elevated bioavailability, have shorter polysaccharide chains and lower molecular weights unlike UFH, with no need in performing regular coagulation tests [52,53]. LMWH can be self-administrated, subcutaneously once a day. If possible, checking out anti Xa levels and testing D-Dimers should be performed monthly during a pregnancy, in order to prevent secondary complications [53,54]. As all heparins, LMWH dosing is based on a patients' weight, but administrating it in accordance to anti Xa levels remains disputed [47]. The optimal therapeutic dose for prophylaxis is not clear, and it has not been demonstrated if dose adaptation in order to maintain clear-cut anti Xa levels increases prophylactic efficacy or safety [47]. On the other hand, UFH may be linked with thrombocytopenia, osteoporosis and maternal bleeding, so LMWH are preferred for a long-term prophylaxis [53]. When extended anticoagulation is needed during pregnancy, maternal complications may occur as well. All anticoagulants are likely to cause bleeding, allergic reactions or pain at the injection's sites—but this should not lead to the interruption of the treatment [52]. While hereditary thrombophilias are mostly linked with an inclination to VTE, acquired forms are associated with both venous and arterial events. APS represents an acquired form of thrombophilia, defined by the presence of antiphospholipid antibodies (aPL), clinically characterized by arterial or venous thrombosis. This is also associated with obstetric complications, the diagnosis being based on the Sydney criteria: one clinical criteria (pregnancy morbidity or arterious or venous thrombosis) and one laboratory criteria (high value of lupus anticoagulant, of anticardiolipin antibodies IgM/IgG or of anti-beta 2 glicoprotein-I antibodies IgM/IgG) [40,49,54,55]. Although antiphospolipid syndrome (APS) was first identified as an autoimmune thrombophilia, we now know that additional mechanisms besides coagulation-mediated thrombosis play a role in various clinical presentations; for example, complement activation may play a role in placental damage, which can result in fetal loss [56]. Even though anticoagulants and thrombolytics are the most administrated drugs in order to prevent pregnancy-related complications in women diagnosed with hereditary thrombophilia (Table 1) [54], at the time of delivery, the risk of haemorrhage may occur in anticoagulated women, but it can be reduced with careful preparation (Table 2) [49].

Table 1. Preferred prophylaxis in order to prevent pregnancy-related complications in women diagnosed with inherited thrombophilia—summary of recommendations (American College of Chest Physicians).

Prevention of Pregnancy-Related Complications	Recommendations
No previous VTE	
HIGH RISK: homozygosity for the mutation of factor V Leiden or the presence of prothrombin gene mutation	
√ Absence of a family history of VTE:	➢ antepartum clinical surveillance ➢ post-delivery prophylaxis up to 6 weeks
√ With a positive family history of VTE:	➢ antepartum prophylaxis ➢ post-delivery prophylaxis
LOW RISK: other forms of thrombophilias	
√ Absence of a family history of VTE:	➢ antepartum and post-delivery clinical surveillance
√ With a positive family history of VTE:	➢ antepartum clinical surveillance ➢ post-delivery prophylaxis up to 6 weeks
Previous VTE	
MODERATE AND HIGH RISK:	➢ antepartum prophylaxis
One or multiple episodes of VTE:	➢ post-delivery prophylaxis up to 6 weeks
LOW RISK:	
One episode of VTE, linked with a temporary risk factor, that is not pregnancy-related:	➢ antepartum clinical surveillance

Information taken from [25,54,55].

Anticoagulants should be started postpartum as soon as proper haemostasis is established [54]. LMWH can be initiated 12–24 h postpartum in deliveries without associated complications. If warfarin is preferred to be used post-delivery, it may be initiated exactly like LMWH. Not only warfarin, but also LMWH is safe for breastfeeding patients. Postpartum prophylaxis is recommended for nearly six weeks, with prophylactic doses of LMWH or UFH, with D-Dimers tested regularly [49,54]. Clinical trials evaluating oral anticoagulants such as direct thrombin and anti Xa inhibitors, as well as apixaban agents, excluded pregnant women from taking part in them, taking into account that potential foetal or maternal complications are not known, so the use of this kind of anticoagulants should be avoided [55].

Table 2. Management at the time of labour.

Administrated Agents—Should Be Interrupted 12–24 h Prior to Elective Induction of Delivery	Recommendations If Unplanned Delivery Happens, Neuroaxial Anaesthesia Should Not Be Performed
UFH	➢ checking activated partial thromboplastin time and considering administrating protamine sulphate in case it is prolonged to reduce the risk of bleeding.
LMWH information taken from [49]	➢ checking out anti Xa levels and testing D-Dimers; ➢ in case of bleeding, protamine sulfate may offer limited neutralization; ➢ major bleeding—recombinant activated factor VII concentrate in case there is lack of response to classic therapy;

4.3.2. Thrombolytics during Pregnancy

Antiplatelets drugs cross the placenta, and a few studies performed on animals showed that thrombolytics may boost the risk of congenital abnormalities, but the information obtained from studies performed on human subjects is contradictory [55,57]. However, aspirin (acetylsalicylic acid) may be administrated in pregnancy for explicit indications, considering that in the course of the second and of the third trimester of pregnancy, it has not been associated with an increased risk of pregnancy loss. A meta-analysis conducted by Kozer [57–59] found no significant risks regarding congenital abnormalities that were linked with aspirin intake, among exposed infants, but it may lead to gastroschisis if taken during the first trimester—five case–control reports confirmed this risk [60]. When questioning if antiplatelets are appropriate to be prescribed in high risk pregnancies, probable risks should be considered as well [57].

4.4. Prevention

Prevention for Adverse Pregnancy-Related Complications

Women who accomplish the APS syndrome criteria, and are also known with three or more recurrent pregnancy losses, are advised to take antepartum prophylactic or intermediate dose of UFH, or prophylactic doses of LMWH associated with aspirin 75 mg up to 100 mg daily [55]. Nonetheless, the results obtained from one multicenter randomized trial, which was based on the association of LMWH with low-dose aspirin, initiated before the 12th week of pregnancy, showed a reduction in early pregnancy losses in women diagnosed with hereditary thrombophilia. Taken together, women known to have hereditary thrombophilia, treated with a combination of prophylactic doses of LMWH and aspirin, initiated before the second trimester of gestation, have had a reduced risk of miscarriage [58].

Treatment choices are questionable. A conventional antithrombotic treatment option for primary and secondary prophylaxis regarding thrombotic events during pregnancy includes anticoagulation LMWHs. Pregnancy raises the risk of VTE, so pharmacological prophylaxis is usually prescribed for women who have had a previous episode of VTE during pregnancy [59]. Heparin and its subsidiaries may strive a helpful effect by limiting gestational vascular complications [60]. Regarding thromboprophylaxis, it has been proven that LMWHs and low dose aspirin (ASA) are really effective in pregnancy, with excellent live birth rates.

4.5. Prognostic Outcomes

Predicting the risk of VTE continues to be challenging and although various efforts have been accomplished in order to establish predictive-biomarkers, only D-dimers remain the most used one [61]. Preeclampsia (PE) is one of the most frequent pregnancy complications that leads to maternal morbidity and mortality globally, and it may be triggered by genetic conditions such as thrombophilia [3,62].

5. Micro RNAs in Pregnancy

The study of micro RNAs (miRNAs) in thrombophilia seeks for a lot of debate. MicroRNAs are small, single-stranded endogenous RNAs that regulate the expression of different target genes post-transcriptionally [63]. The first miRNA, lin-4, was discovered in 1993 as a 22-nucleotide non-coding RNA that controlled the timing of post embryonic development in Caenorhabditis elegans by repressing lin-14 protein expression, and let-7, the second miRNA discovered, was analysed in nematodes. Nowadays, there are known more than one thousand human miRNAs, each likely regulating hundreds of target genes, and they act as valuable gene regulators to regulate different physiological events, including placental development [63].

During pregnancy, the placenta is a transient organ, acting as the junction between maternal and foetal setting. Expanding evidence indicates that miRNAs are important regulators of placental growth [64].

Research on prognosis is significant. More women are now living with hereditary thrombophilia, and nowadays prognosis research seeks to understand and enhance future outcomes, and it provides critical evidence to translate findings from laboratory to human, and from clinical research to clinical practice [65].

In a study conducted in 2020 [66], there were families who had experiences with an idiopathic thrombosis episode—except those with antithrombin deficiency or who have a mutation in factor V Leiden, that volunteered to participate. Patients ceased treatment with oral anticoagulants and antiplatelet medications (slightly 15 days before extraction) as well as heparin medication prior to collection of blood samples (partly 24 h before). This study that analyses the connection between miRNA production and VTE revealed 16 miRNAs of interest that were identified. Therefore, genetic and epigenetic studies are needed to find biomarkers of thrombosis and to identify their clinical applications in the discovery phase, and the internal validation phase showed four of those to be differentially expressed in patients with VTE: hsa-miR-126-3p, hsa-miR-885-5p, hsa-miR-194-5p, and hsamiR-192-5p [66].

Not only did the four validated miRNAs display a big association with VTE, but they are also possible predictors of this pathology, therefore, four differentially expressed plasma miRNAs are described in VTE [66].

It has been estimated that the rate of spontaneous pregnancy loss is 30%; the human placenta has been shown to contain a significant number of miRNAs that are implicated in its growth [67]; as in more, during the peri-implantation cycle, miRNAs control uterine gene expression associated with inflammatory responses and participate in maternal–foetal immune tolerance [67]. The correlation of aberrant miRNA expression with different human diseases linked to reproductive conditions has been seen in various studies [62].

It is important to establish whether genetic polymorphisms display a correlation with idiopathic recurring pregnancy loss in miRNA machinery genes.

High quality research is important in order to define pathways by which polymorphisms of miRNA machinery genes influence the production of RPL, considering these wide potential uses of prognostic factors [67].

The majority of studies on birth cohorts utilizing miRNAs as biomarkers in pregnancy have focused on determining the link between environmental contaminants and alterations in the miRNA-ome in placental samples [68].

6. Conclusions

The main objective of the study was to quantitatively assess the literature data associated with the management of pregnant women with thrombophilia. An essential element would be the rectification of the notion of thrombophilia and an appropriate preventive activity instituted before pregnancy. Since in most cases the pregnant woman is exposed to coagulation disorders occurring during pregnancy, an equally important element is to adapt the general management of the pregnant woman to the particularities generated by thrombophilia. Thus, the following directions of approach to the management of pregnant women with thrombophilia are outlined:

- In screening, the degree of genetic damage that manifests as thrombotic risk is assessed. Depending on this, treatment with anticoagulant and antiaggregant drugs is tailor-made for each patient.
- Following the high degree of risk amplified by the evolution of pregnancy, the frequency of patient monitoring will be increased to avoid any thrombotic event that could endanger pregnancy.
- Postpartum, antithrombotic prevention will be maintained, therapy being adapted to the degree of risk associated with the severity of thrombophilia.

A future direction in the management of pregnant women with thrombophilia will include mandatory microRNA profiling, which will be a useful tool in both diagnosis and monitoring and prognosis.

Author Contributions: Conceptualization, M.S. and A.A.; methodology, R.T. and T.H.; writing—original draft preparation, C.P. and O.P.; writing—review and editing, M.S. and A.A.; supervision, A.A. All authors have read and agreed to the published version of the manuscript.

Funding: This research received no external funding.

Institutional Review Board Statement: Not applicable.

Informed Consent Statement: Not applicable.

Data Availability Statement: Not applicable.

Conflicts of Interest: The authors declare no conflict of interest.

References

1. Campello, E.; Spiezia, L.; Adamo, A.; Simioni, P. Thrombophilia, risk factors and prevention. *Expert Rev. Hematol.* **2019**, *12*, 147–158. [CrossRef] [PubMed]
2. Simcox, L.E.; Ormesher, L.; Tower, C.; Greer, I.A. Thrombophilia and Pregnancy Complications. *Int. J. Mol. Sci.* **2015**, *16*, 28418–28428. [CrossRef] [PubMed]
3. Ahangari, N.; Doosti, M.; Mousavifar, N.; Attaran, M.; Shahrokhzadeh, S.; Memarpour, S.; Ghayoor Karimiani, E. Hereditary thrombophilia genetic variants in recurrent pregnancy loss. *Arch. Gynecol. Obstet.* **2019**, *300*, 777–782. [CrossRef] [PubMed]
4. Pacurar, R.; Ionita, H.; Nicola, D. *Trombofiliile Ereditare*; Editura Victor Babes: Timisoara, Romania, 2010.
5. Middeldorp, S. Inherited thrombophilia: A double-edged sword. *Hematol. Am. Soc. Hematol. Educ. Program* **2016**, *2016*, 1–9. [CrossRef]
6. Bates, S.M.; Rajasekhar, A.; Middeldorp, S.; McLintock, C.; Rodger, M.A.; James, A.H.; Vazquez, S.R.; Greer, I.A.; Riva, J.J.; Bhatt, M.; et al. American Society of Hematology 2018 guidelines for management of venous thromboembolism: Venous thromboembolism in the context of pregnancy. *Blood Adv.* **2018**, *2*, 3317–3359. [CrossRef]
7. Middeldorp, S.; Coppens, M. Evolution of thrombophilia testing. *Hema* **2013**, *7*, 375–382.
8. Friederich, P.W.; Sanson, B.J.; Simioni, P.; Zanardi, S.; Huisman, M.V.; Kindt, I.; Prandoni, P.; Büller, H.R.; Girolami, A.; Prins, M.H. Frequency of pregnancy-related venous thromboembolism in anticoagulant factor-deficient women: Implications for prophylaxis. *Ann. Intern. Med.* **1996**, *125*, 955–960. [CrossRef]
9. Fogerty, A.E.; Connors, J.M. Management of inherited thrombophilia in pregnancy. *Curr. Opin. Endocrinol. Diabetes Obes.* **2009**, *16*, 464–469. [CrossRef]
10. Hellgren, M. Hemostasis during normal pregnancy and puerperium. *Semin. Thromb. Hemost.* **2003**, *29*, 125–130. [CrossRef]
11. Dana, M.; Fibach, E. Fetal Hemoglobin in the Maternal Circulation—Contribution of Fetal Red Blood Cells. *Hemoglobin* **2018**, *42*, 138–140. [CrossRef]
12. Bhave, A.A. Coagulopathies in Pregnancy: What an Obstetrician Ought to Know! *J. Obstet. Gynaecol. India* **2019**, *69*, 479–482. [CrossRef]
13. Giannubilo, S.R.; Tranquilli, A.L. Fetal Thrombophilia. In *Thrombophilia*; IntechOpen: London, UK, 2011. [CrossRef]
14. Lockwood, C.J. Pregnancy-associated changes in the hemostatic system. *Clin. Obstet. Gynecol.* **2006**, *49*, 836–843. [CrossRef]
15. Daugherty, M.M.; Samuelson Bannow, B.T. Hemostasis and Thrombosis in Pregnancy. In *Hemostasis and Thrombosis*; DeLoughery, T., Ed.; Springer: Cham, Switzerland, 2019. [CrossRef]
16. Greer, I.A. Thrombosis in pregnancy: Maternal and fetal issues. *Lancet* **1999**, *353*, 1258–1265. [CrossRef]

17. Siennicka, A.; Kłysz, M.; Chełstowski, K.; Tabaczniuk, A.; Marcinowska, Z.; Tarnowska, P.; Kulesza, J.; Torbe, A.; Jastrzębska, M. Reference Values of D-Dimers and Fibrinogen in the Course of Physiological Pregnancy: The Potential Impact of Selected Risk Factors-A Pilot Study. *Biomed. Res. Int.* **2020**, *2020*, 3192350. [CrossRef]
18. Pinjala, R.K.; Reddy, L.R.; Nihar, R.P.; Praveen, G.V.; Sandeep, M. Thrombophilia—How far and how much to investigate? *Indian J. Surg.* **2012**, *74*, 157–162. [CrossRef]
19. Makris, M. Thrombophilia: Grading the risk. *Blood* **2009**, *113*, 5038–5039. [CrossRef]
20. Găman, A.M.; Găman, G.D. Deficiency Of Antithrombin III (AT III)—Case Report and Review of the Literature. *Curr. Health Sci. J.* **2014**, *40*, 141–143. [CrossRef]
21. Gupta, A.; Patibandla, S. *Protein C Deficiency*; StatPearls Publishing: Treasure Island, FL, USA, 2021.
22. Gupta, A.; Tun, A.M.; Gupta, K.; Tuma, F. *Protein S Deficiency*; StatPearls Publishing: Treasure Island, FL, USA, 2021.
23. Dahlbäck, B.; Hildebrand, B. Inherited resistance to activated protein C is corrected by anticoagulant cofactor activity found to be a property of factor V. *Proc. Natl. Acad. Sci. USA* **1994**, *91*, 1396–1400. [CrossRef]
24. Ridker, P.M.; Miletich, J.P.; Hennekens, C.H.; Buring, J.E. Ethnic distribution of factor V Leiden in 4047 men and women. Implications for venous thromboembolism screening. *JAMA* **1997**, *277*, 1305–1307. [CrossRef]
25. Momot, A.P.; Nikolaeva, M.G.; Yasafova, N.N.; Zainulina, M.S.; Momot, K.A.; Taranenko, I.A. Clinical and laboratory manifestations of the prothrombin gene mutation in women of reproductive age. *J. Blood Med.* **2019**, *10*, 255–263. [CrossRef]
26. Mukhopadhyay, I.; Pruthviraj, V.; Rao, P.S.; Biswas, M. Hyperhomocysteinemia in recurrent pregnancy loss and the effect of folic acid and vitamin B12 on homocysteine levels: A prospective analysis. *Int. J. Reprod. Contracept. Obstet. Gynecol.* **2017**, *6*, 2258–2261. [CrossRef]
27. Pascual, Z.N.; Langaker, M.D. *Physiology, Pregnancy*; StatPearls Publishing: Treasure Island, FL, USA, 2021.
28. Younis, J.S.; Samueloff, A. Gestational vascular complications. *Best Pract. Res. Clin. Haematol.* **2003**, *16*, 135–151. [CrossRef]
29. Szecsi, P.B.; Jørgensen, M.; Klajnbard, A.; Andersen, M.R.; Colov, N.P.; Stender, S. Haemostatic reference intervals in pregnancy. *Thromb. Haemost.* **2010**, *103*, 718–727. [CrossRef]
30. Dobbenga-Rhodes, Y. Shedding Light on Inherited Thrombophilias: The Impact on Pregnancy. *J. Perinat. Neonatal Nurs.* **2016**, *30*, 36–44. [CrossRef]
31. O'Riordan, M.N.; Higgins, J.R. Haemostasis in normal and abnormal pregnancy. *Best Pract. Res. Clin. Obstet. Gynaecol.* **2003**, *17*, 385–396. [CrossRef]
32. Aracic, N.; Roje, D.; Jakus, I.A.; Bakotin, M.; Stefanovic, V. The Impact of Inherited Thrombophilia Types and Low Molecular Weight Heparin Treatment on Pregnancy Complications in Women with Previous Adverse Outcome. *Yonsei Med. J.* **2016**, *57*, 1230–1235. [CrossRef]
33. Lockwood, C.J. Inherited thrombophilias in pregnant patients: Detection and treatment paradigm. *Obstet. Gynecol.* **2002**, *99*, 333–341. [CrossRef]
34. Dossenbach-Glaninger, A.; van Trotsenburg, M.; Oberkanins, C.; Atamaniuk, J. Risk for early pregnancy loss by factor XIII Val34Leu: The impact of fibrinogen concentration. *J. Clin. Lab. Anal.* **2013**, *27*, 444–449. [CrossRef]
35. Ashraf, N.; Visweshwar, N.; Jaglal, M.; Sokol, L.; Laber, D. Evolving paradigm in thrombophilia screening. *Blood Coagul. Fibrinolysis Int. J. Haemost. Thromb.* **2019**, *30*, 249–252. [CrossRef] [PubMed]
36. Lijfering, W.M.; Brouwer, J.L.; Veeger, N.J.; Bank, I.; Coppens, M.; Middeldorp, S.; Hamulyák, K.; Prins, M.H.; Büller, H.R.; van der Meer, J. Selective testing for thrombophilia in patients with first venous thrombosis: Results from a retrospective family cohort study on absolute thrombotic risk for currently known thrombophilic defects in 2479 relatives. *Blood* **2009**, *113*, 5314–5322. [CrossRef] [PubMed]
37. Jennings, I.; Cooper, P. Screening for thrombophilia: A laboratory perspective. *Br. J. Biomed. Sci.* **2003**, *60*, 39–51. [CrossRef] [PubMed]
38. MacCallum, P.; Bowles, L.; Keeling, D. Diagnosis and management of heritable thrombophilias. *BMJ Clin. Res. Ed.* **2014**, *349*, g4387. [CrossRef] [PubMed]
39. Bezgin, T.; Kaymaz, C.; Akbal, Ö.; Yılmaz, F.; Tokgöz, H.C.; Özdemir, N. Thrombophilic Gene Mutations in Relation to Different Manifestations of Venous Thromboembolism: A Single Tertiary Center Study. *Clin. Appl. Thromb. Hemost. Off. J. Int. Acad. Clin. Appl. Thromb. Hemost.* **2018**, *24*, 100–106. [CrossRef] [PubMed]
40. Riva, N.; Gatt, A. Update on the Diagnosis and Anticoagulant Treatment of the Antiphospholipid Syndrome. EMJ. 29 July 2019. Available online: https://www.emjreviews.com/rheumatology/article/update-on-the-diagnosis-and-anticoagulant-treatment-of-the-antiphospholipid-syndrome/ (accessed on 1 March 2022).
41. Merriman, L.; Greaves, M. Testing for thrombophilia: An evidence-based approach. *Postgrad. Med. J.* **2006**, *82*, 699–704. [CrossRef]
42. Bates, S.M.; Middeldorp, S.; Rodger, M.; James, A.H.; Greer, I. Guidance for the treatment and prevention of obstetric-associated venous thromboembolism. *J. Thromb. Thrombolysis* **2016**, *41*, 92–128. [CrossRef]
43. Wu, O.; Robertson, L.; Twaddle, S.; Lowe, G.; Clark, P.; Walker, I.; Brenkel, I.; Greaves, M.; Langhorne, P.; Regan, L.; et al. Thrombosis: Risk and Economic Assessment of Thrombophilia Screening (TREATS) Study Screening for thrombophilia in high-risk situations: A meta-analysis and cost-effectiveness analysis. *Br. J. Haematol.* **2005**, *131*, 80–90. [CrossRef]
44. Colucci, G.; Tsakiris, D.A. Thrombophilia screening revisited: An issue of personalized medicine. *J. Thromb. Thrombolysis* **2020**, *49*, 618–629. [CrossRef]
45. Walker, I.D. Thrombophilia in pregnancy. *J. Clin. Pathol.* **2000**, *53*, 573–580. [CrossRef]

46. Chan, W. Diagnosis of venous thromboembolism in pregnancy. *Thromb. Res.* **2017**, *163*, 221–228. [CrossRef]
47. Bates, S.M. Management of pregnant women with thrombophilia or a history of venous thromboembolism. *Hematol. Am. Soc. Hematol. Educ. Program* **2007**, *2007*, 143–150. [CrossRef]
48. Marino, T. Anticoagulants and Thrombolytics in Pregnancy. Medscape. 30 June 2017. Available online: https://emedicine.medscape.com/article/164069 (accessed on 10 March 2022).
49. Raju, N.; Bates, S.M. Preventing thrombophilia-related complications of pregnancy. *Expert Rev. Hematol.* **2009**, *2*, 183–196. [CrossRef]
50. Bates, S.M.; Greer, I.A.; Middeldorp, S.; Veenstra, D.L.; Prabulos, A.M.; Vandvik, P.O. VTE, thrombophilia, antithrombotic therapy, and pregnancy: Antithrombotic Therapy and Prevention of Thrombosis, 9th ed: American College of Chest Physicians Evidence-Based Clinical Practice Guidelines. *Chest* **2012**, *141* (Suppl. S2), e691S–e736S. [CrossRef]
51. Lagrange, F.; Vergnes, C.; Brun, J.L.; Paolucci, F.; Nadal, T.; Leng, J.J.; Saux, M.C.; Banwarth, B. Absence of placental transfer of pentasaccharide (Fondaparinux, Arixtra) in the dually perfused human cotyledon in vitro. *Thromb. Haemost.* **2002**, *87*, 831–835r.
52. Many, A.; Koren, G. Low-molecular-weight heparins during pregnancy. *Can. Fam. Physician Med. Fam. Can.* **2005**, *51*, 199–201.
53. Dimitrakakis, C.; Papageorgiou, P.; Papageorgiou, I.; Antzaklis, A.; Sakarelou, N.; Michalas, S. Absence of transplacental passage of the low molecular weight heparin enoxaparin. *Haemostasis* **2000**, *30*, 243–248. [CrossRef]
54. Eichinger, S. D-dimer testing in pregnancy. *Semin. Vasc. Med.* **2005**, *5*, 375–378. [CrossRef]
55. Bates, S.M. Preventing thrombophilia-related complications of pregnancy: An update. *Expert Rev. Hematol.* **2013**, *6*, 287–300. [CrossRef]
56. Schreiber, K.; Sciascia, S.; de Groot, P.G.; Devreese, K.; Jacobsen, S.; Ruiz-Irastorza, G.; Salmon, J.E.; Shoenfeld, Y.; Shovman, O.; Hunt, B.J. Antiphospholipid syndrome. *Nat. Rev. Dis. Primers* **2018**, *4*, 17103. [CrossRef]
57. Kozer, E.; Nikfar, S.; Costei, A.; Boskovic, R.; Nulman, I.; Koren, G. Aspirin consumption during the first trimester of pregnancy and congenital anomalies: A meta-analysis. *Am. J. Obstet. Gynecol.* **2002**, *187*, 1623–1630. [CrossRef]
58. De Vries, J.I.; van Pampus, M.G.; Hague, W.M.; Bezemer, P.D.; Joosten, J.H. FRUIT Investigators Low-molecular-weight heparin added to aspirin in the prevention of recurrent early-onset pre-eclampsia in women with inheritable thrombophilia: The FRUIT-RCT. *J. Thromb. Haemost. JTH* **2012**, *10*, 64–72. [CrossRef]
59. Ageno, W.; Crotti, S.; Turpie, A.G. The safety of antithrombotic therapy during pregnancy. *Expert Opin. Drug Saf.* **2004**, *3*, 113–118. [CrossRef] [PubMed]
60. Papadakis, E.; Pouliakis, A.; Aktypi, A.; Christoforidou, A.; Kotsi, P.; Anagnostou, G.; Foifa, A.; Grouzi, E. Low molecular weight heparins use in pregnancy: A practice survey from Greece and a review of the literature. *Thromb. J.* **2019**, *17*, 23. [CrossRef] [PubMed]
61. Morelli, V.M.; Brækkan, S.K.; Hansen, J.B. Role of microRNAs in Venous Thromboembolism. *Int. J. Mol. Sci.* **2020**, *21*, 2602. [CrossRef] [PubMed]
62. Mayor-Lynn, K.; Toloubeydokhti, T.; Cruz, A.C.; Chegini, N. Expression profile of microRNAs and mRNAs in human placentas from pregnancies complicated by preeclampsia and preterm labor. *Reprod. Sci.* **2011**, *18*, 46–56. [CrossRef]
63. Fu, G.; Brkić, J.; Hayder, H.; Peng, C. MicroRNAs in Human Placental Development and Pregnancy Complications. *Int. J. Mol. Sci.* **2013**, *14*, 5519–5544. [CrossRef]
64. Lee, D.C.; Romero, R.; Kim, J.S.; Tarca, A.L.; Montenegro, D.; Pineles, B.L.; Kim, E.; Lee, J.; Kim, S.Y.; Draghici, S.; et al. miR-210 targets iron-sulfur cluster scaffold homologue in human trophoblast cell lines: Siderosis of interstitial trophoblasts as a novel pathology of preterm preeclampsia and small-for-gestational-age pregnancies. *Am. J. Pathol.* **2011**, *179*, 590–602. [CrossRef]
65. Riley, R.D.; Hayden, J.A.; Steyerberg, E.W.; Moons, K.G.; Abrams, K.; Kyzas, P.A.; Malats, N.; Briggs, A.; Schroter, S.; Altman, D.G.; et al. PROGRESS Group Prognosis Research Strategy (PROGRESS) 2: Prognostic factor research. *PLoS Med.* **2013**, *10*, e1001380. [CrossRef]
66. Rodriguez-Rius, A.; Lopez, S.; Martinez-Perez, A.; Souto, J.C.; Soria, J.M. Identification of a Plasma MicroRNA Profile Associated With Venous Thrombosis. *Arterioscler. Thromb. Vasc. Biol.* **2020**, *40*, 1392–1399. [CrossRef]
67. Lee, Y.; Ahn, E.H.; Ryu, C.S.; Kim, J.O.; An, H.J.; Cho, S.H.; Kim, J.H.; Kim, Y.R.; Lee, W.S.; Kim, N.K. Association between microRNA machinery gene polymorphisms and recurrent implantation failure. *Exp. Ther. Med.* **2020**, *19*, 3113–3123. [CrossRef]
68. Barchitta, M.; Maugeri, A.; Quattrocchi, A.; Agrifoglio, O.; Agodi, A. The Role of miRNAs as Biomarkers for Pregnancy Outcomes: A Comprehensive Review. *Int. J. Genom.* **2017**, *2017*, 8067972. [CrossRef]

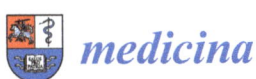

Article

Pregnancy Outcomes in a Cohort of Patients Who Underwent Double-J Ureteric Stenting—A Single Center Experience

Viorel Dragos Radu [1,2], Ingrid-Andrada Vasilache [3,*], Radu-Cristian Costache [1,2], Ioana-Sadiye Scripcariu [3], Dragos Nemescu [3], Alexandru Carauleanu [3], Valentin Nechifor [3], Veaceslav Groza [2], Pavel Onofrei [4], Lucian Boiculese [5] and Demetra Socolov [3]

1 Urology Department, 'Grigore T. Popa' University of Medicine and Pharmacy, 700115 Iasi, Romania; vioreldradu@yahoo.com (V.D.R.); criscostache@hotmail.com (R.-C.C.)
2 Urology Department, 'C.I. Parhon' University Hospital, 700115 Iasi, Romania; grozaveaceslav@yahoo.com
3 Department of Obstetrics and Gynecology, 'Grigore T. Popa' University of Medicine and Pharmacy, 700115 Iasi, Romania; isscripcariu@gmail.com (I.-S.S.); dnemescu@yahoo.com (D.N.); acarauleanu@yahoo.com (A.C.); valentinnechifor60@gmail.com (V.N.); demetrasocolov@gmail.com (D.S.)
4 Morphofunctional Sciences II Department, 'Grigore T. Popa' University of Medicine and Pharmacy, 700115 Iasi, Romania; onofrei.pavel@gmail.com
5 Medical Informatics and Biostatistics Department, 'Grigore T. Popa' University of Medicine and Pharmacy, 700115 Iasi, Romania; lboiculese@gmail.com
* Correspondence: tanasaingrid@yahoo.com

Abstract: *Background and Objectives*: Minimally invasive procedures, such as double-J ureteric stenting, could be a promising therapeutic alternative to conservative management of obstructive urinary tract pathology. We aimed to evaluate the safety and effectiveness of double-J ureteric stenting in pregnant women with ureterohydronephrosis or urolithiasis, along with their infectious complications, and to assess the pregnancy outcomes of this cohort of patients in comparison with a control group. *Materials and Methods*: This observational retrospective study included 52 pregnant patients who underwent double-J ureteric stenting for urologic disorders in the Urology Department of 'C.I. Parhon' University Hospital, and who were followed up at a tertiary maternity hospital- 'Cuza-Voda', Iasi, Romania. The control group (63 patients) was randomly selected from the patient's cohort who gave birth in the same time frame at the maternity hospital, without urinary pathology. Clinical, sonographic, and laboratory variables were examined. Descriptive statistics, non-parametric tests, and a one-to-one propensity score-matched analysis were used to analyze our data. *Results*: The univariate analysis indicated a significant statistical difference between the control group and the interventional group regarding maternal age ($p = 0.018$), previous maternal history of renal colic ($p = 0.005$) or nephrolithiasis ($p = 0.002$). After applying the propensity score-matched analysis, cesarean delivery rates ($p < 0.001$), preterm labour ($p = 0.039$), premature rupture of membranes ($p = 0.026$), preterm birth rates ($p = 0.002$), and post-partum UTI rates ($p = 0.012$) were significantly different between the control group and the matched treatment group. Ureterohydronephrosis, whether simple ($n = 37; 71.2\%$) or infected ($n = 13; 25\%$), was the main indication for double-J ureteric stenting. Complications such as pain ($n = 21; 40.3\%$), stent migration ($n = 3; 5.76\%$) or encrustation ($n = 2; 3.84\%$), as well as reflux pyelonephritis ($n = 2; 3.84\%$) and gross hematuria ($n = 1; 1.92\%$) were recorded during follow-up. *Conclusions*: Our results show that double-J stenting is a safe and effective treatment option for pregnant patients with obstructive urological disorders.

Keywords: double-J stent; ureterohydronephrosis; urolithiasis; pyelonephritis; urosepsis; pregnancy

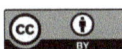

1. Introduction

Ureterohydronephrosis (UHN) is a common maternal adaptation to pregnancy, affecting more than 40% of pregnancies, and is more prevalent in the third trimester [1]. The anatomical changes of the pyelocaliceal system are predominantly encountered in the right side, due to the anatomical relationship of the ureter with iliac and ovarian vessels [2]. Ureterohydronephrosis, along with hormonal and immune changes, predispose pregnant women to infectious complications that range between simple urinary tract infections to urosepsis [3].

Urolithiasis (UL) development during pregnancy is supported by systemic, nephrological and mechanical changes [4], and is associated with important adverse pregnancy outcomes such as preterm birth, preeclampsia or gestational hypertension [5]. If left untreated, obstructive uropathy can lead to urosepsis and renal failure, which could ultimately result in preterm birth, abruptio placentae, stillbirth, or maternal mortality [6–8].

Prenatal management of urinary tract pathology is based on correct diagnosis and individualized treatment. Ultrasonography (USG), magnetic resonance imaging (MRI), complete blood count (CBC), inflammatory markers (C-reactive protein—CRP), renal function tests, urinary analysis, and urine culture are useful diagnostic tools for detection of urinary tract disorders during pregnancy [5,9,10].

Individualized treatment of urinary pathology during pregnancy consists of a conservative (hydration, analgesia, and/or antibiotic treatment) and a surgical approach. The surgical approach is mainly represented by ureteric stent insertion, percutaneous nephrostomy (PCN) and ureteroscopic extraction of the calculus [11–13].

Ureteric stenting is a minimally invasive procedure with a good safety profile during pregnancy that can be used for drainage of the obstructed and/or infected urinary system in patients with symptoms refractory to conservative approaches and/or changes in renal function, pain visual analogue score, obstruction or hydronephrosis grading [14]. The procedure can be easily performed in the lithotomy position, without general anaesthesia [15].

The aim of this study was to evaluate the safety and effectiveness of double-J ureteric stenting in pregnant women with ureterohydronephrosis and renal obstruction due to calculi or physiological obstruction, along with their infectious complications, and to assess the pregnancy outcomes of this cohort of patients in comparison with a control group.

2. Materials and Methods

We conducted an observational retrospective study of all pregnant patients who underwent double-J ureteric stenting for urologic disorders (ureterohydronephrosis, urolithiasis, and their infectious complications) in the Urology Department of 'C.I. Parhon' University Hospital, Iasi, Romania, between January 2014 and December 2020. All patients were followed up at a tertiary maternity hospital- 'Cuza-Voda', Iasi, Romania. The control group was randomly selected from the patient's cohort who gave birth in the same time frame at the maternity hospital, without urinary tract pathology.

Ethical approval for this study was obtained from the Institutional Ethics Committees of 'Cuza-Voda' Maternity Hospital (No. 2871/05.03.2022) and 'C.I. Parhon' University Hospital (No. 1808/04.03.2022). Informed consent was obtained from all participants included in the study. All methods were carried out in accordance with relevant guidelines and regulations.

Medical records of patients were systematically reviewed and data obtained. Exclusion criteria comprised patients who had multiple pregnancies, ectopic pregnancies, first and second trimester abortions, fetal intrauterine demise, fetuses with chromosomal or structural abnormalities, intrauterine infection, incomplete medical records, incorrect/lack of first trimester sonographic pregnancy dating or who were unable to offer informed consent due to various reasons (age less than 18 years old, intellectual deficits, psychiatric disorders, etc.).

A total of 284 pregnant women with urological disorders were admitted at 'C.I. Parhon' University Hospital during our study period. Pregnant patients who underwent double-J ureteric stenting were evaluated, and 52 patients were included in our study. The following variables were recorded: demographic data, the patient's medical history, renal clinical manifestations (febrile syndrome and renal colic) laboratory parameters (CBC, CRP, urinalysis and urine culture), indications for double-J ureteric stenting, duration of the procedure and hospitalization, associated medical treatment, type of complications, and pregnancy outcomes (type of birth, newborn's gender, Apgar score, preterm labour, premature rupture of membranes, preterm birth, fetal growth restriction, preeclampsia, neonatal intensive care unit (NICU) admission, fetal death, and post-partum UTI). The Apgar score, developed by Dr. Virginia Apgar, was used to assess the status of infants after delivery [16]. It comprises 5 components: (1) color; (2) heart rate; (3) reflexes; (4) muscle tone; and (5) respiration [17]. Each of these components is given a score of 0, 1, or 2. An Apgar score less than 7 indicated the need for special neonatal care, while a score between 7 and 10 was considered reassuring.

All pregnancies were dated by an experienced obstetrician with an early ultrasound scan using an E8/E10 (General Electric Healthcare, Zipf, Austria) scanner with a 4.8 MHz transabdominal probe (GE Medical Systems, Milwaukee, WI) between 10 + 0 to 13 + 6 weeks to determine gestational age by measuring the crown-rump length (CRL) [18].

Ultrasound evaluation was also performed by experienced urologists for diagnostic purposes using Siemens ACUSON ×300 or ACUSON REDWOOD (Siemens Healthcare, Erlangen, Germany, gmbH) scanners, with a 3.5 MHz transabdominal probe. At ultrasound evaluation, we could only assess calculi in the pyelocaliceal system, lumbar and pelvic ureter. The patients presenting with UHN without an ultrasound objectification of a calculi were considered as no-lithiasis patients.

UHN grading, adapted after the Society for Fetal Urology (SFU) system, was considered as follows: (a) grade I: minimal changes in urinary stasis; (b) grade II: slight dilation of the renal pelvis involving major calyces; (c) grade III: moderate dilation of the renal pelvis involving major and minor calyces; (d) stage IV: severe dilation with compression on the renal parenchyma [19,20].

In the presence or absence of cystitis symptoms, flank pain, nausea/vomiting, temperature (>38 °C), and/or costovertebral angle tenderness were used as diagnostic criteria for acute pyelonephritis [21] More than 10^5 colony-forming units (CFU)/mL was considered a positive urine culture.

Urosepsis was diagnosed in patients meeting two or more of the following criteria according to the quick sepsis-related organ failure assessment (qSOFA): (1) respiratory rate of ≥ 22 breaths/min; (2) altered consciousness (Glasgow Coma Scale score of <13); (3) systolic blood pressure of ≤ 100 mmHg [22].

The ureter was stented under local anaesthesia, using pregnancy-approved antibiotic prophylaxis. The procedure was conducted using an Olympus rigid cystoscope, 21CH. A 6, 7 or 8CH, 26, 28 cm length, JJ ureteric stent (MEDpro Medical B.V., Fernendal, The Netherlands) was inserted retrogradely over a guidewire. The ureteric stent's location was confirmed by observing the stent markings and distal coiling, as well as intraoperative sonographic stent placement inside the pyelocaliceal system. During the procedure, no fluoroscopy was employed.

When the symptomatology subsided or the urosepsis cleared, the patients were discharged. All recommended antibiotic regimens followed the European Association of Urology guidelines [23].

Statistical analysis was performed using SPSS software (version 28.0.1, IBM Corp, Armonk, NY, USA). Each variable was evaluated with chi-squared and Fisher's exact tests for categorical variables, and T-tests for continuous variables. One-to-one propensity score-matched analysis was performed using Stata SE (version 15, StataCorp LLC), considering demographic characteristics as treatment independent variables, and comparing pregnancy outcomes (type of birth, preterm labour, premature rupture of membranes, preterm birth, neonatal intensive care unit admission rates, and post-partum UTI rates) between the control group (without double-J stent) and treatment group (with double-J stent). A p value less than 0.05 was considered statistically significant.

3. Results

A total of 52 pregnant patients who underwent double-J ureteric stenting were included in our study. A group of 63 patients, who gave birth at 'Cuza Voda' Hospital, without urological illnesses and interventions during pregnancy served as our control group. The demographic characteristics, comorbidities, and pregnancy outcomes of cases and controls are presented in Table 1.

Table 1. Demographic characteristics, comorbidities, and pregnancy outcomes of the evaluated groups.

Variable		Without Double-J Stent (63 Patients)	With Double-J Stent (52 Patients)	p Value
Demographic characteristics	Age	28.7 ± 5.75	26.12 ± 5.74	0.018
	Number of gestations	2.25 ± 1.45	2.40 ± 2.13	0.65
	Parity	1.87 ± 1.28	2.02 ± 1.87	0.62
Comorbidities	Previous cesarean section	No 53 (46.1%) Yes 10 (8.7%)	No 44 (38.3%) Yes 8 (7%)	0.94
	Placenta praevia	No 58 (50.4%) Yes 5 (4.3%)	No 48 (41.7%) Yes 4 (3.5%)	0.96
	Gestational hypertension	No 57 (49.6%) Yes 6 (5.2%)	No 50 (43.5%) Yes 2 (1.7%)	0.23
	Preeclampsia	No 62 (53.9%) Yes 1 (0.8%)	No 49 (42.6%) Yes 3 (2.6%)	0.22
	Previous renal colic	No 61 (53%) Yes 2 (1.7%)	No 42 (36.5%) Yes 10 (8.6%)	0.005
	Previous nephrolithiasis	No 62 (53.9%) Yes 1 (0.8%)	No 43 (37.3%) Yes 9 (7.8%)	0.002
	In vitro fertilization	No 62 (53.9%) Yes 1 (0.9%)	No 51 (44.3%) Yes 1 (0.9%)	0.89
Pregnancy outcomes	Type of birth	Cesarean 28 (24.3%) Vaginal 35 (30.4%)	Cesarean 40 (34.8%) Vaginal 12 (10.4%)	<0.001
	Newborn's gender	Female 31 (27%) Male 32 (27.8%)	Female 26 (22.6%) Male 26 (22.6%)	0.93
	Apgar score	8.73 ± 1.24	8.02 ± 1.56	0.007
	Preterm labour	No 54 (46.9%) Yes 9 (7.8%)	No 36 (31.3%) Yes 16 (13.9%)	0.03
	Premature rupture of membranes	No 62 (53%) Yes 1 (1.7%)	No 44 (33%) Yes 8 (12.1%)	0.006
	Preterm birth	No 61 (53%) Yes 2 (1.7%)	No 38 (33%) Yes 14 (12.1%)	0.002
	Fetal growth restriction	No 61 (53%) Yes 2 (1.7%)	No 47 (40.8%) Yes 5 (4.3%)	0.15
	Preeclampsia	No 62 (53.9%) Yes 1 (0.9%)	No 51 (44.3%) Yes 1 (0.9%)	0.89
	NICU admission	No 59 (51.3%) Yes 4 (3.4%)	No 42 (36.5%) Yes 10 (8.6%)	0.03
	Fetal death	0 (0%)		
	Post-partum UTI	No 61 (53%) Yes 2 (1.7%)	No 40 (34.8%) Yes 12 (10.4%)	<0.001

Our data indicated a significant statistical difference between the control group and the interventional group regarding maternal age ($p = 0.018$), previous maternal history of renal colic ($p = 0.005$) or nephrolithiasis ($p = 0.002$), type of birth ($p < 0.001$), newborn's Apgar score at 5 min ($p = 0.007$), preterm labour rates ($p = 0.03$), premature rupture of membranes ($p = 0.006$), preterm birth ($p = 0.002$), neonatal intensive care unit (NICU) admission rates ($p = 0.03$), and post-partum UTI rates ($p < 0.001$).

After applying the one-to-one propensity score-matched analysis, only cesarean delivery rates ($p < 0.001$), preterm labour ($p = 0.039$), premature rupture of membranes ($p = 0.026$), preterm birth rates ($p = 0.002$), and post-partum UTI rates ($p = 0.012$) were significantly different between the control group and the matched treatment group (Table 2).

Table 2. Results from the propensity score match analysis.

Outcome	Robust Standard Error (RSE)	Coefficient	95% Confidence Interval		p Value
			Lower Limit	Upper Limit	
Type of birth (cesarean)	0.089	0.362	0.186	0.538	<0.001
Preterm labour	0.091	0.160	−0.018	0.340	0.039
Premature rupture of membranes	0.055	0.105	−0.002	0.214	0.026
Preterm birth	0.075	0.236	0.087	0.384	0.002
Fetal growth restriction	0.050	0.056	−0.041	0.15	0.26
Preeclampsia	0.018	−0.008	−0.044	0.027	0.63
NICU admission	0.064	0.086	−0.039	0.213	0.17
Post-partum UTI	0.066	0.166	0.036	0.296	0.012

The most frequent pathogens responsible for post-partum UTI were *Escherichia coli* (interventional vs. control groups, 3:1 cases), *Klebsiella* spp. (interventional vs. control groups, 3:1 cases), *Enterococcus* spp. (interventional vs. control groups, 3:0 cases), followed by *Enterobacter* spp. (interventional vs. control groups, 1:0 cases) and *Staphylococcus* spp. (interventional vs. control groups, 1:0 cases). These UTI were treated with Amoxicillin-clavulanic acid 1 g b.i.d or Cefuroxime 1.5 g b.i.d in the post-partum period for 10–14 days.

A total of 52 pregnant patients underwent double-J ureteric stenting in the Urology Department. The mean gestational age at the moment of the procedure was 23.21 ± 7.11 weeks (Table 3). The majority of the procedures were performed in the second trimester (n = 29, 55.8%), and only five procedures were performed in the first trimester of pregnancy.

The mean values and standard deviations (SDs) of pre-procedural leukocytosis and serum CRP were 15,345.23 ± 2340.4/mm^3 and 123.32 ± 46 mg/L, respectively. We observed a significant reduction in the post-procedural leukocytosis (8650.8 ± 1890.3/mm^3), but we did not evaluate the post-procedural CRP levels due to a slower resolution of the inflammatory syndrome.

The main pathogens that determined urinary tract infection were *Escherichia coli* (n = 19; 36.5%), *Klebsiella* spp. (n = 5; 9.61%), *Enterococcus* spp. (n = 4; 7.6%), followed by *Serratia* spp. (n = 2; 3.8%) and *Staphylococcus* spp. (n = 1; 1.92%). Only 4 cases (7.6%) had UTIs resulting from multidrug resistant *Escherichia coli*, and all of them developed a septic condition.

Antibioprophilaxis, consisting of Ceftriaxone 2 g b.i.d, was administered before procedure, and was continued for 14 days, if the urinary infection was confirmed by a positive culture of urine. Pyelonephritis in pregnancy was treated with either intravenous Amoxicillin Amoxicillin 1 g q.d.s plus Gentamicin 5 mg/kg/day for 14 days or Ceftriaxone 2 g b.i.d. Urosepsis cases were evaluated in the intensive care unit, and received Ceftriaxone 2 g b.i.d, Piperacillin/tazobactam 4.5 g t.i.d or Meropenem 1 g t.i.d (for multiresistant bacteria), along with supportive treatment.

Ureterohydronephrosis, whether simple (n = 37; 71.2%) or infected (n = 13; 25%), was the main indication for double-J ureteric stenting in our cohort of patients. The right side was the most affected, and bilateral occurrence of the simple UHN was encountered in three cases (5.8%), while bilateral infected UHN manifested in two cases. (3.8%)

The mean duration of the procedure was 28.32 ± 13.4 min. Double-J ureteric stent insertion was performed in 46 cases (88.4%), while in six cases (11.6%) double-J stents were replaced because they were in place for at least 6 weeks. We used only local anesthesia for performing these procedures. The mean duration of the hospitalization in the Urology Department was 5.19 ± 1.98 days.

Table 3. Summary of double-J ureteric stenting.

Variable	Mean (±SD) or n (%)
Timing of the procedure (weeks of gestation/trimester of pregnancy)	Mean (SD) 23.21 ± 7.11 First trimester 5 (9.6%) Second trimester 29 (55.8%) Third trimester 18 (34.6%)
Leukocytosis	Pre-procedure 15,345.23 ± 2340.4/mm^3 Post-procedure 8650.8 ± 1890.3/mm^3
CRP	Pre-procedure 123.32 ± 46 mg/l
Urinalysis and urine culture	Leukocyturia 31 (59.6%) *Escherichia coli* 19 (36.5%) *Klebsiella* spp. 5 (9.61%) *Enterococcus* spp. 4 (7.6%) *Serratia* spp. 2 (3.8%) *Staphylococcus* spp. 1 (1.92%)
Indications for double-J stenting	Simple UHN 37 (71.2%) Simple UHN location: • Left 11 (21.2%) • Right 23 (44.2%) • Bilateral 3 (5.8%) Infected UHN 13 (25%) Infected UHN location: • Left 1 (1.9%) • Right 10 (19.2%) • Bilateral 2 (3.8%) UHN grade 1.67 ± 0.51 Urolithiasis 14 (26.9%) Urolithiasis location: • Left 5 (9.6%) • Right 8 (15.4%) • Bilateral 1 (1.9%) Urosepsis 15 (28.8%) Pyelonephritis 3 (5.7%) Pyelonephritis location: • Left 1 (1.9%) • Right 2 (3.8%)
Types of interventions	Double-J ureteric stent insertion n = 46 (88.4%) Double-J ureteric stent replacement n = 6 (11.6%)
Associated procedures	Retrograde ureteroscopy with lithotripsy 1 (1.92%) Endoscopic lithotripsy 1 (1.92%)
Complications	Pain/ urinary discomfort 21 (40.3%) Stent migration 3 (5.76%) Stent encrustation 2 (3.84%) Reflux pyelonephritis 2 (3.84%) Gross hematuria 1 (1.92%)
Duration of hospitalization	5.19 ± 1.98 days
Duration of the procedure	28.32 ± 13.4 min

In two cases, additional procedures were required. In one case, retrograde ureteroscopy with lithotripsy (n = 1; 1.92%) was performed for a pelvic ureteral calculus, followed by double-J stent insertion. Because a wire could not be passed through the cystoscope and the obstructive calculus was smaller than 10 mm in diameter, we performed retrograde ureteroscopy with lithotripsy. In another case, due to significant calcification of the distal end of the double-stent, endoscopic lithotripsy ($n = 1$; 1.92%) was performed in order to retrieve the stent for replacement. Intravenous general anesthesia without oro-tracheal intubation was performed in these two cases.

A total of 21 patients (40.3%) reported pain or urinary discomfort after the procedure, and we administered intravenous Acetaminophen 1 g b.i.d, Metamizole 1 g b.i.d or Drotaverine hydrochloride 40 mg b.i.d. Stent migration ($n = 3$; 5.76%) or encrustation ($n = 2$; 3.84%), as well as reflux pyelonephritis ($n = 2$; 3.84%) and gross hematuria ($n = 1$; 1.92%) were other complications recorded during follow-up. No maternal or fetal death was recorded following the procedure.

4. Discussion

In this retrospective study, we assessed the safety and effectiveness of double-J ureteric stenting in pregnant women with ureterohydronephrosis, renal obstruction due to calculi or physiological ureteral obstruction, and their infectious complications, as well as the pregnancy outcomes of this cohort of patients in comparison with a control group.

Our results showed that the double-J stenting is a safe and effective treatment option for pregnant patients. Most of the procedures were performed during the second trimester. It was reported that double-J ureteric stenting can be difficult in the third trimester due to the tortuosity of the ureter [24]. However, we did not confirm this aspect because all our patients had successful stenting, regardless of the trimester of pregnancy.

The main indication for these procedures was UHN, simple (71.2%) or complicated with infection (25%). Right ureterohydronephrosis was the most frequently encountered in our cohort of patients. This aspect can be explained by the dextrorotation of the uterus during pregnancy with subsequent vascular compression, and by the anatomical relationship of the ureter with iliac and ovarian vessels [25,26]. All patients had complete resolution of the hydronephrosis on follow-up renal ultrasound and regression of hydronephrosis and urinary symptoms after ureteral stenting.

Escherichia coli, *Klebsiella* spp., and *Enterococcus* spp. were the main determinants of infectious complications in our cohort of patients. This bacterial spectrum corresponds to the pathogenic microorganisms associated with UTI in pregnancy [27–29]. All patients underwent antibioprophilaxis with a third-generation cephalosporin, Ceftriaxone, which was continued for 14 days if an UTI was confirmed by urine culture.

Complicated UTIs such as pyelonephritis were treated with either a combination of intravenous Amoxicillin plus Gentamicin or Ceftriaxone for two weeks. The use of an aminoglycoside was considered after weighting the risks and benefits of this drug during pregnancy, and all patients agreed with its administration after a proper counseling. Current literature data, although limited, does not support an association between Gentamicin use and increased risk of birth defects or audiologic deficits [30–32].

In the case of urosepsis, supplementary antibiotic options included Piperacillin/tazobactam and Meropenem along with supportive treatment, as recommended by current guidelines [23,33]. Meropenem was reserved for the treatment of severe infections caused by extended-spectrum β-lactamases (ESBL) positive *Escherichia coli*.

The mean duration of the procedure was 28.32 ± 13.4 min. Unilateral placement of the double-J ureteric stent was performed in the majority of cases ($n = 46$; 88.4%), and in 12 cases (23%) double-J stents were replaced because they were in place for at least 6 weeks. The mean duration of the hospitalization was 5.19 ± 1.98 days. We must emphasize that all procedures of double-J insertion were made in an emergency regime due to the known fact that lumbar pain secondary to physiologic ureteral obstruction, symptomatic lithiasis, and ascending urinary infections carry a higher risk for poor maternal and fetal outcomes [34–36]. We preferred to rapidly solve the urinary stasis and avoid the prolonged conservative approach reported in other studies [37–39]. Furthermore, we postponed ureteroscopy or percutaneous nephrolithotomy until after birth.

In two cases, additional procedures were required. Retrograde ureteroscopy with lithotripsy was performed for a pelvic ureteral calculus, followed by double-J stent insertion.

Due to significant calcification of the distal end of the double-J stent, endoscopic lithotripsy was performed for another case in order to retrieve the stent for replacement. In our study, we replaced 12 double-J stents that were placed for more than 6 weeks. It has been reported that if a double-J stent is indwelled for 6 weeks, 6–12 weeks, or greater than 12 weeks, the rates of stent encrustation are 9.2 percent, 47.5 percent, and 76.3 percent, respectively [40]. The general opinion is that within 6 weeks to 6 months, the stent should be replaced or removed [40–42]. After birth, the stents were removed, and we performed a urography to identify calculi.

In our cohort of patients, the complication rates were low, and no fetal or maternal morbidity was recorded. Similar rates of stent migration, stent encrustation, reflux pyelonephritis, and hematuria were reported in other series of pregnant patients [15,43].

As for pregnancy outcomes, it appeared that the cesarean rate was significantly higher in the interventional group compared to the control group (34.8% vs. 24.3%), and the Apgar score at birth appeared to be significantly lower in the interventional group (8.02 ± 1.56 vs. 8.73 ± 1.24).

Preterm labour, as well as premature rupture of membrane rates, were significantly higher in the interventional group. Tocolysis included calcium channel blockers (Nifedipine), magnesium sulphate (also used for neuroprotection) or betamimetics (Hexoprenaline). The results from the univariate analysis showed that preterm birth rates, as well as NICU admission rates, were significantly higher in the interventional group. However, the propensity score match analysis did not support the higher NICU admission rates in the control group. No neonatal death was recorded. Similar findings were outlined in pregnant patients with a urologic pathology [44,45].

Postpartum UTIs were more frequently encountered in the interventional group, and the bacterial spectrum responsible for postpartum UTIs was similar to that described in the pre-procedural urine culture, with *Escherichia coli*, *Klebsiella* spp., and *Enterococcus* spp. being the most prevalent. The higher risk of postpartum urinary infection can be explained by the presence of double-J stents, which increase this risk, and by low patient compliance, persistent infections, or reinfections.

The main limitation of our study was that we could not include the majority of pregnant patients operated on at 'Parhon Hospital' during the selected period due to the lack of data about obstetrical outcomes. Other limitations included the retrospective and unicentric study design. A greater cohort of patients recruited from multiple centers would allow a more comprehensive picture of the issue.

5. Conclusions

In this study, we provided consistent data that support our approach of urologic emergencies during pregnancy. Double-J stenting is a safe and effective procedure that can be easily performed throughout pregnancy using only local anesthesia.

Further research is needed to evaluate larger cohorts of patients with various poor obstetrical outcomes possibly associated with the double-J ureteric stenting procedure.

Author Contributions: Conceptualization, V.D.R. and I.-A.V.; methodology, D.S., R.-C.C., V.G., V.N. and I.-A.V.; formal analysis, V.D.R., L.B., D.N., A.C. and I.-S.S.; investigation, P.O.; data curation, V.N. and V.G.; writing, original draft preparation, V.D.R., I.-A.V. and D.S.; writing, review and editing, V.D.R. and I.-A.V.; supervision, D.S. All authors have read and agreed to the published version of the manuscript.

Funding: This research received no external funding.

Institutional Review Board Statement: The study was conducted in accordance with the Declaration of Helsinki, and approved by the Institutional Ethics Committee of Ethical approval for this study was obtained from the Institutional Ethics Committees of 'Cuza-Voda' Maternity Hospital (No. 2871/05.03.2022) and 'C.I. Parhon' University Hospital (No. 1808/04.03.2022).

Informed Consent Statement: Informed consent was obtained from all subjects involved in the study.

Data Availability Statement: The data presented in this study are available on request from the corresponding author. The data are not publicly available due to local policies.

Conflicts of Interest: The authors declare no conflict of interest.

References

1. Faúndes, A.; Brícola-Filho, M.; Pinto e Silva, J.L. Dilatation of the urinary tract during pregnancy: Proposal of a curve of maximal caliceal diameter by gestational age. *Am. J. Obstet. Gynecol.* **1998**, *178*, 1082–1086. [CrossRef]
2. Schulman, A.; Herlinger, H. Urinary tract dilatation in pregnancy. *Br. J. Radiol.* **1975**, *48*, 638–645. [CrossRef] [PubMed]
3. Connolly, A.; Thorp, J.M. Urinary Tract Infections in Pregnancy. *Urol. Clin. N. Am.* **1999**, *26*, 779–787. [CrossRef]
4. Semins, M.J.; Matlaga, B.R. Kidney stones during pregnancy. *Nat. Rev. Urol.* **2014**, *11*, 163–168. [CrossRef] [PubMed]
5. Zhou, Q.; Chen, W.Q.; Xie, X.S.; Xiang, S.L.; Yang, H.; Chen, J.H. Maternal and neonatal outcomes of pregnancy complicated by urolithiasis: A systematic review and meta-analysis. *J. Nephrol.* **2021**, *34*, 1569–1580. [CrossRef] [PubMed]
6. D'Elia, F.L.; Brennan, R.E.; Brownstein, P.K. Acute renal failure secondary to ureteral obstruction by a gravid uterus. *J. Urol.* **1982**, *128*, 803–804. [CrossRef]
7. vanSonnenberg, E.; Casola, G.; Talner, L.B.; Wittich, G.R.; Varney, R.R.; D'Agostino, H.B. Symptomatic renal obstruction or urosepsis during pregnancy: Treatment by sonographically guided percutaneous nephrostomy. *AJR Am. J. Roentgenol.* **1992**, *158*, 91–94. [CrossRef]
8. Liu, Y.; Ma, X.; Zheng, J.; Liu, X.; Yan, T. Pregnancy outcomes in patients with acute kidney injury during pregnancy: A systematic review and meta-analysis. *BMC Pregnancy Childbirth* **2017**, *17*, 235. [CrossRef]
9. Krajewski, W.; Wojciechowska, J.; Dembowski, J.; Zdrojowy, R.; Szydełko, T. Hydronephrosis in the course of ureteropelvic junction obstruction: An underestimated problem? Current opinions on the pathogenesis, diagnosis and treatment. *Adv. Clin. Exp. Med.* **2017**, *26*, 857–864. [CrossRef]
10. Mervak, B.M.; Altun, E.; McGinty, K.A.; Hyslop, W.B.; Semelka, R.C.; Burke, L.M. MRI in pregnancy: Indications and practical considerations. *J. Magn. Reson. Imaging* **2019**, *49*, 621–631. [CrossRef]
11. Shrotri, K.N.; Morrison, I.D.; Shrotri, N.C. Urological conditions in pregnancy: A diagnostic and therapeutic challenge. *J. Obstet. Gynaecol.* **2007**, *27*, 648–654. [CrossRef] [PubMed]
12. Demir, M.; Yagmur, İ.; Pelit, E.S.; Katı, B.; Ördek, E.; Çiftçi, H. Urolithiasis and Its Treatment in Pregnant Women: 10-Year Clinical Experience from a Single Centre. *Cureus* **2021**, *13*, e13752. [CrossRef] [PubMed]
13. González-Padilla, D.A.; González-Díaz, A.; García-Rojo, E.; Abad-López, P.; Santos-Pérez de la Blanca, R.; Hernández-Arroyo, M.; Teigell-Tobar, J.; Peña-Vallejo, H.; Rodríguez-Antolín, A.; Cabrera-Meirás, F. Analgesic refractory colic pain: Is prolonged conservative management appropriate? *Am. J. Emerg. Med.* **2021**, *44*, 137–142. [CrossRef] [PubMed]
14. Cheriachan, D.; Arianayagam, M.; Rashid, P. Symptomatic urinary stone disease in pregnancy. *Aust. N. Z. J. Obstet. Gynaecol.* **2008**, *48*, 34–39. [CrossRef] [PubMed]
15. Ngai, H.Y.; Salih, H.Q.; Albeer, A.; Aghaways, I.; Buchholz, N. Double-J ureteric stenting in pregnancy: A single-centre experience from Iraq. *Arab. J. Urol.* **2013**, *11*, 148–151. [CrossRef]
16. Apgar, V. A proposal for a new method of evaluation of the newborn infant. *Curr. Res. Anesth. Analg.* **1953**, *32*, 260–267. [CrossRef]
17. Apgar, V.; Holaday, D.A.; James, L.S.; Weisbrot, I.M.; Berrien, C. Evaluation of the newborn infant; second report. *J. Am. Med. Assoc.* **1958**, *168*, 1985–1988. [CrossRef]
18. Salomon, L.J.; Alfirevic, Z.; Bilardo, C.M.; Chalouhi, G.E.; Ghi, T.; Kagan, K.O.; Lau, T.K.; Papageorghiou, A.T.; Raine-Fenning, N.J.; Stirnemann, J.; et al. ISUOG practice guidelines: Performance of first-trimester fetal ultrasound scan. *Ultrasound Obs. Gynecol.* **2013**, *41*, 102–113. [CrossRef]
19. Onen, A. Grading of Hydronephrosis: An Ongoing Challenge. *Front. Pediatr.* **2020**, *8*, 458. [CrossRef]
20. Szkodziak, P. Ultrasound screening for pyelectasis in pregnant women. Clinical necessity or "art for art's sake"? *J. Ultrason.* **2018**, *18*, 152–157. [CrossRef]
21. Colgan, R.; Williams, M.; Johnson, J.R. Diagnosis and treatment of acute pyelonephritis in women. *Am. Fam. Physician* **2011**, *84*, 519–526. [PubMed]
22. Singer, M.; Deutschman, C.S.; Seymour, C.W.; Shankar-Hari, M.; Annane, D.; Bauer, M.; Bellomo, R.; Bernard, G.R.; Chiche, J.D.; Coopersmith, C.M.; et al. The Third International Consensus Definitions for Sepsis and Septic Shock (Sepsis-3). *JAMA* **2016**, *315*, 801–810. [CrossRef] [PubMed]
23. Urology, E.A.O. *EAU Guidelines*; Edn. Presented at the EAU Annual Congress Amsterdam, The Netherlands; EAU Guidelines Office: Arnhem, The Netherlands, 2022; ISBN 978-94-92671-16-5.
24. Drago, J.R.; Rohner, T.J., Jr.; Chez, R.A. Management of urinary calculi in pregnancy. *Urology* **1982**, *20*, 578–581. [CrossRef]
25. Stothers, L.; Lee, L.M. Renal colic in pregnancy. *J. Urol.* **1992**, *148*, 1383–1387. [CrossRef]
26. Vendola, N.; Giumelli, P.; Galdini, R.; Bennici, S. Ureteral drainage with double-J catheters in obstructive uropathy during pregnancy. A report of 3 cases. *Gynecol. Obstet. Investig.* **1995**, *40*, 274–275. [CrossRef] [PubMed]
27. Sheiner, E.; Mazor-Drey, E.; Levy, A. Asymptomatic bacteriuria during pregnancy. *J. Matern. Fetal. Neonatal. Med.* **2009**, *22*, 423–427. [CrossRef]

28. Balachandran, L.; Jacob, L.; Al Awadhi, R.; Yahya, L.O.; Catroon, K.M.; Soundararajan, L.P.; Wani, S.; Alabadla, S.; Hussein, Y.A. Urinary Tract Infection in Pregnancy and Its Effects on Maternal and Perinatal Outcome: A Retrospective Study. *Cureus* **2022**, *14*, e21500. [CrossRef]
29. Geerlings, S.E. Clinical Presentations and Epidemiology of Urinary Tract Infections. *Microbiol. Spectr.* **2016**, *4*, 4–5. [CrossRef]
30. Kirkwood, A.; Harris, C.; Timar, N.; Koren, G. Is gentamicin ototoxic to the fetus? *J. Obstet. Gynaecol. Can.* **2007**, *29*, 140–145. [CrossRef]
31. Leung, J.C.; Cifra, C.L.; Agthe, A.G.; Sun, C.-C.J.; Viscardi, R.M. Antenatal factors modulate hearing screen failure risk in preterm infants. *Arch. Dis. Child.-Fetal Neonatal Ed.* **2016**, *101*, 56–61. [CrossRef]
32. Czeizel, A.E.; Rockenbauer, M.; Olsen, J.; Sørensen, H.T. A teratological study of aminoglycoside antibiotic treatment during pregnancy. *Scand. J. Infect. Dis.* **2000**, *32*, 309–313. [PubMed]
33. Napolitano, L.M. Sepsis 2018: Definitions and Guideline Changes. *Surg. Infect.* **2018**, *19*, 117–125. [CrossRef] [PubMed]
34. Ciciu, E.; Pașatu-Cornea, A.-M.; Petcu, L.C.; Tuță, L.-A. Early diagnosis and management of maternal ureterohydronephrosis during pregnancy. *Exp. Ther. Med.* **2022**, *23*, 1–6. [CrossRef] [PubMed]
35. Korkes, F.; Rauen, E.C.; Heilberg, I.P. Urolithiasis and pregnancy. *J. Bras. Nefrol.* **2014**, *36*, 389–395. [CrossRef] [PubMed]
36. Szweda, H.; Jóźwik, M. Urinary tract infections during pregnancy—An updated overview. *Dev. Period Med.* **2016**, *20*, 263–272. [PubMed]
37. Parulkar, B.; Hopkins, T.; Wollin, M.; Howard, P.; Lal, A. Renal colic during pregnancy: A case for conservative treatment. *J. Urol.* **1998**, *159*, 365–368. [CrossRef]
38. Blanco, L.T.; Socarras, M.R.; Montero, R.F.; Diez, E.L.; Calvo, A.O.; Gregorio, S.A.; Cansino, J.R.; Galan, J.A.; Rivas, J.G. Renal colic during pregnancy: Diagnostic and therapeutic aspects. Literature review. *Cent. Eur. J. Urol.* **2017**, *70*, 93.
39. Andreoiu, M.; MacMahon, R. Renal colic in pregnancy: Lithiasis or physiological hydronephrosis? *Urology* **2009**, *74*, 757–761. [CrossRef]
40. Bultitude, M.F.; Tiptaft, R.C.; Glass, J.M.; Dasgupta, P. Management of encrusted ureteral stents impacted in upper tract. *Urology* **2003**, *62*, 622–626. [CrossRef]
41. Borboroglu, P.G.; Kane, C.J. Current management of severely encrusted ureteral stents with a large associated stone burden. *J. Urol.* **2000**, *164*, 648–650. [CrossRef]
42. Kawahara, T.; Ito, H.; Terao, H.; Yamagishi, T.; Ogawa, T.; Uemura, H.; Kubota, Y.; Matsuzaki, J. Ureteral stent retrieval using the crochet hook technique in females. *PLoS ONE* **2012**, *7*, e29292. [CrossRef] [PubMed]
43. Delakas, D.; Karyotis, I.; Loumbakis, P.; Daskalopoulos, G.; Kazanis, J.; Cranidis, A. Ureteral drainage by double-J-catheters during pregnancy. *Clin. Exp. Obstet. Gynecol.* **2000**, *27*, 200–202. [PubMed]
44. Ordon, M.; Dirk, J.; Slater, J.; Kroft, J.; Dixon, S.; Welk, B. Incidence, Treatment, and Implications of Kidney Stones During Pregnancy: A Matched Population-Based Cohort Study. *J. Endourol.* **2020**, *34*, 215–221. [CrossRef] [PubMed]
45. Lewis, D.F.; Robichaux, A.G., 3rd; Jaekle, R.K.; Marcum, N.G.; Stedman, C.M. Urolithiasis in pregnancy. Diagnosis, management and pregnancy outcome. *J. Reprod. Med.* **2003**, *48*, 28–32. [CrossRef] [PubMed]

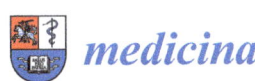

Article

The Impact of Ethnicity on Fetal and Maternal Outcomes of Gestational Diabetes

Tiziana Filardi [1,*], Maria Cristina Gentile [1], Vittorio Venditti [1], Antonella Valente [1], Enrico Bleve [1], Carmela Santangelo [2] and Susanna Morano [1]

[1] Department of Experimental Medicine, "Sapienza" University, Viale del Policlinico 155, 00161 Rome, Italy
[2] Center for Gender-Specific Medicine, Gender Specific Prevention and Health Unit, Istituto Superiore di Sanità, 00161 Rome, Italy
* Correspondence: tiziana.filardi@uniroma1.it; Tel.: +39-064-997-0567

Abstract: *Background and Objectives*: The prevalence of gestational diabetes mellitus (GDM) significantly varies across different ethnic groups. In particular, Africans, Latinos, Asians and Pacific Islanders are the ethnic groups with the highest risk of GDM. The aim of this study was to evaluate the impact of ethnicity on pregnancy outcomes in GDM. *Patients and Methods*: n = 399 patients with GDM were enrolled, n = 76 patients of high-risk ethnicity (HR-GDM), and n = 323 of low-risk ethnicity (LR-GDM). Clinical and biochemical parameters were collected during pregnancy until delivery. Fetal and maternal short-term outcomes were evaluated. *Results*: HR-GDM had significantly higher values of glycosylated hemoglobin checked at 26–29 weeks of gestation ($p < 0.001$). Gestational age at delivery was significantly lower in HR-GDM ($p = 0.03$). The prevalence of impaired fetal growth was significantly higher in HR-GDM than LR-GDM ($p = 0.009$). In logistic regression analysis, the likelihood of impaired fetal growth was seven times higher in HR-GDM than in LR-GDM, after adjustment for pre-pregnancy BMI and gestational weight gain (OR = 7.1 [2.0–25.7] 95% CI, $p = 0.003$). *Conclusions*: HR-GDM had worse pregnancy outcomes compared with LR-GDM. An ethnicity-tailored clinical approach might be effective in reducing adverse outcomes in GDM.

Keywords: gestational diabetes mellitus; GDM; race; ethnicity; pregnancy; pregnancy outcomes; pregnancy complications; large for gestational age

1. Introduction

Gestational diabetes mellitus (GDM) refers to "diabetes diagnosed in the second or third trimester of pregnancy that was not clearly overt diabetes prior to gestation" [1]. This condition is broadly diffused worldwide, even though its prevalence is largely influenced by race or ethnicity, as well as by the heterogeneity of the diagnostic criteria adopted in different countries.

It is well known that belonging to specific ethnicities significantly increases the risk of developing GDM. Specifically, high-risk ethnic groups are South and East Asians, Africans, Hispanics, Native Americans and Pacific Islanders [2–5]. Adverse fetal and maternal outcomes are recognized to be associated with GDM. Perinatal complications encompass impaired fetal growth, which include large for gestational age (LGA, neonatal weight > 90th percentile) and, to a lesser extent, small for gestational age (SGA, neonatal weight < 10th percentile) newborns [6]. Moreover, offspring of women with GDM have increased risk of fetal malformations, rendering antenatal and perinatal management mandatory [7,8]. Maternal short-term complications include preterm delivery, gestational hypertension, preeclampsia and increased rate of caesarean section [9,10]. As for long-term complications, both mothers and infants have an increased likelihood of developing type 2 diabetes (T2D), metabolic syndrome, obesity, and cardiovascular disease (CVD) later in life [9–11]. In light of this, prompt diagnosis and appropriate management of GDM, together with long-term follow-up of patients and infants might effectively limit the burden of GDM-related adverse outcomes.

In recent years, the volume of human migration to high income countries has been increasing due to political issues and economic crises. Migration flow includes a large number of women of childbearing age, markedly influencing the patterns of reproductive health in receiving countries [12]. Ethnic minorities carry with them their genetic background and lifestyle habits, which inevitably merge with high income countries' cultures, increasing the risk of developing cardiovascular and metabolic diseases [13,14]. Although pregnancy and birth are physiological events, migrants might experience substantial language and cultural barriers that limit their access to maternal and neonatal care in destination countries [15]. There is growing concern about the high risk of pregnancy complications and adverse outcomes in ethnic minorities, which urges the adoption of pregnancy monitoring schedules and health policies tailored for ethnic-specific characteristics, in order to reduce the impact of the increased burden of these diseases on healthcare systems.

The understanding of the differences between specific ethnic groups helps in managing pregnancy complications and might considerably limit the burden of GDM. Several retrospective cohort studies have observed ethnic disparities in short-term and long-term outcomes of GDM, reporting conflicting results. In particular, an increased risk of adverse fetal outcomes has been reported in high-risk ethnicities compared to low-risk counterparts [16,17]. However, other studies showed only a modest impact or no effect of race or ethnicity on pregnancy outcomes [18–20]. Of note, not all high-risk ethnic groups have been linked to adverse outcomes. Specifically, Asians were consistently reported to have the lowest risk of LGA and macrosomia compared with other ethnicities [21–23].

The aim of this study was to evaluate the impact of ethnicity on short-term pregnancy complications, in order to identify relevant risk factors for adverse perinatal outcomes in patients with GDM.

2. Patients and Methods

2.1. Patients

This study involved $n = 399$ patients with GDM, $n = 76$ of high-risk ethnicity (HR-GDM), and $n = 323$ of low-risk ethnicity (LR-GDM), recruited in the outpatient clinics of Policlinico Umberto I, "Sapienza" University Hospital of Rome, between 2015 and 2021. LR-GDM were all Caucasian, while HR-GDM were 71.1% Asian, 15.8% African, 13.1% Hispanic. All subjects gave their informed consent for inclusion before they participated in the study. The study was conducted in accordance with the Declaration of Helsinki, and the protocol was approved by the Hospital Ethics Committee of "Sapienza" University of Rome (project identification code 3830, date of approval 22 October 2015).

Current recommendations were applied to diagnose GDM [24]. Exclusion criteria were: age < 18 years; pre-pregnancy diabetes (T2D and Type 1 diabetes); alcohol or drug abuse; psychiatric diseases; multiple pregnancy. The patients were evaluated monthly from diagnosis until delivery. A detailed medical history was collected (age, ethnicity, family history, physiological, obstetrical, pharmacological anamnesis, previous diseases). Anthropometric and vital parameters were obtained (weight, BMI, blood pressure, and heart rate). The following laboratory parameters were collected: fasting plasma glucose (FPG), 1-h and 2-h PG after 75-g oral glucose tolerance test (OGTT), glycated haemoglobin (HbA1c), total cholesterol [TC], triglycerides [TG], high density lipoprotein cholesterol [HDL-c], calculated low density lipoprotein cholesterol [LDL-c]), complete blood count. Information about therapy for GDM (diet or insulin) and other therapies (antihypertensive, other drugs) was also collected. Fetal ultrasound parameters at third trimester and delivery outcomes were obtained (gestational week at delivery, type of delivery, neonatal weight, Apgar index, maternal and fetal complications).

A follow-up visit 6–12 weeks after delivery was performed to check post-partum OGTT results.

2.2. Statistical Analysis

Mean values ± standard deviations are reported for continuous variables. Frequencies are reported for categorical variables. Kolmogorov–Smirnov testing was used to check for normal distribution of variables. Differences between groups were tested with unpaired sample *t*-testing or Mann–Whitney U testing, according to normal or skewed distribution, respectively. Categorical variables were compared with Fisher's exact test. Differences between groups were evaluated with a linear model, adjusting for covariates. Univariable and multivariable regression analyses were performed to evaluate the association between the variables of interest, adjusting for confounding factors. A *p*-value < 0.05 was considered statistically significant. Statistical analysis was performed with IBM SPSS Statistics software version 23 (Chicago, IL, USA).

3. Results

The clinical and laboratory parameters of the enrolled population are reported in Tables 1 and 2, respectively. The fetal US parameters at the third trimester are shown in Table 3.

Table 1. Clinical parameters.

	HR-GDM n = 76	LR-GDM n = 399	*p*-Value
Age (years)	31.6 ± 5.0	34.8 ± 5.4	<0.001 *
Gestational week at enrolment (n)	27.4 ± 6.1	27.6 ± 5.3	0.78
Pre-pregnancy BMI (kg/m^2)	26.6 ± 6.0	26.6 ± 6.7	0.97
3rd trimester BMI (kg/m^2)	29.9 ± 6.6	30.0 ± 6.3	0.92
Family history of T2D (%)	60.6	36.1	<0.001 *
Previous GDM (%)	20.5	9.0	0.012 *
Nulliparity (%)	26.0	34.3	0.21
Previous miscarriages (%)	24.7	37.6	0.17 ‡
Insulin therapy (%)	50.0	40.1	0.15
Gestational hypertension (%)	5.4	8.1	0.63

HR-GDM: High-risk ethnicity; LR-GDM: low-risk ethnicity; BMI: body mass index; T2D: type 2 diabetes; SBP: systolic blood pressure; DBP: diastolic blood pressure; * $p < 0.05$; ‡ Adjusted for age. Data are expressed as mean ± standard deviation or as frequencies.

Table 2. Laboratory parameters.

	HR-GDM n = 76	LR-GDM n = 399	*p*-Value
FPG (mg/dL)	99.6 ± 16.3	92.5 ± 14.7	0.18
Gestational week OGTT (n)	23.1 ± 5.6	24.6 ± 4.7	0.035 *
Glycaemia T0 16–18 w (mg/dL)	94.9 ± 14.8	92.9 ± 11.1	0.55
Glycaemia T60 16–18 w (mg/dL)	188.1 ± 31.3	171.7 ± 40.6	0.14
Glycaemia T120 16–18 w (mg/dL)	146.6 ± 34.9	144.8 ± 36.7	0.85
Glycaemia T0 24–28 w (mg/dL)	91.3 ± 11.8	88.0 ± 11.5	0.09
Glycaemia T60 24–28 w (mg/dL)	177.6 ± 35.0	176.9 ± 32.5	0.90
Glycaemia T120 24–28 w (mg/dL)	153.9 ± 30.7	149.4 ± 34.5	0.42
HbA1c (26–29 w) (%)	5.6 ± 0.4	5.3 ± 0.5	<0.001 *
TC (mg/dL)	230.2 ± 46.9	252.5 ± 57.5	0.06
LDL-c (mg/dL)	120.4 ± 43.6	140.3 ± 49.4	0.056
HDL-c (mg/dL)	63.2 ± 16.7	72.0 ± 26.4	0.13
Triglycerides (mg/dL)	233.5 ± 60.1	222.5 ± 101.8	0.59

HR-GDM: High-risk ethnicity; LR-GDM: low-risk ethnicity; w: weeks; FPG: fasting plasma glucose; OGTT: oral glucose tolerance test; HbA1c: glycated hemoglobin; TC: total cholesterol; LDL-c: LDL-cholesterol; HDL-c: HDL-cholesterol; * $p < 0.05$; Data are expressed as mean ± standard deviation.

Table 3. Fetal ultrasound parameters (third trimester).

	HR-GDM $n = 76$	LR-GDM $n = 399$	p-Value
Gestational week (n)	29.2 ± 4.9	30.1 ± 4.3	0.34
BPD (mm)	72.6 ± 13.6	76.6 ± 14.0	0.24
HC (mm)	255.3 ± 52.0	280.8 ± 38.8	0.06
AC (mm)	247.1 ± 66.1	264.6 ± 61.0	0.24
FL (mm)	55.4 ± 12.5	58.4 ± 9.8	0.24
HL (mm)	49.1 ± 11.7	52.5 ± 7.5	0.16
EFW (g)	2033.2 ± 467.0	1911.8 ± 564.0	0.48

HR-GDM: High-risk ethnicity; LR-GDM: low-risk ethnicity; BPD: biparietal diameter; HC: head circumference; AC: abdominal circumference; FL: femur length; HL: humeral length; EFW: estimated fetal weight; data are expressed as mean ± standard deviation.

Mean age was significantly lower in HR-GDM than in LR-GDM (31.6 ± 5.0 vs. 34.8 ± 5.4 years, $p < 0.001$)

The prevalence of first-degree family history of T2D was significantly higher in the HR-GDM group than in the LR-GDM group (60.6% vs. 36.1% $p < 0.001$).

A greater percentage of patients in the HR-GDM group had previous GDM, compared with the LR-GDM patients (20.5% vs. 9.0%, $p = 0.012$).

HbA1c values checked at 26–29 weeks of gestation were higher in HR-GDM patients compared with LR-GDM patients (5.6 ± 0.4 vs. 5.3 ± 0.5%, $p < 0.001$).

Delivery data were available for n.28 HR-GDM patients and n.83 LR-GDM patients (Table 4). Gestational age at delivery was significantly lower in HR-GDM than in LR-GDM (37.1 ± 1.3 vs. 38.3 ± 1.8 weeks, $p = 0.03$).

Table 4. Neonatal parameters and pregnancy outcomes.

	HR-GDM $n = 28$	LR-GDM $n = 83$	p-Value
Gestational week delivery (n)	37.1 ± 1.3	38.3 ± 1.8	0.009 *
Caesarean section (%)	72.2	66.7	0.78
Impaired growth	35.7	12.0	0.009 *
LGA (%)	21.4	7.2	-
SGA (%)	14.3	4.8	-
Apgar score	8.6 ± 0.6	9.0 ± 0.9	0.07
Hypoglycemia (%)	16.7	2.4	0.13
Jaundice (%)	8.3	2.5	0.41
ARDS (%)	0	2.4	1.00

HR-GDM: High-risk ethnicity; LR-GDM: low-risk ethnicity; LGA: large for gestational age; SGA: small for gestational age; ARDS: acute respiratory distress syndrome; * $p < 0.05$; Data are expressed as mean ± standard deviation or as frequencies.

The prevalence of impaired fetal growth was 18% in the whole population (LGA 10.8% and SGA 7.2%), and was significantly higher in HR-GDM (35.7% vs. 12.0%, $p = 0.009$).

According to logistic regression analysis, the likelihood of impaired fetal growth was four times higher in HR-GDM patients than in LR-GDM patients (OR = 4.1 [1.5–11.2] 95% CI, $p = 0.007$). In the multivariate model, HR-GDM was an independent predictor of impaired fetal growth, after adjustment for pre-pregnancy BMI and gestational weight gain (OR = 7.1 [2.0–25.7] 95% CI, $p = 0.003$).

Only 16.1% of patients adhered to the follow-up visit 6–12 weeks after delivery.

4. Discussion

GDM can lead to severe pregnancy complications and has become a major public health problem worldwide.

In this study, a sample of pregnant women with GDM were followed-up until delivery and pregnancy outcomes were compared according to ethnicity.

Relevant differences emerged between patients belonging to ethnic groups considered high-risk and low-risk for GDM, both in the baseline risk factors, and in pregnancy outcomes. In particular, the HR-GDM group were significantly younger than LR-GDM patients, despite the comparable prevalence of nulliparity between the two groups. This aspect might mirror relevant cultural differences in approaches to pregnancy across different ethnic groups. Furthermore, a greater proportion of HR-GDM patients had first-degree family history of T2D, which is another major risk factor for GDM. These findings are in line with previous evidence indicating diverse background characteristics between Caucasian and non-Caucasian women with GDM [20,25,26]. Specifically, in a retrospective analysis conducted in Italy, Caucasian GDM patients were significantly older than non-Caucasians [20]. In another study, non-Caucasian women with GDM were younger and had higher prevalence of family history of T2D compared with Caucasian women [26].

It is well established that previous history of GDM markedly increases the incidence of GDM in subsequent pregnancies [27]. In this study, the percentage of women with recurrent GDM was higher in the HR-GDM group compared with the LR-GDM group (20.5% vs. 9%), despite the younger age of HR-GDM patients. Accordingly, although the rate of GDM recurrence is not yet well defined, studies in which the majority of patients belonged to high risk ethnic groups reported higher GDM recurrence rates than studies involving mostly low-risk populations [28].

Although it remained in the normal range, HbA1c measured at GDM diagnosis in the early third trimester was significantly higher in HR-GDM compared with LR-GDM, reflecting higher mean glycemic levels in the previous three months in the high-risk patients. Although OGTT is the gold standard for GDM diagnosis due to its high sensitivity and specificity, it has been observed that HbA1c values in the first trimester of pregnancy are predictive of GDM and postpartum T2D [29–32]. In addition, several studies have suggested an association between different cut-off levels of HbA1c during pregnancy and adverse outcomes in GDM [29,33–36]. The mean value of HbA1c decreases by 0.5% in pregnancy compared with pre-pregnancy values, mainly due to the shorter half-life of erythrocytes [37]. In light of this, some studies have tried to define a pregnancy-specific normal range of HbA1c, which seems to stand between 4.3 and 5.4% [38]. Values above this range have previously been associated with poor pregnancy outcomes in GDM [29,33–36]. Accordingly, compared with LR-GDM women in this study, HR-GDM had mean values of HbA1c above this range and a more frequent occurrence of birth weight impairment. In light of this, further studies are necessary to define the role of HbA1c in predicting GDM and adverse outcomes. In particular, a pregnancy-specific HbA1c cut-off might have clinical usefulness for identifying at an early stage pregnancies with increased risk of GDM complications, helping physicians in tailoring GDM management according to risk stratification.

In this study, impaired fetal growth was more frequent in HR-GDM patients than in LR-GDM patients, even after adjustment for confounding factors. In recent decades, a growing number of studies have reported ethnic disparities in the development of GDM complications. Most of these studies showed that high-risk ethnicities were associated with a greater risk of poor pregnancy outcomes, compared with low-risk ethnicities. In particular, Silva et al. observed that Pacific Islanders and Filipinos had increased prevalence of macrosomia compared with Japanese, Chinese, and Caucasian women [17]. Similarly, in another retrospective study, non-Caucasian patients had more frequent occurrence of macrosomia and LGA, regardless of confounding factors such as BMI and maternal glycemic control [39]. Of note, the risk of adverse perinatal outcomes seems to vary substantially even across high-risk ethnicities. In particular, Asian women with GDM, especially South Asians, have been consistently reported to have lower risk of LGA and macrosomia compared with other ethnic groups [21,23,30,40]. Some studies have found that non-Hispanic black women with GDM had the highest risk of LGA [21,23,30,40]. Meanwhile, in another study, the highest risk of Caesarean section and perinatal complications (LGA, neonatal hypoglycemia) was associated with Hispanic ethnicity compared with other groups, including African patients [16]. However, the proportion of black patients included in the latter analysis was relatively low. On the other hand, not all studies have observed relevant differences in perinatal outcomes among different ethnic groups [19,20].

Several studies have focused on other outcomes such as incident diabetes after GDM, reporting conflicting results. Specifically, Shen et al. observed that Chinese women with previous GDM had the greatest risk of T2D in the following 10 years, whereas African American and Caucasian women had intermediate and low risk, respectively [41]. Conversely, in a recent meta-analysis including more than 80,000 women with previous GDM, the highest incidence of T2D after GDM was associated with black ethnicity [42,43]. In our study, only a small proportion of women underwent post-partum screening (16.1%). Due to the lack of data about OGTT 6–12 weeks after delivery, the incidence of post-partum diabetes in this population could not be estimated. Overall, rates of recommended post-partum screening are reportedly low (around 40–50%) [42–44] and seem to be associated with several socio-cultural factors, including education, parity, and race or ethnicity [44]. These results suggest the need for urgent strategies to increase post-partum follow-up adherence, in order to reduce the burden of long-term maternal and fetal complications of GDM, namely T2D and cardiovascular diseases, through appropriate preventive intervention programs.

Overall, in light of these findings, specific ethnic groups that are at high risk of complications might benefit from more tailored education and intervention strategies and follow-up programs in the management of GDM. Moreover, the monitoring of HbA1c might be of clinical utility to avoid poor maternal and fetal outcomes in pregnant women with GDM.

The main limitations of this study were the retrospective nature of the analysis and the small number of patients included in the evaluation at term and after delivery, which calls for cautious interpretation. Future studies with larger sample sizes and longer follow-ups are mandatory to confirm these findings.

5. Conclusions

Ethnic groups at high risk of developing GDM had worse glycemic control at GDM diagnosis, lower gestational age at delivery, and increased risk of impaired fetal growth.

Given the implications of poor perinatal outcomes associated with GDM, the adoption of ethnic-specific management strategies might be useful in clinical practice.

Author Contributions: Conceptualization, S.M. and T.F.; Methodology, S.M. and T.F.; Formal Analysis, T.F., M.C.G., V.V. and E.B.; Investigation, T.F., S.M., M.C.G., V.V., E.B. and A.V.; Data Curation, T.F., M.C.G., V.V., E.B. and A.V.; Writing—Original Draft Preparation, T.F.; Writing—Review & Editing, S.M. and C.S.; Supervision, S.M. and C.S. All authors have read and agreed to the published version of the manuscript.

Funding: This research received no external funding.

Institutional Review Board Statement: The study was conducted in accordance with the Declaration of Helsinki, and approved by the Hospital Ethics Committee of "Sapienza" University of Rome (project identification code 3830, date of approval 22 October 2015).

Informed Consent Statement: Informed consent was obtained from all subjects involved in the study.

Data Availability Statement: The data presented in this study are available on request from the corresponding author.

Conflicts of Interest: The authors declare no conflict of interest.

References

1. American Diabetes Association Professional Practice Committee; Draznin, B.; Aroda, V.R.; Bakris, G.; Benson, G.; Brown, F.M.; Freeman, R.; Green, J.; Huang, E. 2. Classification and Diagnosis of Diabetes: Standards of Medical Care in Diabetes-2022. *Diabetes Care* **2022**, *45*, S17–S38. [CrossRef]
2. Berkowitz, G.S.; Lapinski, R.H.; Wein, R.; Lee, D. Race/ethnicity and other risk factors for gestational diabetes. *Am. J. Epidemiol.* **1992**, *135*, 965–973. [CrossRef] [PubMed]

3. Dornhorst, A.; Paterson, C.M.; Nicholls, J.S.; Wadsworth, J.; Chiu, D.C.; Elkeles, R.S.; Johnston, D.G.; Beard, R.W. High prevalence of gestational diabetes in women from ethnic minority groups. *Diabet. Med.* **1992**, *9*, 820–825. [CrossRef] [PubMed]
4. Metzger, B.E.; Coustan, D.R. Summary and recommendations of the Fourth International Workshop-Conference on Gestational Diabetes Mellitus. The Organizing Committee. *Diabetes Care* **1998**, *21* (Suppl. S2), B161–B167.
5. Yuen, L.; Wong, V.W.; Simmons, D. Ethnic Disparities in Gestational Diabetes. *Curr. Diab. Rep.* **2018**, *18*, 68. [CrossRef]
6. Hapo Study Cooperative Research Group; Metzger, B.E.; Lowe, L.P.; Dyer, A.R.; Trimble, E.R.; Chaovarindr, U.; Coustan, D.R.; Hadden, D.R.; McCance, D.R.; Hod, M.; et al. Hyperglycemia and adverse pregnancy outcomes. *N. Engl. J. Med.* **2008**, *358*, 1991–2002. [CrossRef]
7. Zhang, T.N.; Huang, X.M.; Zhao, X.Y.; Wang, W.; Wen, R.; Gao, S.Y. Risks of specific congenital anomalies in offspring of women with diabetes: A systematic review and meta-analysis of population-based studies including over 80 million births. *PLoS Med.* **2022**, *19*, e1003900. [CrossRef]
8. Quaresima, P.; Homfray, T.; Greco, E. Obstetric complications in pregnancies with life-limiting malformations. *Curr. Opin. Obstet. Gynecol.* **2019**, *31*, 375–387. [CrossRef]
9. Pintaudi, B.; Fresa, R.; Dalfra, M.; Dodesini, A.R.; Vitacolonna, E.; Tumminia, A.; Sciacca, L.; Lencioni, C.; Marcone, T.; Lucisano, G.; et al. The risk stratification of adverse neonatal outcomes in women with gestational diabetes (STRONG) study. *Acta Diabetol.* **2018**, *55*, 1261–1273. [CrossRef]
10. Xiang, A.H.; Li, B.H.; Black, M.H.; Sacks, D.A.; Buchanan, T.A.; Jacobsen, S.J.; Lawrence, J.M. Racial and ethnic disparities in diabetes risk after gestational diabetes mellitus. *Diabetologia* **2011**, *54*, 3016–3021. [CrossRef] [PubMed]
11. Kelstrup, L.; Damm, P.; Mathiesen, E.R.; Hansen, T.; Vaag, A.A.; Pedersen, O.; Clausen, T.D. Insulin resistance and impaired pancreatic beta-cell function in adult offspring of women with diabetes in pregnancy. *J. Clin. Endocrinol. Metab.* **2013**, *98*, 3793–3801. [CrossRef] [PubMed]
12. Balaam, M.C.; Haith-Cooper, M.; Parizkova, A.; Weckend, M.J.; Fleming, V.; Roosalu, T.; Vrzina, S.S. A concept analysis of the term migrant women in the context of pregnancy. *Int. J. Nurs. Pract.* **2017**, *23*, e12600. [CrossRef]
13. Tillin, T.; Forouhi, N.; Johnston, D.G.; McKeigue, P.M.; Chaturvedi, N.; Godsland, I.F. Metabolic syndrome and coronary heart disease in South Asians, African-Caribbeans and white Europeans: A UK population-based cross-sectional study. *Diabetologia* **2005**, *48*, 649–656. [CrossRef]
14. Satia-Abouta, J.; Patterson, R.E.; Neuhouser, M.L.; Elder, J. Dietary acculturation: Applications to nutrition research and dietetics. *J. Am. Diet. Assoc.* **2002**, *102*, 1105–1118. [CrossRef]
15. Song, J.E.; Ahn, J.A.; Kim, T.; Roh, E.H. A qualitative review of immigrant women's experiences of maternal adaptation in South Korea. *Midwifery* **2016**, *39*, 35–43. [CrossRef]
16. Hernandez-Rivas, E.; Flores-Le Roux, J.A.; Benaiges, D.; Sagarra, E.; Chillaron, J.J.; Paya, A.; Puig-de Dou, J.; Goday, A.; Lopez-Vilchez, M.A.; Pedro-Botet, J. Gestational diabetes in a multiethnic population of Spain: Clinical characteristics and perinatal outcomes. *Diabetes Res. Clin. Pract.* **2013**, *100*, 215–221. [CrossRef]
17. Silva, J.K.; Kaholokula, J.K.; Ratner, R.; Mau, M. Ethnic differences in perinatal outcome of gestational diabetes mellitus. *Diabetes Care* **2006**, *29*, 2058–2063. [CrossRef]
18. Seghieri, G.; Di Cianni, G.; Seghieri, M.; Lacaria, E.; Corsi, E.; Lencioni, C.; Gualdani, E.; Voller, F.; Francesconi, P. Risk and adverse outcomes of gestational diabetes in migrants: A population cohort study. *Diabetes Res. Clin. Pract.* **2020**, *163*, 108128. [CrossRef]
19. Mocarski, M.; Savitz, D.A. Ethnic differences in the association between gestational diabetes and pregnancy outcome. *Matern. Child Health J.* **2012**, *16*, 364–373. [CrossRef]
20. Caputo, M.; Bullara, V.; Mele, C.; Sama, M.T.; Zavattaro, M.; Ferrero, A.; Daffara, T.; Leone, I.; Giachetti, G.; Antoniotti, V.; et al. Gestational Diabetes Mellitus: Clinical Characteristics and Perinatal Outcomes in a Multiethnic Population of North Italy. *Int. J. Endocrinol.* **2021**, *2021*, 9474805. [CrossRef]
21. Wan, C.S.; Abell, S.; Aroni, R.; Nankervis, A.; Boyle, J.; Teede, H. Ethnic differences in prevalence, risk factors, and perinatal outcomes of gestational diabetes mellitus: A comparison between immigrant ethnic Chinese women and Australian-born Caucasian women in Australia. *J. Diabetes* **2019**, *11*, 809–817. [CrossRef]
22. Kwong, W.; Ray, J.G.; Wu, W.; Feig, D.S.; Lowe, J.; Lipscombe, L.L. Perinatal Outcomes Among Different Asian Groups With Gestational Diabetes Mellitus in Ontario: A Cohort Study. *Can. J. Diabetes* **2019**, *43*, 606–612. [CrossRef] [PubMed]
23. Esakoff, T.F.; Caughey, A.B.; Block-Kurbisch, I.; Inturrisi, M.; Cheng, Y.W. Perinatal outcomes in patients with gestational diabetes mellitus by race/ethnicity. *J. Matern. Fetal Neonatal Med.* **2011**, *24*, 422–426. [CrossRef] [PubMed]
24. Associazione Medici Diabetologi—Società Italiana di Diabetologia. Standard Italiani per La Cura Del Diabete Mellito 2018. Available online: http://www.siditalia.it/clinica/standard-di-cura-amd-sid (accessed on 23 July 2022).
25. Bordin, P.; Dotto, L.; Battistella, L.; Rosso, E.; Pecci, L.; Valent, F.; Collarile, P.; Vanin, M. Gestational diabetes mellitus yesterday, today and tomorrow: A 13 year italian cohort study. *Diabetes Res. Clin. Pract.* **2020**, *167*, 108360. [CrossRef] [PubMed]
26. Read, S.H.; Wu, W.; Ray, J.G.; Lowe, J.; Feig, D.S.; Lipscombe, L.L. Characteristics of Women with Gestational Diabetes From Non-Caucasian Compared With Caucasian Ethnic Groups. *Can. J. Diabetes* **2019**, *43*, 600–605. [CrossRef]
27. Morikawa, M.; Yamada, T.; Saito, Y.; Noshiro, K.; Mayama, M.; Nakagawa-Akabane, K.; Umazume, T.; Chiba, K.; Kawaguchi, S.; Watari, H. Predictors of recurrent gestational diabetes mellitus: A Japanese multicenter cohort study and literature review. *J. Obstet. Gynaecol. Res.* **2021**, *47*, 1292–1304. [CrossRef]

28. Egan, A.M.; Enninga, E.A.L.; Alrahmani, L.; Weaver, A.L.; Sarras, M.P.; Ruano, R. Recurrent Gestational Diabetes Mellitus: A Narrative Review and Single-Center Experience. *J. Clin. Med.* **2021**, *10*, 569. [CrossRef]
29. Kattini, R.; Hummelen, R.; Kelly, L. Early Gestational Diabetes Mellitus Screening with Glycated Hemoglobin: A Systematic Review. *J. Obstet. Gynaecol. Can.* **2020**, *42*, 1379–1384. [CrossRef]
30. Kwon, S.S.; Kwon, J.Y.; Park, Y.W.; Kim, Y.H.; Lim, J.B. HbA1c for diagnosis and prognosis of gestational diabetes mellitus. *Diabetes Res. Clin. Pract.* **2015**, *110*, 38–43. [CrossRef]
31. Renz, P.B.; Chume, F.C.; Timm, J.R.T.; Pimentel, A.L.; Camargo, J.L. Diagnostic accuracy of glycated hemoglobin for gestational diabetes mellitus: A systematic review and meta-analysis. *Clin. Chem. Lab. Med.* **2019**, *57*, 1435–1449. [CrossRef] [PubMed]
32. Valadan, M.; Bahramnezhad, Z.; Golshahi, F.; Feizabad, E. The role of first-trimester HbA1c in the early detection of gestational diabetes. *BMC Pregnancy Childbirth* **2022**, *22*, 71. [CrossRef] [PubMed]
33. Arbib, N.; Shmueli, A.; Salman, L.; Krispin, E.; Toledano, Y.; Hadar, E. First trimester glycosylated hemoglobin as a predictor of gestational diabetes mellitus. *Int. J. Gynaecol. Obstet.* **2019**, *145*, 158–163. [CrossRef] [PubMed]
34. Fong, A.; Serra, A.E.; Gabby, L.; Wing, D.A.; Berkowitz, K.M. Use of hemoglobin A1c as an early predictor of gestational diabetes mellitus. *Am. J. Obstet. Gynecol.* **2014**, *211*, 641.e1–641.e7. [CrossRef] [PubMed]
35. Hughes, R.C.; Moore, M.P.; Gullam, J.E.; Mohamed, K.; Rowan, J. An early pregnancy HbA1c >/=5.9% (41 mmol/mol) is optimal for detecting diabetes and identifies women at increased risk of adverse pregnancy outcomes. *Diabetes Care* **2014**, *37*, 2953–2959. [CrossRef]
36. Mane, L.; Flores-Le Roux, J.A.; Pedro-Botet, J.; Gortazar, L.; Chillaron, J.J.; Llaurado, G.; Paya, A.; Benaiges, D. Is fasting plasma glucose in early pregnancy a better predictor of adverse obstetric outcomes than glycated haemoglobin? *Eur. J. Obstet. Gynecol. Reprod. Biol.* **2019**, *234*, 79–84. [CrossRef] [PubMed]
37. Radder, J.K.; van Roosmalen, J. HbA1c in healthy, pregnant women. *Neth. J. Med.* **2005**, *63*, 256–259. [PubMed]
38. O'Connor, C.; O'Shea, P.M.; Owens, L.A.; Carmody, L.; Avalos, G.; Nestor, L.; Lydon, K.; Dunne, F. Trimester-specific reference intervals for haemoglobin A1c (HbA1c) in pregnancy. *Clin. Chem. Lab. Med.* **2011**, *50*, 905–909. [CrossRef]
39. Aulinas, A.; Biagetti, B.; Vinagre, I.; Capel, I.; Ubeda, J.; Maria, M.A.; Garcia-Patterson, A.; Adelantado, J.M.; Ginovart, G.; Corcoy, R. Gestational diabetes mellitus and maternal ethnicity: High prevalence of fetal macrosomia in non-Caucasian women. *Med. Clin.* **2013**, *141*, 240–245. [CrossRef]
40. Xiang, A.H.; Black, M.H.; Li, B.H.; Martinez, M.P.; Sacks, D.A.; Lawrence, J.M.; Buchanan, T.A.; Jacobsen, S.J. Racial and ethnic disparities in extremes of fetal growth after gestational diabetes mellitus. *Diabetologia* **2015**, *58*, 272–281. [CrossRef]
41. Shen, Y.; Hou, L.; Liu, H.; Wang, L.; Leng, J.; Li, W.; Hu, G. Racial differences of incident diabetes postpartum in women with a history of gestational diabetes. *J. Diabetes Complicat.* **2019**, *33*, 107472. [CrossRef]
42. Herrick, C.J.; Puri, R.; Rahaman, R.; Hardi, A.; Stewart, K.; Colditz, G.A. Maternal Race/Ethnicity and Postpartum Diabetes Screening: A Systematic Review and Meta-Analysis. *J. Womens Health* **2020**, *29*, 609–621. [CrossRef] [PubMed]
43. Wang, Y.; Chen, L.; Horswell, R.; Xiao, K.; Besse, J.; Johnson, J.; Ryan, D.H.; Hu, G. Racial differences in the association between gestational diabetes mellitus and risk of type 2 diabetes. *J. Womens Health* **2012**, *21*, 628–633. [CrossRef] [PubMed]
44. Brown, S.D.; Hedderson, M.M.; Zhu, Y.; Tsai, A.L.; Feng, J.; Quesenberry, C.P.; Ferrara, A. Uptake of guideline-recommended postpartum diabetes screening among diverse women with gestational diabetes: Associations with patient factors in an integrated health system in USA. *BMJ Open Diabetes Res. Care* **2022**, *10*, e002726. [CrossRef] [PubMed]

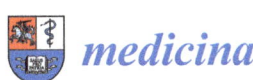

Article

The Hematopoietic Effect of Ninjinyoeito (TJ-108), a Traditional Japanese Herbal Medicine, in Pregnant Women Preparing for Autologous Blood Storage

Eriko Fukuda, Takuya Misugi *, Kohei Kitada, Megumi Fudaba, Yasushi Kurihara, Mie Tahara, Akihiro Hamuro, Akemi Nakano, Masayasu Koyama and Daisuke Tachibana

Department of Obstetrics and Gynecology, Graduate School of Medicine, Osaka Metropolitan University, 1-4-3 Asahimachi Abeno-ku Osaka, Osaka 545-8585, Japan
* Correspondence: t-misugi@omu.ac.jp; Tel.: +81-6-6645-3862

Abstract: *Background and Objectives:* There are no reports showing the hematopoietic effect of TJ-108 on pregnant women. The aim of this study was to investigate the effect of TJ-108 on the hemoglobin and hematocrit levels, and white blood cell and platelet counts of pregnant women complicated with placenta previa who were managed with autologous blood storage for cesarean section. *Materials and Methods:* We studied two groups of patients who were complicated with placenta previa and who underwent cesarean delivery. Group A consisted of women who were treated with oral iron medication (100 mg/day), and Group B consisted of women who were treated with TJ-108 at a dose of 9.0 g per day, in addition to oral iron medication, from the first day of blood storage until the day before cesarean delivery. To evaluate the effect of TJ-108, the patients' red blood cell (RBC); Hb; hematocrit (Ht); white blood cell (WBC); and platelet count (PLT) levels were measured 7 days after storage and at postoperative days (POD) 1 and 5. *Results:* The study included 65 individuals, 38 in group A and 27 in group B. At the initial storage, a 0.2 g/dL reduction in Hb levels was observed, as compared to the initial Hb levels, in the TJ-108 treated patients, whereas a 0.6 g/dL reduction in Hb levels was observed in the non-TJ-108 treated group. On the other hand, regarding the second and subsequent storages, no significant difference was found in the decrease in the Hb levels of both groups. *Conclusions:* This study is the first report showing the effect of TJ-108 on improving anemia in pregnant women, presumably by its boosting effect on myelohematopoiesis. Therefore, the combined administration of both iron and TJ-108 is effective as a strategy for pregnant women at a high risk of PPH due to complications such as placenta previa.

Keywords: Ninjinyoeito; autologous blood storage; postpartum hemorrhage; hematopoiesis; pregnancy; placenta previa

1. Introduction

Postpartum hemorrhage (PPH) is one of the leading causes of maternal death. Multidisciplinary treatment, including blood transfusion, should be set up beforehand, especially for pregnant women at a high risk of PPH due to such conditions as placenta previa or placenta accreta [1]. Hemorrhage during cesarean section that is associated with placenta previa is highly correlated with the need for allogenic blood transfusion [2]. Despite the markedly improved safety of allogenic blood transfusion, the risk of transmission of viral or bacterial infection cannot be completely eliminated [3]. Placenta previa is one of the most serious complications during pregnancy and is associated with increased blood loss at delivery; it is also an important cause of serious fetal and maternal morbidity and mortality [4]. Prenatal diagnosis, followed by the careful planning of cesarean delivery and preparation for possible blood loss by a multidisciplinary team, reduces the risk of fetal and maternal morbidity and mortality [5]. Allogeneic blood transfusion has been used for postpartum hemorrhage, although there are substantial risks, such as viral infection, allergy, posttransfusion immune suppression and graft versus host disease [6]. The usefulness of autologous blood transfusion has been previously reported [7–9]; however, this method of blood storage can lead to preoperative anemia.

As an alternative to allogenic blood transfusion, preoperative autologous blood storage is useful [10], although the process can induce anemia.

Ninjinyoeito (TJ-108) (Tsumura Co., Tokyo, Japan) is a Japanese herbal medicine that has been used to improve anemia in patients for several years [11]. TJ-108 is composed of 12 unrefined ingredients in fixed proportion: 3.0 g of ginseng; 4.0 g of Japanese angelica root; 2.0 g of peony root; 4.0 g of rehmannia root; 4.0 g of atractylodes rhizome; 4.0 g of poria sclerotium; 2.5 g of cinnamon bark; 1.5 g of astragalus root; 1.5 g of unshiu peel; 2.0 g of polygala root; 1.0 g of schisandra fruit; and 1.0 g of glycyrrhiza. However, to our knowledge, there have been no reports showing the hematopoietic effect of TJ-108 on pregnant women until now.

The aim of this study was to investigate the effect of TJ-108 on the hemoglobin and hematocrit levels, and white blood cell and platelet counts of pregnant women complicated with placenta previa who were managed with autologous blood storage for cesarean section.

2. Materials and Methods

This retrospective observational study was approved by the institutional review board (Approved Number: 2022-030, 13 June 2022). Between January 2016 and December 2020, pregnant women who underwent cesarean delivery with the indication of placenta previa were selected for this study. Patients whose hemoglobin (Hb) level was less than 10.0 g/dL were excluded from this study. Cesarean delivery was performed at 36 or 37 gestational weeks. Data of each patient were retrospectively obtained from medical records.

Autologous blood storage was performed when the patient's Hb level was above 10.0 g/dL and canceled at less than 10.0 g/dL. All patients had 300 mL of blood stored each time for a maximum of 1200 mL (4 times). The initial storage was scheduled according to the gestational weeks. The storage was scheduled every week until 7 days before the scheduled day of cesarean delivery. All patients took a daily oral iron medication (100 mg per day) from the day of the initial storage until the day before the cesarean delivery. From 2019, TJ-108 prescriptions in addition to iron administration were initiated for all women who performed autologous blood storage.

We studied two groups of patients. Group A consisted of women who underwent cesarean delivery between January 2016 and December 2018 who did not take TJ-108. Group B consisted of women who underwent cesarean delivery between January 2019 and December 2020 who were treated with TJ-108 at a dose of 9.0 g per day, in addition to the oral iron medication, from the first day of blood storage until the day before the cesarean delivery. Informed consent for the research was obtained from all patients. We informed the patients of their choice to opt-out.

To evaluate the effect of TJ-108, red blood cell (RBC); Hb; hematocrit (Ht); white blood cell (WBC); and platelet count (PLT) levels were measured after 7 days of storage and at postoperative days (POD) 1 and 5. For laboratory tests, serum aspartate aminotransferase (AST); alanine aminotransferase (ALT); creatinine; blood urea nitrogen; sodium; potassium; and chlorine were measured on the day of storage and at POD 1.

Cesarean delivery was performed on the scheduled day for non-eventful patients, and emergency cesarean delivery was performed in cases with bleeding or uterine contraction. All patients were allowed to take clear liquid until 3 h before the scheduled operation and were administered a continuous infusion of lactate Ringers' solution (200 mL/h). The intraoperative loss of blood (including amniotic fluid) was estimated by measuring the amount of blood in the suction collection unit and by weighting the used surgical gauzes.

Continuous variables were expressed as median (range), and categorical variables were expressed as a number (%). Statistical analyses were examined using the Mann–Whitney U-test and Fisher's exact test performed with BellCurve for Excel (Social Survey

Research Information Co., Ltd., Tokyo, Japan). A *p*-value of < 0.05 was considered to indicate significance.

3. Results

During the survey period, 38 patients were treated without TJ-108 (Group A), and 27 patients were treated with TJ-108 (Group B). Table 1 shows the clinical characteristics of the participants in both groups, and the characteristics were not significantly different between the two.

Table 1. Clinical characteristics of participants.

Variables	Group A n = 38 Number or Median (Range)	Group B n = 27 Number or Median (Range)	p Value
Age (year)	35 (28–44)	34 (24–44)	0.310
Height (cm)	160 (140–165)	160 (151–169)	0.329
Body weight before pregnancy (kg)	52 (41–65)	51 (44–87)	0.669
BMI at before pregnancy (kg/m^2)	20.7 (16.4–27.8)	20.4 (17.5–32.7)	0.926
Body weight at birth (kg)	61 (47–72)	59 (50–89)	0.680
BMI at birth (kg/m^2)	24 (21.0–28.5)	24.2 (19.3–33.5)	0.963
Gestational age (week)	37.0 (34.4–37.3)	37 (32.4–37.7)	0.942
Primigravida (%)	15 (39.5)	15 (55.6)	0.200
ART (%)	6 (15.8)	7 (25.9)	0.314
Emergency cesarean delivery (%)	7 (18.4)	6 (22.2)	0.706
Apgar score 1 min	8 (1–9)	8 (3–9)	0.660
Apgar score 5 min	9 (5–9)	9 (6–9)	0.225
Birth weight (g)	2643 (1966–3440)	2500 (1917–3035)	0.250
Male (%)	24 (63.2)	11 (40.7)	0.074
Female (%)	14 (36.8)	16 (59.3)	0.074

BMI: body mass index; ART: assisted reproductive technology.

The characteristics of maternal and neonatal outcomes data are shown in Table 2. Allogeneic transfusion during cesarean delivery was not significantly different between the two groups, and there was no significant difference between the two in the total amount of blood storage. The median autologous transfusion was 300 mL in both groups, and the frequency of transfusion during cesarean section or blood loss wase not significantly different between the two groups.

Table 3 shows the results of the patients' complete blood count before and 7 days after the initial blood storage of both groups. Hb levels were significantly higher in Group B at 7 days after the initial storage (Group A: 10.0 g/dL; Group B: 10.6 g/dL. $p = 0.001$, 95% confidence interval, 0.13–1.01) (Figure 1a,b). Moreover, the Hb level in Group B was reduced by 0.2 g/dL, as compared to the initial Hb level before storage, whereas the Hb level was reduced by 0.6 g/dL in Group A ($p = 0.012$). The cancellation rate of blood storage in the next instance was significantly lower in group B due to the reduced decrease in hemoglobin levels.

Table 2. Operative outcomes of both groups.

Variables		Group A n = 38 Number or Median (Range)	Group B n = 27 Number or Median (Range)	p Value
Total of autologous blood storage (mL)		600 (300–1200)	600 (300–1200)	0.589
Blood transfusion during cesarean section	Autologous transfusion (mL)	300 (0–1200)	300 (0–1200)	0.336
	Allogeneic transfusion (%)	8 (21.1)	8 (29.7)	0.121
	RBC (unit)	0 (0–10)	0 (0–8)	0.729
	FFP (unit)	0 (0–10)	0 (0–6)	0.779
	PC (unit)	0 (0–10)	0 (0–0)	0.919
Infusion (mL)		1950 (850–4300)	1450 (700–3400)	0.186
Blood loss (mL)		1835 (340–7500)	1760 (895–5500)	0.863
Urine output (mL)		110 (0–550)	80 (0–500)	0.105
Operation time (min)		65 (39–148)	68 (41–104)	0.739

RBC: red blood cell; FFP: fresh frozen plasma; PC: platelet concentrates.

Table 3. Blood cell counts and differences in the initial autologous blood storage.

	Group A 38 Storage (n = 38) Median (Range)	Group B 27 Storage (n = 27) Median (Range)	p Value
Cancellation rate of next storage (%)	17 (44.7)	3 (11.1)	0.004 *
Hb level before storage (g/dL)	10.5 (10.0–12.6)	10.8 (10.2–12.1)	0.070
Hb level after 7 days of storage (g/dL)	10.0 (8.3–11.6)	10.6 (9.5–12.3)	0.001 **
Amount of change in Hb (g/dL)	−0.6 (−2.1–0.4)	−0.2 (−1.5–0.6)	0.012 *
Ht level before storage (%)	31.9 (29.6–39.5)	32.3 (29.8–36.3)	0.394
Ht level after 7 days of storage (%)	30.5 (27.7–36.5)	32.1 (28.4–36.4)	0.015 *
Amount of change in Ht (%)	−1.8 (−5.8–1.9)	−0.7 (−2.5–1.2)	0.015 *
RBC level before storage ($\times 10^4/\mu L$)	356 (296–433)	354 (318–430)	0.730
RBC level after 7 days of storage ($\times 10^4/\mu L$)	333 (270–396)	349 (299–398)	0.125
Amount of change in RBC ($\times 10^4/\mu L$)	−24 (−69–12)	−11.5 (−45–12)	0.003 **

Hb: hemoglobin; Ht: hematocrit; RBC: red blood cell. * $p < 0.05$, ** $p < 0.0$.

Table 4 shows the results of the parameters after the second and subsequent storages in both groups. There were no significant differences in Hb and Ht levels (Hb: 10.7 vs. 10.5; $p = 1.000$, Ht: 32.2 vs. 31.8; $p = 0.259$, respectively) (Figure 1c,d).

No significant differences were found between the two groups regarding white blood cell and platelet levels after 7 days of blood storage, and regarding Hb, Ht and RBC on POD 1 and 5. Blood tests on POD 1 showed elevated AST and ALT in two cases in group A and two cases in group B. No other abnormalities were found in other laboratory values.

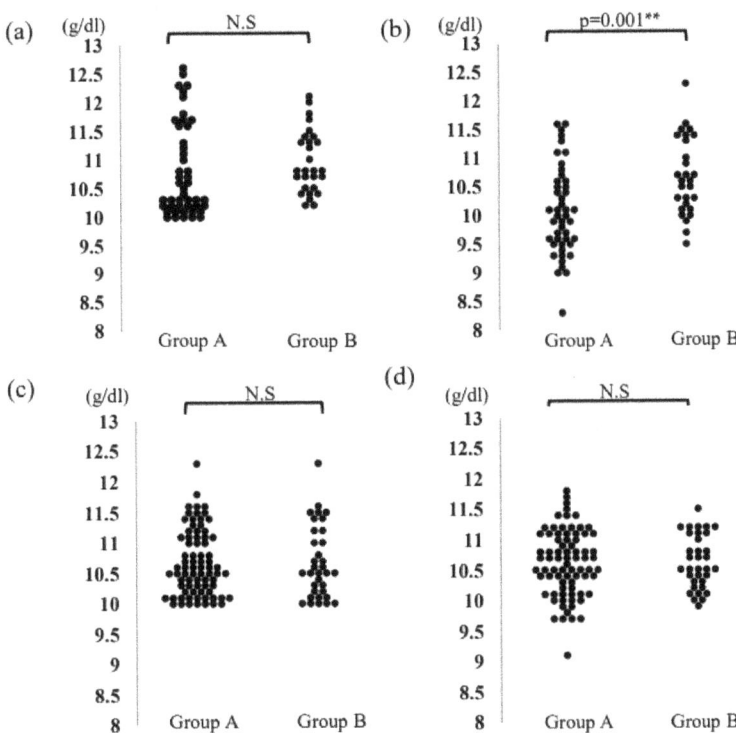

Figure 1. The dot-plot diagram shows the distribution of hemoglobin values (**a**) before the initial storage; (**b**) seven days after the initial storage; (**c**) before the second or subsequent storage; (**d**) seven days after the second or subsequent storage. ** $p < 0.01$, N.S: not significant.

Table 4. Blood cell counts and differences in the second and subsequent storages.

	Group A	Group B	
	55 Storage ($n = 38$)	38 Storage ($n = 27$)	p Value
	Median (Range)	Median (Range)	
Cancel rate of next storage (%)	6 (10.9)	1 (2.7)	0.137
Hb level before storage (g/dL)	10.6 (10.0–11.8)	10.5 (10.0–12.3)	0.769
Hb level after 7 days of storage (g/dL)	10.7 (9.1–11.8)	10.5 (9.9–11.5)	1.000
Amount of change in Hb (g/dL)	−0.1 (−1.0–1.1)	0.0 (−1.4–0.6)	0.692
Ht level before storage (%)	32.2 (29.0–37.2)	31.8 (28.9–36.4)	0.367
Ht level after 7 days of storage (%)	32.2 (28.8–37.2)	31.7 (28.6–34.1)	0.259
Amount of change in Ht (%)	0.2 (−3.4–3.2)	−0.1 (−3.1–2.7)	0.629
RBC level before storage ($\times 10^4/\mu L$)	343 (305–404)	337 (298–398)	0.205
RBC level after 7 days of storage ($\times 10^4/\mu L$)	344 (292–392)	332 (297–384)	0.082
Amount of change in RBC ($\times 10^4/\mu L$)	−4 (−36–24)	−8 (−34–18)	0.841

Hb: hemoglobin; Ht: hematocrit; RBC: red blood cell.

4. Discussion

The present study first revealed that the reduction in Hb levels in the TJ-108 treated patients was significantly less than that observed in the non-TJ-108 treated patients 7 days after storage. At the initial storage, a 0.2 g/dL reduction in Hb levels was observed, as compared to the initial Hb levels in the TJ-108 treated patients, whereas a 0.6 g/dL reduction in Hb levels was observed in the non-TJ-108 treated group. On the other hand, regarding the second and subsequent storages, no significant difference was found in the decrease in Hb levels of both groups.

Takano et al. reported that an oral administration of TJ-108 protected against hematotoxicity in mice treated with 5-fluorouracil (5-FU), which causes severe anemia [12]. They showed that TJ-108 inhibited 5-FU-induced decreases in peripheral reticulocyte and bone marrow cell counts on day 10, and markedly hastened their recovery on day 20 in a dose-dependent manner. Erythroid progenitor colonies, such as colony forming units-erythroid (CFU-E) and burst forming units-erythroid (BFU-E) formed by marrow cells from mice treated with 5-FU were significantly increased by an oral administration of TJ-108 [13].

In the differentiation of erythroblastic cells, BFU-E becomes CFU-E cells, and they then differentiate into erythroblasts. During the late stage of erythroid differentiation, proerythroblasts undergo mitosis to produce basophilic, polychromatic and orthochromatic erythroblasts, and these orthochromatic erythroblasts expel their nuclei to generate reticulocytes. Finally, the reticulocytes mature into RBC, initially in bone marrow, and then in the circulation [14]. In these processes of RBC differentiation, EFU-E or CFU-E are in an earlier stage of differentiation dependent on erythropoietin, and erythroblast or normoblasts are in a later stage of differentiation dependent on iron. [15]. In our study, TJ-108 showed a significant potentiate effect in hematogenesis at the initial storage, yet it had no effect at the second and subsequent blood storages. This may be because TJ-108 stimulated BFU-E, CFU-E or the upper stream of differentiation of erythroblasts and showed a synergistically boosting effect on myelohematopoiesis with iron preparation. Promoting hematopoiesis after blood storage takes some time, and the TJ-108-treated group showed an early effect due to boosting. Therefore, it showed a difference from the non-treated group. However, after the second and subsequent storage, the hematopoiesis of the non-treated group caught up, and no difference was observed.

Hatano et al. reported that angelica roots, one of the components of TJ-108, increase the recovery of erythrocytopenia and stimulates the differentiation of erythroid progenitors without promoting erythropoietin synthesis. They also reported that TJ-108 lowered plasma interferon-γ levels, which may suppress the activity of erythroid progenitor cells. They considered the possibility that the polysaccharides in angelica roots promote hematopoiesis by activating immature erythroid cells, in part, by suppressing cytokine secretion [16].

Presently, complementary and alternative medicines, such as traditional Japanese Kampo medicines, are frequently used together with Western medicines for the treatment of various diseases, including anemia. Motoo et al. showed a randomized controlled trial with TJ-108 for patients complicated with hepatitis C and receiving ribavirin, which is known to cause severe anemia. They reported that a maximal decrease in Hb in the TJ-108 group was significantly smaller than that in the control group (TJ-108: 2.59 g/dL vs. non-TJ-108: 3.71 g/dL, respectively). They also concluded that TJ-108 could be used as a supportive remedy to reduce the ribavirin-induced anemia in the treatment of chronic hepatitis C [13].

In Japan, the current health insurance system covers the prescription of Kampo medicines including TJ-108, available as both herbs for decoctions and extract formulations. It has been reported that herbal medicines are widely used worldwide to treat a variety of ailments during pregnancy [17–19]. Though there have been no reports of TJ-108 being administered to pregnant women, the herbal medicines that comprise TJ-108 have been reported to be safe for use in pregnant women [20].

There were some limitations to this study. Firstly, as we did not evaluate the condition of iron or related inspection items (reticulocytes, ferritin, transferrin saturation, vitamin B12 and folates), we were unable to determine the effect of TJ-108 on bone marrow's ability to produce new blood cells. Secondly, we retrospectively reviewed a relatively small number of patients. Further studies are needed to elucidate the effect of TJ-108 on bone marrow activity in autologous blood storage.

5. Conclusions

This study is the first report showing the effect of TJ-108 on improving anemia in pregnant women, presumably with a boosting effect on myelohematopoiesis. It is suggested that the combined administration of iron and TJ-108 is an effective strategy for pregnant women at a high risk of PPH such as placenta previa.

Author Contributions: Conceptualization, E.F., T.M. and D.T.; methodology, M.K.; software, T.M.; validation, K.K., M.T. and A.N.; formal analysis, A.H.; investigation, E.F. and T.M.; resources, T.M.; data curation, T.M., M.F., Y.K., M.T., A.H. and A.N.; writing—original draft preparation, E.F.; writing—review and editing, T.M.; visualization, E.F. and T.M.; supervision, D.T.; project administration, D.T. All authors have read and agreed to the published version of the manuscript.

Funding: This research received no external funding.

Institutional Review Board Statement: The study was approved by the Institutional Review Board of Osaka Metropolitan University (Approved Number: 2022-030, 13 June 2022).

Informed Consent Statement: We informed the patients of their choice to opt-out.

Data Availability Statement: The datasets used and/or analyzed during the current study are available from the corresponding author on reasonable request.

Acknowledgments: We are sincerely grateful to the clinical staff at the Department of Obstetrics and Gynecology who contributed to the present work. The authors thank Brian C. Nolan for English proofreading.

Conflicts of Interest: The authors declare no conflict of interest.

References

1. Say, L.; Chou, D.; Gemmill, A.; Tuncalp, O.; Moller, A.B.; Daniels, J.; Gulmezoglu, A.M.; Temmerman, M.; Alkema, L. Global causes of maternal death: A WHO systematic analysis. *Lancet Glob. Health* **2014**, *2*, e323–e333. [CrossRef]
2. Chua, S.C.; Joung, S.J.; Aziz, R. Incidence and risk factors predicting blood transfusion in caesarean section. *Aust. New Zealand J. Obstet. Gynaecol.* **2009**, *49*, 490–493. [CrossRef] [PubMed]
3. Vetter, T.R.; Adhami, L.F.; Porterfield, J.R., Jr.; Marques, M.B. Perceptions about blood transfusion: A survey of surgical patients and their anesthesiologists and surgeons. *Anesth. Analg.* **2014**, *118*, 1301–1308. [CrossRef] [PubMed]
4. Silver, R.M. Abnormal Placentation: Placenta Previa, Vasa Previa, and Placenta Accreta. *Obstet. Gynecol.* **2015**, *126*, 654–668. [CrossRef] [PubMed]
5. Oyelese, Y.; Smulian, J.C. Placenta previa, placenta accreta, and vasa previa. *Obstet. Gynecol.* **2006**, *107*, 927–941. [CrossRef] [PubMed]
6. Billote, D.B.; Glisson, S.N.; Green, D.; Wixson, R.L. Efficacy of preoperative autologous blood donation: Analysis of blood loss and transfusion practice in total hip replacement. *J. Clin. Anesth.* **2000**, *12*, 537–542. [CrossRef]
7. Dinsmoor, M.J.; Hogg, B.B. Autologous blood donation with placenta previa: Is it feasible? *Am. J. Perinatol.* **1995**, *12*, 382–384. [CrossRef]
8. Fruchart, M.F.; Rolland, E.; Courtois, F.; Meier, F.; Besse-Moreau, M.; Foucher, E.; Engelmann, P. Programmed autologous transfusion in obstetrics. Blood samples in 100 patients in the last month of pregnancy. *J. Gynecol. Obstet. Biol. Reprod.* **1995**, *24*, 204–208.
9. Yamada, T.; Mori, H.; Ueki, M. Autologous blood transfusion in patients with placenta previa. *Acta Obstet. Gynecol. Scand* **2005**, *84*, 255–259. [CrossRef] [PubMed]
10. Spahn, D.R.; Casutt, M. Eliminating blood transfusions: New aspects and perspectives. *Anesthesiology* **2000**, *93*, 242–255. [CrossRef] [PubMed]
11. Miyano, K.; Nonaka, M.; Uzu, M.; Ohshima, K.; Uezono, Y. Multifunctional Actions of Ninjinyoeito, a Japanese Kampo Medicine: Accumulated Scientific Evidence Based on Experiments With Cells and Animal Models, and Clinical Studies. *Front. Nutr.* **2018**, *5*, 93. [CrossRef] [PubMed]
12. Takano, F.; Ohta, Y.; Tanaka, T.; Sasaki, K.; Kobayashi, K.; Takahashi, T.; Yahagi, N.; Yoshizaki, F.; Fushiya, S.; Ohta, T. Oral Administration of Ren-Shen-Yang-Rong-Tang 'Ninjin'yoeito' Protects Against Hematotoxicity and Induces Immature Erythroid Progenitor Cells in 5-Fluorouracil-induced Anemia. *Evid. Based Complement Alternat. Med.* **2009**, *6*, 247–256. [CrossRef] [PubMed]

13. Motoo, Y.; Mouri, H.; Ohtsubo, K.; Yamaguchi, Y.; Watanabe, H.; Sawabu, N. Herbal medicine Ninjinyoeito ameliorates ribavirin-induced anemia in chronic hepatitis C: A randomized controlled trial. *World J. Gastroenterol.* **2005**, *11*, 4013–4017. [CrossRef] [PubMed]
14. Waugh, R.E.; Mantalaris, A.; Bauserman, R.G.; Hwang, W.C.; Wu, J.H. Membrane instability in late-stage erythropoiesis. *Blood* **2001**, *97*, 1869–1875. [CrossRef] [PubMed]
15. Muckenthaler, M.U.; Rivella, S.; Hentze, M.W.; Galy, B. A Red Carpet for Iron Metabolism. *Cell* **2017**, *168*, 344–361. [CrossRef]
16. Hatano, R.; Takano, F.; Fushiya, S.; Michimata, M.; Tanaka, T.; Kazama, I.; Suzuki, M.; Matsubara, M. Water-soluble extracts from *Angelica acutiloba* Kitagawa enhance hematopoiesis by activating immature erythroid cells in mice with 5-fluorouracil-induced anemia. *Exp. Hematol.* **2004**, *32*, 918–924. [CrossRef] [PubMed]
17. Kennedy, D.A.; Lupattelli, A.; Koren, G.; Nordeng, H. Herbal medicine use in pregnancy: Results of a multinational study. *BMC Complement Altern. Med.* **2013**, *13*, 355. [CrossRef] [PubMed]
18. John, L.J.; Shantakumari, N. Herbal medicines use during pregnancy: A review from the Middle East. *Oman. Med. J.* **2015**, *30*, 229–236. [CrossRef] [PubMed]
19. Ahmed, M.; Hwang, J.H.; Choi, S.; Han, D. Safety classification of herbal medicines used among pregnant women in Asian countries: A systematic review. *BMC Complement Altern. Med.* **2017**, *17*, 489. [CrossRef] [PubMed]
20. Suzuki, S.; Obara, T.; Ishikawa, T.; Noda, A.; Matsuzaki, F.; Arita, R.; Ohsawa, M.; Mano, N.; Kikuchi, A.; Takayama, S.; et al. Prescription of Kampo Formulations for Pre-natal and Post-partum Women in Japan: Data From an Administrative Health Database. *Front. Nutr.* **2021**, *12*, 762895. [CrossRef] [PubMed]

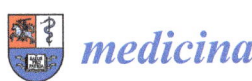 medicina

Article

In Vitro Toxicological Profile of Labetalol-Folic Acid/Folate Co-Administration in H9c2(2-1) and HepaRG Cells

Robert Rednic [1], Iasmina Marcovici [2,3], Razvan Dragoi [1,*], Iulia Pinzaru [2,3,*], Cristina Adriana Dehelean [2,3], Mirela Tomescu [1], Diana Aurora Arnautu [1], Marius Craina [1], Adrian Gluhovschi [1], Mihaela Valcovici [1] and Aniko Manea [1]

[1] Faculty of Medicine, "Victor Babes" University of Medicine and Pharmacy Timisoara, Eftimie Murgu Square No.2, 300041 Timisoara, Romania; rednic.robert@umft.ro (R.R.); tomescu.mirela@umft.ro (M.T.); aurora.bordejevic@umft.ro (D.A.A.); craina.marius@umft.ro (M.C.); gluhovschi.adrian@umft.ro (A.G.); mvalcovici@cardiologie.ro (M.V.); aniko180798@yahoo.com (A.M.)

[2] Faculty of Pharmacy, "Victor Babes" University of Medicine and Pharmacy Timisoara, Eftimie Murgu Square No.2, 300041 Timisoara, Romania; iasmina.marcovici@umft.ro (I.M.); cadehelean@umft.ro (C.A.D.)

[3] Research Center for Pharmaco-Toxicological Evaluations, Faculty of Pharmacy, "Victor Babes" University of Medicine and Pharmacy Timisoara, Eftimie Murgu Square No.2, 300041 Timisoara, Romania

* Correspondence: dragoi.razvan@umft.ro (R.D.); iuliapinzaru@umft.ro (I.P.)

Citation: Rednic, R.; Marcovici, I.; Dragoi, R.; Pinzaru, I.; Dehelean, C.A.; Tomescu, M.; Arnautu, D.A.; Craina, M.; Gluhovschi, A.; Valcovici, M.; et al. In Vitro Toxicological Profile of Labetalol-Folic Acid/Folate Co-Administration in H9c2(2-1) and HepaRG Cells. *Medicina* **2022**, *58*, 784. https://doi.org/10.3390/medicina58060784

Academic Editor: Masafumi Koshiyama

Received: 6 May 2022
Accepted: 7 June 2022
Published: 10 June 2022

Publisher's Note: MDPI stays neutral with regard to jurisdictional claims in published maps and institutional affiliations.

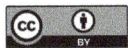

Copyright: © 2022 by the authors. Licensee MDPI, Basel, Switzerland. This article is an open access article distributed under the terms and conditions of the Creative Commons Attribution (CC BY) license (https://creativecommons.org/licenses/by/4.0/).

Abstract: *Background and Objectives:* The consumption of dietary supplements has increased over the last decades among pregnant women, becoming an efficient resource of micronutrients able to satisfy their nutritional needs during pregnancy. Furthermore, gestational drug administration might be necessary to treat several pregnancy complications such as hypertension. Folic acid (FA) and folate (FT) supplementation is highly recommended by clinicians during pregnancy, especially for preventing neural tube birth defects, while labetalol (LB) is a β-blocker commonly administered as a safe option for the treatment of pregnancy-related hypertension. Currently, the possible toxicity resulting from the co-administration of FA/FT and LB has not been fully evaluated. In light of these considerations, the current study was aimed at investigating the possible in vitro cardio- and hepatotoxicity of LB-FA and LB-FT associations. *Materials and Methods:* Five different concentrations of LB, FA, FT, and their combination were used in myoblasts and hepatocytes in order to assess cell viability, cell morphology, and wound regeneration. *Results:* The results indicate no significant alterations in terms of cell viability and morphology in myoblasts (H9c2(2-1)) and hepatocytes (HepaRG) following a 72-h treatment, apart from a decrease in the percentage of viable H9c2(2-1) cells (~67%) treated with LB 150 nM–FT 50 nM. Additionally, LB (50 and 150 nM)–FA (0.2 nM) exerted an efficient wound regenerating potential in H9c2(2-1) myoblasts (wound healing rates were >80%, compared to the control at 66%), while LB-FT (at all tested concentrations) induced no significant impairment to their migration. *Conclusions:* Overall, our findings indicate that LB-FA and LB-FT combinations lack cytotoxicity in vitro. Moreover, beneficial effects were noticed on H9c2(2-1) cell viability and migration from LB-FA/FT administration, which should be further explored.

Keywords: labetalol; folic acid; folate; dietary supplements; cytotoxicity

1. Introduction

The last few decades have seen extensive growth in the consumption of dietary supplements (DTs), which can be defined as oral products administered with the purpose of correcting one's dietary deficiencies. DTs containing micronutrients (e.g., vitamins and minerals) play a vital role in satisfying maternal nutritional requirements during pregnancy, which are insufficiently met through their daily diets [1]. Furthermore, micronutrient deficiency during pregnancy has been correlated with serious maternal and fetal health issues, such as congenital malformations and pre-eclampsia [1,2]. Thus, in order to prevent possible nutrient inadequacies during pregnancy, DTs are highly recommended by clinicians, becoming a common practice among pregnant women worldwide [1,3]. In particular, folic acid (FA) supplementation (at intake levels of 400 μg to 5 mg/day) is recommended for all women of reproductive age both in the periconceptional period and up until the 12th week of pregnancy [4,5].

FA is a synthetic dietary supplement belonging to a family of water-soluble vitamins typically referred to as "folates" or "vitamin B9" [6,7]. FA plays an essential role in DNA synthesis, repair, and methylation [8], and its maternal supplementation has been correlated with a reduced risk of developing neural tube birth defects [5]. However, FA needs to undergo several transformations within the human body in order to become metabolically active [9]. This process includes the reduction of FA to dihydrofolate (DHF) and tetrahydrofolate (THF), followed by its conversion to the biologically active 5-methyltetrahydrofolate (5-MTHF) [6]. 5-MTHF represents the predominant form found in plasma (>90% of total folate) and the main active metabolite of the ingested FA [9].

Many physiological changes occur during pregnancy to enable proper placental and fetal development. Unfortunately, these changes might affect preexisting maternal diseases or even result in pregnancy-related disorders [10]. Hypertension represents the most commonly encountered medical complication during pregnancy (up to 10% of pregnancies) and is the leading cause of maternal, fetal, and neonatal morbidity and mortality worldwide [11–13]. Pregnancy-related hypertensive disorders, which have been associated with an increased risk of developing maternal type 2 diabetes and cardiovascular disease in later life [14,15], cover a broad spectrum of conditions, including chronic hypertension, gestational hypertension, pre-eclampsia, and pre-eclampsia superimposed on chronic hypertension [16,17]. While the definitive treatment for acute hypertensive syndromes occurring during pregnancy is delivery, antihypertensive medication is one of the most employed management strategies in preventing maternal cerebrovascular and cardiac complications. Antihypertensive agents that are widely recommended to control maternal hypertension during pregnancy should not impair the uteroplacental and fetal circulation, and present limited toxicity to the fetus [16]. In current practice, the first-line pharmacological treatment of pregnancy-related hypertensive disorders is based on antihypertensive drugs, such as methyldopa and labetalol, while the second-line strategy includes nifedipine, verapamil, clonidine, and hydrochlorothiazide [18].

Labetalol (LB) is a β-blocker medication commonly recommended as a safe option for the treatment of maternal hypertension during pregnancy [19,20]. Compared to other β-blockers, LB contains both selective α-adrenergic and non-selective β-adrenergic blocking activities in a single agent and preserves the uteroplacental blood flow. However, despite its favorable safety profile, LB has been associated with several side effects, including hypotension, bradycardia, cardiac impairment, and maternal hepatotoxicity [21,22].

The leading hypothesis of this study was that labetalol-folic acid or folate co-administration during pregnancy might result in deleterious side effects, which, to the best of our knowledge, lack any investigation so far. Thereafter, the aim of the current paper was to portray an in vitro toxicological profile of labetalol associated with folic acid and folate using healthy myoblasts and hepatocytes as models for compound-induced cardio- and hepato-toxicity.

2. Materials and Methods

2.1. Reagents

Labetalol hydrochloride (LB), folic acid, folate (as 5-Methyltetrahydrofolic acid), trypsin-EDTA solution, phosphate saline buffer (PBS), dimethyl sulfoxide (DMSO), fetal calf serum (FCS), penicillin/streptomycin, insulin from bovine pancreas, hydrocortisone 21-hemisuccinate sodium salt, and MTT (3-(4,5 dimethylthiazol2-yl)-2,5-diphenyltetrazolium bromide) reagent were purchased from Sigma Aldrich, Merck KgaA (Darmstadt, Germany). Dulbecco's Modified Eagle Medium (DMEM; ATCC® 30-2002™) was purchased from ATCC (American Type Cell Collection, Lomianki, Poland), and William's E Medium was purchased from Gibco Waltham, MA, USA.

2.2. Cell Culture

Myoblast (heart, myocardium) immortalized cell line (H9C2(2-1); code CRL-1446™) was provided as a frozen vial by ATCC. The cells were cultured in their specific media (DMEM). Hepatic immortalized cell line (HepaRG; code HPRGC10) was purchased from ThermoFisher Scientific (Gibco Waltham, MA, USA) and cultured in William's E Medium enriched with insulin and hydrocortisone 21-hemisuccinate sodium salt at final concentrations of 4 μg/mL and 50 μM, respectively. Both media contained a 10% FCS and 1% penicillin (100 U/mL)/streptomycin (100 μg/mL) mixture. The cells were kept in an incubator at 37 °C and 5% CO_2 during the experiments.

2.3. Cellular Viability

To evaluate the impact of LB, FA, and FT on the viability of myoblasts and hepatocytes, the MTT technique was applied. Briefly, H9c2(2-1) and HepaRG cells were cultured in 96-well plates (10^4 cells/well) and stimulated for 72 h with LB (10, 25, 50, 100, and 150 nM), FA, and FT (0.2, 1, 10, 25, and 50 nM). The stock solution of LB was prepared by dissolving the substance in distilled water, while the FA and FT stock solutions were prepared in DMSO. The FA and FT solutions were further diluted in distilled water and culture media for in vitro testing. At the end of the treatment, fresh media (100 μL) and MTT reagent (10 μL) were added to the wells, and the plates were incubated at 37 °C for another 3 h. Finally, the solubilization solution (100 μL/well) was added to each well. The plates were kept at room temperature for 30 min, protected from light, and the absorbance values were measured at two wavelengths (570 and 630 nm) using Cytation 5 (BioTek Instruments Inc., Winooski, VT, USA).

2.4. Cellular Morphology and Confluence

To verify the influence of LB-FA and LB-FT associations on the morphology and confluence of H9c2(2-1) and HepaRG cells, a bright field microscopic examination was performed. The cells were photographed at the end of the 72-h treatment period using Cytation 1 (BioTek Instruments Inc., Winooski, VT, USA). The obtained pictures were processed using the Gen5™ Microplate Data Collection and Analysis Software (BioTek Instruments Inc., Winooski, VT, USA).

2.5. Wound Regeneration

The regenerating potential of LB, FA, FT, and their combinations on healthy H9c2(2-1) and HepaRG cells following wounding was evaluated by applying the wound healing (scratch) assay. In brief, the cells (10^5 cells/mL/well) were cultured in 12-well plates, and a manual scratch was made in the middle of each well. The cells were treated with the test compounds for 24 h, and representative images were taken at 0 h and 24 h using an Olympus IX73 inverted microscope equipped with a DP74 camera. The wound widths were measured at the end of the treatment with CellSense Dimension 1.17 (Olympus, Tokyo, Japan). The quantification of the effects in terms of cell migration was performed by calculating the wound healing rates (%) according to a formula used in our previous work [23,24].

2.6. Statistical Analysis

All data are expressed as the means ± SD, and the differences were compared by one-way ANOVA analysis followed by Dunnett's multiple comparisons post-test. The used software was GraphPad Prism version 9.2.0 for Windows (GraphPad Software, San Diego, CA, USA, www.graphpad.com). The statistically significant differences among the data are marked with * (* $p < 0.05$; ** $p < 0.01$; *** $p < 0.001$; **** $p < 0.0001$).

3. Results

3.1. Cellular Viability

The effects of LB, FA, FT, and their combinations on the viability of healthy myoblasts were evaluated following a prolonged treatment (72 h). LB induced a dose-dependent decrease in the viability of H9c2(2-1) cells, the most prominent effect being recorded at 150 nM (~79%) (Figure 1A). Similarly, FA lowered the cell viability in a concentration-dependent manner up to ~82% at 50 nM (Figure 1B). FT determined a significant increase in the percentage of viable cells at the lowest concentration of 0.2 nM (~127%), while at the highest concentration of 50 nM, the viability was reduced to ~83%. A similar trend was noticed in the HepaRG cells (Figure 1B), their viability being dose-dependently reduced following the single treatments. The lowest cell viability percentages were registered at the highest concentrations tested, as follows: LB 150 nM—88%, FA 50 nM—81%, and FT 50 nM—84%.

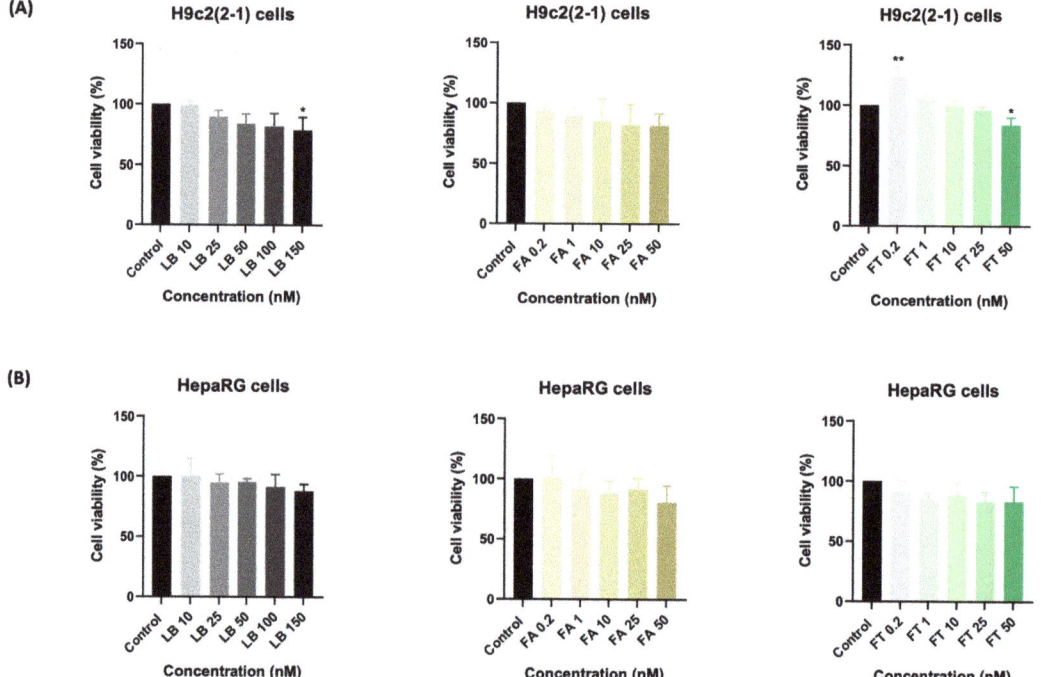

Figure 1. The impact of a 72-h treatment with labetalol (LB), folic acid (FA), and folate (FT) on the viability of (**A**) H9c2(2-1) and (**B**) HepaRG cells. The data are expressed as the mean values ± SD of three independent experiments performed in triplicate ($n = 3$). The statistical differences between the control and the treated group were quantified by one-way ANOVA analysis followed by Dunnett's multiple comparisons post-test (* $p < 0.05$; ** $p < 0.01$).

The impact of the LB–FT combination on the myoblasts' viability was concentration-dependent. The addition of LB 50 nM to the FT treatment exerted a stimulatory effect (138% for FT 25 nM, and 106% for FT 50 nM). On the other hand, LB 150 nM combined with FT 25 and 50 nM reduced the cell viability to ~96% and ~68%, respectively. The impact of LB combined with FA on the viability of H9c2(2-1) cells was insignificant (compared to the control) (Figure 2A). In the case of the HepaRG cells (Figure 2B), a reduction in cell viability was observed following the combination of LB 50 and 150 with FA 0.2 nM (~91%, and ~87%, respectively) and FT 50 nM (~92% and ~86%, respectively). The other treatment regimens led to cell viabilities that were similar to untreated cells (around the value of 100%).

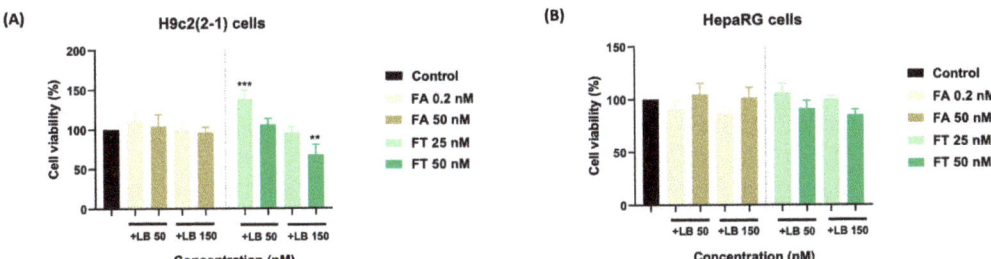

Figure 2. The impact of a 72-h treatment with LB–FA and LB–FT on the viability of (**A**) H9c2(2-1) cells and (**B**) HepaRG cells. The data are expressed as the mean values ± SD of three independent experiments performed in triplicate ($n = 3$). The statistical differences between the control and the treated group were quantified by one-way ANOVA analysis followed by Dunnett's multiple comparisons post-test (** $p < 0.01$; *** $p < 0.001$).

3.2. Cellular Morphology and Confluence

The morphological evaluation (Figures 3 and 4) indicated no significant confluence changes in the H9c2(2-1) and HepaRG cells following the 72 h treatment with LB–FA and LB–FT. However, the addition of LB 150 nM induced a slight decrease in the cell confluence (most visible for FT 50 nM in the H9c2(2-1) cells and FA 50 nM in the HepaRG cells).

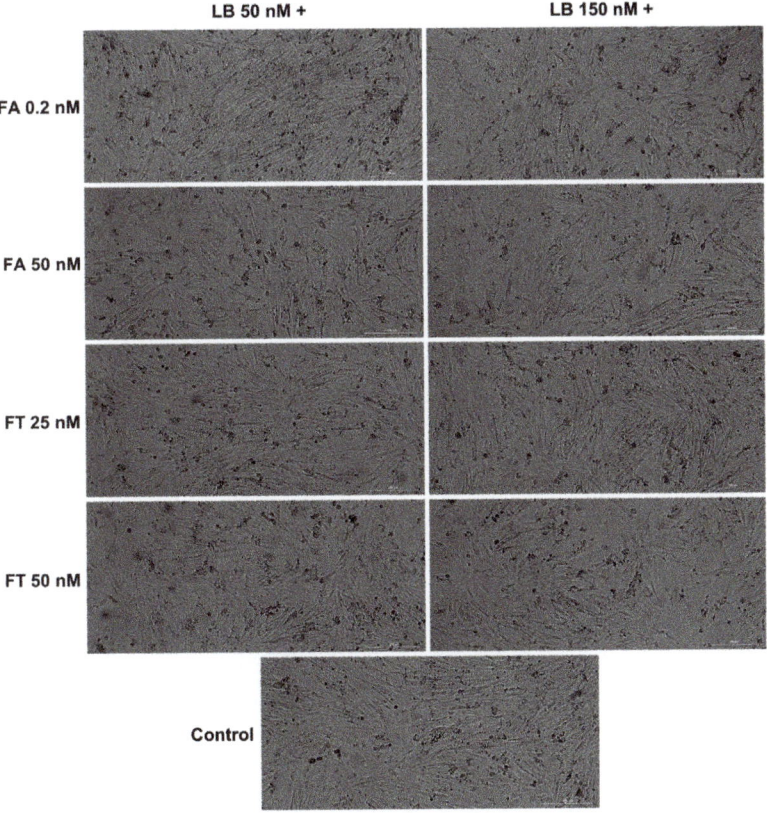

Figure 3. Morphological analysis of H9c2(2-1) myoblasts following the 72-h combined treatment of LB 50 and 150 nM with FA (0.2 and 50 nM) and FT (25 and 50 nM).

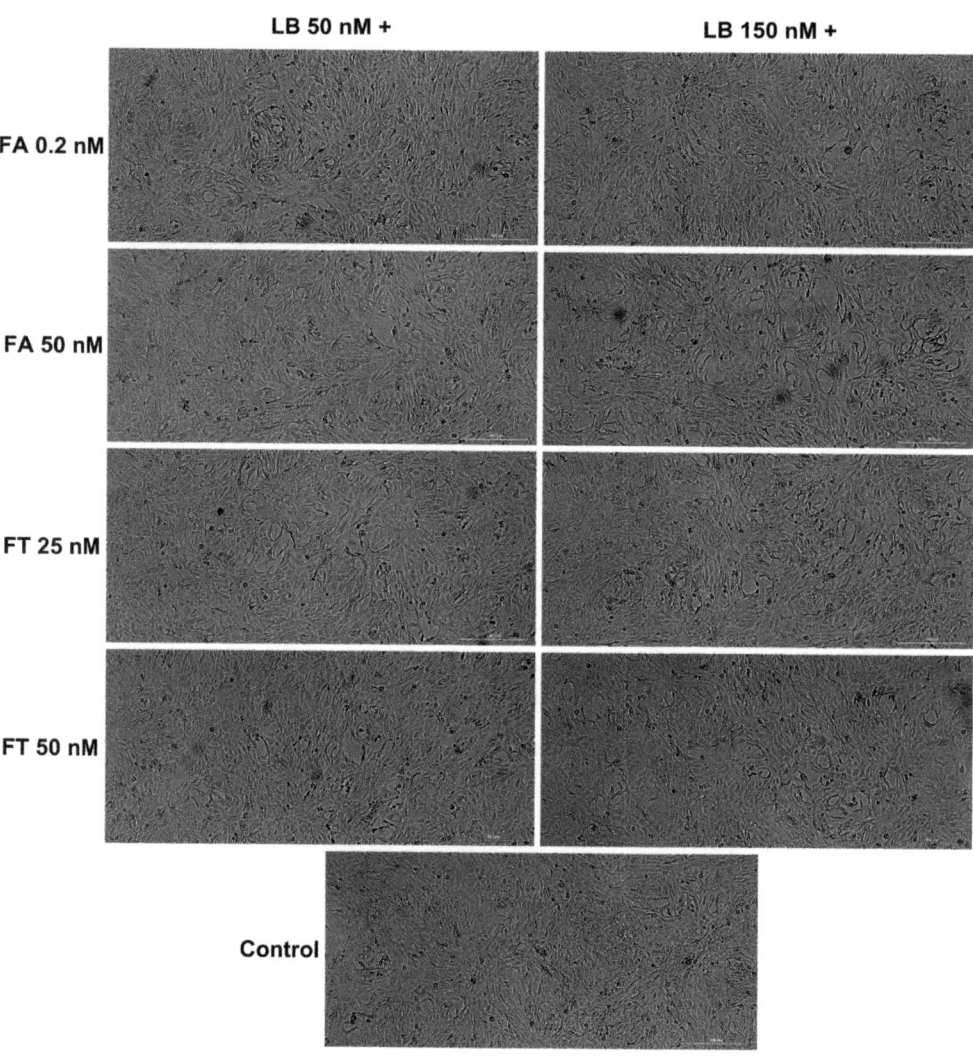

Figure 4. Morphological analysis of HepaRG hepatocytes following the 72-h combined treatment of LB 50 and 150 nM with FA (0.2 and 50 nM) and FT (25 and 50 nM).

3.3. Wound Regeneration

In order to assess whether LB, FA, FT, and their combinations interfere with the migration of H9c2(2-1) cells, a wound healing assay was performed. The wound healing rate of untreated H9c2(2-1) cells (control) reached the value of ~66% (out of 100%, indicating full scratch closure) following 24 h. Compared to the control, the single treatment of the H9c2(2-1) cells with LB and FA inhibited wound healing at both tested concentrations following 24 h of treatment. FT, on the other hand, exerted an inhibitory effect at 25 nM, while slightly stimulating wound regeneration at 50 nM with a wound healing rate of ~70%. The results also suggest that all combinations, except for LB 150 nM–FA 50 nM (wound healing rate = ~53%), stimulate cell migration and wound healing following 24 h of treatment. Compared to untreated cells, the strongest stimulatory effects were recorded when LB (at concentrations of 50 and 150 nM) was combined with FA 0.2 nM with wound healing rates of ~85% and ~88%, respectively. The results are presented in Figure 5.

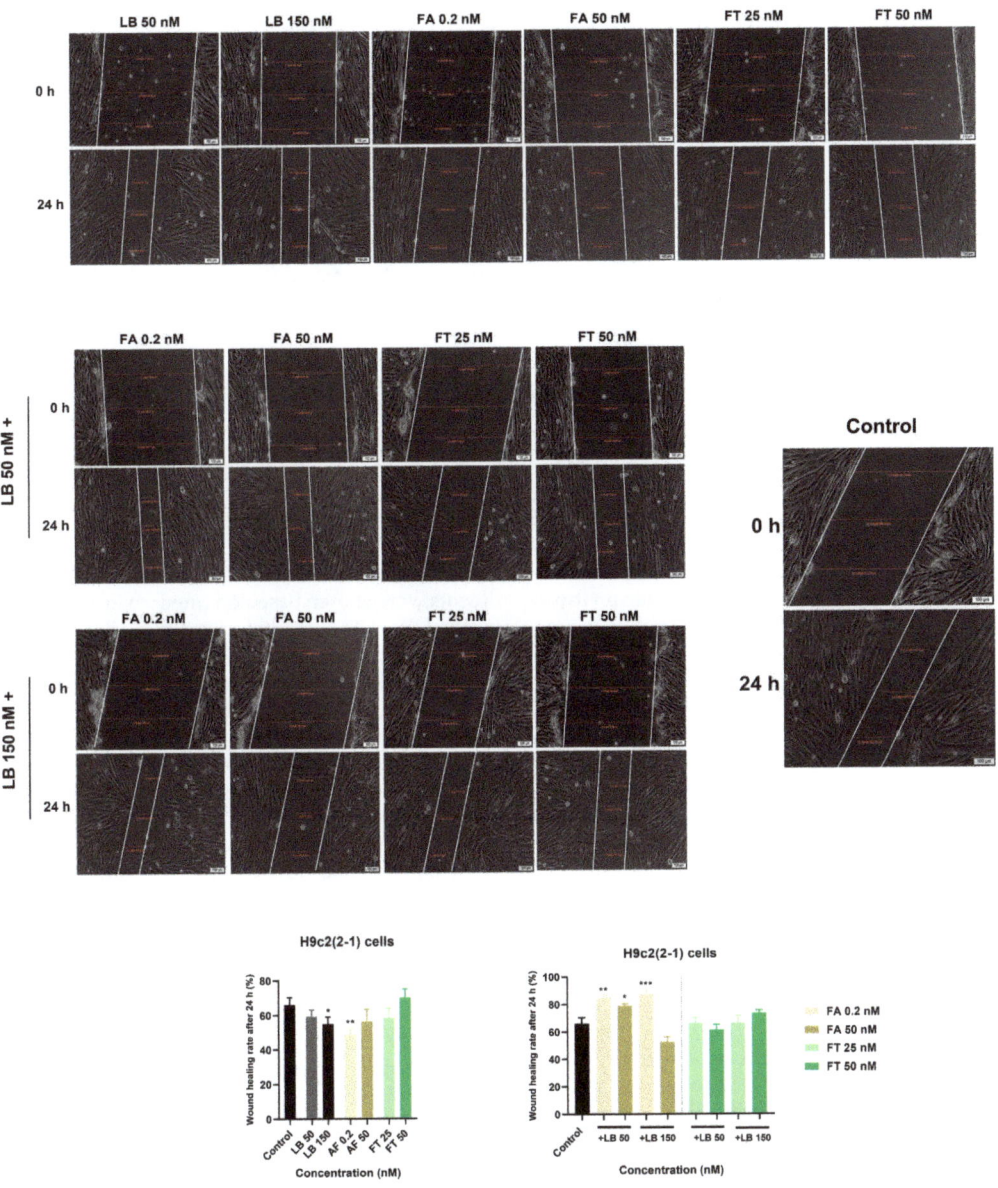

Figure 5. Representative images highlighting the impact of LB, FA, FT, and their combinations on wound regeneration in H9c2(2-1) cells following a 24 h treatment, and graphic representations of the calculated wound healing rates for each treatment regimen (single and combined). The white lines indicate the wound area. The scale bars indicate 100 μm. The data are expressed as the mean values ± SD of three independent experiments performed in triplicate. The statistical differences between the control and the treated group were quantified by one-way ANOVA analysis followed by Dunnett's multiple comparisons post-test (* $p < 0.05$; ** $p < 0.01$; *** $p < 0.001$).

4. Discussion

The safety of the individual administration of folic acid/folate and labetalol during pregnancy has already been documented in the literature [5,25]; however, studies regarding the possible toxicity caused by their co-administration are scarce. Driven by the lack of data on this subject, the current study was designed to examine the potential in vitro cardio- and hepato-toxicity resulting from drug (LB)–dietary supplement (FA/FT) association that might occur during pregnancy. This study was conducted using two immortalized healthy cell lines—H9c2(2-1) myoblasts and HepaRG hepatocytes. The selected cardiac cells have proliferated well in vitro and have been used as an in vitro model in cardiotoxicity analyses, studies regarding the metabolic activity of the heart and mechanisms involved in myocyte damage, as well as in evaluations of compound-induced toxic effects [26,27]. In particular, their applicability in various in vitro studies results from the close morphological resemblance of H9c2 cells to immature embryonic cardiomyocytes. The cardiotoxicity of a given drug can be assessed through the evaluation of cell parameters such as morphology and proliferation. According to a recent study by Witek et al., the response of H9c2 cells to cytotoxic agents is highly dependent on the number of cell passages, this in vitro model being reliable if only cultured at low passages [26]. Thereafter, the cells employed for this study were cultured at low passages to avoid any lack of reliability. HepaRG is an immortalized human hepatic progenitor cell line recently emerging as a useful in vitro model for toxicological evaluations, representing one of the most employed cell lines for the study of drug-induced toxicity [28–30]. Compared to primary hepatocytes, HepaRG cells are more advantageous in terms of availability and reproducibility [28].

Considering that pregnancy has been associated with profound physiological changes affecting drugs' pharmacokinetics [31], the LB, FA, and FT concentrations (expressed as nM) used for the in vitro experiments were chosen based on previous studies illustrating their blood levels in pregnant women following oral administration [32,33]. Thereafter, the concentrations of interest for this study were as follows: LB—50 and 150 nM; FA—0.2 nM; FT—25 nM. Additionally, we tested high concentrations of FA and FT (50 nM).

First, the possible cytotoxicity caused by a prolonged treatment (72 h) of H9c2(2-1) and HepaRG cells with LB, FA, FT, and their combinations was evaluated. The results indicate a dose-dependent decrease in the percentages of viable H9c2(2-1) and HepaRG cells following their individual treatments with LB, FA, and FT (Figure 1). LB produced no significant alterations in terms of cell viability—the H9c2(2-1) and HepaRG percentages were up to 79% and 88%, respectively—while FA exerted a similar effect (cell viabilities of 82% and 81%, respectively) at the highest concentration tested (50 nM), which exceeds physiological FA blood levels [33]. FT, on the other hand, showed a stimulatory effect on the viability of H9c2(2-1) at 0.2 nM, which might be linked to the currently available reports indicating the benefits of FT supplementation during pregnancy in preventing congenital heart defects [34–36]. Furthermore, observational studies have suggested the ameliorative property of FT intake on cardiovascular morbidity and mortality [37].

The impact of the association of LB with FA on the viability of H9c2(2-1) and HepaRG cells was statistically non-significant (Figure 2A,B). Similarly, the viability of the HepaRG cells following the LB–FT treatments was comparable to the control (Figure 2B), suggesting good biocompatibility. Interestingly, the individual treatments with LB 50 nM and FT 25 nM led to viability values of 84% and 96% in the H9c2(2-1) cells, while their combination improved cell viability up to 127%. The in vivo administration of FA, which is known to be subsequently converted into active folate [9], has been found to mitigate the cardiotoxicity induced by several drugs, including celecoxib and doxorubicin [38,39]. Thereafter, our in vitro results suggest that FT treatment can alleviate the viability-reducing effects exerted by LB on healthy myoblasts. However, this protective property exerted by FT has been noticed only at low concentrations, while at high concentrations (LB 150 nM and FT 50 nM), their association led to cardiac cytotoxicity, with cell viability of ~68% (Figure 2A). Regarding cellular morphology analysis, in comparison to the control, no significant morphological changes were noticed at the end of the combined 72 h treatment, apart from a slight confluence reduction in the H9c2(2-1) cells (Figure 3) treated with LB 150 nM–FT 50 nM and in the HepaRG cells (Figure 4) treated with LB 150 nM–FA 50 nM, data that are in correlation with the viability results.

Further, the influence of LB, FA, FT, LB–FA, and LB–FT on wound regeneration was assessed using the H9c2(2-1) cell line. As can be seen in our results (Figure 5), the individual treatment of the H9c2(2-1) cells with LB (50 and 150 nM), FA (0.2 and 50 nM), and FT 25 nM inhibited wound healing following 24 h of treatment, while FT 50 nM slightly stimulated the motility of myoblasts. To the best of our knowledge, the effect of LB on wound healing has not been evaluated so far. However, other β-blockers were included in similar studies. One such example is the study conducted by Cuesta et al. showing that propranolol treatment delayed wound healing in vitro in primary human umbilical vein endothelial HUVEC cells [40]. Regarding the wound healing properties of FA, Pakdemirli et al. highlighted in a recent in vitro study on HUVEC cells that FA (at μM concentrations) is effective for improving endothelial damage [41]. According to our data showing a better healing property of FA at 50 nM compared to 0.2 nM, it can be assumed that high concentrations of FA are required to promote wound regeneration. The association between LB (50 and 150 nM) and FA 0.2 nM proved beneficial for the wound regeneration of myoblasts, a significant increase in cell migration being recorded at the end of the treatment (wound healing rates > 80%). The combined LB–FT treatment induced no significant impairment during the cardiac healing process in vitro.

5. Conclusions

The current study was proposed to evaluate the possible toxicity induced by labetalol association with folic acid and folate on cardiac and hepatic cells, considering their possible association in clinical practice. The main conclusion of the study is that in vitro LB–FA and LB–FT exerted no cardio- or hepato-toxicity at known plasmatic concentrations. On the contrary, LB–FT improved the viability of H9c2(2-1) myoblasts, while LB–FA demonstrated cardiac healing properties, suggesting a possible benefit for cardiac function resulting from their co-administration, which should be explored in future studies.

Author Contributions: Conceptualization, R.R. and C.A.D.; Data curation, R.R., D.A.A. and M.V.; Formal analysis, R.D., I.P., M.T., D.A.A. and A.G.; Funding acquisition, R.D., M.T. and M.C.; Investigation, I.M., D.A.A. and A.G.; Methodology, I.M., C.A.D., M.T. and M.V.; Project administration, R.R., I.P., M.C. and A.M.; Resources, R.D., M.C. and A.M.; Software, I.M., M.T. and M.V.; Supervision, I.P.; Validation, R.D., C.A.D. and A.G.; Visualization, I.M., C.A.D., D.A.A., M.C., A.G. and A.M.; Writing—original draft, R.R. and M.V.; Writing—review and editing, I.P. and A.M. All authors have read and agreed to the published version of the manuscript.

Funding: This research received no external funding.

Institutional Review Board Statement: Not applicable.

Informed Consent Statement: Not applicable.

Data Availability Statement: The data presented in this study are available upon request from the corresponding author.

Conflicts of Interest: The authors declare no conflict of interest.

References

1. Xiang, C.; Luo, J.; Yang, G.; Sun, M.; Liu, H.; Yang, Q.; Ouyang, Y.; Xi, Y.; Yong, C.; Khan, M.J.; et al. Dietary Supplement Use during Pregnancy: Perceptions versus Reality. *Int. J. Environ. Res. Public Health* **2022**, *19*, 4063. [CrossRef] [PubMed]
2. Ballestín, S.S.; Campos, M.I.G.; Ballestín, J.B.; Bartolomé, M.J.L. Is Supplementation with Micronutrients Still Necessary during Pregnancy? A Review. *Nutrients* **2021**, *13*, 3134. [CrossRef] [PubMed]
3. Jun, S.; Gahche, J.J.; Potischman, N.; Dwyer, J.T.; Guenther, P.M.; Sauder, K.A.; Bailey, R.L. Dietary Supplement Use and Its Micronutrient Contribution During Pregnancy and Lactation in the United States. *Obstet. Gynecol.* **2020**, *135*, 623–633. [CrossRef] [PubMed]
4. Barbour, R.S.; Macleod, M.; Mires, G.; Anderson, A.S. Uptake of folic acid supplements before and during pregnancy: Focus group analysis of women's views and experiences. *J. Hum. Nutr. Diet.* **2012**, *25*, 140–147. [CrossRef]

5. Field, M.S.; Stover, P.J. Safety of folic acid. *Ann. N. Y. Acad. Sci.* **2018**, *1414*, 59–71. [CrossRef]
6. Greenberg, J.A.; Bell, S.J.; Guan, Y.; Yu, Y.H. Folic Acid supplementation and pregnancy: More than just neural tube defect prevention. *Rev. Obstet. Gynecol.* **2011**, *4*, 52–59.
7. Shulpekova, Y.; Nechaev, V.; Kardasheva, S.; Sedova, A.; Kurbatova, A.; Bueverova, E.; Kopylov, A.; Malsagova, K.; Dlamini, J.C.; Ivashkin, V. The Concept of Folic Acid in Health and Disease. *Molecules* **2021**, *26*, 3731. [CrossRef]
8. Duthie, S.J. Folate and cancer: How DNA damage, repair and methylation impact on colon carcinogenesis. *J. Inherit. Metab. Dis.* **2011**, *34*, 101–109. [CrossRef]
9. Scaglione, F.; Panzavolta, G. Folate, folic acid and 5-methyltetrahydrofolate are not the same thing. *Xenobiotica* **2014**, *44*, 480–488. [CrossRef]
10. Feghali, M.; Venkataramanan, R.; Caritis, S. Pharmacokinetics of drugs in pregnancy. *Semin. Perinatol.* **2015**, *39*, 512–519. [CrossRef]
11. Xu, B.; Charlton, F.; Makris, A.; Hennessy, A. Antihypertensive drugs methyldopa, labetalol, hydralazine, and clonidine improve trophoblast interaction with endothelial cellular networks in vitro. *J. Hypertens.* **2014**, *32*, 1075–1083. [CrossRef] [PubMed]
12. Wang, W.; Xie, X.; Yuan, T.; Wang, Y.; Zhao, F.; Zhou, Z.; Zhang, H. Epidemiological trends of maternal hypertensive disorders of pregnancy at the global, regional, and national levels: A population-based study. *BMC Pregnancy Childbirth* **2021**, *21*, 364. [CrossRef] [PubMed]
13. Kintiraki, E.; Papakatsika, S.; Kotronis, G.; Goulis, D.G.; Kotsis, V. Pregnancy-Induced hypertension. *Hormones (Athens)* **2015**, *14*, 211–223. [CrossRef]
14. Li, Q.; Xu, S.; Chen, X.; Zhang, X.; Li, X.; Lin, L.; Gao, D.; Wu, M.; Yang, S.; Cao, X.; et al. Folic Acid Supplement Use and Increased Risk of Gestational Hypertension. *Hypertension* **2020**, *76*, 150–156. [CrossRef]
15. Liu, C.; Liu, C.; Wang, Q.; Zhang, Z. Supplementation of folic acid in pregnancy and the risk of preeclampsia and gestational hypertension: A meta-analysis. *Arch. Gynecol. Obstet.* **2018**, *298*, 697–704. [CrossRef] [PubMed]
16. Kattah, A.G.; Garovic, V.D. The Management of Hypertension in Pregnancy. *Adv. Chronic Kidney Dis.* **2013**, *20*, 229–239. [CrossRef]
17. Khedagi, A.M.; Bello, N.A. Hypertensive Disorders of Pregnancy. *Cardiol. Clin.* **2021**, *39*, 77–90. [CrossRef]
18. Brown, C.M.; Garovic, V.D. Drug treatment of hypertension in pregnancy. *Drugs* **2014**, *74*, 283–296. [CrossRef]
19. Magee, L.A.; Namouz-Haddad, S.; Cao, V.; Koren, G.; von Dadelszen, P. Labetalol for hypertension in pregnancy. *Expert Opin. Drug Saf.* **2015**, *14*, 453–461. [CrossRef]
20. El-Borm, H.T.; Gobara, M.S.; Badawy, G.M. Ginger extract attenuates labetalol induced apoptosis, DNA damage, histological and ultrastructural changes in the heart of rat fetuses. *Saudi J. Biol. Sci.* **2021**, *28*, 440–447. [CrossRef]
21. Odigboegwu, O.; Pan, L.J.; Chatterjee, P. Use of Antihypertensive Drugs During Preeclampsia. *Front. Cardiovasc. Med.* **2018**, *5*, 50. [CrossRef] [PubMed]
22. Whelan, A.; Izewski, J.; Berkelhammer, C.; Walloch, J.; Kay, H.H. Labetalol-Induced Hepatotoxicity during Pregnancy: A Case Report. *AJP Rep.* **2020**, *10*, e210–e212. [CrossRef] [PubMed]
23. Maghiari, A.L.; Coricovac, D.; Pinzaru, I.A.; Macașoi, I.G.; Marcovici, I.; Simu, S.; Navolan, D.; Dehelean, C. High Concentrations of Aspartame Induce Pro-Angiogenic Effects in Ovo and Cytotoxic Effects in HT-29 Human Colorectal Carcinoma Cells. *Nutrients* **2020**, *12*, 3600. [CrossRef] [PubMed]
24. Kis, A.M.; Macasoi, I.; Paul, C.; Radulescu, M.; Buzatu, R.; Watz, C.G.; Cheveresan, A.; Berceanu, D.; Pinzaru, I.; Dinu, S.; et al. Methotrexate and Cetuximab-Biological Impact on Non-Tumorigenic Models: In Vitro and In Ovo Assessments. *Medicina (Kaunas)* **2022**, *58*, 167. [CrossRef]
25. Clark, S.M.; Dunn, H.E.; Hankins, G.D. A review of oral labetalol and nifedipine in mild to moderate hypertension in pregnancy. *Semin. Perinatol.* **2015**, *39*, 548–555. [CrossRef]
26. Witek, P.; Korga, A.; Burdan, F.; Ostrowska, M.; Nosowska, B.; Iwan, M.; Dudka, J. The effect of a number of H9C2 rat cardiomyocytes passage on repeatability of cytotoxicity study results. *Cytotechnology* **2016**, *68*, 2407–2415. [CrossRef]
27. Zordoky, B.N.M.; EL-Kadi, A.O.S. H9c2 cell line is a valuable in vitro model to study the drug metabolizing enzymes in the heart. *J. Pharmacol. Toxicol. Methods* **2007**, *56*, 317–322. [CrossRef]
28. Hu, L.; Wu, F.; He, J.; Zhong, L.; Song, Y.; Shao, H. Cytotoxicity of safrole in HepaRG cells: Studies on the role of CYP1A2-mediated ortho-quinone metabolic activation. *Xenobiotica* **2019**, *49*, 1504–1515. [CrossRef]
29. Blidisel, A.; Marcovici, I.; Coricovac, D.; Hut, F.; Dehelean, C.A.; Cretu, O.M. Experimental models of hepatocellular carcinoma—A preclinical perspective. *Cancers* **2021**, *13*, 3651. [CrossRef]
30. Han, W.; Wu, Q.; Zhang, X.; Duan, Z. Innovation for hepatotoxicity in vitro research models: A review. *J. Appl. Toxicol.* **2019**, *39*, 146–162. [CrossRef]
31. Ayad, M.; Costantine, M.M. Epidemiology of medications use in pregnancy. *Semin. Perinatol.* **2015**, *39*, 508–511. [CrossRef] [PubMed]
32. Uematsu, K.; Kobayashi, E.; Katsumoto, E.; Sugimoto, M.; Kawakami, T.; Terajima, T.; Maezawa, K.; Kizu, J. Umbilical cord blood concentrations of labetalol hydrochloride administered to patients with pregnancy induced hypertension, and subsequent neonatal findings. *Hypertens. Res. Pregnancy* **2013**, *1*, 88–92. [CrossRef]
33. Obeid, R.; Kasoha, M.; Kirsch, S.H.; Munz, W.; Herrmann, W. Concentrations of unmetabolized folic acid and primary folate forms in pregnant women at delivery and in umbilical cord blood. *Am. J. Clin. Nutr.* **2010**, *92*, 1416–1422. [CrossRef] [PubMed]

34. Obeid, R.; Holzgreve, W.; Pietrzik, K. Folate supplementation for prevention of congenital heart defects and low birth weight: An update. *Cardiovasc. Diagn. Ther.* **2019**, *9* (Suppl. 2), S424–S433. [CrossRef] [PubMed]
35. Feng, Y.; Wang, S.; Chen, R.; Tong, X.; Wu, Z.; Mo, X. Maternal folic acid supplementation and the risk of congenital heart defects in offspring: A meta-analysis of epidemiological observational studies. *Sci. Rep.* **2015**, *5*, 8506. [CrossRef]
36. Garbern, J.C.; Lee, R.T. Mitochondria and metabolic transitions in car-diomyocytes: Lessons from development for stem cell-derived cardiomyocytes. *Stem Cell Res. Ther.* **2021**, *12*, 177. [CrossRef]
37. Xu, X.; Wei, W.; Jiang, W.; Song, Q.; Chen, Y.; Li, Y.; Zhao, Y.; Sun, H.; Yang, X. Association of folate intake with cardiovascular-disease mortality and all-cause mortality among people at high risk of cardiovascular-disease. *Clin. Nutr.* **2022**, *41*, 246–254. [CrossRef]
38. Ahmad, S.; Panda, B.P.; Kohli, K.; Fahim, M.; Dubey, K. Folic acid ameliorates celecoxib car-diotoxicity in a doxorubicin heart failure rat model. *Pharm. Biol.* **2017**, *55*, 1295–1303. [CrossRef]
39. Octavia, Y.; Kararigas, G.; de Boer, M.; Chrifi, I.; Kietadisorn, R.; Swinnen, M.; Duimel, H.; Verheyen, F.K.; Brandt, M.M.; Fliegner, D.; et al. Folic acid reduces doxorubicin-induced cardiomyopathy by modulating endothelial nitric oxide synthase. *J. Cell. Mol. Med.* **2017**, *21*, 3277–3287. [CrossRef]
40. Cuesta, A.M.; Albiñana, V.; Gallardo-Vara, E.; Recio-Poveda, L.; de Rojas, P.I.; de Las Heras, K.V.G.; Aguirre, D.T.; Botella, L.M. The β2-adrenergic receptor antagonist ICI-118,551 blocks the constitutively activated HIF signalling in hemangioblastomas from von Hippel-Lindau disease. *Sci. Rep.* **2019**, *9*, 10062. [CrossRef]
41. Pakdemirli, A.; Toksöz, F.; Karadağ, A.; Mısırlıoğlu, H.K.; Başpınar, Y.; Ellidokuz, H.; Açıkgöz, O. Role of mesenchymal stem cell-derived soluble factors and folic acid in wound healing. *Turk. J. Med. Sci.* **2019**, *49*, 914–921. [CrossRef] [PubMed]

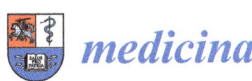

Article

Perineal Massage during Pregnancy for the Prevention of Postpartum Urinary Incontinence: Controlled Clinical Trial

María Álvarez-González [1], Raquel Leirós-Rodríguez [2,*], Lorena Álvarez-Barrio [1] and Ana F. López-Rodríguez [1]

[1] Faculty of Health Sciences, University of León, Astorga Ave. 15, 24401 Ponferrada, Spain
[2] SALBIS Research Group, Faculty of Health Sciences, University of León, Astorga Ave. 15, 24401 Ponferrada, Spain
* Correspondence: rleir@unileon.es

Abstract: *Background and objectives*: Urinary incontinence is any involuntary loss of urine. It may result in anxiety, depression, low self-esteem and social isolation. Perineal massage has spread as a prophylactic technique for treating complications during labor. Acknowledged effects of perineal massage are reduction of incidence and severity of perineal tear and use of equipment directly related to the intrapartum perineal trauma. The aim of this study was to determine the effectiveness of massage in urinary incontinence prevention and identification of possible differences in its form of application (self-massage or by a physiotherapist), with the previous assumption that it is effective and that there are differences between the different forms of application. *Materials and Methods*: A controlled clinical trial with a sample of 81 pregnant women was conducted. The participants were divided into three groups: a group that received the massage applied by a specialized physiotherapist, another group that applied the massage to themselves, and a control group that only received ordinary obstetric care. *Results*: No differences were identified in the incidence or severity of urinary incontinence among the three groups. The severity of the incontinence was only affected by the body mass index and the weight of the baby at the time of delivery. *Conclusions*: A relationship between perineal massage interventions and development of urinary incontinence has not been observed.

Keywords: musculoskeletal manipulations; primary prevention; perineum; obstetric labor complications; physical therapy modalities

1. Introduction

Urinary incontinence (UI) is defined by the International Continence Society as any involuntary loss of urine [1]. It may result in anxiety, depression, low self-esteem and social isolation [2]. There are three types of UI: stress UI—loss of urine upon effort or physical exertion (jumping) or sneezing or coughing due to the lacking capacity of the musculoskeletal system to compensate the increase in intra-abdominal pressure; urgency UI—loss of urine associated with a sudden and urgent need of urinating due to spasms of the bladder detrusor muscle; and mixed UI, when the patient shows a combination of both stress and urgency UI [3,4]. All cases are an important medical, social and economic problem that has an impact of the quality of life of women and that shows a growing tendency (though their prevalence is very different among different geographic regions and dependent on age) [5].

In recent years, perineal massage has spread as a prophylactic technique for complications during labor [6]. Acknowledged effects of perineal massage are reduction of incidence and severity of perineal tear and use of equipment directly related to the intrapartum perineal trauma [7,8]. In addition, the incidence of the two conditions (perineal tear and use of equipment) has been associated with the duration of delivery (especially the second phase). This has been related to the greater incidence of postpartum complications [9,10].

Therefore, we conclude that perineal massage has preventive effects on UI development in postpartum. The present investigation was consequently considered necessary in order to determine the effectiveness of massage in UI prevention and identification of possible differences in its form of application (self-massage or by a physiotherapist).

2. Materials and Methods

2.1. Design and Sample

A controlled non-randomized study was conducted with a sample of women selected from the maternity unit of their primary care center (first obstetric consultation with matron and/or gynecologist or through information leaflets, handed at the care attention center). Recruitment was carried out through three primary care centers served by the same hospital for six months. The women were selected through their interest in participating in the study by the information provided to them in their Primary Care Center (first obstetric consultation with a midwife and/or gynecologist or by notice through information brochures in their own clinic).

The sample was calculated using the G Power software package. The effect size was set as 0.5; $\alpha = 0.05$; sample size = 81; actual power = 0.95 or 95%.

The inclusion criteria for participation were the following: (a) being aged between 18 and 40; (b) expecting a full-term delivery (week 37 or later); (c) expecting a singleton pregnancy; (d) expecting uncomplicated gestation and delivery; (e) not participating in any other psychoprophylaxis intervention; (f) delivering at Hospital Nuestra Señora de Sonsoles (Spain); (g) giving informed consent of participation in the study and attending to all intervention and or evaluation sessions. The exclusion criteria defined were: (a) any counter indication for perineal massage; (b) medical diagnosis of any pelvi-perineal pathology prior to becoming pregnant; (c) any records on cesarean delivery (in the present or previous deliveries); and (d) presence of UI prior to delivery identified through International Consultation on Incontinence Questionnaire-Short Form (ICIQ-SF) [11].

The sample consisted of 81 women (Figure 1). Throughout the course of the investigation, there was no sample loss.

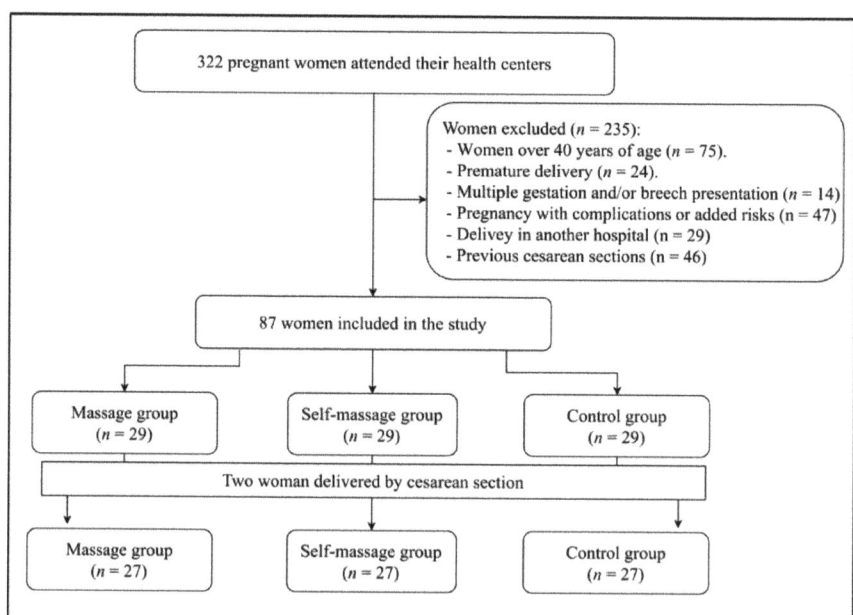

Figure 1. CONSORT flow diagram.

2.2. Procedure

The research protocol was registered in ClinicalTrials.gov (ID: NCT05114811) on 10 November 2021. Participants were divided into three groups according to their personal preference: perineal massage ($n = 27$); self-massage group ($n = 27$), and a control group ($n = 27$) which had regular obstetric attention (regular medical control and information sessions with matron).

All participants signed an informed consent form according to Declaration of Helsinki (rev. 2013) and were also informed on the confidentiality of their personal data. Study had been previously approved by the Ethics Committee of the University of León, Spain (code: 021-2018).

Data collection took place in one evaluation session on the 5th or 6th postpartum week through a self-informed questionnaire where participants registered: characteristics of delivery (week of gestation, weight of the baby, duration of labor, posture, tear, episiotomy, use of equipment and/or analgesia), quality of life through the King's Health Questionnaire (KHQ), and UI incidence through ICIQ-SF (punctuation higher than 0) and description (quantity of loss of urine and how this affects to their daily life), identified in the items included in the questionnaire.

The ICIQ-SF is a condition-specific questionnaire that assesses the subjective symptoms and quality of life of women with urinary incontinence [12,13]. The questionnaire consists of four items pertaining to the frequency of leakage, amount of leakage, interference with everyday life, and the perceived cause of leakage. For the first three questions, the patients were asked to rate their answers on a Likert scale where the maximum scores possible (corresponding to the greatest severity of the condition) were 5, 6, and 10, respectively. For the last question, the purpose of which was to diagnose the type of incontinence, the patients were asked to indicate all the circumstances under which urine leakage occurred. The scores for the frequency of leakage, amount of leakage, and interference with everyday life were added up to obtain the total score. The total score ranged from 0 to 21, and the higher the score, the more severe the condition [14]. The internal consistency of the Spanish version of this questionnaire is 0.89 for its Cronbach's alpha score [15].

Finally, the KHQ is a condition-specific questionnaire that assesses the quality of life of women with urinary incontinence [16]. The KHQ consists of 21 items in the following nine domains: general health perceptions, incontinence impact, role limitations, physical limitations, social limitations, personal relationships, emotions, sleep/energy, and incontinence severity. Each KHQ domain provided a score, and the scores ranged from 0 to 100, the higher scores indicating poorer quality of life. The internal consistency of the different dimensions included in this questionnaire as well as its complete structure in its Spanish version is Good ($0.65 <$ Cronbach's alpha score > 0.92) [17].

2.3. Interventions Applied

(a) Perineal self-massage intervention. As described in a previous publication [16], self-massage group received standing instructions on perineal massage during pregnancy: it should be performed at least twice a week (on alternate days) for 10 min using a water-base lubricant from the 34th gestation week until delivery.

(b) Perineal massage intervention. Perineal massage was applied by a physiotherapist expert in Urogynecol. and obstetrics over 6–10 sessions (from 34th gestation week until delivery) of 30 min each on a weekly basis. The intervention protocol has been used previously [16]. The procedure included direct manual techniques, the use of the EPI-NO® device (Northampton, UK), and another external manual technique [18].

2.4. Statistical Analysis

The statistical analysis was carried out by an investigator blinded to experimental groups (unaware of the meaning of codification of the database of the three sample subgroups). The sample was described by descriptive statistical descriptions (frequency, percentages, media and typical deviation).

Kolmogorov–Smirnov tests and Levene's test for equality of variances were applied to check the distribution of the data for the pretreatment measure of the outcome variables in the three experimental conditions. Since the results confirmed normal distribution and equality of variances, in categorical variables independent samples Chi-square test and Fisher exact test were used to verify the homogeneity of the groups, using Cramer's V as measure of the effect sizes. The three groups' repeated measure analyses of variance (ANOVA) were used to assess changes in clinical variables and psychosocial functioning, computing pairwise differences using Bonferroni correction, and partial eta-squared (η^2_p) was calculated to assess effect sizes. All effect sizes were interpreted using the benchmarks provided by Cohen [19] (η^2_p: small <0.06, medium >0.06 and <0.14, and large >0.14; Cramer's V: small <0.3; medium >0.3 and <0.6, and large >0.6).

A correlation analysis was conducted between the impact of the quality of life due to UI and the quantity of loss of urine and other obstetric variables to find out the relationship between them. Moreover, we applied linear regression models using both the dependent variable and the independent, obstetric variables adjusted by age. R^2 statistic was used to evaluate the fit in the linear regression models. Omega squared was calculated to evaluate the size of the effect of the models. All calculations were performed using the STATA software v.13 (Stata Corp., College Station, TX, USA). The significance level was set at $p < 0.05$.

3. Results

Descriptive analysis of the sample (Table 1) identified significant differences in the age variable between the control and massage subgroups ($p < 0.01$; $\eta^2_p = 0.11$). Obstetric characteristics (Table 2) were statistically different only in relation to the incidence of episiotomy ($X^2 = 23$; $p < 0.001$; $V = 0.53$).

Table 1. Descriptive data of the sample (mean ± standard deviation).

	All (n = 81)	Control (n = 27)	Self-Massage (n = 27)	Massage (n = 27)
Age (years)	32.6 ± 4	30.7 ± 4.3 [a]	33.2 ± 3.2	33.8 ± 3.8 [a]
Height (cm)	164 ± 6.2	163.4 ± 6.3	163.8 ± 5.5	164.7 ± 6.9
Weight (kg)	58 ± 8.3	58.2 ± 9.3	59.1 ± 8.9	56.8 ± 6.5
Body Mass Index (kg/m^2)	21.6 ± 2.8	21.8 ± 2.8	22 ± 2.9	21.2 ± 2.9
Weight gain (kg)	12 ± 4	12.6 ± 4.8	11.9 ± 3.4	11.5 ± 3.8
Deliveries (n°)	1.3 ± 0.5	1.4 ± 0.5	1.2 ± 0.4	1.4 ± 0.6
Labor week (n°)	39.3 ± 1.7	39 ± 2.3	39.4 ± 1.6	39.5 ± 1.2
Baby weight (kg)	3.3 ± 0.4	3.3 ± 0.5	3.2 ± 0.2	3.4 ± 0.3
Duration of labor (hours)	10.9 ± 8.1	9.3 ± 6.6	13 ± 9.3	10.4 ± 8.2

ANOVA significant results: [a] $p < 0.05$; control vs. massage.

A correlation analysis was conducted between the duration of labor and the weight of the baby and did not result statistically significative ($p > 0.05$). The association of quality of life and age, weight of the mother, body mass index (BMI), weight gained during pregnancy, duration of labor ($p > 0.05$) was also analyzed. Quality of life was only significantly correlated inversely with the week of delivery ($r = -0.6$; $p = 0.006$) and the weight of the baby ($r = -0.6$; $p = 0.005$) and directly with the quantity of urine loss ($r = 0.7$; $p = 0.005$). Quantity or loss of urine was only correlated to the BMI ($r = 0.6$; $p = 0.03$).

The linear regressions used as dependent variables were the following: number of deliveries, BMI, weight gained during pregnancy, week of delivery, severity of tear, duration of labor and weight of the baby (Table 3). The quality of life was only affected by the week of delivery and the weight of the baby at the time of delivery ($-0.61 < B > -0.25$; $p < 0.01$; $0.25 < \omega^2 > 0.26$) and the quantity of urine loss was only affected by the BMI and the weight of the baby at the time of delivery ($B = 0.04$; $p < 0.05$; $0.04 < \omega^2 > 0.2$).

Table 2. Delivery and urinary incontinence characteristics [data provided: n (percentage)].

	All (n = 81)	Control (n = 27)	Self-Massage (n = 27)	Massage (n = 27)
Episiotomy *	35 (43.2%)	19 (70.4%)	14 (51.9%)	2 (7.4%)
Perineal tear:				
No	57 (70.4%)	15 (55.6%)	20 (74.1%)	22 (81.5%)
Mild	17 (21%)	8 (29.6%)	5 (18.5%)	4 (14.8%)
Moderate/severe	7 (8.6%)	4 (14.8%)	2 (7.4%)	1 (3.7%)
Position:				
Lithotomy	63 (77.8%)	25 (92.6%)	21 (77.8%)	17 (63%)
Sideways	5 (6.2%)	1 (3.7%)	3 (11.1%)	1 (3.7%)
Sit/squat	11 (13.6%)	1 (3.7%)	2 (7.4%)	8 (29.6%)
Standing	2 (2.5%)	0 (0%)	1 (3.7%)	1 (3.7%)
Instrumental:				
No	64 (71.9%)	17 (63%)	23 (85.2%)	24 (88.9%)
Vacuum	10 (12.4%)	6 (22.2%)	1 (3.7%)	3 (11.1%)
Forceps	7 (8.6%)	4 (14.8%)	3 (11.1%)	0 (0%)
Analgesia:				
No	16 (19.8%)	4 (14.8%)	5 (18.5%)	7 (25.9%)
Local	2 (2.5%)	1 (3.7%)	1 (3.7%)	0 (0%)
Epidural	63 (77.8%)	22 (81.5%)	21 (77.8%)	20 (74.1%)
Urinary incontinence:				
No	56 (69.1%)	18 (66.7%)	15 (55.6%)	23 (85.2%)
Yes	25 (30.9%)	9 (33.3%)	12 (44.4%)	4 (14.8%)
Severity of urinary incontinence (perception of amount of urine from leaks):				
Nothing	56 (69.1%)	18 (66.7%)	15 (55.6%)	23 (85.2%)
Little	24 (29.6%)	8 (29.6%)	12 (44.4%)	4 (14.8%)
Moderate	1 (1.2%)	1 (3.7%)	0 (0%)	0 (0%)
A lot	0 (0%)	0 (0%)	0 (0%)	0 (0%)
Quality of life (mean ± standard deviation):				
0–100 points	39.6 ± 20.1	31.4 ± 34.1	57.3 ± 13.4	50 ± 18.9

Chi-squared significant results: * $p < 0.001$.

Table 3. Linear regression models of impact of urinary incontinence on quality of life and severity of urinary incontinence in relation to obstetrics variables (continuous variables) adjusted by age.

Variable	Quality of Life			UI Severity		
	B	SE	R^2	B	SE	R^2
Number of deliveries	−0.27	1	0.003	0.02	0.11	0.001
Body Mass Index	0.02	0.18	0.001	0.04 *	0.02	0.05
Weight gain	0.04	0.16	0.003	0.01	0.01	0.002
Labor week	−0.61 **	0.2	0.286	−0.01	0.03	0.99
Perineal tear	−0.97	0.99	0.04	0.08	0.121	0.005
Duration of labor	0.01	0.06	0.002	0.01	0.007	0.002
Baby weight	−0.25 **	0.01	0.3	0.04 **	0.001	0.005

UI: urinary incontinence; B: regression coefficient; SE: standard error; R^2: coefficient of determination. * $p < 0.05$; ** $p < 0.001$.

4. Discussion

The objective of the present investigation was to determine the effectiveness of massage in UI prevention and identification of possible differences between its mode of application (self-massage or by a physiotherapist). After analysis of the results obtained, this intervention seems to have no influence on UI postpartum nor the severity of its consequences.

Prevalence of postpartum UI was not related with the distinction among the sample subgroups. This phenomenon was also identified by Eason et al. [20] with the peculiarity that it was identified three months postpartum; in the present study, such relation was discarded even in the early puerperium. Though perineal massage has been associated with a lower incidence in and use of equipment in labor, and these two phenomena have been repeatedly related to UI prevalence [21,22], we have not been able to establish a relationship between applied interventions and development of UI in the present study.

Severity of UI was also associated with the mother's BMI (registered during the first trimester of pregnancy). This association is consistent with previous publications and has been thoroughly studied [23,24]. Previous studies have associated the weight of the baby with the incidence of UI postpartum [25,26], but this is the first investigation that associates it only with severity.

In the massage group, we identified that an incidence of episiotomy was statistically lower than in the control group and the self-massage group. However, no relevant differences were identified between the latter two groups. Such findings were consistent with previous investigations which had already identified the preventive effect of perineal massage on episiotomy [27–29], although this is the first time that a lower efficiency of auto-applied massage is stated, despite the fact that auto-applied massage has been a popular recommendation of professional obstetricians, especially during the recent months when health care assistance was generally not on-site due to the COVID-19 pandemic [30].

Duration of labor was not significantly associated with the weight of the newborns; this contradicts what has been published by a recent paper [31]. In any case, it is an association which has hardly been investigated in scientific literature. It has been established that active labor lasts for less than 12 h [32]; the only group that lasted longer was the self-massage group, and the group that lasted the least amount of time on delivery on average was the control group. Consequently, the present study discarded the influence of perineal massage on duration of delivery, regardless of its application mode. Therefore, the physiological mechanism by which perineal massage reduces the development of intrapartum perineal trauma appears to have no correlation with its influence on duration of delivery.

The authors must recognize that this research has methodological limitations. Fundamentally, the sample size (although representative and with proven statistical power) is small. Furthermore, the fact that the information analyzed was obtained through questionnaires means that the data could be biased or unreliable. It would have been an added value to the present investigation to include long-term follow-up of the characteristics of the participants' urine leakage. Finally, the authors must acknowledge the implicit bias in the way the women were divided into the three subgroups: the fact that the women themselves decided whether or not to undergo perineal intervention could mask some extraneous variable that was not taken into account.

In any case, this investigation also presents strengths such as being the first with this research objective and containing a multitude of obstetric variables that act as extraneous variables not considered on other occasions. Furthermore, it should be the fruit of future research to assess whether the interventions evaluated here could have more significant or better effects on maternal perineal health if applied for a longer period of time (not only in the last weeks of gestation).

5. Conclusions

We have not been able to establish a relationship between applied interventions and development of UI in the present study. In the massage group, we identified an incidence of episiotomy statistically lower than in the other two. However, there were no differences in the incidence of episiotomy between the control and self-massage groups.

The results presented should be taken into account by health care professionals specializing in obstetrics; though prepartum perineal massage has physical and psychological benefits for women, there is no evidence that such procedure decreases incidence of postpartum UI. It is necessary to carry out more investigations studying the specific effects and benefits of perineal massage during pregnancy.

Author Contributions: M.Á.-G., R.L.-R., L.Á.-B., A.F.L.-R. conceptualized and designed the study, drafted the initial manuscript, designed the data collection instruments, collected data, carried out the initial analyses, and critically reviewed the manuscript for important intellectual content. All authors have read and agreed to the published version of the manuscript.

Funding: This research received no external funding.

Institutional Review Board Statement: The study was conducted according to the guidelines of the Declaration of Helsinki (rev. 2013) and approved by the Ethics Committee of the University of León, Spain (code: 021-2018). The data were treated confidentially, and an informed consent was obtained from all subjects involved in the study.

Informed Consent Statement: Informed consent was obtained from all subjects involved in the study.

Data Availability Statement: The dataset used and analyzed during the current study are available from the corresponding author.

Conflicts of Interest: The authors declare no conflict of interest.

References

1. Lukacz, E.S.; Santiago-Lastra, Y.; Albo, M.E.; Brubaker, L. Urinary incontinence in women: A review. *JAMA* **2017**, *318*, 1592–1604. [CrossRef] [PubMed]
2. Frigerio, M.; Barba, M.; Cola, A.; Braga, A.; Celardo, A.; Munno, G.M.; Schettino, M.T.; Vagnetti, P.; de Simone, F.; di Lucia, A.; et al. Quality of life, psychological wellbeing, and sexuality in women with urinary incontinence-Where are we now: A narrative review. *Medicina* **2022**, *58*, 525. [CrossRef] [PubMed]
3. Leirós-Rodríguez, R.; Romo-Pérez, V.; García-Soidán, J. Prevalence of urinary incontinence and its relation with sedentarism in Spain. *Act. Urol. Esp.* **2017**, *41*, 624–630. [CrossRef] [PubMed]
4. Yuaso, D.R.; Santos, J.L.; Castro, R.A.; Duarte, Y.A.O.; Girão, M.J.B.C.; Berghmans, B.; Tamanini, J.T.N. Female double incontinence: Prevalence, incidence, and risk factors from the SABE (health, wellbeing and aging) study. *Int. Urogynecol. J.* **2018**, *29*, 265–272. [CrossRef] [PubMed]
5. Hage-Fransen, M.A.; Wiezer, M.; Otto, A.; Wieffer-Platvoet, M.S.; Slotman, M.H.; Nijhuis, M.W.G.; Pool-Goudzwaard, A.L. Pregnancy-and obstetric-related risk factors for urinary incontinence, fecal incontinence, or pelvic organ prolapse later in life: A systematic review and meta-analysis. *Acta Obstet. Gynecol. Scand.* **2021**, *100*, 373–382. [CrossRef] [PubMed]
6. Graziottin, A.; Murina, F. Vulvar pain during pregnancy and after childbirth. In *Vulvar Pain*; Graziottin, A., Murina, F., Eds.; Springer: Geneva, Switzerland, 2017; pp. 109–127.
7. Dieb, A.S.; Shoab, A.Y.; Nabil, H.; Gabr, A.; Abdallah, A.A.; Shaban, M.M.; Attia, A.H. Perineal massage and training reduce perineal trauma in pregnant women older than 35 years: A randomized controlled trial. *Int. Urogynecol. J.* **2020**, *31*, 613–619. [CrossRef]
8. Akhlaghi, F.; Baygi, Z.S.; Miri, M.; Najafi, M.N. Effect of Perineal Massage on the Rate of Episiotomy. *J. Fam. Reprod. Health* **2019**, *13*, 160–166. [CrossRef]
9. Djusad, S.; Purwosunu, Y.; Hidayat, F. Relationship between Perineal Body Length and Degree of Perineal Tears in Primigravidas Undergoing Vaginal Delivery with Episiotomy. *Obstet. Gynecol. Int.* **2021**, *2021*, 2621872. [CrossRef]
10. Laughon, S.K.; Berghella, V.; Reddy, U.M.; Sundaram, R.; Lu, Z.; Hoffman, M.K. Neonatal and Maternal Outcomes With Prolonged Second Stage of Labor. *Obstet. Gynecol.* **2014**, *124*, 57–67. [CrossRef]
11. Hajebrahimi, S.; Corcos, J.; Lemieux, M. International consultation on incontinence questionnaire short form: Comparison of physician versus patient completion and immediate and delayed self-administration. *Urology* **2004**, *63*, 1076–1078. [CrossRef]
12. Avery, K.; Donovan, J.; Peters, T.J.; Shaw, C.; Gotoh, M.; Abrams, P. ICIQ: A brief and robust measure for evaluating the symptoms and impact of urinary incontinence. *Neurourol. Urodyn.* **2004**, *23*, 322–330. [CrossRef] [PubMed]
13. Gotoh, M. Scored ICIQ-SF (International Consultation on Incontinence Questionnaire-Short Form) for symptoms and quality of life assessment in patients with urinary incontinence. *JNBS* **2001**, *12*, 227–231.
14. Gotoh, M.; Homma, Y.; Funahashi, Y.; Matsukawa, Y.; Kato, M. Psychometric validation of the Japanese version of the International Consultation on Incontinence Questionnaire-Short Form. *Int. J. Urol.* **2009**, *16*, 303–306. [CrossRef] [PubMed]
15. Espuña, M.; Rebollo, P.; Puig, M. Validación de la versión española del International Consultation on Incontinence Questionnaire-Short Form: Un cuestionario para evaluar la incontinencia urinaria [Validation of the Spanish versión of the International Consultation on Incontinence Questionnaire-Short Form: A questionnaire for assessing the urinary incontinence]. *Med. Clin.* **2004**, *122*, 288–292.
16. Hebbar, S.; Pandey, H.; Chawla, A. Understanding King's Health Questionnaire (KHQ) in assessment of female urinary incontinence. *Int. J. Res. Med. Sci.* **2015**, *3*, 531–538. [CrossRef]
17. Badia, X.; Castro, D.; Conejero, J.; King's Group. Validez del cuestionario King's Health para la evaluación de la calidad de vida en pacientes con incontinencia urinaria [Validity of the King's Health Questionnaire in the assessment of quality of life in patients with urinary incontinence]. *Med. Clin.* **2000**, *114*, 647–652. [CrossRef]

18. Álvarez-González, M.; Leirós-Rodríguez, R.; Álvarez-Barrio, L.; López-Rodríguez, A.F. Prevalence of Perineal Tear Peripartum after Two Antepartum Perineal Massage Techniques: A Non-Randomised Controlled Trial. *J. Clin. Med.* **2021**, *10*, 4934. [CrossRef]
19. Cohen, J. *Statistical Power Analysis for the Behavioural Sciences*; Laurence Erlbaum Associates: Mahwah, NJ, USA, 1988.
20. Eason, E.; Labrecque, M.; Marcoux, S.; Mondor, M. Effects of carrying a pregnancy and of method of delivery on urinary incontinence: A prospective cohort study. *BMC Pregnancy Childbirth* **2004**, *4*, 4. [CrossRef]
21. Beta, J.; Khan, N.; Fiolna, M.; Khalil, A.; Ramadan, G.; Akolekar, R. Maternal and neonatal complications of fetal macrosomia: Cohort study. *Ultrasound Obstet. Gynecol.* **2019**, *54*, 319–325. [CrossRef]
22. Shinozaki, K.; Suto, M.; Ota, E.; Eto, H.; Horiuchi, S. Postpartum urinary incontinence and birth outcomes as a result of the pushing technique: A systematic review and meta-analysis. *Int. Urogynecol. J.* **2022**, *33*, 1435–1449. [CrossRef]
23. Liang, C.C.; Chao, M.; Chang, S.D.; Chiu, S.Y.H. Impact of prepregnancy body mass index on pregnancy outcomes, incidence of urinary incontinence and quality of life during pregnancy—An observational cohort study. *Biomed. J.* **2020**, *43*, 476–483. [CrossRef] [PubMed]
24. Can, Z.; Şahin, S. The prevalence of urinary incontinence in obese women and its effect on quality of life. *Health Care Women Int.* **2022**, *43*, 207–218. [CrossRef] [PubMed]
25. Siahkal, S.F.; Iravani, M.; Mohaghegh, Z.; Sharifipour, F.; Zahedian, M. Maternal, obstetrical and neonatal risk factors' impact on female urinary incontinence: A systematic review. *Int. Urogynecol. J.* **2020**, *31*, 2205–2224. [CrossRef] [PubMed]
26. Wesnes, S.L.; Hannestad, Y.; Rortveit, G. Delivery parameters, neonatal parameters and incidence of urinary incontinence six months postpartum: A cohort study. *Acta Obstet. Gynecol. Scand.* **2017**, *96*, 1214–1222. [CrossRef]
27. Abdelhakim, A.M.; Eldesouky, E.; Elmagd, I.A.; Mohammed, A.; Farag, E.A.; Mohammed, A.E.; Hamam, K.M.; Hussein, A.S.; Ali, A.S.; Keshta, N.H.A.; et al. Antenatal perineal massage benefits in reducing perineal trauma and postpartum morbidities: A systematic review and meta-analysis of randomized controlled trials. *Int. Urogynecol. J.* **2020**, *31*, 1735–1745. [CrossRef]
28. Demirel, G.; Golbasi, Z. Effect of perineal massage on the rate of episiotomy and perineal tearing. *Int. J. Gynecol. Obstet.* **2015**, *131*, 183–186. [CrossRef]
29. Zare, O.; Pasha, H.; Faramarzi, M. Effect of perineal massage on the incidence of episiotomy and perineal laceration. *Health* **2014**, *6*, 10–14. [CrossRef]
30. Boelig, R.C.; Manuck, T.; Oliver, E.A.; Di Mascio, D.; Saccone, G.; Bellussi, F.; Berghella, V. Labor and delivery guidance for COVID-19. *Am. J. Obstet. Gynecol. MFM* **2020**, *2*, 100110. [CrossRef]
31. Favilli, A.; Tiburzi, C.; Gargaglia, E.; Cerotto, V.; Bagaphou, T.C.; Checcaglini, A.; Bini, V.; Gori, F.; Torrioli, D.; Gerli, S. Does epidural analgesia influence labor progress in women aged 35 or more? *J. Matern.-Fetal Neonatal Med.* **2022**, *35*, 1219–1223. [CrossRef]
32. World Health Organization. *Managing Prolonged and Obstructed Labor*; World Health Organization: Geneva, Switzerland, 2008.

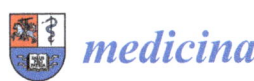

Article

The Risk of Obstetrical Hemorrhage in Placenta Praevia Associated with Coronavirus Infection Antepartum or Intrapartum

Irina Pacu [1,2], Nikolaos Zygouropoulos [2], Alina Elena Cristea [2], Cristina Zaharia [2], George-Alexandru Rosu [1,2], Alexandra Matei [1,2], Liana-Tina Bodei [1,3], Adrian Neacsu [1,3,*] and Cringu Antoniu Ionescu [1,2]

1. Department of Obstetrics and Gynecology—"Carol Davila" University of Medicine and Pharmacy, 050474 Bucharest, Romania; irinapacu@hotmail.com (I.P.); george.rosu@drd.umfcd.ro (G.-A.R.); alexandra.matei@drd.umfcd.ro (A.M.); liana.tina.bodei@rez.umfcd.ro (L.-T.B.); cringu.ionescu@umfcd.ro (C.A.I.)
2. "St. Pantelimon" Emergency Clinical Hospital, 021623 Bucharest, Romania; nz@zitaquality.ro (N.Z.); alina.elena.cristea@rez.umfcd.ro (A.E.C.); cristina.zaharia@rez.umfcd.ro (C.Z.)
3. Bucur Maternity "Saint Ioan" Clinical Hospital, Strada Bucur nr. 6, 012363 Bucharest, Romania
* Correspondence: adrianneacsu2006@yahoo.com

Abstract: *Background and Objectives*: The aim was to evaluate the severity of obstetrical bleeding in the third trimester associated with COVID infection in placenta previa and accreta. *Materials and Methods*: A retrospective study was conducted to compare the risk of obstetrical bleeding in the case of placenta previa with or without associated SARS-CoV-2 infection. Patients presenting with placenta previa before labor were classified into three groups: group A (control) as no infection throughout their pregnancy, group B as confirmed infection during the 1st trimester, and group C as confirmed infection at the time of delivery. Infected patients were stratified according to the severity of signs and symptoms. The severity of obstetrical hemorrhage at birth was assessed quantitatively and qualitatively. All placentas were analyzed histologically to identify similarities. *Results*: Prematurity and pregnancy-induced hypertension appear significantly related to SARS-CoV-2 infection during the 3rd trimester. Placenta accreta risk increases significantly with infection during the 1st trimester. No statistically significant differences in the severity of hemorrhage associated with childbirth in cases with placenta previa between groups A and C but increased obstetrical bleeding mainly due to emergency hemostatic hysterectomy in group B driven by placenta accrete were detected. Obstetrical hemorrhage at birth in the case of coexistence of the infection was found not to correlate with the severity of the viral disease. Meanwhile, the number of days of hospitalization after birth is related to the specific treatment of COVID infection and not related to complications related to birth. *Conclusions*: The study finds an increased incidence of placenta accreta associated with placenta previa in cases where the viral infection occurred in the first trimester of pregnancy, associated with an increased incidence of hemostasis hysterectomies in these patients. Placental histological changes related to viral infection are multiple and more important in patients who had COVID infection in the first trimester.

Keywords: obstetrical bleeding; SARS-CoV-2; placenta previa; placenta accreta

1. Introduction

The COVID-19 pandemic is a reality of the last few years that has created important medical problems that were unforeseen and difficult to control, evaluate, and solve in absolutely all medical fields. Some of the most frequently encountered and controversial pathologies are related to the spectrum of coagulopathies, thrombosis, and bleeding associated with infection with the SARS-CoV-2 virus, with specific complications [1].

The impact of SARS-CoV-2 infection on the pregnant woman, fetus, and newborn is still little known, both regarding the short-term consequences during pregnancy, at the time of birth, or the long-term, distant consequences. The histopathological changes at

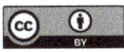

the placental level during pregnancy are already known: changes that are nonspecific but are responsible for the increased rate of premature birth and hypertension induce pregnancy [2]. Although the syncytiotrophoblast is an effective barrier to viral infections, the existence of infection at the placental level and transplacental transmission to the fetus during pregnancy by aspiration of amniotic fluid has been demonstrated [2–4].

Numerous clinical data suggest that exacerbation of the immune response in pregnancy associated with cytokine storm caused by infection with the SARS-CoV-2 virus could more easily trigger varying degrees of consumption coagulopathy [5,6]. There are currently insufficient data on the severity of obstetrical bleeding in the third trimester associated with COVID infection.

In recent years, the incidence of hemorrhages in the third trimester is increasing especially because of the increased incidence of births by cesarean section in the context of practicing defensive obstetrics, the increasing maternal age at first birth, and the use of assisted human reproduction techniques [7]. We can already observe the negative consequences related to this aspect by the increasing number of pregnant women with non-intact uteri (due to prior delivery by cesarean section) which also leads to an increased incidence of low-lying placenta and abnormal adhesions to the placenta in the following pregnancies. We can currently say that placenta previa is the main cause of obstetrical bleeding in the third trimester of pregnancy [8].

2. Materials and Methods

We conducted a retrospective study whose objective is to compare the risk of obstetrical bleeding in the case of placenta previa associated with SARS-CoV-2 infection with the risk of obstetrical bleeding related to the placenta previa unrelated to the SARS-CoV-2 infection. The study included patients who gave birth in the St. Pantelimon Obstetrics and Gynecology Clinic in Bucharest and Bucur Maternity of Saint Johns' Hospital in Bucharest between January 2018 and December 2021. During the 2020–2022 period, Bucur Maternity acted as a support maternity unit for pregnant women with SARS-CoV-2 infection.

The study was carried out with the agreement of the Ethics Council of the Hospital of Obstetrics and Gynecology "Saint Pantelimon", Bucharest, and of the Ethics Committee of the Bucur Maternity "Saint John's" Clinical Hospital, Bucharest.

Three study groups were considered:
- Group A—patients with placenta previa who do not have SARS-CoV-2 infection diagnosed from the moment of conception until birth;
- Group B—patients with placenta previa who have a history of SARS-CoV-2 infection in the first trimester of pregnancy and who are negative at the time of birth;
- Group C—positive SARS-CoV-2 patients at the time of birth only.

Patients that were diagnosed positive for SARS-CoV-2 at the time of birth and were also positive in the first trimester and/or second trimester of pregnancy were decided to be excluded from the study to isolate the effects of infection per trimester. No patients were found to fit in the above-mentioned situation. Similarly, in the case that patients were found to be positive during the second trimester but not during delivery, it was decided that they should form a group of their own. Again, no such patients were identified.

The demographic, obstetrical, birth method, and status/history of SARS-CoV-2 infection were obtained from the patients' observation sheet. Positive SARS-CoV-2 infection was diagnosed based on the results of the nasopharyngeal sample collected at the time of hospital admission and a positive result validated by an accredited laboratory; either PCR tests for the SARS-CoV-2 virus or antigenic tests were considered. Only patients for whom there was a positive PCR test result or an antigen test performed at an accredited laboratory during the first or second trimesters were considered as having reliable evidence of past infections.

SARS-CoV-2 infection at the time of birth was classified in the following categories [1,9]:
- Asymptomatic if the PCR test is positive but without respiratory or general symptoms;
- Mild if there were any of the following signs or symptoms: fever, chills, mild cough, headache, etc., but without shortness of breath, chest pain, or breathlessness;
- Moderate if there are respiratory difficulties, suggestive pulmonary imaging, and/or $SpO_2 > 94\%$;
- Severe if the respiratory rate is over 30 breaths per minute, $SpO_2 < 94\%$, severe breathlessness, cough, altered general condition, and severe respiratory failure.

The severity of obstetrical hemorrhage at birth was assessed according to the preoperative and postoperative values of hemoglobin and the calculated percentage loss of blood volume taking into consideration the effect of the number of blood units (erythrocyte concentrates) that were transfused. The average duration of the days of hospitalization and the intra- and post-operative complications were used as a qualitative aspect of the severity of obstetrical hemorrhage according to the data from the specialized literature [1,10,11]. All these aspects were retrospectively recorded from the patients' observation sheets.

The diagnosis of placenta previa was made based on the preoperative ultrasound examination performed during the evolution of pregnancy after 20 weeks of amenorrhea, with the classification of the anatomical variants of placenta previa being made as follows [12,13]:
- Grade I: low-lying placenta: placenta lies in the lower uterine segment, but its lower edge does not abut the internal cervical orifice (lower edge 0.5–2.0 cm from the internal orifice);
- Grade II: marginal previa: placental tissue reaches the margin of the internal cervical orifice, but does not cover it;
- Grade III: partial previa: placenta partially covers the internal cervical orifice;
- Grade IV: complete previa: placenta completely covers the internal cervical orifice.

The groups were compared with descriptive and bivariate statistics using Student's *t*-test for continuous variables. Chi-square test or Fisher's test were used for categorical variables. ANOVA test was used to determine if there is a statistically significant difference between two or more categorical groups. All analyses were completed using Addinsoft (2022) and XLSTAT statistical and data analysis solution, New York, NY, USA.

We analyzed macroscopic and histopathological aspects of all the placentas with the help of the Department of Pathological Anatomy within the two clinics. Ultrasound examination was performed before birth, and the diagnosis of placenta accreta was suspected in all cases. The definite diagnosis of placenta accreta was made only after the histopathological evaluation of postoperative certainty. In all cases with placenta accreta, an emergency hemostatic hysterectomy was performed.

3. Results

Between January 2018 and December 2022, the number of births in the two clinics was 10,026. The study group includes 154 patients who gave birth in these two maternity wards between January 2018 and December 2021, namely 87 (56.49%) cases during 2018–2020 and 67 (43.51%) cases during 2020–2021 with the diagnosis of placenta previa.

Group A includes 120 negative cases during pregnancy and childbirth for COVID infection (77.92%), group B includes 15 cases that presented the infection in the first trimester (9.74%), and group C includes 19 positive cases for COVID at birth (12.34%).

Demographic data and aspects related to SARS-CoV-2 infection are presented in Table 1. *p*-values shown in the tables are derived using one-way ANOVA testing between all three different groups unless otherwise stated, where groups were tested in pairs using *t*-test. In some cases, *p*-value was not calculated on the basis that either it was not significant, or comparisons between the related groups were considered either out of the scope of this research or not clinically significant.

Table 1. Demographic, obstetrical, and related characteristics of SARS-CoV-2 infection. Percentages quoted are based on specific categories expressed in comparison to the respective group.

	Group A COVID-Negative (n = 120)	Group B COVID-Positive in Trimester I (n = 15)	Group C COVID-Positive during Labor (n = 19)	p-Value (a = 0.05)
Age (in years)	25.7 ± 5.9	27.2 ± 6.0	25.6 ± 5.7	0.680
Body mass index	24.5 ± 6.1	25.9 ± 7.2	25.1 ± 5.7	0.679
Tobacco consumption				
• None	85 (70.83%)	11 (73.3%)	13 (68.42%)	0.785
• Smoker	35 (29.17%)	4 (26.7%)	6 (31.58%)	
Parity				0.885
• Nulliparous	73 (60.83%)	9 (60.00%)	12 (63.16%)	
• Multiparous	47 (39.17%)	6 (40.00%)	7 (36.84%)	
Gestational age (in weeks) at the time of delivery				Between: Group A and B: 0.0675 Group A and C: 0.0345
• Preterm, < 37 weeks	29 (24.16%)	4 (26.67%)	7 (36.84%)	
• At term ≥ 37 weeks	91 (75.84%)	11 (73.33%)	12 (63.15%)	
Placenta previa				
• Grade I	23 (19.10%)	3 (20.00%)	3 (15.79%)	$p \gg 0.05$
• Grade II	41 (34.17%)	3 (20.00%)	5 (26.32%)	
• Grade III	32 (26.67%)	4 (26.67%)	6 (31.57%)	
• Grade IV	24 (20.06%)	5 (33.33%)	5 (26.32%)	
Placenta accreta spectrum (PAS)	12 (10.00%)	5 (33.33%)	3 (15.79%)	0.496
Fetal weight (g)	2759 ± 352	2899 ± 458	2650 ± 424	
Apgar Score at 1 min postpartum	8 ± 1	9 ± 1	8 ± 1	
Mode of delivery				$\gg 0.05$
• Vaginal	23 (19.17%)	3 (20.00%)	3 (15.79%)	
• Cesarean section	97 (80.83%)	12 (80.00%)	16 (84.21%)	
Anesthesia type				
• None	12 (10.00%)	2 (13.33%)	2 (10.52%)	
• Spinal/epidural	86 (71.67%)	10 (66.66%)	10 (52.63%)	
• General	22 (18.33%)	3 (20.00%)	7 (36.84%)	
The severity of SARS-CoV-2 infection				
• Asymptomatic	0	3 (20.00%)	4 (21.05%)	
• Mild	0	7 (46.67%)	9 (47.37%)	
• Moderate	0	5 (33.33%)	5 (26.31%)	
• Severe	0	0	1 (5.27%)	

Table 2 includes comparative data on the severity of obstetrical hemorrhage between the three study groups.

We also performed a comparative analysis between the severity of obstetrical hemorrhage and the clinical form of the COVID infection, with data presented in Table 3.

Table 4 presents the analysis of the causes of hysterectomy of hemostasis in the study groups.

From the histopathological point of view, placental changes were analyzed in all groups, comparatively analyzing (Table 5) the incidence of abnormalities associated with COVID infection in pregnancy, according to the studies carried out so far [2,4].

Table 2. Comparison between the three groups on the severity of obstetrical hemorrhage and postoperative morbidity.

	Group A (n = 120)	Group B (n = 15)	Group C (n = 19)	p
Preoperative/Prelabor hemoglobin (g/dL)	11.3 ± 0.7	11.7 ± 1.2	11.5 ± 0.9	>>0.05
Postoperative/Postpartum hemoglobin (g/dL)	10.2 ± 0.6	9.7 ± 1.1	10.2 ± 0.8	Between: Group A and B: 0.022 Group A and C: >>0.05
Decrease in hemoglobin (%)	11.2 ± 3.5	17.8 ± 4.1	13.5 ± 3.9	Between: Group A and B: 0.023 Group A and C: 0.065
Blood transfusion—erythrocytes concentrate (IU)	2.3 ± 1.1	3.9 ± 2.2	2.1 ± 1.2	
Hospitalization (days)				
• 3–5 days	45 (37.5%)	3 (20.00%)	5 (26.31%)	
• 6–7 days	59 (49.16%)	7 (46.67%)	10 (52.63%)	
• >7 days	16 (13.30%)	5 (33.33%)	4 (21.05%)	
No complications	87 (72.5%)			
Complications				
• Bladder injury	5 (4.17%)	2 (13.3%)	1 (5.26%)	
• Coagulopathy	1 (0.83%)	1 (6.66%)	0	
• Uterine relaxation	5 (4.17%)	0	1 (5.26%)	
• Infection	0	1 (6.66%)	1 (5.26%)	
• Hysterectomy	12 (10%)	4 (26.67%)	3 (15.79%)	
• Re-exploration	1 (0.83%)	0	0	
• Thrombosis	0	1 (6.66%)	1 (5.26%)	

Table 3. Comparison between the severity of obstetrical bleeding and the clinical form of SARS-CoV-2 infection.

	Asymptomatic Form (n = 7)	Mild Form (n = 16)	Moderate Form (n = 8)	Severe Form (n = 1)	p-Value (a = 0.05)
Preoperative/Prelabor hemoglobin (g/dL)	11.2 ± 1.2	11.4 ± 1.1	10.5 ± 2.1	9.8 ± 1.5	
Postoperative/Prelabor hemoglobin (g/dL)	10.1 ± 0.9	10.7 ± 1.5	9.8 ± 1.8	9.7 ± 1.2	
Decrease in hemoglobin (%)	10.1 ± 0.5	9.5 ± 1.7	11.5 ± 1.6	6.5 ± 1.9	$p > 0.05$
Blood transfusion—erythrocytes concentrate (IU)	1.6 ± 1.0	1.8 ± 1.6	2.2 ± 2.0	2.1 ± 1.8	
Hospitalization (days)					
• 3–5 days	5 (71.42%)	10 (62.50%)	5 (62.50%)	0	
• 6–7 days	1 (14.29%)	3 (18.75%)	1 (12.50%)	0	
• >7 days	1 (14.29%)	3 (18.75%)	2 (25.00%)	1 (100.00%)	
No complications					
Complications					
• Bladder injury	0	1 (6.25%)	1 (12.50%)	1 (100.00%)	
• Coagulopathy	0	0	0	1 (100.00%)	
• Uterine relaxation	1 (14.2%)	0	1 (12.50%)	0	
• Infection	0	1	0	1 (100.00%)	
• Hysterectomy	1	3	2 (25.00%)	0	
• Re-exploration	0	0	0	0	
• Thrombosis	0	0	1 (12.50%)	1 (100.00%)	

Table 4. Causes of hysterectomy of hemostasis per group. Percentages quoted to indicate the percentage of hysterectomy cases per group.

Cause	Group A (n = 120)	Group B (n = 15)	Group C (n = 19)	p-value (a = 0.05)
PAS	3 (2.50%)	3 (20.00%)	1 (5.26%)	0.0243
Uterine relaxation	4 (3.33%)	0	1 (5.26%)	
Uterine myoma	2 (1.67%)	1 (6.67%)	0	
Other	1 (0.83%)	0	1 (5.26%)	
Total per group	10 (8.33%)	4 (26.67%)	3 (20.0%)	0.0126

Table 5. Comparison of placenta microscopic features of COVID-19 versus the control group A (non-COVID placenta previa group).

Microscopic Features	Group A (n = 120), Control Group	Group B (n = 15)	Group C (n = 19)
Increased microcalcifications	15 (12.50%)	5 (33.33%)	5 (26.31%)
Chorangiosis	5 (4.17%)	4 (26.66%)	3 (15.79%)
Villous agglutination	3 (2.50%)	3 (20.00%)	3 (15.79%)
Increased fibrin deposits	11 (9.17%)	4 (26.67%)	5 (26.31%)
Local thrombosis	13 (10.83%)	5 (33.33%)	4 (21.05%)
Increased syncytial knotting	2 (1.67%)	5 (33.33%)	2 (10.53%)
Delayed villous maturity	4 (3.33%)	3 (20.00%)	2 (10.53%)

4. Discussion

Regarding the demographic data, there are no statistically significant differences in terms of age, parity, BMI, or tobacco consumption between group A and group B or C as proven when testing for homogeneity.

There are no statistically significant differences between the obstetrical data, but still, the patients who had COVID in the first or third trimester during pregnancy have an increased rate of premature birth, independent of the coexistence of the placenta previa. This increase premature birth is only found to be statistically significant for group C ($p = 0.0345$, < 0.05) and not for group B ($p = 0.0675$, < 0.05). These data are similar to those in the literature that attests to the increased incidence of premature birth and the association with pregnancy-induced hypertension in the 3rd trimester (17% vs. 8.7% for preterm birth, 18.9% vs. 7.8% for preeclampsia) [1,14,15]. When analyzing using unadjusted odds ratios, it was found that it is 45.4% for group C and only 12.4% for group B more likely in comparison to group A to deliver prematurely.

Concerning the fetal outcome, as defined by fetal weight and Apgar score, homogeneity was confirmed between group A and group B or C. There are no statistically significant differences in fetal prognosis (weight, Apgar score). The birth was performed in 125 cases (81.17%) by cesarean section and in only 29 cases (18.83%) vaginally, with these being the cases with minimal bleeding and 1st degree placenta previa. There are no significant differences in the mode of delivery between groups, and correlation testing proved that COVID infection, albeit in the 1st trimester or active irrespective of severity, did not significantly influence delivery mode.

There are no statistically significant differences ($p >> 0.05$ using one-way ANOVA) between the three groups regarding the type of placenta previa.

An increased incidence of placenta accreta is observed in the group of patients who had SARS-CoV-2 infection in the first trimester of pregnancy (weeks 5–14 of amenorrhea) at the time of trophoblast formation. The odds ratio (OR) for placentation not to be accreta in group B was calculated at 0.22 (0.065–0.759, CI 95%) and 0.592 in group C (0.151–2.332, CI 95%).

Most COVID infections are asymptomatic and mild, without statistically significant differences between the three groups. There was only one serious case with respiratory failure that required hospitalization in the intensive care unit, with the birth being performed by emergency cesarean section surgery for maternal purposes at 35 weeks of amenorrhea. Maternal and fetal evolution was favorable, with an increased number of days of hospitalizations (27 days).

It is worth noting an increased incidence of pregnancies with placenta previa (154 cases out of the total of 10,026 births, 1.536%) compared to the data from the specialized literature, (0.15–1.1%) [16,17], which is explained by the framing of the two centers in which the study was conducted in the category of grade III maternity wards, with a significantly increased addressability of pregnancies with high obstetrical risk. In addition, between 2020–2021, Bucur Maternity Hospital was the only unit in Bucharest and the surrounding areas dedicated to childbirth assistance exclusively for patients with COVID infection. There are no differences in the incidence of pregnancies with placenta previa in the period 2018–2019 (1.5%) compared to the period 2020–2012 (1.582%).

To date, there are very few studies to try to evaluate blood loss at birth and postoperative morbidity in obstetrical bleeding associated with COVID infection, and the studies that have been conducted include a small number of cases [1]. For the non-pregnant population, there are studies and case presentations that report morbidity and mortality associated with COVID infection, and the data are still controversial due to the heterogeneity of laboratory data and the difficulty of unitary quantification of blood loss. More data are needed in this regard, and the present study aims to guide the public and anesthesiologists in establishing as correctly as possible the hemorrhagic risk for these pregnant women, especially when it is associated with other obstetrical causes of severe hemorrhage.

4.1. Hemostasis Changes in COVID Infection

Abnormalities of blood clotting are characteristic of COVID infection, directly proportional to the severity of the disease. Starting from an altered inflammatory response, the balance between pro and anticoagulant factors changes and endothelial dysfunction plays a major role [18]. Changes in blood growth during the COVID infection proved to be the main prognostic factor regarding the evolution of the disease [19].

There is also thrombocyte hyperactivity that is more pronounced in severe cases and that participates in thrombotic complications [18]. Patients with increased platelet/lymphocyte ratio have an increased duration of the disease [19,20]. The SARS-CoV-2 virus inhibits hemopoiesis via CD-13 receptors, which leads to the possibility of thrombocytopenia, especially in the case of increased bleeding in other coexisting pathologies. [18]

The initial procoagulant status was initially considered to be part of the first phase of the disseminated intravascular coagulation (DIC) process but is currently considered not to meet the DIC criteria of the International Society of Thrombosis and Haemostasis [18].

4.2. Hemostasis in Pregnancy

Pregnancy is a procoagulant diathesis with the increase of prothrombotic factors VII, VIII, X, XI, von Willebrand, and fibrinogen and the decrease of the S protein and the alteration of the fibrinolysis. It is mandatory to recognize all prothrombotic risk factors for pregnant women to establish thromboprophylaxis in pregnancy and postpartum [21], with COVID infection being part of this category.

4.3. Impact of COVID on Blood Clotting during Pregnancy

Since the first trimester of pregnancy, COVID association increases thrombotic risk, with the risk being maximum in the third trimester, in association with maternal obesity, thrombotic history, thrombophilia, age over 35 years, and diabetes mellitus [3]. The risk is directly proportional to the severity of the viral infection, with the condition of bed immobilization of the pregnant woman adding to the additional factors related to prolonged venous stasis [19,20].

Under the conditions of association of severe obstetrical bleeding in the third trimester with COVID infection, all these factors cause an increased risk of developing DIC [18–20].

In our study, initial preoperative/prelabor hemoglobin levels had no significance difference between the three groups ($p \gg 0.05$), while postoperative/postpartum hemoglobin levels were significantly different between group A and B ($p = 0.022$) and not between A and C ($p = 0.0045$). Similarly, when blood loss during delivery was expressed as a percentage decrease of hemoglobin during labor, groups A and B had a significant difference ($p = 0.023$), and groups A and C did not ($p = 0.065$). All in all, values of paraclinical analyses and postoperative morbidity did not yield statistically significant differences in the severity of hemorrhage associated with childbirth in cases with placenta previa between groups A and C but did between groups A and B, primarily driven by an increased incidence of obstetrical bleeding and emergency hemostatic hysterectomy in group B of patients who had SARS-CoV-2 infection in the first trimester ($p = 0.0243$, CI 95%). This result is related to a significantly increased incidence ($p = 0.496$, CI 95%) of abnormal adhesions of the placenta (Table 1) and an increased rate of hysterectomies of hemostasis ($p < 0.05$), as shown in Table 2.

General anesthesia by orotracheal intubation (IOT) predominates in the group of patients with placenta accreta (Table 1), but this is mainly driven by operative considerations rather than COVID status.

The results overlap with the data of other studies [1,21] that do not identify an increased risk of obstetrical hemorrhage at birth in the case of coexistence of the infection, and there is no correlation with the severity of the viral disease (Table 3). One-way ANOVA proved no significant differences between groups.

The number of days of hospitalization after birth is increased for medium and severe cases related to the specific treatment of COVID infection and not related to complications related to placenta previa. A correlation study between hospitalization days and infection severity yielded an r^2 value of 0.886 in comparison to hospitalization days and complications directly linked to PAS of 0.456.

Intraoperative lesions of the bladder, coagulopathy, and reinterventions were more common in group B and related to hysterectomies of hemostasis, but again, statistically, no significance could be proven ($p \gg 0.05$). There are no statistically significant differences between uterine relaxation, postoperative infection, or thrombotic complications. It should be mentioned that in all cases, postoperative antithrombotic prophylaxis with low-molecular-weight heparin preparations was performed.

According to the data from the literature [1,3,5], the incidence of emergency hemostatic hysterectomies in pregnancies associated with the placenta previa is increased (4, 4–5, 9%). Further, a statistically significant increase in the incidence of emergency hysterectomies was found between group A and groups B and C cumulatively ($p = 0.0126$, CI 95%), while no significant difference was found between groups B and C.

Table 4 presents the analysis of the causes of hysterectomy of hemostasis in the study groups. It provides the insight that the increased incidence of hysterectomies is mainly driven by PAS in group B. with a significant difference in comparison to groups A and C ($p = 0.0243$, $p < 0.05$, CI 95%), while in group C, there is not a specific cause predominating, and in group A, PAS and uterine relaxation remain the predominant causes.

The necessity of hemostasis hysterectomy was achieved mainly for abnormal adhesions of the placenta (placenta accreta), their incidence being superior in the group of patients who had SARS-CoV-2 infection in the first trimester of pregnancy ($p = 0.243$, $a = 0.05$), without there being statistically significant differences between the main risk factors of the placenta accreta between the three groups (Table 4). The highest incidence of placenta accreta associated with placenta previa was found in group B of the study, between groups A and C. The OR for placentation not to be accreta in group B was calculated at 0.22 (0.065–0.759, CI 95%) and 0.592 in group C (0.151–2.332, CI 95%). There is an increased risk of placental changes for group B of the patients who had COVID infection in the first trimester of pregnancy compared to those who were positive at the time of birth, i.e., those who presented the infection in the third trimester.

However, analyzing all the cases with placenta previa, we identified that study group B of the patients with a history of SARS-CoV-2 infection in the first trimester of pregnancy and who, compared to the positive patients in the third trimester or those who have no history of COVID infection, had a statistically significant difference regarding the possibility of a severe obstetrical hemorrhage at birth. No testing for COVID-19 has been done at the placental level under any circumstances. No case of COVID infection was registered in newborns in the case of maternal infection at the time of birth; all newborns with COVID-positive mothers were tested at the time of birth. Group B recorded the highest loss of blood volume, on average $17.1 \pm 3.5\%$, followed by group C with $13.5 \pm 3.9\%$ in comparison to group A at $11.2 \pm 3.5\%$, with statistical significance when comparing group A with B or C ($p = 0.0234$ and $p = 0.0445$, respectively, for CI 95%) and having considered transfusions. In terms of transfusions, group B had the largest average with 3.9 ± 2.2 units in comparison to group A or B with 2.3 ± 1.1 or 2.1 ± 1.2, respectively. Statistical significance was identified only between groups B and A but not for groups A and C. The average number of days of hospitalization was maximum, where most intra- and postoperative complications occurred. In this regard, it is worth noting the statistically significant difference regarding the hysterectomies of hemostasis, the maximum percentage being in the group of patients who had COVID infection in the first trimester, with most of them having as an indication the placenta accreta. The increased incidence of hysterectomies is mainly driven by PAS in group B with a significant difference in comparison to groups A and C ($p = 0.0243$, $p < 0.05$, CI 95%), while in group C, there is not a specific cause predominating, and in group A, PAS and uterine relaxation remain the predominant causes.

There are no statistically significant differences between the three groups related to the risk factors known for PAS.

Starting from these statistical results, we analyzed data from the specialized literature related to the placental histopathological changes in the COVID infection that could explain the practical clinical aspects revealed by the present study [22–24].

It is well-known that the immune status in pregnancy is modified in the sense of adapting to accept an allograft that is the product of conception, leading to a specific immune maternal response to the different types of infections that may occur during pregnancy [25,26]. During the COVID infection, the functionality of the NK cells is also altered, which overlaps with the reduction of their number that occurs physiologically during pregnancy [25,26]. In pregnancy, there are alterations of the CD4+ population, predominantly of the phenotype T-Helper-2 compared to T-Helper-1, which explains maternal immune tolerance [25].

In the task, there is a special pattern of recognition of Toll-like receptors (TLRs), especially TLR4. Three levels of activation of these receptors shall be described. The first level is represented by the activation from the first trimester at the time of implantation of the blastocyst, the second occurs in the second trimester to reduce the pro-inflammatory phenomena that would be physiologically stimulated by fetal growth, and the last is represented by the increased activation in the third trimester to support labor and delivery [26,27]. Infection with the SARS-CoV-2 virus prevents the release of proteins that become ligands for TLR molecules, which exacerbates the immune response from the moment of implantation and formation of the placenta. Further studies will determine whether these phenomena are the basis of the increased susceptibility to infection of the pregnant woman or are protective against infection during pregnancy [26].

The SARS-CoV-2 virus penetrates the nasal mucosa by binding to the angiotensin-converting enzyme 2 receptors (ACE2), which is also found in the digestive tract, placenta, ovary, uterus, and vagina. Intracellular penetration is facilitated by the spike protein at the viral level via trans-serine membranes protease 2 (TMPRSS2) [26]. The cells with the highest susceptibility to being virally infected are those that express both ACE2 and TMPRSS2 [26]. The cells of syncytio- and cyto-trophoblasts express ACE2 from week 7, and thus, there is the possibility of transplacental transmission from the onset of pregnancy.

There are no studies that identify placental pathological changes at the macroscopic level. From the microscopic point of view, non-specific changes such as old or recent microthrombi, infarcts, and fibrin deposits that move the villi of the spines towards the periphery have been described [27]. In cases with reduced maternal-traumatic infusion, the characteristic lesions were those of chorangiosis (the presence of over 10 terminal villi with over 10 capillaries in over three different placental areas), delay in villous maturation [27], and increased syncytial knotting [28]. Chorangiosis is an adaptive response to reduce blood infusion that causes hypoxia and is associated in most cases with maternal desaturation [23]. Increased syncytial knotting appears to be related to the state of hypercoagulability in the COVID infection [29].

Inflammatory lesions at the placental level have been suggested by the increased number of Hoffbauer cells at this level, which is known to be involved in the vertical transmission of viral infections [28]. These are macrophages localized since the beginning of pregnancy at the level of the chorionic villi, being involved in phagocytosis of the apoptotic material and antigen presentation in response to infectious agents.

The starting point of PAS is an incorrect decidualization, which leads to an abnormal invasion of the trophoblast from the moment of its formation. From the histopathological point of view, there is an increased incidence of placental basal chorionic inflammation, maternal vascular changes that lead to abnormalities of maternal circulation, and placental intervillous hemorrhages. Microscopic examination of the placenta will reveal in all cases the presence at the level of the placental basal plaque of myometrial fibers [28].

The development of the placenta is a multifactorial complex and incompletely known process. Hypotheses related to placental abnormal adhesions converge on a combination of the absence of basal plaque, exaggerated extravillous trophoblastic invasion, and abnormal maternal vascular proliferation [24,26,28]. Multiple parallels were made between the abnormal placental invasion in PAS and the tumor proliferation model, in both cases being an increased ability of trophoblastic cells to overcome the local immune systems, induce exaggerated angiogenesis, and activate tissue invasion, often associating a localized inflammatory process [28].

A long-studied aspect is the association between PAS and chronic basal inflammation. It is not known exactly which lymphocytic subpopulations [22] are involved and what their contributions are. Ernst et al. [24] demonstrated that there is an increased lymphocytic infiltrate at the level of the placental implantation site in the case of PAS compared to other pathologies. There appears to be a low number of CD4+ T lymphocytes and an increase in CD25+ lymphocytes compared to normal pregnancy, suggesting a suppression of the immune response mediated by T cells. Increased trophoblastic invasion without differences in cellular dendritic density suggests an immunological dysfunction at the deciduous level [1,22]. In addition, natural killer deciduous cells (dNK), which are the only natural killer cells that play an important role in the early stages of pregnancy, are significantly reduced in the placentas of PAS [22].

There is an obvious overlap between the local and general uterine disturbances that lead to the appearance of PAS in general and the placental changes generated by the COVID infection, which could explain the increased incidence of PAS in cases where the viral infection occurred in the first trimester of pregnancy.

The histological analysis of the placenta previa of the patients included in the present study identifies in the case of patients with infection in the I and II trimesters of the increased prevalence of microcalcifications, fibrin deposits, chorioangiosis lesions, syncial knotting, and local villous inflammation towards patients who did not have the infection in pregnancy. These lesions have significantly increased incidence for patients who had the infection in the first trimester of pregnancy and who present PAS; the group of patients with COVID infection at birth has an increased incidence of local thrombosis. These changes could be in the context of the procoagulant status given by the viral infection or represent a pattern of abnormal proliferation of the trophoblast.

The study makes an important contribution to placental histopathological changes related to SARS-CoV-2 virus infection and the increased risk for abnormal placenta adhesions even in conditions of mild or symptomatic infections. Cesarian is important to be performed in a third-degree maternity ward with addressability for high obstetrical risk cases, including SARS-CoV-2 infection.

The limit of the study is given by the fact that there may be cases of asymptomatic COVID infections, so the number of patients who presented the infection in the first trimester can be changed. These preliminary data should be confirmed by more extensive studies that include a larger number of patients, but the present results may be a starting point for future research.

5. Conclusions

SARS-CoV-2 is the pathogen responsible for the current pandemic situation, and there is still no complete data on all the pathophysiological aspects related to this infection. Its implications on pregnancy and maternal and fetal prognosis in the long term is further researched, as the complete discovery of these can be useful in the correct evaluation of many infectious pathologies in pregnancy. There are certain data related to the increased incidence of hypertension induced by pregnancy, premature birth, and low fetal birth weight in pregnant women with COVID infection in pregnancy. There are not yet enough, and complete studies related to hemorrhages in pregnancy associated with this infection and this study can complete these data. The results of the study confirm the data from the specialized literature that do not report an increased incidence and severity of bleeding in the third trimester under the conditions of COVID infection at birth in patients with placenta previa. However, the study finds an increased incidence of PAS associated with placenta previa in cases where the viral infection occurred in the first trimester of pregnancy, associated with an increased incidence of hemostasis hysterectomies in these patients. Consequently, we consider that a perspective study should be pursued regarding timeliness of COVID infection during pregnancy and PAS-associated placenta previa. Further, we wish to draw attention to medical professionals that timeliness of past COVID infections is another parameter that perhaps needs to be taken into consideration while probing for a patients personal history. Lastly, placental histological changes related to viral infection are multiple and more important in patients who had COVID infection in the first trimester.

Author Contributions: Conceptualization, I.P., C.A.I. and A.N.; methodology, C.Z., G.-A.R. and A.M.; software, L.-T.B., A.E.C. and A.N.; validation, I.P., A.N. and N.Z.; formal analysis, N.Z., G.-A.R. and A.M.; investigation, C.A.I., I.P., N.Z. and A.E.C.; resources, A.N, G.-A.R. and A.M.; data curation, I.P., N.Z., A.E.C. and C.A.I.; writing—original draft preparation, A.M, A.N., N.Z. and G.-A.R.; writing—review and editing, I.P. and C.A.I.; visualization, L.-T.B., C.Z. and A.E.C.; supervision, I.P., A.N. and C.A.I.; project administration, I.P., C.A.I. and A.M. All authors have read and agreed to the published version of the manuscript.

Funding: This research received no external funding.

Institutional Review Board Statement: Patients provided signed informed consent regarding the experimental treatment. They were allowed to terminate their participation at any stage without prejudice.

Informed Consent Statement: Patients provided a signed informed consent regarding the use, storage, and manipulation of the data collected and agreed to be published anonymously.

Data Availability Statement: All data (except actual experimental data) and information were collected through open or paid databases containing published journals. Experimental raw data collected during the study are available on request in accordance with the provisions stipulated in the patient consent for publication.

Conflicts of Interest: The authors declare that they have no conflict interest that would prejudice the impartiality of the research reported.

References

1. Wang, M.J.; Schapero, M.; Iverson, R.; Yarrington, C.D.; Wang, J. Obstetric Hemorrhage Risk Associated with Novel COVID-19 Diagnosis from a Single-Institution Cohort in the United States. *Am. J. Perinatol.* **2020**, *37*, 1411–1416. [CrossRef]
2. Hecht, J.L.; Quade, B.; Deshpande, V.; Mino-Kenudson, M.; Ting, D.T.; Desai, N.; Dygulska, B.; Heyman, T.; Salafia, C.; Shen, D.; et al. SARS-CoV-2 Can Infect the Placenta and Is Not Associated with Specific Placental Histopathology: A Series of 19 Placentas from COVID-19-Positive Mothers. *Mod. Pathol.* **2020**, *33*, 1. [CrossRef]
3. Liu, Y.; Chen, H.; Tang, K.; Guo, Y. Withdrawn: Clinical Manifestations and Outcome of SARS-CoV-2 Infection during Pregnancy. *J. Infect.* **2020**. Epub ahead of print. [CrossRef]
4. Hosier, H.; Farhadian, S.F.; Morotti, R.A.; Deshmukh, U.; Lu-Culligan, A.; Campbell, K.H.; Yasumoto, Y.; Vogels, C.B.F.; Casanovas-Massana, A.; Vijayakumar, P.; et al. SARS-CoV-2 Infection of the Placenta. *J. Clin. Investig.* **2020**, *130*, 4947–4953. [CrossRef]
5. Koumoutsea, E.V.; Vivanti, A.J.; Shehata, N.; Benachi, A.; Gouez, A.L.; Desconclois, C.; Whittle, W.; Snelgrove, J.; Malinowski, A.K. COVID-19 and Acute Coagulopathy in Pregnancy. *J. Thromb. Haemost. JTH* **2020**, *18*, 1648–1652. [CrossRef]
6. Liao, J.; He, X.; Gong, Q.; Yang, L.; Zhou, C.; Li, J. Analysis of Vaginal Delivery Outcomes among Pregnant Women in Wuhan, China during the COVID-19 Pandemic. *Int. J. Gynecol. Obstet.* **2020**, *150*, 53–57. [CrossRef]
7. Zhou, C.; Zhao, Y.; Li, Y. Clinical Analysis of Factors Influencing the Development of Placenta Praevia and Perinatal Outcomes in First-Time Pregnant Patients. *Front. Surg.* **2022**, *9*, 862655. [CrossRef]
8. Park, H.-S.; Cho, H.-S. Management of Massive Hemorrhage in Pregnant Women with Placenta Previa. *Anesth. Pain Med.* **2020**, *15*, 409–416. [CrossRef]
9. National Institute for Health and Care Excellence (NICE); Scottish Intercollegiate Guidelines Network (SIGN); Royal College of General Practitioners (RCGP). COVID-19 Rapid Guideline: Managing the Longterm Effects of COVID-19. Last Updated 11 November 2021. Available online: https://www.nice.org.uk/guidance/ng188 (accessed on 15 January 2022).
10. Bose, P.; Regan, F.; Paterson-Brown, S. Improving the Accuracy of Estimated Blood Loss at Obstetric Haemorrhage Using Clinical Reconstructions. *BJOG Int. J. Obstet. Gynaecol.* **2006**, *113*, 919–924. [CrossRef]
11. Kerr, R.S.; Weeks, A.D. Postpartum Haemorrhage: A Single Definition is No Longer Enough. *BJOG Int. J. Obstet. Gynaecol.* **2017**, *124*, 723–726. [CrossRef]
12. Quant, H.S.; Friedman, A.M.; Wang, E.; Parry, S.; Schwartz, N. Transabdominal Ultrasonography as a Screening Test for Second-Trimester Placenta Previa. *Obstet. Gynecol.* **2014**, *123*, 628–633. [CrossRef] [PubMed]
13. Kollmann, M.; Gaulhofer, J.; Lang, U.; Klaritsch, P. Placenta Praevia: Incidence, Risk Factors and Outcome. *J. Matern. Fetal Neonatal Med.* **2016**, *29*, 1395–1398. [CrossRef] [PubMed]
14. Jang, D.G.; We, J.S.; Shin, J.U.; Choi, Y.J.; Ko, H.S.; Park, I.Y.; Shin, J.C. Maternal Outcomes According to Placental Position in Placental Previa. *Int. J. Med. Sci.* **2011**, *8*, 439–444. [CrossRef]
15. Ahmed, S.R.; Aitallah, A.; Abdelghafar, H.M.; Alsammani, M.A. Major Placenta Previa: Rate, Maternal and Neonatal Outcomes Experience at a Tertiary Maternity Hospital, Sohag, Egypt: A Prospective Study. *J. Clin. Diagn. Res. JCDR* **2015**, *9*, QC17–QC19. [CrossRef] [PubMed]
16. Lockwood, C.J.; Russo-Steiglitz, K. Placenta Praevia: Epidemiology, Clinical Features, Diagnosis, Morbidity and Mortality. Uptodate. Available online: https://www.medilib.ir/uptodate/show/6772 (accessed on 15 January 2022).
17. Jauniaux, E.; Grønbeck, L.; Bunce, C.; Langhoff-Roos, J.; Collins, S.L. Epidemiology of Placenta Previa Accreta: A Systematic Review and Meta-Analysis. *BMJ Open* **2019**, *9*, e031193. [CrossRef]
18. Daru, J.; White, K.; Hunt, B.J. COVID-19, Thrombosis and Pregnancy. *Thromb. Update* **2021**, *5*, 100077. [CrossRef]
19. D'Souza, R.; Malhamé, I.; Teshler, L.; Acharya, G.; Hunt, B.J.; McLintock, C. A Critical Review of the Pathophysiology of Thrombotic Complications and Clinical Practice Recommendations for Thromboprophylaxis in Pregnant Patients with COVID-19. *Acta Obstet. Gynecol. Scand.* **2020**, *99*, 1110–1120. [CrossRef]
20. Servante, J.; Swallow, G.; Thornton, J.G.; Myers, B.; Munireddy, S.; Malinowski, A.K.; Othman, M.; Li, W.; O'Donoghue, K.; Walker, K.F. Haemostatic and Thrombo-Embolic Complications in Pregnant Women with COVID-19: A Systematic Review and Critical Analysis. *BMC Pregnancy Childbirth* **2021**, *21*, 108. [CrossRef]
21. Guidance, 13th Feburary 2021. Available online: https://www.rcog.org.uk/globalassets/documents/guidelines/2021-02-19-coronavirus-covid-19-infection-in-pregnancy-v13.pdf (accessed on 9 July 2021).
22. Gelany, S.E.; Mosbeh, M.H.; Ibrahim, E.M.; Mohammed, M.; Khalifa, E.M.; Abdelhakium, A.K.; Yousef, A.M.; Hassan, H.; Goma, K.; Alghany, A.A.; et al. Placenta Accreta Spectrum (PAS) Disorders: Incidence, Risk Factors and Outcomes of Different Management Strategies in a Tertiary Referral Hospital in Minia, Egypt: A Prospective Study. *BMC Pregnancy Childbirth* **2019**, *19*, 313. [CrossRef]
23. Menter, T.; Mertz, K.D.; Jiang, S.; Chen, H.; Monod, C.; Tzankov, A.; Waldvogel, S.; Schulzke, S.M.; Hösli, I.; Bruder, E. Placental Pathology Findings during and after SARS-CoV-2 Infection: Features of Villitis and Malperfusion. *Pathobiol. J. Immunopathol. Mol. Cell. Biol.* **2021**, *88*, 69–77. [CrossRef]
24. Shanes, E.D.; Mithal, L.B.; Otero, S.; Azad, H.A.; Miller, E.S.; Goldstein, J.A. Placental Pathology in COVID-19. *Am. J. Clin. Pathol.* **2020**, *154*, 23–32. [CrossRef] [PubMed]
25. Racicot, K.; Mor, G. Risks Associated with Viral Infections during Pregnancy. *J. Clin. Invest.* **2017**, *127*, 1591. [CrossRef] [PubMed]

26. Rad, H.S.; Röhl, J.; Stylianou, N.; Allenby, M.C.; Bazaz, S.R.; Warkiani, M.E.; Guimaraes, F.S.F.; Clifton, V.L.; Kulasinghe, A. The Effects of COVID-19 on the Placenta during Pregnancy. *Front. Immunol.* **2021**, *12*, 743022. [CrossRef] [PubMed]
27. Baergen, R.N.; Heller, D.S. Placental Pathology in COVID-19 Positive Mothers: Preliminary Findings. *Pediatr. Dev. Pathol. Off. J. Soc. Pediatr. Pathol. Paediatr. Pathol. Soc.* **2020**, *23*, 177–180. [CrossRef] [PubMed]
28. Singh, N.; Buckley, T.; Shertz, W. Placental Pathology in COVID-19: Case Series in a Community Hospital Setting. *Cureus* **2021**, *13*, e12522. [CrossRef]
29. Giordano, G.; Petrolini, C.; Corradini, E.; Campanini, N.; Esposito, S.; Perrone, S. COVID-19 in Pregnancy: Placental Pathological Patterns and Effect on Perinatal Outcome in Five Cases. *Diagn. Pathol.* **2021**, *16*, 88. [CrossRef]

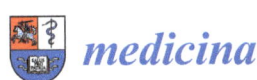

Case Report

Management of Postpartum Extensive Venous Thrombosis after Second Pregnancy

Andreea Taisia Tiron [1,2,†], Anca Filofteia Briceag [2,†], Liviu Moraru [3,*], Lavinia Alice Bălăceanu [1,4], Ion Dina [1,5] and Laura Caravia [6]

1. Faculty of Medicine, "Carol Davila" University of Medicine and Pharmacy, 050474 Bucharest, Romania; taisia_andreea@yahoo.com (A.T.T.); alicebalaceanu@yahoo.com (L.A.B.); ion.dina@umfcd.ro (I.D.)
2. Department of Cardiology, "St. John" Emergency Hospital, 13 Vitan Barzesti Street, 042122 Bucharest, Romania; briceag_anca@yahoo.ro
3. Department of Anatomy, "George Emil Palade" University of Medicine, Pharmacy, Sciences and Technology, 540142 Targu Mures, Romania
4. Department of Internal Medicine, "St. John" Emergency Hospital, 13 Vitan Barzesti Street, 042122 Bucharest, Romania
5. Department of Gastroenterology, "St. John" Emergency Hospital, 13 Vitan Barzesti Street, 042122 Bucharest, Romania
6. Division of Cellular and Molecular Biology and Histology, Department of Morphological Sciences "Carol Davila" University of Medicine and Pharmacy, 050474 Bucharest, Romania; laura.caravia@umfcd.ro
* Correspondence: liviu.moraru@umfst.ro
† These authors contributed equally to this work.

Abstract: *Background*: Pregnancy induces a physiological prothrombotic state. The highest risk period for venous thromboembolism and pulmonary embolism in pregnant women is during the postpartum period. *Materials and Methods*: We present the case of a young woman who gave birth 2 weeks before admission and was transferred to our clinic for edema. She had an increased temperature in her right limb, and a venous Doppler of the limb confirmed thrombosis of the right femoral vein. From the paraclinical examination, we obtained a CBC with leukocytosis, neutrophilia, and thrombocytosis, and a positive D-dimer test. Thrombophilic tests were negative for AT III, lupus anticoagulant negative, and protein S and C, but were positive for heterozygous PAI-1, heterozygous MTHFR A1298C, and EPCR with A1/A2 alleles. After 2 days of UFH with therapeutic APTT, the patient had pain in her left thigh. We performed a venous Doppler, which revealed bilateral femoral and iliac venous thrombosis. During the computed tomography examination, we assessed the venous thrombosis extension on the inferior cava, common iliac, and bilateral common femoral veins. Thrombolysis was initiated with 100 mg of Alteplase given at a rate of 2 mg/h; however, this did not lead to a considerable reduction in the thrombus. Additionally, the treatment with UFH was continued under therapeutic APTT. After 7 days of UFH and triple antibiotic therapy for genital sepsis, the patient had a favorable evolution with remission of venous thrombosis. *Results*: Alteplase is a thrombolytic agent that is created with recombinant DNA technology, and it was successfully used to treat thrombosis that occurred in the postpartum period. *Conclusions*: Thrombophilias are associated with a high VTE risk but also with adverse pregnancy outcomes, including recurrent miscarriages and gestational vascular complications. In addition, the postpartum period is associated with a higher VTE risk. A thrombophilic status with heterozygous PAI-1, heterozygous MTHFR A1298C, and EPCR with A1/A2 positive alleles is associated with a high risk of thrombosis and cardiovascular events. Thrombolysis can be successfully used postpartum to treat VTEs. Thrombolysis can be used successfully in VTE developed in the postpartum period.

Keywords: postpartum; venous thrombosis; pregnancy; management

Citation: Tiron, A.T.; Briceag, A.F.; Moraru, L.; Bălăceanu, L.A.; Dina, I.; Caravia, L. Management of Postpartum Extensive Venous Thrombosis after Second Pregnancy. *Medicina* 2023, *59*, 871. https://doi.org/10.3390/medicina59050871

Academic Editors: Marius L. Craina and Elena Bernad

Received: 10 March 2023
Revised: 18 April 2023
Accepted: 26 April 2023
Published: 30 April 2023

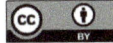

Copyright: © 2023 by the authors. Licensee MDPI, Basel, Switzerland. This article is an open access article distributed under the terms and conditions of the Creative Commons Attribution (CC BY) license (https://creativecommons.org/licenses/by/4.0/).

1. Introduction

Pregnancy induces a physiological prothrombotic state. The highest risk period for venous thromboembolisms is during the postpartum period [1]. Pregnancy increases the risk of thrombosis due to the hormonal, biological changes in the body. These changes occur in the blood flow via venous stasis from a pregnant uterus; changes in the vascular wall and coagulation factors (increased levels of factor II, V, VII, VIII, IX, X, von Willebrand factor); and increased D-dimer, fibrinogen, activation of platelets, and activity levels of natural anticoagulants (protein C, protein S, and plasminogen activator inhibitor-1). All these changes persist for another 6 weeks postpartum [2–4]. The VTE risk is higher in the third trimester, but the highest risk is observed postpartum. Thus, the relative risk is 20 times higher in the first six weeks postpartum, and 80% of these thrombotic events occur in the first three weeks postpartum [2]. Compared with the nonpregnant state, the 6-week postpartum period is associated with increases in stroke risk by a factor of 3 to 9, in myocardial infarction risk by a factor of 3 to 6, and in venous thromboembolism risk by a factor of 9 to 22 [5]. The risk can persist up to 12 weeks after delivery, but it is higher in the first 6 weeks. Guidelines recommend LMWH (Low Molecular Heparin) 6 weeks postpartum [6]. The obstetric complications associated with VTE are pregnancy loss, IUGR (Intrauterine Growth Retard), fetal death, abruptio placentae, and PE (Preeclampsia) [7,8]. Women experience five times more frequent DVT during pregnancy due to their hypercoagulability state, which is a defense mechanism against excess bleeding in the case of a miscarriage and childbirth [7,8]. In developing countries, postpartum hemorrhage is a frequent cause of death in pregnancy. The frequency of the risk of thrombosis increases in trimester III and postpartum, presenting the following clinical characteristics limb edema, skin changes, ulcerations, and recurrent thrombosis. Frequent associations with DVT are inherited thrombophilia, acquired thrombophilia, a history of thrombosis, heart disease, and sickle cell disease. To this, we add obesity, age over 35 years old, multiparity, nulliparity, immobilization in bed or sedentary lifestyle, smoking, assisted reproduction procedures, diabetes, infections, and caesarean sections. Virchov's triad is an essential pathogenic mechanism as it involves venous stasis, endothelial damage, and hypercoagulability [3]. Antiphospholipid syndrome [APS] and autoimmune diseases are also responsible for recurrent thrombosis. APS promotes a hypercoagulation state during pregnancy. APS is an autoimmune disease characterized by the presence of antiphospholipid antibodies that promote recurrent arterial and venous thrombosis, which is accompanied by important complications during pregnancy; these complications are sometimes catastrophic and can lead to the failure of multiple organs [9]. Clarifying the pathogenic mechanism is essential when providing therapy for the disease [9]. The antibodies that must be tested to confirm the disease are the lupus anticoagulant, antibodies against cardiolipin, and antibodies against beta 2 glycoprotein [10]. They are sources of procoagulant cell activation. They activate the complement cascade, which leads to an increase in the capillary permeability, the activation of platelets and neutrophils, and the release of cytokines and TNF alpha from monocytes, which accelerate inflammation and trigger the coagulation cascade. They activate endothelial cells that produce prothrombotic molecules via the activating complement [11].

The management consists of administering anticoagulants, among which the preferred one is LMWH; with the necessary precautions, anticoagulants produce HIT syndrome with thrombocytopenia and are administered with caution in renal diseases, depending on molecular weight and the chain, being cleared from the body by the kidneys. Warfarin transplacentally passes, which causes fetal bleeding, neurological damage, stillbirths, and low intelligence, which is why it is not used during pregnancy. In the case of Direct Factor Xa inhibitors, we do not know their side effects during pregnancy [3].

Identifying patients at risk of thrombosis and using anticoagulant prophylaxis in those patients during pregnancy and 6 weeks postpartum is important. In total, 15% of the population has thrombophilia, and thrombophilia is associated with DVT in proportions up to 50% in certain conditions [3]. The most serious form is that with homozygous Leyden

Factor V. Protein C and S deficiencies, as well as prothrombin G20210A or antithrombin deficiencies are also important. The American College of Chest Physicians recommends prophylaxis with LMWH in all pregnant women with a history of VTE and thrombophilia or in those with a history of more than two DVT episodes, without consensus regarding the dose. For those with thrombophilia without VTE, prophylaxis with LMWH is not recommended until postpartum [3,12,13]. In recent years, VTE risk has increased [14].

Pregnancy with thrombophilia induces a high-risk state for VTE, and sepsis only increases the risk. Assisted human reproduction methods also increase the VTE risk to a lesser extent [15]. A series of pathological conditions besides APS and hereditary thrombophilia can be associated with thrombotic risk: von Willebrand disease, sickle cell, inflammatory bowel disease, heart disease, smoking, immobilization, maternal age, obesity, and being African American. The recommended prophylaxis is LMWH [16,17].

Inherited bleeding disorders are pathological conditions that are also accompanied by VTE and determine mortality with a 6% prevalence [16]. The most common inherited bleeding disease is hemophilia, but it is very rare, not specific to pregnancy, and can appear in newborns who have thrombotic and hemorrhage disorders. In pregnancy, diagnosing bleeding disorders is difficult due to the lack of specific laboratory tests [18]. Thrombotic microangiopathy (TMA) consists of TTP (Thrombotic Thrombocytopenic Purpura) and HUS (Hemolytic Uremic Syndrome), which is associated with increased mortality and is difficult to diagnose [16]. Cardiac valvulopathies with valve prostheses, especially mechanical, are associated with a state of increased hypercoagulability, which requires management with a multidisciplinary team of cardiologists, obstetricians, anesthesiologists, neonatologists, and radiologists [16].

Thromboses are 75–82% venous and 20–25% arterial. VTEs occur during pregnancy in 0.5–2/1000 women. VTEs are responsible for 1.5 deaths per 100,000 deliveries in the USA [17].

In pregnant women, most thrombotic events occur in the left iliofemoral and inferior vena cava because of the increased venous stasis and compression by the pregnant uterus [5,19].

This manuscript is about the progression of thrombosis under LMWH treatment in a 20-year-old postpartum woman without prothrombotic risk factor and which evolved unexpectedly aggressively, so thrombolysis was necessary.

2. Case Report

We present the case of a 20 year old woman giving birth 2 weeks before admission. This was her second pregnancy; her first pregnancy was carried out to term without complications, and she had no family history of VTEs and no other known risk factors. The delivery occurred without complications, and the baby had an Apgar score of 10. During the pregnancy, the patient gained 30 kg in weight. At the time of the delivery the risk of VTE was low and prophylaxis was not indicated.

Two weeks after the delivery, the patient was admitted to the gynecology ward for right limb edema with erythema and a local increased temperature. After conducting a venous Doppler evaluation, right femoral and popliteal vein thrombosis was confirmed. The patient was transferred to the cardiology department for treatment and further investigations.

On admission, she was hemodynamically stable, and at the physical exam, she presented with right limb erythema, edema, and warm skin, with a positive Homans sign and normal pulmonary murmur without lung crackles. Her respiratory rate was 22 breaths/min, and her $SaO_2 = 94\%$, and she had a normal cardiac rhythm with no added heart sounds, an arterial blood pressure of 110/60 mmHg, a heart rate of 76 bpm, and no other remarkable findings on the clinical exam. The gynecological examination revealed a normal appearance and physiological involution of the uterus without signs of bleeding.

From the paraclinical examination, we obtained a CBC with leukocytosis, neutrophilia, $WBC = 14.71 \times 10^3/\mu L$ and $NEU = 11.61 \times 10^3/\mu L$, anemia with $Hb = 11.5$ g/dL, $HT = 35\%$, $MCH = 24.63$ pg, thrombocytosis with $PLT = 439 \times 10^3/\mu L$, $CRP = 35.42$ mg/L, fibrinogen = 558.99 mg/dL, and D-dimer = 760 μg/mL. The thrombophilic tests were conducted with AT III in normal ranges, a negative lupus anticoagulant, and S and C proteins in normal ranges. Following the investigation for hereditary thrombophilia, the tests were positive for the heterozygous PAI-1, MTHFR A1298C, EPCR with A1/A2 alleles, and homozygous 4G/4G genotype, which corresponds to minor thrombophilia. These associations decrease the plasma levels of inhibitor activator plasminogen and the fibrinolytic activity with a high thrombosis risk. With this new information, adding sepsis and thrombophilia, the patient's risk score for VTE increased to high risk. The results of the ECG at admission demonstrated the following: a sinus rhythm with 130 bpm and an QRS axis +60 degrees without other changes in the ST segment (Figure 1).

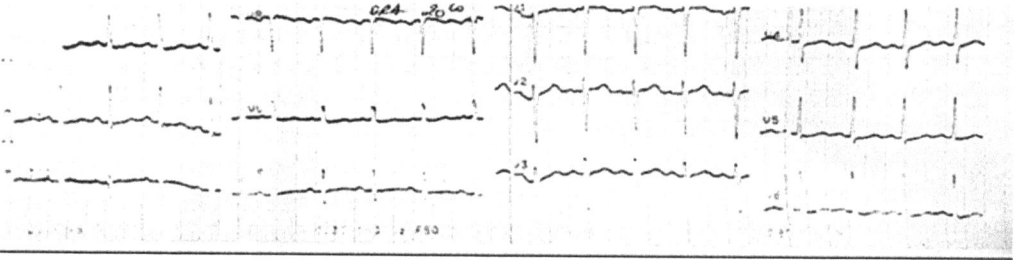

Figure 1. Sinus tachycardia, no pathological changes.

Echocardiography was performed, and the results revealed normal cardiac cavities, a normal LV ejection fraction, and diastolic dysfunction grade I without valvular dysfunction or pericardial effusion.

In our clinic, the patient received treatment with UFH (Unfractioned Heparin), therapeutic APTT, and analgesics for 2 days, and she experienced no reduction in the edema of her limbs. The patient was treated with heparin to treat an intense pain in her left thigh, and a venous Doppler was performed, which confirmed the bilateral iliac and femoral vein thrombosis. We decided to initiate thrombolysis on a central venous catheter with Alteplase, which did not lead to a considerable reduction in the thrombus, followed by UHF therapy by using therapeutic APTT.

The results of the abdominal and pelvic computed tomography examination revealed venous thrombosis in the inferior cava vein with an extension to both the common iliac veins and internal and external iliac veins, and it also extended to the bilateral femoral veins (Figure 2). The pulmonary artery and its branches were completely opacified without signs of pulmonary thromboembolism. Additionally, minimal basal right pleural fluid was observed.

Her general condition was worsening with important inflammatory syndrome and important leukocytosis with neutrophilia, and the anemia was also worsening with Hb = 9.6 g/dL, HT = 30.9%, MCH = 23.83 pg, MCV = 76.52 fL, and low seric iron at 13 ug/dL. We combined biological cultures with negative blood cultures and a positive culture from pharyngeal and nasal exudate to treat the Pseudomonas. Antibiotic therapy with 1 g/8 h of meropenem, 2 g/24 h of vancomycin, and 2 g/24 h of metronidazole was administered for 10 days to treat genital sepsis, and the patient experienced clinical improvements.

Post-thrombolysis, the patient received UFH for 7 days under the therapeutic control of APTT, triple antibiotic therapy, beta blockers, gastric antisecretory, and parenteral hydration, which resulted in a favorable evolution and a remission of the limb edema and inflammatory syndrome. The patient was discharged with an order to undergo an anticoagulant treatment of 15 mg of Rivaroxaban twice a day for 14 days and 20 mg/twice a day for the antiaggregant therapy. During the follow-up 2 months later, we found that the patient had partial right superficial vein thrombosis without other thromboses, but due to a genetic mutation, the patient was advised to take long-term oral anticoagulation medications. After long-term follow-up, at the Doppler ultrasound one year later, the partial right superficial vein thrombosis persisted. In this situation, it is recommended to continue the anticoagulation with aspenter and take into account the other procoagulant pathologies that could be triggered during a new pregnancy.

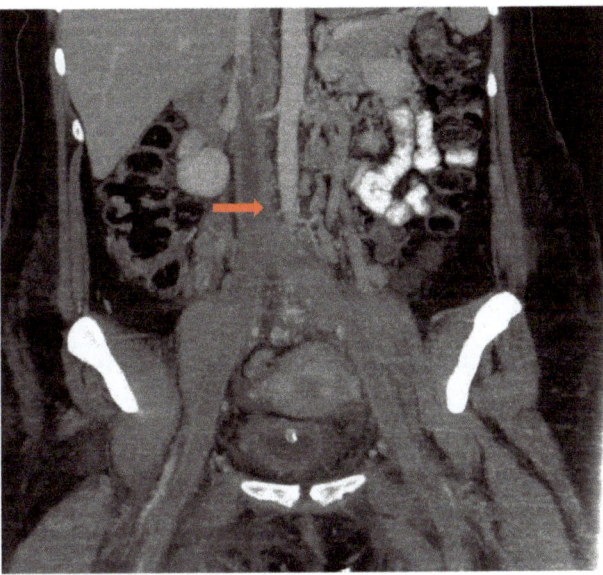

Figure 2. Venous thrombosis in inferior cava vein with extension to the common iliac veins and bilateral femoral veins (red arrow).

3. Discussion

The thrombophilia, postpartum status, and sepsis were the factors that induced DVT in our young patient after her second pregnancy.

The highest risk period for venous thromboembolisms and pulmonary embolisms in pregnant women is during the postpartum period. Any prophylaxis against these events should be particularly targeted for postpartum women. Risk factors to be considered include prior VTE, familial VTE history, the presence of known thrombophilia, caesarean delivery, prolonged antepartum immobilization, increased body mass index (BMI), considerable pregnancy complications, and medical comorbidities [19].

Data, largely from retrospective cohorts and case–control studies, have shown that inherited thrombophilias are not only associated with VTE but also with adverse pregnancy outcomes, including recurrent miscarriage and gestational vascular complications. The most common inherited thrombophilias are Factor V Leiden (FVL) and Factor II (prothrombin) G20210A, which affect 3–11% of the population; less prevalent (<1%) are inherited thrombophilias, including protein C, protein S, an antithrombin deficiency, dysfibrinogenemia, and hyperhomocysteinemia [12,20,21].

A thrombophilic status with heterozygous PAI-1 and MTHFR A1298C and EPCR with A1/A2 positive alleles together are associated with decreasing plasma levels of inhibitor activator plasminogens and a decrease in fibrinolytic activity with a high thrombosis risk [22].

The results of prospective and retrospective studies have demonstrated a modest association of homocysteine with venous thrombosis, but when associated with other mutations such as PAI-1 heterozygous, homocysteine increases the cardiovascular and VTE risks. Heparins, UFH, and LMWH are the preferred agents for anticoagulation in pregnancy because they show no transplacental passage. Both heparins and warfarin are safe for the infant during breastfeeding. Under DOACs (Direct acting oral anticoagulants), breastfeeding is not recommended as no evidence of its safety exists [23].

Because anticoagulant treatment is proposed in 91% of cases, the preferred treatment would be LMWH as it has a strong safety profile, does not cross the placenta, and lowers the risk of preeclampsia; intra-arterial thrombolysis is used in 20% of cases, and a thrombectomy with thrombolysis is used in 8% of cases, with excellent outcomes if the diagnosis is correct [13,24]. DVT in pregnancy is associated with high morbidity and mortality. Pulmonary embolisms cause maternal death. DVT leads to long-term complications. Women develop DVT five times more frequently during pregnancy. Apart from the standard treatment, which is anticoagulation, an endovascular inferior cava filter can be installed, and the pharmacomechanical catheter for directed thrombolysis is only used in pregnancy or in the case of massive life-threatening situations as it has been associated with abruptio placentae, premature birth, and fetal damage [3,4]. When administering LMWH, antiFactor Xa dosage is not necessary in pregnancy and coumarins are contraindicated, but elastic compression is beneficial [4,13]. In the case of APS resistant to treatment, new therapeutic strategies should also be searched [25].

The signs used to provide a DVT diagnosis are swelling of the legs, discomfort, erythema, abdominal or pelvic pain, edema, and dyspnea [3,4]. D dimers are not measured because they are increased in pregnancy anyway. The diagnosis consists of imaging by CT, MRI, and a color Doppler with intraluminal echoes [3,26]. Compression duplex ultrasonography is also indicated in deep thrombosis and pulmonary imaging for possible pulmonary embolisms, and EKG shows tachycardia and nonspecific features that suggest pulmonary embolisms, oxygen saturation, or angiography in nonpregnant/postpartum patients, in addition to the leg circumference being 2 cm larger [4]. A Doppler velocimetry is essential in fetal assessment [25].

In inherited bleeding disorders, the management, as well as the diagnosis, is more complicated. Two types of TMA thrombotic microangiopathies exist: Thrombotic thrombocytopenic purpura (TTP) and hemolytic uremic syndrome (HUS). They can appear during pregnancy or postpartum. TTP can be acquired or can be a congenital deficiency of ADAMTS 13, and this especially occurs in the second and third trimester of pregnancy. The treatment consists of restoring ADAMTS 13 activity with plasmapheresis and immunosuppressive agents [27]. A HUS atypical complement is triggered by pregnancy. The treatment consists of the anti-C5 humanized monoclonal antibody eculizumab. We found that both situations were associated with pre-eclampsia and HELLP syndrome. We identified that the von Willebrand cleaving protease ADAMTS 13 is a major factor in TTP pathogenesis and clinically determined neurological damage, renal failure, and thrombosis. In HUS, we found that the dysregulation of the alternate complement pathway was a mechanism of HUS occurrence, and in this case, ADAMTS 13 was over 10% [18,27].

Only a few available sensitive laboratory tests exist, and the current ones are insufficient to make a diagnosis. This results in diagnostic challenges, problems in the current treatment, and the need for guidelines for more efficient management [11]. In some pregnancy complications associated with thrombosis or hemorrhage, the proteins that control blood clotting become overactive, and DIC sets in. From this point of view, the DIC disseminated intravascular coagulation score would be useful in predicting uncontrolled coagulopathy [18]. It consists of determining the complete blood cell count, prothrombin time (PT), partial thromboplastin time (APTT), fibrinogen, and D dimers. However, the DIC score is modified during pregnancy and cannot be used because fibrinogen increases, platelets decrease, and the PT and PTT do not change during pregnancy. Only modified PTs are used as DIC indicators. DIC indicators are present during uncontrolled bleeding at birth, abruptio placentae, placenta previa, uterine rupture, cervical and vaginal laceration, infections, surgical techniques, and HELLP syndrome. Corrected by surgery and blood transfusions, DIC is associated with thrombocytopenia below 50,000, prolonged PT, increased dimers, and low fibrinogen. Additionally, an algorithm that compares the types of bleeding and thrombosis that can appear in pregnancy with the laboratory tests specific to each disease would also be useful in terms of making life-saving diagnoses and management [18].

Von Willebrand disease seems to affect 0.01–1.3% of the general population, and it is the most common inherited mild bleeding condition. Because a high risk of bleeding is present at birth, F VIII must be restored. Blood-product administration is performed to manage PPH, and therefore it requires massive transfusion protocols, laboratory monitoring, and a multidisciplinary approach [16].

Pregnancy failure is prevented by conventional therapy in women with APS. Various treatment strategies are leading to remarkably higher live birth rates. Conventional therapy consists of a prophylactic dose of heparin plus a low dose of aspirin to prevent pregnancy loss, and for those with a history of thrombosis, a therapeutic dose of heparin with LDA is provided instead. Here, we add intravenous immunoglobulin, low-dose prednisolone, plasmapheresis, and immunoadsorption. New clinical studies are needed. During diagnosis, in addition to antibody dosing, a Doppler velocimetry showing notch on the uterine arteries suggests a poor prognosis. The activation of complement cascades and inflammation are involved in trophoblast invasion disorder [28]. An innovative treatment would be the slow infusion of the tissue-type plasminogen activator in the case of thrombosed mechanical valves [29]. A risk of hemorrhage and preterm birth exists.

Choosing contraceptives after venous thromboembolism (VTE) is challenging because hormonal contraceptives may increase the risk of recurrent VTE. Estrogen contraceptives are usually contraindicated in women with a personal VTE history, and the use of oral progestin-only contraceptives is still being studied. Nonhormonal contraceptives are recommended [30]. For the next pregnancy of this patient, and to reduce the associated risks, we recommend using LMWH after conception.

A multidisciplinary team that includes a cardiologist, hematologist, and gynecologist is required to prevent thrombotic events in the future, especially if a third pregnancy is desired, as her VTE risk score is high, even in the absence of an infection. Considering the long-term follow-up with the presence of residual thrombosis at such a young age with minor thrombophilia, which does not explain the dramatic evolution of VTE that appeared in this case, we suggest future investigation of all conditions presented here as possible procoagulant pathologies.

4. Conclusions

Thrombophilias are associated with a high VTE risk but also with adverse pregnancy outcomes, and the postpartum period is associated with a higher VTE risk. One's thrombophilic status is associated with a high risk of thrombosis and cardiovascular events in the postpartum period. Thrombolysis can be successfully used in this situation, and Alteplase is a thrombolytic agent that is created with recombinant DNA technology and was effective in this case, along with LMWH.

Author Contributions: Conceptualization, A.T.T. and L.A.B.; software, A.T.T., L.C. and L.A.B.; validation, A.T.T., L.C. and L.M.; investigation, A.T.T., L.C. and I.D.; writing—original draft preparation, A.T.T. and L.A.B.; writing—review and editing, A.T.T., L.C., A.F.B. and L.M. All authors have read and agreed to the published version of the manuscript.

Funding: This research received no external funding.

Institutional Review Board Statement: Not applicable.

Informed Consent Statement: Written informed consent to publish this paper was obtained from the patient.

Data Availability Statement: Data supporting reported results can be found in the Department of Cardiology database, "St. John" Emergency Hospital, 13 Vitan Barzesti Street, 042122 Bucharest, Romania.

Conflicts of Interest: The authors declare no conflict of interest.

References

1. Chan, W.S.; Rey, E.; Kent, N.E.; Chan, W.S.; Kent, N.E.; Rey, E.; Corbett, T.; David, M.; Douglas, M.J.; Gibson, P.S.; et al. Venous thromboembolism and antithrombotic therapy in pregnancy. *J. Obstet. Gynaecol. Can.* 2014, *36*, 527–553. [CrossRef] [PubMed]
2. Sultan, A.A.; West, J.; Tata, L.J.; Fleming, K.M.; Nelson-Piercy, C.; Grainge, M.J. Risk of first venous thromboembolism in and around pregnancy: A population-based cohort study. *Br. J. Haematol.* 2012, *156*, 366–373. [CrossRef] [PubMed]
3. Devis, P.; Knuttinen, M.G. Deep venous thrombosis in pregnancy: Incidence, pathogenesis and endovascular management. *Cardiovasc. Diagn. Ther.* 2017, *7*, S309–S319. [CrossRef] [PubMed]
4. Greer, I.A. CLINICAL PRACTICE. Pregnancy Complicated by Venous Thrombosis. *N. Engl. J. Med.* 2015, *373*, 540–547. [CrossRef]
5. Abdul Sultan, A.; Grainge, M.J.; West, J.; Fleming, K.M.; Nelson-Piercy, C.; Tata, L.J. Impact of risk factors on the timing of first postpartum venous thromboembolism: A population-based cohort study from England. *Blood* 2014, *124*, 2872–2880. [CrossRef]
6. De Carolis, S.; Tabacco, S.; Rizzo, F.; Giannini, A.; Botta, A.; Salvi, S.; Garufi, C.; Benedetti Panici, P.; Lanzone, A. Antiphospholipid syndrome: An update on risk factors for pregnancy outcome. *Autoimmun. Rev.* 2018, *17*, 956–966. [CrossRef]
7. Mitranovici, M.I.; Puscasiu, L.; Craina, M.; Iacob, D.; Chiriac, V.D.; Ionita, I.; Moleriu, R.D.; Furau, G.; Sisu, A.; Petre, I. The Role of Low Molecular Weight Heparin in Pregnancies of Patients with Inherited Thrombophilia that Have Presented (and) Thrombotic Complications During Previous Pregnancies. *Rev. Chim.* 2017, *68*, 2970–2973. [CrossRef]
8. Othman, M.; Santamaría Ortiz, A.; Cerdá, M.; Erez, O.; Minford, A.; Obeng-Tuudah, D.; Blondon, M.; Bistervels, I.; Middeldorp, S.; Abdul-Kadir, R. Thrombosis and hemostasis health in pregnancy: Registries from the International Society on Thrombosis and Haemostasis. *Res. Pract. Thromb. Haemost.* 2019, *3*, 607–614. [CrossRef]
9. Xie, H.; Sheng, L.; Zhou, H.; Yan, J. The role of TLR4 in pathophysiology of antiphospholipid syndrome-associated thrombosis and pregnancy morbidity. *Br. J. Haematol.* 2014, *164*, 165–176. [CrossRef]
10. Andreoli, L.; Chighizola, C.B.; Banzato, A.; Pons-Estel, G.J.; Ramire de Jesus, G.; Erkan, D. Estimated frequency of antiphospholipid antibodies in patients with pregnancy morbidity, stroke, myocardial infarction, and deep vein thrombosis: A critical review of the literature. *Arthritis Care Res.* 2013, *65*, 1869–1873. [CrossRef]
11. Oku, K.; Nakamura, H.; Kono, M.; Ohmura, K.; Kato, M.; Bohgaki, T.; Horita, T.; Yasuda, S.; Amengual, O.; Atsumi, T. Complement and thrombosis in the antiphospholipid syndrome. *Autoimmun. Rev.* 2016, *15*, 1001–1004. [CrossRef]
12. Khan, S.; Dickerman, J.D. Hereditary thrombophilia. *Thromb. J.* 2006, *4*, 15. [CrossRef]
13. Croles, F.N.; Nasserinejad, K.; Duvekot, J.J.; Kruip, M.J.; Meijer, K.; Leebeek, F.W. Pregnancy, thrombophilia, and the risk of a first venous thrombosis: Systematic review and bayesian meta-analysis. *BMJ* 2017, *359*, j4452. [CrossRef]
14. Kane, E.V.; Calderwood, C.; Dobbie, R.; Morris, C.; Roman, E.; Greer, I.A. A population-based study of venous thrombosis in pregnancy in Scotland 1980–2005. *Eur. J. Obstet. Gynecol. Reprod. Biol.* 2013, *169*, 223–229. [CrossRef]
15. Villani, M.; Dentali, F.; Colaizzo, D.; Tiscia, G.L.; Vergura, P.; Petruccelli, T.; Petruzzelli, F.; Ageno, W.; Margaglione, M.; Grandone, E. Pregnancy-related venous thrombosis: Comparison between spontaneous and ART conception in an Italian cohort. *BMJ Open* 2015, *5*, e008213. [CrossRef]
16. Othman, M.; McLintock, C.; Kadir, R. Thrombosis and Hemostasis Related Issues in Women and Pregnancy. *Semin. Thromb. Hemost.* 2016, *42*, 693–695. [CrossRef]
17. James, A.H. Thrombosis in pregnancy and maternal outcomes. *Birth Defects Res. Part C Embryo Today Rev.* 2015, *105*, 159–166. [CrossRef]
18. Mitranovici, M.I.; Pușcașiu, L.; Oală, I.E.; Petre, I.; Craina, M.L.; Mager, A.R.; Vasile, K.; Chiorean, D.M.; Sabău, A.H.; Turdean, S.G.; et al. A Race against the Clock: A Case Report and Literature Review Concerning the Importance of ADAMTS13 Testing in Diagnosis and Management of Thrombotic Thrombocytopenic Purpura during Pregnancy. *Diagnostics* 2022, *12*, 1559. [CrossRef]
19. Pomp, E.R.; Lenselink, A.M.; Rosendaal, F.R.; Doggen, C.J. Pregnancy, the postpartum period and prothrombotic defects: Risk of venous thrombosis in the MEGA study. *J. Thromb. Haemost.* 2008, *6*, 632–637. [CrossRef]
20. Fiengo, L.; Bucci, F.; Patrizi, G. Postpartum deep vein thrombosis and pulmonary embolism in twin pregnancy: Undertaking of clinical symptoms leading to massive complications. *Thromb. J.* 2013, *4*, 11. [CrossRef]
21. Arachchillage, D.J.; Mackillop, L.; Chandratheva, A.; Motawani, J.; MacCallum, P.; Laffan, M. Thrombophilia testing: A British Society for Haematology guideline. *Br. J. Haematol.* 2022, *198*, 443–458. [CrossRef] [PubMed]
22. Den Heijer, M.; Lewington, S.; Clarke, R. Homocysteine, MTHFR and risk of venous thrombosis: A meta-analysis of published epidemiological studies. *J. Thromb. Haemost.* 2005, *3*, 292–299. [CrossRef] [PubMed]
23. Tang, A.W.; Greer, I. A systematic review on the use of new anticoagulants in pregnancy. *Obstet. Med.* 2013, *6*, 64–71. [CrossRef] [PubMed]
24. Kashkoush, A.I.; Ma, H.; Agarwal, N.; Panczykowski, D.; Tonetti, D.; Weiner, G.M.; Ares, W.; Kenmuir, C.; Jadhav, A.; Jovin, T.; et al. Cerebral venous sinus thrombosis in pregnancy and puerperium: A pooled, systematic review. *J. Clin. Neurosci.* 2017, *39*, 9–15. [CrossRef]
25. Latino, J.O.; Udry, S.; Aranda, F.M.; Perés Wingeyer, S.D.A.; Fernández Romero, D.S.; de Larrañaga, G.F. Pregnancy failure in patients with obstetric antiphospholipid syndrome with conventional treatment: The influence of a triple positive antibody profile. *Lupus* 2017, *26*, 983–988. [CrossRef]
26. Sharma, N.; Sharma, S.R.; Hussain, M. An audit of cerebral venous thrombosis associated with pregnancy and puerperium in teaching hospital in North Eastern India. *J. Fam. Med. Prim. Care* 2019, *8*, 1054–1057. [CrossRef]

27. Fakhouri, F. Pregnancy-related thrombotic microangiopathies: Clues from complement biology. *Transfus. Apher. Sci.* **2016**, *54*, 199–202. [CrossRef]
28. Ruffatti, A.; Salvan, E.; Del Ross, T.; Gerosa, M.; Andreoli, L.; Maina, A.; Alijotas-Reig, J.; De Carolis, S.; Mekinian, A.; Bertero, M.T.; et al. Treatment strategies and pregnancy outcomes in antiphospholipid syndrome patients with thrombosis and triple antiphospholipid positivity. A European multicentre retrospective study. *Thromb. Haemost.* **2014**, *112*, 727–735. [CrossRef]
29. Özkan, M.; Çakal, B.; Karakoyun, S.; Gürsoy, O.M.; Çevik, C.; Kalçık, M.; Oğuz, A.E.; Gündüz, S.; Astarcioglu, M.A.; Aykan, A.Ç.; et al. Thrombolytic therapy for the treatment of prosthetic heart valve thrombosis in pregnancy with low-dose, slow infusion of tissue-type plasminogen activator. *Circulation* **2013**, *128*, 532–540. [CrossRef]
30. Nguyen, K.; Prasad, P.; Pare, E.; Chadderdon, S.; Khan, A. Thrombolytic therapy for mechanical aortic valve thrombosis in pregnancy: Case report. *Eur. Heart J. Case Rep.* **2022**, *6*, ytac461. [CrossRef]

Disclaimer/Publisher's Note: The statements, opinions and data contained in all publications are solely those of the individual author(s) and contributor(s) and not of MDPI and/or the editor(s). MDPI and/or the editor(s) disclaim responsibility for any injury to people or property resulting from any ideas, methods, instructions or products referred to in the content.

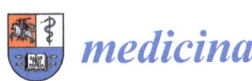

Case Report

The Very First Romanian Unruptured 13-Weeks Gestation Tubal Ectopic Pregnancy

Ciprian Ilea [1,2], Ovidiu-Dumitru Ilie [3,*], Olivia-Andreea Marcu [4], Irina Stoian [1,*] and Bogdan Doroftei [1,2,5]

1. Faculty of Medicine, University of Medicine and Pharmacy "Grigore T. Popa", University Street, no 16, 700115 Iasi, Romania
2. Clinical Hospital of Obstetrics and Gynecology "Cuza Voda", Cuza Voda Street, no 34, 700038 Iasi, Romania
3. Department of Biology, Faculty of Biology, "Alexandru Ioan Cuza" University, Carol I Avenue, no 20A, 700505 Iasi, Romania
4. Department of Preclinics, Faculty of Medicine and Pharmacy, University of Oradea, December 1 Market Street, no 10, 410068 Oradea, Romania
5. Origyn Fertility Center, Palace Street, no 3C, 700032 Iasi, Romania
* Correspondence: ovidiuilie90@yahoo.com (O.-D.I.); stoian.irinalv@yahoo.com (I.S.)

Abstract: Tubal ectopic pregnancies remain a challenging and life-threatening obstetric condition in the early stages that unavoidably lead to abortion or rupture, further reflected by the associated maternal mortality. Therefore, in the present case report, we report the experience of a 36-year-old woman who presented to our Emergency Department with a history of moderate hypogastric pain, mild vaginal bleeding, and bilateral mastalgia, symptoms that started 20 days ago after uterine curettage for a declarative eight-week pregnancy. On admission, a physical examination showed regular standard signs. The ultrasound examination revealed in the left abdominal flank a gestational sac with a live fetus corresponding to the gestational age of 13 weeks. Given the position of the gestational sac, we suspected a possible abdominal pregnancy. Independently on her human chorionic gonadotropin (hCG) of 33.980 mIU/mL and hemoglobin (Hb) of 13.4 g/dL, the exact location of the pregnancy following ultrasound was hard to establish. Magnetic resonance imaging (MRI) examination was requested, after which we suspected the diagnosis of ovarian pregnancy. Given the paraclinical and clinical context of the worsening of painful symptoms, we decided to perform an exploratory laparoscopy in the multidisciplinary team (digestive and vascular surgeon) that showed the existence of a tubal pregnancy.

Keywords: tubal pregnancy; ectopic pregnancy; live fetus; first trimester

1. Introduction

According to the Centers for Disease Control and Prevention (CDC), ectopic pregnancy is a life-threatening condition in the early stages. Per current figures, it accounts for 2% of all cases, oscillating from 1.3% to 2.4% [1]. In terms of the actual incidence, the evidence is contradictory since studies are lacking [2].

An ectopic pregnancy defines the implantation outside the endometrial cavity [3] of the fertilized ovum found in the blastocyst stage. In 70–90% of cases, it takes place in the fallopian tubes within the ampulla. However, numerous other sites were described over the years, surrounding the fimbrial, isthmic, and interstitial segments. There are also data referring to the ovary, the myometrium, the cervix, the abdomen, and cesarean (C)-section scar [4,5], with most ectopic pregnancies diagnosed between 6 and 10 weeks of gestation [6]. Circumstances that describe cases in advanced stages also exist in the literature.

Moreover, a rupture might occur between the 5th to 9th week of pregnancy in situations of ectopic pregnancy, leading to abdominal or pelvic pain, amenorrhea, and in limited scenarios, vaginal bleeding [7]. It is rare for an ectopic pregnancy to advance into the 2nd trimester without the presence of symptoms, and a proper diagnosis can avert rupture.

Therefore, this manuscript aims to further provide evidence to the literature with a rare case report of a live 13-week ectopic tubal pregnancy, the sole documented occurrence in Romania, uncomplicated at this age of gestation.

2. Case Presentation

2.1. Patient Information

A 36-year-old female (T.I.), gravida 1, para 0, presented to our Emergency Department reporting moderate hypogastric pain, mild vaginal bleeding, and bilateral mastalgia. During the interview, she declared that symptoms started 20 days ago, despite her medical record without registration. On admission, a physical examination showed typical vital signs.

2.2. Clinical History

Retrospectively, she had amenorrhea for eight weeks with a positive pregnancy test result but decided to follow an elective curettage in another medical center. She stated that, before the curettage, she did not undergo a pelvic ultrasound examination.

2.3. Diagnostic Assessment and Investigations

The transvaginal pelvic ultrasound examination showed, in the left abdominal flank, a gestational sac with a live fetus corresponding to the gestational age of 13 weeks and an empty uterine cavity with no fluid in the pouch of Douglas (Figures 1–3). Given the position of the gestational sac, we suspected a possible abdominal pregnancy, but the exact anatomical location of the pregnancy following ultrasound was hard to establish. The physical examination of the breast and ultrasound excluded noncylic mastalgia. The patient's serum hCG was 33.980 mIU/mL with no signs of anemia, having a Hb of 13.4 g/dL. The results of the other paraclinical tests (blood and urine biochemistry) were within normal limits.

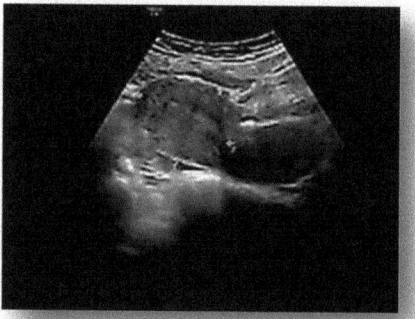

Figure 1. Transvaginal ultrasound from a 36-year-old woman with a left ectopic tubal pregnancy of 13 weeks of gestation. Ultrasound showed uterine body with linear endometrium and no gestational sac.

We conducted the MRI exam that showed a suspicion of ovarian pregnancy according to the description: on the left ovarian topography, there is a suggestive aspect for the gestational sac, inside which a living fetus was seen (spontaneous movements during the examination), and a placenta developed at the level of the lower wall; the gestational sac with global dimensions of ~53/64/65 mm (a-p/t/c-c) and with localization in the front of external iliac vascular bundles; on the right side, the gestational sac comes into contact with the sigmoid, without signs of invasion; venous dilatations of the utero–ovarian plexus developed perilesionally around the formation; uterus in anteroversion/anteroflexion without expansive formations; the linear endometrium (5 mm), empty uterine cavity, cervix without expansive formations; right ovary with normal follicular appearance; no free fluid in the abdominal cavity; no pelvic lymphadenopathy (Figure 4a–c).

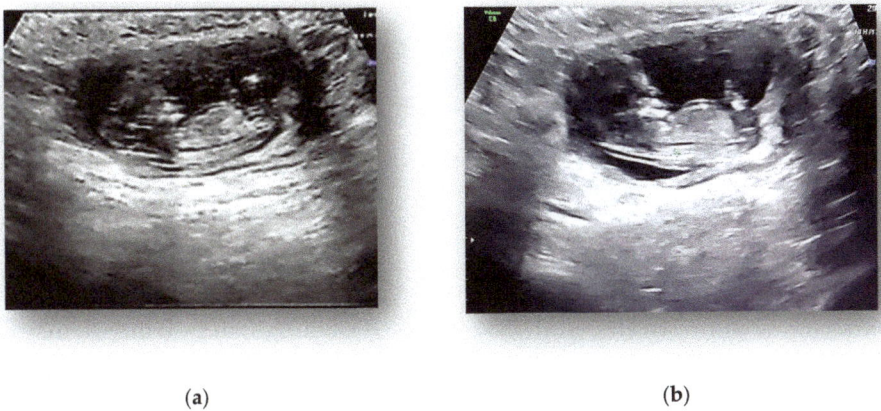

(a) (b)

Figure 2. (**a**) Ultrasound showed in the left abdominal flank a gestational sac with a live fetus corresponding to the gestational age of 13 weeks. (**b**) Ultrasound showed gestational sac with fetus corresponding to 13 weeks.

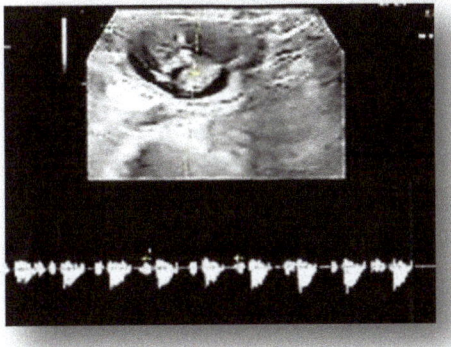

Figure 3. Ultrasound examination of the fetus cardiac activity.

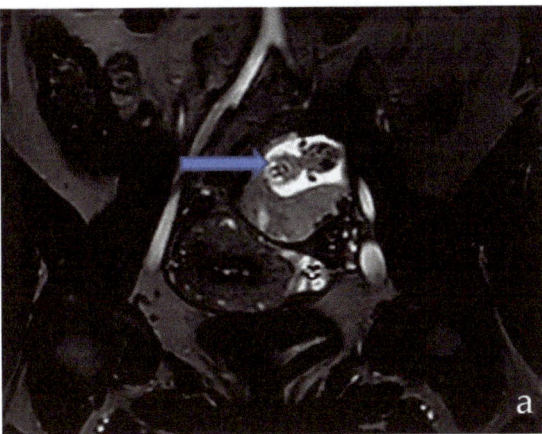

Figure 4. *Cont.*

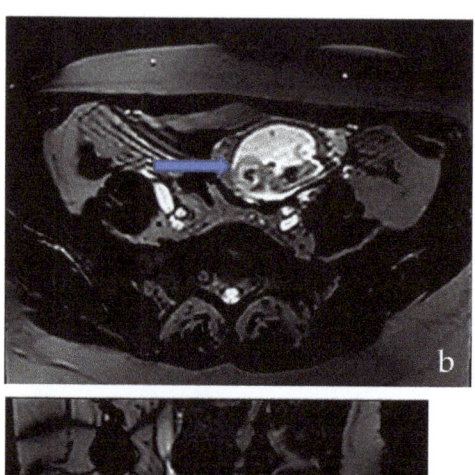
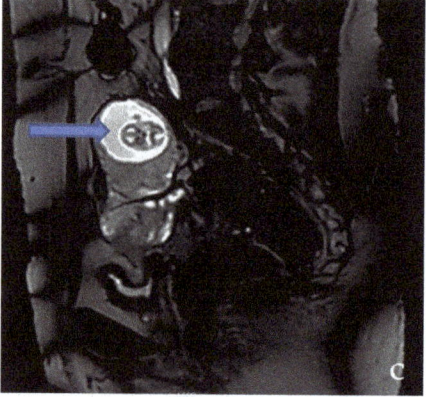

Figure 4. MRI examination: coronal T2-weighted (**a**), axial T2-weighted (**b**) sagittal T2-weighted (**c**)—show the ectopic pregnancy on the left ovarian topography.

Given the paraclinical and clinical context—the uncertainty of the positive diagnosis of the exact anatomical location of the pregnancy and accentuation of the abdominal pain—we decided to perform an exploratory laparoscopy in the multidisciplinary team (digestive and vascular surgeons) after obtaining informed consent. We actually found that it was a tubal pregnancy localized in the intestinal portion of the fallopian tubes, not an ovarian pregnancy (according to MRI) or abdominal pregnancy (according to ultrasound) (Figure 5a,b). The right ovary, fallopian tube, and the left ovary looked normal. In this context, we decided to perform a left salpingectomy (Figure 6). Her postoperative outcome was favorable, and the serum hCG levels decreased to <50 mIU/mL on the fourth day after surgery. Following the salpingectomy, the specimen (fetus and fetal annexes) were sent for anatomopathological examination (Figure 7a,b).

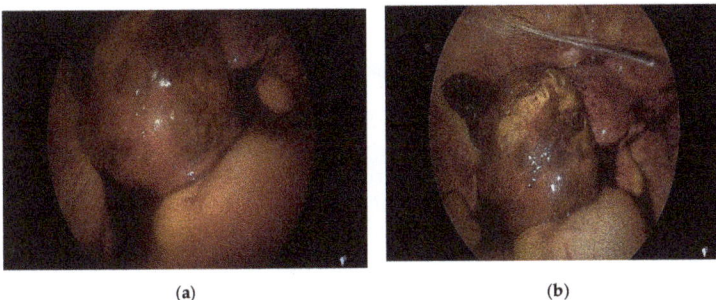

Figure 5. (a) Intra-operative image indicating the gestational sac on the left fallopian tube. (b) Intra-operative image indicating the gestational sac on the left fallopian tube.

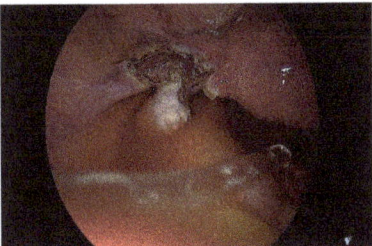

Figure 6. Intra-operative image after left salpingectomy.

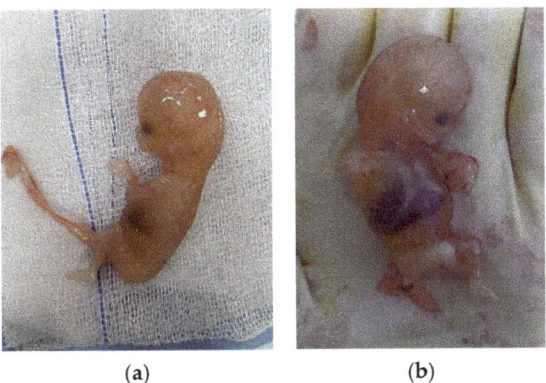

Figure 7. Anatomopathological specimen with the fetus after the removal of the tubal pregnancy from two distinct perspectives (a,b).

3. Discussion

Ectopic pregnancy is an obstetric first-trimester pregnancy complication [8] with a vast repertoire of locations (ampulla—70% [5], isthmus—12%, fimbria—11.1%, and interstitium—2.4%) [9]. The estimated prevalence oscillates at around 18%, while morbidity and mortality accounting for 9% and 13% of all related deaths [1]. The cases of ectopic pregnancy reaching the second trimester are rare [2].

A tubal pregnancy may emerge to a most symptomatic phase as a consequence of the lack of submucosal layer within the fallopian tube wall. It enables ovum implantation within the muscular wall, considering that trophoblasts rapidly proliferate and erode this muscularis layer. Such a phenomenon usually causes tubal rupture and might occur at 7.2 weeks ± 2.2 with significant hemodynamic consequences. As already mentioned, in some rare cases, the fallopian tubes dilate to accommodate a pregnancy until the second or third trimester of pregnancy [9]. The possible factors responsible for this situation can be represented by the tubal structural anomalies that cause an increase in the elasticity of the fallopian tube and the abnormalities of the trophoblastic invasion that does not penetrate the entire tubal wall. This argument emphasizes the risk of missing the early diagnosis of ectopic pregnancy. On two previous occasions from the literature, the authors reported ectopic pregnancies at an advanced gestational age [10,11]. In our case, the fact that a standard pelvic ultrasound (with its limitations) was not performed to locate the pregnancy before the curettage increased the risk of not diagnosing the tubal pregnancy, with possibly important implications for the final diagnosis.

Three distinct management procedures are currently applied to target an ectopic pregnancy. Thus, clear documentation is mandatory considering the fulminant attendance to an outpatient department for a proper diagnosis. It is imperative to remember the threats since the correct method relies on the ongoing examination based on a series of clinical factors [12]. In the case of a ruptured ectopic pregnancy, surgery is compulsory. A laparoscopy is preferred when the patient is hemodynamically stable, which is a procedure associated with shorter operative times and hospital stays reflected in the intra-operative blood loss and analgesia requirements [13–15]. On the other hand, a laparotomy should be provided to patients when presenting with a rupture and in a state of hypovolemic shock and compromised. A salpingectomy is reserved for cases where the contralateral tube is healthy; where the fallopian tube or the concerned fragment that contains the ectopic gestation is removed, a salpingostomy involves the removal of the ectopic pregnancy by dissecting the tube and fallopian tube, in situ, to preserve the fertility status [16]. Three teams performed systematic reviews whose objective was to report the reproductive outcomes in patients with a healthy contralateral tube, including studies evaluating the patient selection, surgical procedure, and follow-up period [17–19], but several manuscripts declare conflicting results [20,21].

Moreover, it is known that the chance of an intrauterine pregnancy is not increased after salpingostomy in contrast to salpingectomy, conservative surgical techniques without exposing women to significant tubal bleeding shortly post-operation, and the need for further treatment of persistent trophoblast [16] and supports current guidelines regarding the laparoscopic salpingectomy as the method of choice when there is a healthy contralateral tube [22].

As already mentioned, a laparoscopic salpingostomy should be conducted in the presence of contralateral tubal disease to preserve the fertility potential. Serum β-hCG levels following tubal bleeding are pointers, where the size of the ectopic pregnancy when >2 cm or β-hCG concentrations are >3000 IU/L or higher shortly before the surgery [23]. In such circumstances, women should undergo serial β-hCG measurements and methotrexate (MTX). Despite salpingostomy implications on costs, post-operative follow-up, and treatment of persistent trophoblast [24], it will surpass salpingectomy in terms of assisted conception avoidance [21].

The second alternative is medical treatment involving the usage of MTX [25–27], a folic acid antagonist associated with rapid cell division and mitosis arrest [16,28]. MTX is required when the patients are hemodynamically stable with unruptured tubal ectopic pregnancy with insignificant manifestations and diminished volume of free intraperitoneal fluid on ultrasound scan. Presently, intramuscular MTX is extensively used because of its efficiency when administered in a single dose [24,29].

Congruent with the previous aspects regarding patient suitability, several indexes such as weight and height alongside blood count correlated with other standard tests for kidney and liver functionality are needed. Although the cases are limited, the regime might cause hair loss or lead to toxicity of the bone marrow or of the liver. The most common symptoms include abdominal discomfort and bloating for approximately half a week [30].

While 14–20% of the women that underwent a single dose will need to repeat the process [31,32] due to the β-hCG concentration not dropping below 15% on day 4–7 after treatment, 10% must undergo surgery [33]. A less common approach for patients who have β-hCG levels > 5000 IU/L constitutes the direct injection of MTX into the ectopic pregnancy as a multi-dose protocol (day 1, 3, 5, and 7) and leucovorin (0.1 mg/kg on day 2, 4, 6, and 8) [34].

The last approach rotating around ectopic pregnancies is when they spontaneously resolve without any intervention via regression or tubal abortion as a conservative strategy [29]. The individual must not portray indications or symptoms of a ruptured ectopic pregnancy and be stable, with a consistent drop of serum β-hCG or progesterone and assessment of β-hCG (<1000 IU/L) [35] up to 3 times per week and ultrasonography with relatively high success rates in between [36].

Unfortunately, some results indicate a risk of recurrence of 10% in women with a known history of ectopic pregnancy and may increase to 25%. The most common risk factors are advanced maternal age (AMA), smoking, in vitro fertilization (IVF), and infertility due to previous abdominopelvic surgery or adhesions caused by infections or pelvic inflammatory disease [37–39]. It is possible that women who achieve pregnancy via assisted reproductive technology (ART), among which multiple embryo transfers (ETs) and tubal factor, have an increased risk of ectopic pregnancy [40].

The incidence might increase mainly because of sexually transmitted diseases (STDs) [5]. This is why patients must undergo transvaginal ultrasonography and measurement of serum β-hCG as per the guidelines issued [6]. Women using an intrauterine device (IUD) are at a lower risk of suffering an ectopic pregnancy in comparison to women not using contraception. However, in 53% of cases, an ectopic pregnancy might occur despite the presence of an IUD [41]. Implicitly, there are also numerous non-related ectopic pregnancy factors, counting C-section, oral contraceptives (COCs), or emergency contraception failure [42].

In our case, there was no associated risk factor. The anatomopathological report revealed, besides the classical representative aspects of tubal ectopic pregnancy (chorionic villi within the lumen of the tube), the presence of an important chronic inflammatory infiltrate at the level of the remaining tubal wall, possibly having to do with a history of pelvic inflammatory disease. However, it is essential to specify that the patient comes from a disadvantaged socioeconomic area with limited access to medical diagnostic services. A chronological overview of the previous case reports that report 13-week tubal ectopic pregnancies are discussed below (Table 1). Although numerous references concerning ectopic pregnancies can be found in the literature, those highlighting a 13-week tubal ectopic pregnancy are relatively limited.

Table 1. A retrospective overview of 13-week tubal ectopic pregnancies.

Year of Publication	Age of Patient	Common Clinical Signs, Intervention and Weeks of Gestation	Reference
2018	31-year-old	amenorrhea for three months and one week; abdominal pain; Hb 8.5 g/dL; β-hCG 80.427, 9 mIU/mL; salpingo-oophorectomy	[43]
2019	39-year-old	abdominal pain; vaginal bleeding; Hb 8.7 g/dL; β-hCG 55.713 mIU/mL; salpingectomy	[44]
2020	38-year-old	amenorrhea for three months; abdominal pain; Hb 3.2 g/L; β-hCG 11.300 IU/mL; salpingectomy	[45]

Hamura et al. [46] performed a retrospective case review study over 56 months, analyzing the medical records of 73 women from Papua New Guinea. They reveal a rate of ectopic pregnancy of 6.3 per 1000 deliveries, with no maternal death, from which 85%

were parous, 67% rural dwellers, and 62% with a documented history of sub-fertility, all following salpingectomy. Davenport et al. [47] conducted a retrospective cohort study between 2004 and 2018 in which they assessed 216 patients who received a single dose of intramuscular MTX (50 mg/m^2) for the diagnosis of tubal ectopic pregnancy. Thus, aiming to investigate the time to resolution when the serum hCG < 5 IU/L, respectively, the need for rescue surgery, they noted a median time of 22 days to resolution with rescue surgery. For an hCG < 1000 IU/L, the median was 20 days, but when hCG > 2000 IU/L, the median was 34.5 days.

Based on all aspects, bedside point-of-care ultrasound (POCUS) is crucial for physicians since it reflects the time of diagnosis and patient and detects ruptures of ectopic pregnancies and ongoing abdominal bleeding. Thus, POCUS retains the sensitivity for ruptured ectopic pregnancies to detect an empty uterus, free fluid, gestational sac(s), and extrauterine masses [48].

Given the dimensions of the tubal pregnancy, in some cases, a transvaginal ultrasound (TVS) alone may not be the appropriate approach to differentiate between an abdominal and a tubal pregnancy, an MRI being necessary. However, TVS) and the assessment of β-hCG have both sensitivity and specificity compared with transabdominal ultrasound (TUS) in ectopic pregnancy diagnosis [49].

4. Conclusions

We presented a rare case of a 36-year-old woman with a live ectopic left tubal pregnancy corresponding to 13 weeks of gestation. To the authors' best knowledge, this is the sole documented evolving tubal ectopic pregnancy in Romania, uncomplicated at this age. The diagnosis of such a pregnancy is an imaging challenge due to its rarity and location, and despite MRI examination, the diagnosis was certainly possible only after laparoscopy. The other peculiarity of the case is the failure to diagnose the ectopic pregnancy before performing the curettage on request. Therefore, an ectopic pregnancy diagnosis should always be ruled out in the first trimester of a pregnancy before an elective curettage. In addition, the diagnosis of a tubal pregnancy at 13 weeks of gestation using imaging remains a challenge.

Author Contributions: C.I., O.-D.I. and I.S. (conceptualization, data curation, investigation, formal analysis, methodology, writing—original draft), O.-A.M. and B.D. (formal analysis, writing—review and editing, supervision, validation, project administration). All authors have read and agreed to the published version of the manuscript.

Funding: This research received no external funding.

Institutional Review Board Statement: The design of this study was approved by the Ethical Committee of the Clinical Hospital of Obstetrics and Gynecology "Cuza Voda" from Iasi (no 9320/20/07/2022). It must be stated that the present study respected the Helsinki Declaration on Human Rights, concomitantly with National and European legislation regarding Biomedical Research.

Informed Consent Statement: Written informed consent was obtained from the patient(s) to publish this paper.

Data Availability Statement: The datasets used and analyzed in this study are available from the corresponding author on reasonable request.

Conflicts of Interest: The authors declare no conflict of interest.

References

1. Taran, F.-A.; Kagan, K.-O.; Hübner, M.; Hoopmann, M.; Wallwiener, D.; Brucker, S. The Diagnosis and Treatment of Ectopic Pregnancy. *Dtsch. Arztebl. Int.* **2015**, *112*, 693–704. [CrossRef]
2. Mhaskar, R.; Harish, M.; Jaiprakash, T. Unruptured Ampullary Ectopic Pregnancy at 16-week Period of Gestation with Live Fetus. *J. Obstet. Gynaecol. India* **2014**, *64*, 73–74. [CrossRef]
3. Committee on Practice Bulletins—Gynecology. ACOG Practice Bulletin No. 191: Tubal Ectopic Pregnancy. *Obstet. Gynecol.* **2018**, *131*, e65–e77. [CrossRef] [PubMed]
4. Panelli, D.M.; Phillips, C.H.; Brady, P.C. Incidence, diagnosis and management of tubal and nontubal ectopic pregnancies: A review. *Fertil. Res. Pract.* **2015**, *1*, 15. [CrossRef] [PubMed]

5. Bouyer, J.; Coste, J.; Fernandez, H.; Pouly, J.L.; Job-Spira, N. Sites of ectopic pregnancy: A 10 year population-based study of 1800 cases. *Hum. Reprod.* **2002**, *17*, 3224–3230. [CrossRef]
6. Murray, H.; Baakdah, H.; Bardell, T.; Tulandi, T. Diagnosis and treatment of ectopic pregnancy. *Can. Med. Assoc. J.* **2005**, *173*, 905–912. [CrossRef] [PubMed]
7. Cunningham, F.G.; Leveno, K.J.; Bloom, S.L.; Spong, C.Y.; Dashe, J.S.; Hoffman, B.L. Ectopic Pregnancy. *Williams Obstetretics*, 24th ed.; McGraw-Hill Education: New York, NY, USA, 2013.
8. Grimes, D.A. The morbidity and mortality of pregnancy. Still risky business. *Am. J. Obstet. Gynecol.* **1994**, *170*, 1489–1494.
9. Khalil, M.M.; Badran, E.Y.; Ramadan, M.F.; Shazly, S.A.-E.M.; Ali, M.K.; Abdel Badee, A.Y. An advanced second trimester tubal pregnancy: Case report. *Middle East Fertil. Soc. J.* **2012**, *17*, 136–138. [CrossRef]
10. Nkwabong, E.; Tincho, E. A case of a 26 weeks ampullary pregnancy mimicking IUD. *Anatol. J. Obs. Gynecol.* **2012**, *1*, 422–424.
11. Sachan, R.; Gupta, P.; Patel, M. Second trimester unruptured ampullary ectopic pregnancy with variable presentations: Report of two cases. *Int. J. Case Reports Images* **2012**, *3*, 1–4.
12. Kumar, V.; Gupta, J. Tubal ectopic pregnancy. *BMJ Clin. Evid.* **2015**, *2015*, 1406. [PubMed]
13. Parker, J.; Bisits, A. Laparoscopic Surgical Treatment of Ectopic Pregnancy: Salpingectomy or Salpingostomy? *Aust. N. Z. J. Obstet. Gynaecol.* **1997**, *37*, 115–117. [CrossRef] [PubMed]
14. Clausen, I. Conservative versus radical surgery for tubal pregnancy. *Acta Obstet. Gynecol. Scand.* **1996**, *75*, 8–12. [CrossRef] [PubMed]
15. Thornton, K.L.; Diamond, M.P.; DeCherney, A.H. Linear salpingostomy for ectopic pregnancy. *Obstet. Gynecol. Clin. N. Am.* **1991**, *18*, 95–109. [CrossRef]
16. Nama, V.; Manyonda, I. Tubal ectopic pregnancy: Diagnosis and management. *Arch. Gynecol. Obstet.* **2009**, *279*, 443–453. [CrossRef]
17. Bangsgaard, N.; Lund, C.O.; Ottesen, B.; Nilas, L. Improved fertility following conservative surgical treatment of ectopic pregnancy. *BJOG An. Int. J. Obstet. Gynaecol.* **2003**, *110*, 765–770. [CrossRef]
18. Mol, B.W.; Matthijsse, H.C.; Tinga, D.J.; Huynh, T.; Hajenius, P.J.; Ankum, W.M.; Bossuyt, P.M.; van der Veen, F. Fertility after conservative and radical surgery for tubal pregnancy. *Hum. Reprod.* **1998**, *13*, 1804–1809. [CrossRef]
19. Kelly, A.J.; Sowter, M.C.; Trinder, J. *The Management of Tubal Pregnancy*; Royal College of Obstetricians and Gynaecologists: London, UK, 2004.
20. Gracia, C.; Barnhart, K.T. Diagnosing ectopic pregnancy: Decision analysis comparing six strategies. *Obstet. Gynecol.* **2001**, *97*, 464–470. [CrossRef]
21. Rulin, M.C. Is salpingostomy the surgical treatment of choice for unruptured tubal pregnancy? *Obstet. Gynecol.* **1995**, *86*, 1010–1013.
22. Mukul, L.V.; Teal, S.B. Current Management of Ectopic Pregnancy. *Obstet. Gynecol. Clin. North Am.* **2007**, *34*, 403–419. [CrossRef]
23. Goodman, L.S.; Gilman, A. *The Pharmacological Basis of Therapeutics*; The Macmillan: Stuttgart, Germany, 1955.
24. Stovall, T.G.; Ling, F.W.; Gray, L.A. Single-dose methotrexate for treatment of ectopic pregnancy. *Obstet. Gynecol.* **1991**, *77*, 754–757. [PubMed]
25. Lipscomb, G.H.; McCord, M.L.; Stovall, T.G.; Huff, G.; Portera, S.G.; Ling, F.W. Predictors of Success of Methotrexate Treatment in Women with Tubal Ectopic Pregnancies. *N. Engl. J. Med.* **1999**, *341*, 1974–1978. [CrossRef] [PubMed]
26. Lipscomb, G.H.; Bran, D.; McCord, M.L.; Portera, J.C.; Ling, F.W. Analysis of three hundred fifteen ectopic pregnancies treated with single-dose methotrexate. *Am. J. Obstet. Gynecol.* **1998**, *178*, 1354–1358. [CrossRef]
27. Sowter, M.C.; Farquhar, C.M.; Petrie, K.J.; Gudex, G. A randomised trial comparing single dose systemic methotrexate and laparoscopic surgery for the treatment of unruptured tubal pregnancy. *BJOG An. Int. J. Obstet. Gynaecol.* **2001**, *108*, 192–203. [CrossRef]
28. Barnhart, K.T.; Gosman, G.; Ashby, R.; Sammel, M. The medical management of ectopic pregnancy: A meta-analysis comparing "single dose" and "multidose" regimens. *Obstet. Gynecol.* **2003**, *101*, 778–784. [CrossRef]
29. Condous, G.; Timmerman, D.; Goldstein, S.; Valentin, L.; Jurkovic, D.; Bourne, T. Pregnancies of unknown location: Consensus statement. *Ultrasound Obstet. Gynecol.* **2006**, *28*, 121–122. [CrossRef]
30. Yuk, J.-S.; Lee, J.H.; Park, W.I.; Ahn, H.S.; Kim, H.J. Systematic review and meta-analysis of single-dose and non-single-dose methotrexate protocols in the treatment of ectopic pregnancy. *Int. J. Gynecol. Obstet.* **2018**, *141*, 295–303. [CrossRef]
31. Shalev, E.; Peleg, D.; Tsabari, A.; Romano, S.; Bustan, M. Spontaneous resolution of ectopic tubal pregnancy: Natural history. *Fertil. Steril.* **1995**, *63*, 15–19. [CrossRef]
32. Lozeau, A.-M.; Potter, B. Diagnosis and management of ectopic pregnancy. *Am. Fam. Physician* **2005**, *72*, 1707–1714.
33. Butts, S.; Sammel, M.; Hummel, A.; Chittams, J.; Barnhart, K. Risk factors and clinical features of recurrent ectopic pregnancy: A case control study. *Fertil. Steril.* **2003**, *80*, 1340–1344. [CrossRef]
34. Alur-Gupta, S.; Cooney, L.G.; Senapati, S.; Sammel, M.D.; Barnhart, K.T. Two-dose versus single-dose methotrexate for treatment of ectopic pregnancy: A meta-analysis. *Am. J. Obstet. Gynecol.* **2019**, *221*, 95–108. [CrossRef]
35. Murphy, A.A.; Nager, C.W.; Wujek, J.J.; Michael Kettel, L.; Torp, V.A.; Chin, H.G. Operative laparoscopy versus laparotomy for the management of ectopic pregnancy: A prospective trial. In Proceedings of the 46th Annual Meeting of The American Fertility Society, Washington, DC, USA, 13–18 October 1990.

36. Abdulkareem, T.A. *Ectopic Pregnancy: Diagnosis, Prevention and Management*; Abduljabbar, H.S., Ed.; IntechOpen: Rijeka, Croatia, 2017; p. 3. [CrossRef]
37. Ankum, W.M.; Mol, B.W.J.; van der Veen, F.; Bossuyt, P.M.M. Risk factors for ectopic pregnancy: A meta-analysis. in part by grant OG 93/007 from the Ziekenfonds-Raad, Amstelveen, The Netherlands. *Fertil Steril* **1996**, *65*, 1093–1099. [CrossRef]
38. Gueye, M.D.N.; Gueye, M.; Thiam, I.; Mbaye, M.; Gaye, A.M.; Diouf, A.A.; Niang, M.M.; Moreau, J.C. Unruptured tubal pregnancy in the second trimester. *South Sudan Med. J.* **2013**, *6*, 95–96.
39. Radaelli, T.; Bulfamante, G.; Cetin, I.; Marconi, A.M.; Pardi, G. Advanced tubal pregnancy associated with severe fetal growth restriction: A case report. *J. Matern. Neonatal. Med.* **2003**, *13*, 422–425. [CrossRef] [PubMed]
40. Perkins, K.M.; Boulet, S.L.; Kissin, D.M.; Jamieson, D.J.; Group for the NARTS (NASS). Risk of Ectopic Pregnancy Associated With Assisted Reproductive Technology in the United States, 2001–2011. *Obstet. Gynecol.* **2015**, *125*, 70. [CrossRef]
41. Backman, T.; Rauramo, I.; Huhtala, S.; Koskenvuo, M. Pregnancy during the use of levonorgestrel intrauterine system. *Am. J. Obstet. Gynecol.* **2004**, *190*, 50–54. [CrossRef]
42. American College of Obstetricians and Gynecologists' Committee on Practice Bulletins—Gynecology. ACOG Practice Bulletin No. 193 Summary: Tubal Ectopic Pregnancy. *Obstet. Gynecol.* **2018**, *131*, e91–e103. [CrossRef]
43. Zacharis, K.; Kravvaritis, S.; Charitos, T.; Fouka, A. Ectopic Pregnancy at 13-week Period of Gestation with Live Fetus. *HJOG* **2018**, *17*, 99–102. [CrossRef]
44. Kim, M.; Hiramatsu, K.; Fukui, K.; Amemiya, K. Unexpected Tubal Pregnancy at 13 Weeks' Gestation that Was Treated with Laparoscopic Surgery Under Massive Hemoperitoneum. *Gynecol. Minim. Invasive Ther.* **2019**, *8*, 30–32. [CrossRef]
45. Gari, R.; Abdulgader, R.; Abdulqader, O. A Live 13 Weeks Ruptured Ectopic Pregnancy: A Case Report. *Cureus* **2020**, *12*, e10993. [CrossRef]
46. Hamura, N.N.; Bolnga, J.W.; Wangnapi, R.; Horne, A.W.; Rogerson, S.J.; Unger, H.W. The impact of tubal ectopic pregnancy in Papua New Guinea—A retrospective case review. *BMC Pregnancy Childbirth* **2013**, *13*, 86. [CrossRef]
47. Davenport, M.J.; Lindquist, A.; Brownfoot, F.; Pritchard, N.; Tong, S.; Hastie, R. Time to resolution of tubal ectopic pregnancy following methotrexate treatment: A retrospective cohort study. *PLoS ONE* **2022**, *17*, e0268741. [CrossRef] [PubMed]
48. Richardson, A.; Gallos, I.; Dobson, S.; Campbell, B.K.; Coomarasamy, A.; Raine-Fenning, N. Accuracy of first-trimester ultrasound in diagnosis of tubal ectopic pregnancy in the absence of an obvious extrauterine embryo: Systematic review and meta-analysis. *Ultrasound Obstet. Gynecol.* **2016**, *47*, 28–37. [CrossRef] [PubMed]
49. Kirk, E.; Bottomley, C.; Bourne, T. Diagnosing ectopic pregnancy and current concepts in the management of pregnancy of unknown location. *Hum. Reprod. Update* **2014**, *20*, 250–261. [CrossRef] [PubMed]

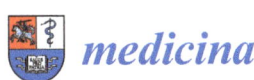

Case Report

Trophoblastic Tissue Reimplantation below the Spleen Following Laparoscopic Bilateral Salpingectomy for Ectopic Tubal Pregnancy: A Case Report

Dominyka Surgontaitė [1,*], Artūras Sukovas [1], Dalia Regina Railaitė [1], Tautvydas Jankauskas [2], Arnoldas Bartusevičius [1] and Eglė Bartusevičienė [1]

1. Department of Obstetrics and Gynaecology, Lithuanian University of Health Sciences, 50161 Kaunas, Lithuania
2. Department of Interventional Radiology, Lithuanian University of Health Sciences, 50161 Kaunas, Lithuania
* Correspondence: dominyka.surgontaite@gmail.com; Tel.: +37-064-469-864

Abstract: Background: Trophoblastic tissue reimplantation after laparoscopic salpingectomy is a very rare complication. These cases may present a diagnostic challenge and the majority of patients need a surgical treatment. Case presentation: A 31-year-old patient came to a tertiary referral center for nausea and pain in the upper left abdominal quadrant. Ultrasound and abdominal CT scan showed a $68 \times 60 \times 87$ mm size heterogenic mass below the spleen with arterial extravasation from the lower spleen pole. Recent history of surgery for ectopic pregnancy and serum hCG testing allowed to diagnose extratubal secondary trophoblastic tissue reimplantation below the spleen. Embolization of the bleeding vessel and successful treatment with methotrexate was achieved. Conclusions: In cases of a nondisseminated trophoblastic tissue reimplantation, consider embolization and treatment with methotrexate if the patient is hemodynamically stable; thus, secondary surgical treatment is preventable.

Keywords: trophoblastic tissue reimplantation; embolization; methotrexate

Citation: Surgontaitė, D.; Sukovas, A.; Railaitė, D.R.; Jankauskas, T.; Bartusevičius, A.; Bartusevičienė, E. Trophoblastic Tissue Reimplantation below the Spleen Following Laparoscopic Bilateral Salpingectomy for Ectopic Tubal Pregnancy: A Case Report. *Medicina* **2023**, *59*, 701. https://doi.org/10.3390/medicina59040701

Academic Editors: Marius L. Craina and Elena Bernad

Received: 14 March 2023
Revised: 30 March 2023
Accepted: 31 March 2023
Published: 3 April 2023

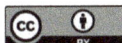

Copyright: © 2023 by the authors. Licensee MDPI, Basel, Switzerland. This article is an open access article distributed under the terms and conditions of the Creative Commons Attribution (CC BY) license (https://creativecommons.org/licenses/by/4.0/).

1. Introduction

Ectopic pregnancy occurs in 1–2% of all pregnancies [1,2]. The rate of persistent ectopic pregnancy after expectant management, surgical or methotrexate treatment is reported in 4–15% of the cases [3,4]. Ectopic pregnancy tissue reimplantation is a very rare complication. A total of 25 cases of reimplantation of trophoblastic tissue following laparoscopic removal of ectopic pregnancy have been reported in the period from January 1989 to January 2018, and only a few of these cases describe peritoneal trophoblastic implantation following laparoscopic salpingectomy [5–9]. To our knowledge, only two similar cases have been reported since 2019 [10,11].

In the latest ectopic pregnancy treatment guidelines, there is no necessary follow-up after salpingectomy, as it is considered a definitive treatment for tubal pregnancy [3]. In this report, we present a clinical case of trophoblastic tissue reimplantation below the spleen following laparoscopic bilateral salpingectomy.

2. Clinical Case

A 31-year-old woman was sent to the emergency department of a tertiary referral center due to an unknown diagnosis. The patient was feeling nauseous and complained of intensifying pain in the upper left abdominal quadrant.

The woman was hemodynamically stable. During physical examination, abdominal muscle tension was observed, and there was no rebound tenderness. Ultrasound revealed a mass in the upper left side of the abdomen and a small amount of unclear fluid around the intestines. In the blood test, only leukocytosis of 17.3×10^9/L was abnormal.

Three weeks earlier, in a regional hospital, she was diagnosed with ectopic pregnancy (7 weeks of gestation) in her left fallopian tube. Left laparoscopic salpingostomy was planned, although salpingectomy was performed due to heavy bleeding. Data on ultrasound findings before surgery was not available. The serum human chorionic gonadotropin (hCG) concentration was not tested. Histological reports showed no chorionic villus, and only several trophoblasts were seen in the surgically removed material. In the past, the woman had had two normal deliveries, pelvic inflammatory disease and one more ectopic pregnancy in her right fallopian tube. Therefore, she underwent laparoscopic right salpingectomy.

A computed tomography (CT) scan was performed to differentiate the mass found on ultrasound. Abdominal and pelvic CT showed a 68 × 60 × 87 mm heterogenic mass, likely a hematoma, which was below the spleen. Pelvis was filled with hemorrhagic fluid, and the uterus was enlarged. Arterial extravasation was spotted from the lower spleen pole. Conventional angiography of the splenic artery was performed, and extravasation was identified in the region below the spleen. The vessel was embolized (Figure 1A–E). Due to the unknown origin of the hematoma and the recent history of surgery for ectopic pregnancy, and gynecologist consultation was sought. The gynecologist ordered a urine pregnancy test, which was positive. The serum human chorionic gonadotropin (hCG) concentration was 3363.6 U/L. The clinical case was considered a rare pathology of extratubal secondary trophoblastic tissue reimplantation. As the bleeding was stopped with embolization, a conservative two-dose methotrexate (MTX) treatment protocol with MTX 50 mg per square meter of body surface area intramuscularly (mg/m^2 BSA i/m) on day 1 and day 4 was administered. Abdominal pain did not intensify; subjectively, the woman started feeling better. The decrease in serum hCG concentration between days 4 and 7 was 24.1% (i.e., more than 15%); thus, hCG testing was repeated weekly (Chart 1). Menstruation renewed 29 days after the first dose of MTX. Seven months later, the CT scan showed that the size of the heterogenic mass below the spleen decreased to 18 × 14 × 16 mm (Figure 1F).

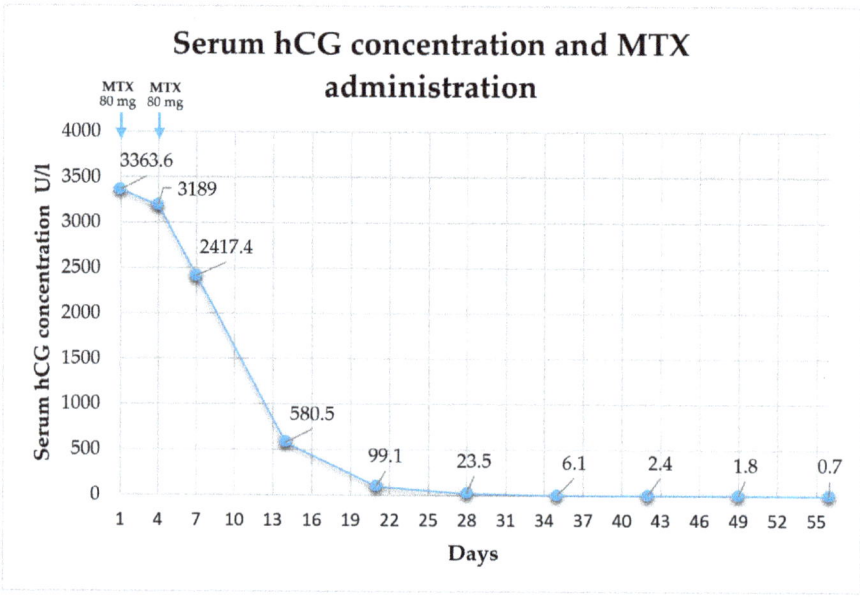

Chart 1. Serum hCG concentration drop and methotrexate administration.

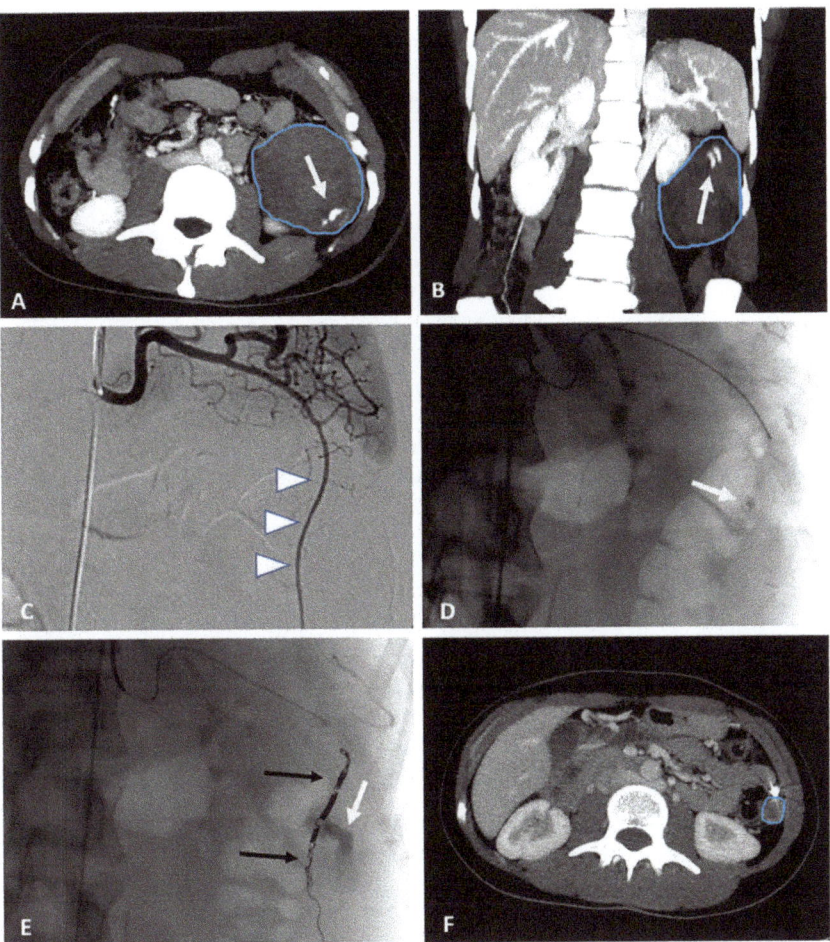

Figure 1. Axial and coronal 15 mm maximum intensity projections (contrast-enhanced computed tomography (CE-CT) in the emergency department, prior to embolization), large hematoma is seen in the upper left abdomen (blue outline) with active arterial extravasation (white arrow) (**A**,**B**). Digital subtraction angiography of coeliac trunk shows unusual large arterial branch (white arrowheads) descending from the splenic artery to lower abdomen—most likely hypertrophied left epiploic artery (**C**). Selective angiography with micro catheter shows slow arterial extravasation (white arrow) (**D**). Post-embolization image (**E**) with embolizing coils (black arrows) above and below extravasation site, also stagnated contrast medium in hematoma can be seen (white arrow). Significant size reduction of hematoma is seen at 7 month follow-up CT image (blue outline) (**F**).

3. Discussion

The extratubal secondary trophoblastic tissue reimplantation following surgical removal of an ectopic pregnancy is estimated to be found in 1–1.9% of the cases, and it seems that there is an equal distribution between salpingostomy and salpingectomy [9]. Given that these cases may present a diagnostic challenge and are usually detected via sudden abdominal pain and acute hemoperitoneum, it is necessary to prevent and diagnose such cases in the early period after the primary surgery [10]. Current guidelines state that hCG follow-up after laparoscopic salpingostomy should be made 7 days after the surgery, then one measurement per week until a negative result is obtained. A subsequent urine pregnancy test could be performed 3 weeks after salpingectomy [2,3].

In our clinical case, salpingostomy was considered first, because the patient previously had an ectopic pregnancy and underwent contralateral laparoscopic salpingectomy. When the bleeding began, salpingectomy was performed, and there was a possible dissemination of trophoblastic tissue. Our case supports the recommendation of some authors regarding postoperative hCG monitoring if the specimen was fragmented during salpingectomy and if there could have been spillage of the trophoblastic tissue [11,12]. It would have been reasonable to have performed serial hCG measurements given the attempted salpingostomy. In addition, it is important to avoid iatrogenic dissemination of trophoblast tissue through surgery. It is recommended to limit the use of the Trendelenburg position thorough suction and the removal of blood clots, abundant irrigation of the abdominal cavity, and careful removal of the pregnancy tissue [5,9].

To diagnose the peritoneal reimplantation of trophoblastic tissue can be very difficult. The symptoms vary from abdominal pain and vaginal bleeding to hemorrhagic shock. The time period from the first operation until the patient returned to the hospital varied from 7 to 51 days. Therefore, it is important to consider the possibility of persistent or reimplanted trophoblastic tissue even though weeks have passed since the primary operation [9,11]. In our case, the patient was hospitalized 21 days after the surgery for ectopic pregnancy due to abdominal pain and intra-abdominal bleeding. These cases are hard to interpret through ultrasound, and often auxiliary examinations (abdominal, pelvic CT and/or magnetic resonance imaging (MRI)) are requested. MRI could be the key diagnostic method if hCG continues to rise. It also assists in determining the location of the possible reimplantation and helps to plan surgical steps [13,14]. In the presented case, trophoblastic tissue reimplantation diagnosis was not easily made. The patient was thoroughly investigated by an emergency physician and a surgeon. After a CT scan, hemorrhage of an unknown origin was considered; accordingly, the bleeding was managed with embolization. A certain diagnosis of extratubal secondary trophoblastic tissue reimplantation was made only after a gynecologist's consultation, urine pregnancy test, and serum hCG testing.

The treatment of trophoblastic tissue reimplantation depends on whether the patient is hemodynamically stable [8,9]. Schyum AC et al. presented a literature review of trophoblastic tissue reimplantation in which all patients needed surgical treatment: laparoscopy in 40% (10/25) and laparotomy in 28% (7/25). The surgical method was not stated in eight of the twenty-five cases. MTX was only used as an additional treatment during or after the second operation [9]. However, MTX can be one of the primary treatment options for hemodynamically stable patients [10]. Our clinical case suggests that if a nondisseminated trophoblastic tissue implant after salpingectomy is diagnosed in a hemodynamically stable patient, embolization of the bleeding vessel and treatment with MTX can be considered. After embolization, MTX concentrations in trophoblastic tissue were appropriate as the serum hCG count continued to fall.

4. Conclusions

The diagnosis of the peritoneal reimplantation of trophoblastic tissue can be very challenging; thus, it is very important to avoid iatrogenic dissemination of trophoblast tissue through operation and to follow up serum hCG even after salpingectomy, especially when the conditions of trophoblastic tissue removal are questionable. If a nondisseminated trophoblastic tissue implant after salpingectomy is diagnosed prior to the development of massive intra-abdominal hemorrhage, we suggest considering embolization of the bleeding vessel and treatment with methotrexate.

Author Contributions: D.S., A.S., T.J. and E.B. writing—original draft preparation, D.R.R., A.B. and E.B. writing—review and editing, D.S. and T.J. visualization. All authors have read and agreed to the published version of the manuscript.

Funding: This research received no external funding.

Institutional Review Board Statement: Not applicable.

Informed Consent Statement: Patient consent was waived due to the anonymous presentation of the case. There is no possibility to identify the patient described in this article.

Data Availability Statement: Not applicable.

Conflicts of Interest: The authors declare no conflict of interest.

References

1. Farquhar, C.M. Ectopic pregnancy. *Lancet* **2005**, *366*, 583. [CrossRef]
2. Elson, C.J.; Salim, R.; Potdar, N.; Chetty, M.; Ross, J.A.; Kirk, E.J. Diagnosis and management of ectopic pregnancy. *BJOG Int. J. Obstet. Gynaecol.* **2016**, *123*, e15–e55.
3. NICE Guideline. *Ectopic Pregnancy and Miscarriage: Diagnosis and Initial Management*; NICE: London, UK, 2019; pp. 1–36. Available online: https://www.nice.org.uk/guidance/ng126/resources/ectopic-pregnancy-and-miscarriage-diagnosis-and-initial-management-pdf-66141662244037 (accessed on 1 June 2022).
4. Tulandi, T. Ectopic Pregnancy: Surgical Treatment. 2022. Available online: https://www.uptodate.com/contents/ectopic-pregnancy-surgical-treatment?search=Ectopic%20pregnancy:&source=search_result&selectedTitle=5~150&usage_type=default&display_rank=5 (accessed on 1 June 2022).
5. Ben-Arie, A.; Goldchmit, R.; Dgani, R.; Hazan, Y.; Ben-Hur, H.; Open, M.; Hagay, Z. Trophoblastic peritoneal implants after laparoscopic treatment of ectopic pregnancy. *Eur. J. Obstet. Gynecol. Reprod. Biol.* **2001**, *96*, 113–115. [CrossRef]
6. Ali, C.R.; Fitzgerald, C. Omental and peritoneal secondary trophoblastic implantation—An unusual complication after IVF. *Reprod. Biomed. Online* **2006**, *12*, 776–778. [CrossRef]
7. Bucella, D.; Buxant, F.; Anaf, V.; Simon, P.; Fayt, I.; Noël, J.C. Omental trophoblastic implants after surgical management of ectopic pregnancy. *Arch. Gynecol. Obstet.* **2009**, *280*, 115–117. [CrossRef]
8. Humphreys, C.A.; Ragnarsdottir, B.; Brown, P.; Jack, S. Acute hemoperitoneum 6 weeks post-laparoscopic salpingectomy—A rare case of secondary peritoneal trophoblast implantation. *Gynecol. Surg.* **2012**, *9*, 457–460. [CrossRef]
9. Schyum, A.C.; Rosendal, B.M.B.; Andersen, B. Peritoneal reimplantation of trophoblastic tissue following laparoscopic treatment of ectopic pregnancy: A case report and review of literature. *J. Gynecol. Obstet. Hum. Reprod.* **2019**, *48*, 213–216. [CrossRef]
10. Robson, D.; Lusink, V.; Campbell, N. Persistent omental trophoblastic implantation following salpingostomy, salpingectomy and methotrexate for ectopic pregnancy: A case report. *Case Rep. Womens Health* **2019**, *21*, e00095. [CrossRef]
11. Wang, T.; Li, Q. Extratubal secondary trophoblastic implants (ESTI) following laparoscopic bilateral salpingectomy for ectopic pregnancy: Problems that have been neglected for a long time. *Gynecol. Endocrinol.* **2022**, *38*, 608–611. [CrossRef]
12. Cartwright, P.S. Peritoneal trophoblastic implants after surgical management of tubal pregnancy. *J. Reprod. Med.* **1991**, *36*, 523–524.
13. Trail, C.E.; Watson, A.; Schofield, A.M. Case of hepatic flexure ectopic pregnancy medically managed with methotrexate. *BMJ Case Rep.* **2018**, *2018*, bcr2017220480. [CrossRef]
14. Yi, K.W.; Yeo, M.K.; Shin, J.H.; Kim, K.A.; Oh, M.-J.; Lee, J.K.; Hur, J.-Y.; Saw, H.-S. Laparoscopic management of early omental pregnancy detected by magnetic resonance imaging. *J. Minim. Invasive Gynecol.* **2008**, *15*, 231–234. [CrossRef]

Disclaimer/Publisher's Note: The statements, opinions and data contained in all publications are solely those of the individual author(s) and contributor(s) and not of MDPI and/or the editor(s). MDPI and/or the editor(s) disclaim responsibility for any injury to people or property resulting from any ideas, methods, instructions or products referred to in the content.

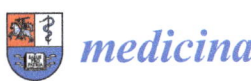

Case Report

Interstitial Ectopic Pregnancy—Case Reports and Medical Management

Małgorzata Kampioni *, Karolina Chmaj-Wierzchowska, Katarzyna Wszołek * and Maciej Wilczak

Department of Maternal and Child Health, Poznan University of Medical Sciences, Polna 33, 69-535 Poznan, Poland
* Correspondence: iubesc@poczta.onet.pl (M.K.); katarzyna.wszolek@ump.edu.pl (K.W.)

Abstract: The term intramural (interstitial) ectopic pregnancy refers to a pregnancy developing outside the uterine cavity, with a gestational sac implanted into the interstitial part of the Fallopian tube, surrounded by a layer of the myometrium. The prevalence rate of interstitial pregnancy (IP) is 2–4% of all ectopic pregnancies. Surgery is the primary treatment for interstitial ectopic pregnancy; the pharmacological management of ectopic pregnancy, including IP, in asymptomatic patients includes systemic administration of methotrexate. In this report, we present two cases of this rare pregnancy type, reviewing our management technique and treatment ways presented in the literature. In our patients, the management was initially conservative and included methotrexate, administered as intravenous bolus injection, regular beta-human chorionic gonadotropins (β-HCG) level measurements in peripheral blood, and monitoring of the patient's general condition. Due to signs of intra-abdominal bleeding in patient A and inadequate β-HCG level reduction in patient B, both patients eventually underwent laparoscopic cornual resection. Pregnancy, implanted into the interstitial part of the Fallopian tube and surrounded by myometrial tissue with myometrial invasion of the trophoblast, poses a serious diagnostic challenge to modern gynecology due to particularly low sensitivity and specificity of symptoms, and may require both pharmacological and surgical treatment.

Keywords: pregnancy; ectopic; laparoscopy; clinical decision making

Citation: Kampioni, M.; Chmaj-Wierzchowska, K.; Wszołek, K.; Wilczak, M. Interstitial Ectopic Pregnancy—Case Reports and Medical Management. *Medicina* 2023, 59, 233. https://doi.org/10.3390/medicina59020233

Academic Editors: Marius L. Craina, Elena Bernad and Edgaras Stankevičius

Received: 28 September 2022
Revised: 21 January 2023
Accepted: 23 January 2023
Published: 26 January 2023

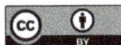

Copyright: © 2023 by the authors. Licensee MDPI, Basel, Switzerland. This article is an open access article distributed under the terms and conditions of the Creative Commons Attribution (CC BY) license (https://creativecommons.org/licenses/by/4.0/).

1. Introduction

The term intramural (interstitial) ectopic pregnancy refers to pregnancy developing outside the uterine cavity, with a gestational sac implanted into the interstitial part of the Fallopian tube, surrounded by a layer of the myometrium, i.e., the middle uterine wall layer, composed mainly of smooth muscle cells (myocytes), as well as the supporting interstitial and vascular tissue [1–3]. The interstitial part of the Fallopian tube is approximately 1–2 cm long and 0.7 mm wide [1]. According to the literature, cornual pregnancy specifically refers to the presence of a gestational sac within a rudimentary uterine horn, a unicornuate uterus, the cornua of a bicornuate uterus, or a septate uterus [4,5].

The prevalence rate of interstitial pregnancy (IP) is estimated to be 2–4% of all ectopic pregnancies by most authors [2,3,5–9] and may range from 6–8%, according to some studies [10]. Due to particularly low sensitivity and specificity of symptoms, it poses one of the largest diagnostic and treatment challenges in modern gynecology. The symptoms, including pelvic, abdominal, or chest pain, vaginal bleeding, intra-abdominal bleeding, hypovolemic shock or uterine rupture are only manifested after 12 gestational weeks in over 20% of cases. They can be life-threatening, and the condition has a mortality rate of up to 2% [1]. The classic clinical triad of ectopic pregnancy, including abdominal pain, vaginal bleeding, and amenorrhea, is only present in 40% of cornual pregnancies [1,3,4,8,11]. Implantation into the tubal wall and myometrial invasion of the trophoblast significantly impede ultrasound-based differential diagnosis of intrauterine or cornual pregnancy [3,8,12–14].

The ultrasound diagnostic criteria, developed to identify intramural pregnancy, include [3,8,12–15]:
- An empty uterine cavity;
- A chorionic sac located eccentrically and at >1 cm from the lateral edge of the uterine cavity;
- A thin (<5 mm) myometrial layer surrounding the chorionic sac;
- The interstitial line sign;
- No double decidual sac sign, typically seen in the intrauterine pregnancy.

The treatment strategies should be individualized, but surgery is still the main treatment of interstitial ectopic pregnancy [9,14]. A number of laparoscopic or laparotomic techniques are available, including cornual resection, salpingectomy, cornuostomy, or hysterectomy. Due to significant advances in endoscopic surgery in recent years, laparoscopic techniques are currently the treatment of choice in the IP [9,10,16] and is preferable to an open approach [15] with laparoscopic cornuotomy or cornual wedge resection [17]. The choice depends on the patient's condition, availability of medical equipment, and surgical skills of a gynecologist [9,18,19], but laparoscopy has replaced surgical treatments used previously, which included uterine horn resection or even hysterectomy [20].

The pharmacological management of an ectopic pregnancy, including IP, in asymptomatic patients includes the systemic administration of methotrexate (MTX). However, in cases of an IP > 5 cm in diameter, this method fails in 9–65% of cases [19]. In the general population, the failure percentage is estimated to be 25% and additional, surgical treatment is often needed [18]. MTX can also be administered directly into the gestational sac during a local hysteroscopic injection in patients diagnosed at an early stage of IP [21]. This method is described as effective and allows patients to avoid a surgical scar on the uterine muscle [18].

The aim of this study is to present two cases of uterine horn pregnancy to discuss the complexity of the issue and to share our experience in this field as well as review the literature to gain an indication of the different treatment methods.

2. Presentation of Case Reports

2.1. Case 1 (Patient A)

Patient A, a 17-year-old primiparous woman (G0P0A0), was admitted to the Department of Maternal and Child Health, Obstetrics and Gynecology University Hospital, Poznan University of Medical Sciences on 31 July 2019. She was referred by her gynecologist, with an ambulatory diagnosis of 10 weeks of ectopic IP located within the right uterine horn. This diagnosis was confirmed during hospitalization. The β-HCG level on admission was 22,344 mIU/mL. On admission, the patient reported blood-stained vaginal discharge and the absence of other symptoms. The vaginal examination carried out following her giving consent and in the presence of her legal guardian yielded the following findings: ectocervix small, clear and smooth with a punctuate os; moderate amount of dark bloody discharge; uterine body anteroflexed, round, normal in size and mobility; ovaries and Fallopian tubes normal on palpation; no pelvic masses; negative peritoneal signs. A transvaginal ultrasound revealed a uterine body sized 56 × 32 mm, homogeneity in echotexture, and endometrium thickness up to 10 mm. A gestational sac (GS) (15.5 mm in diameter—4w6d, with an embryo crown rump length—CRL = 12 mm − 7w3d) was located interstitially in the right uterine corn, near to the right proximal tubal ostium. Fetal heart rate was 120 bpm. The ovaries appeared normal. There was no free fluid within the cul-de-sac (Figure 1A,B).

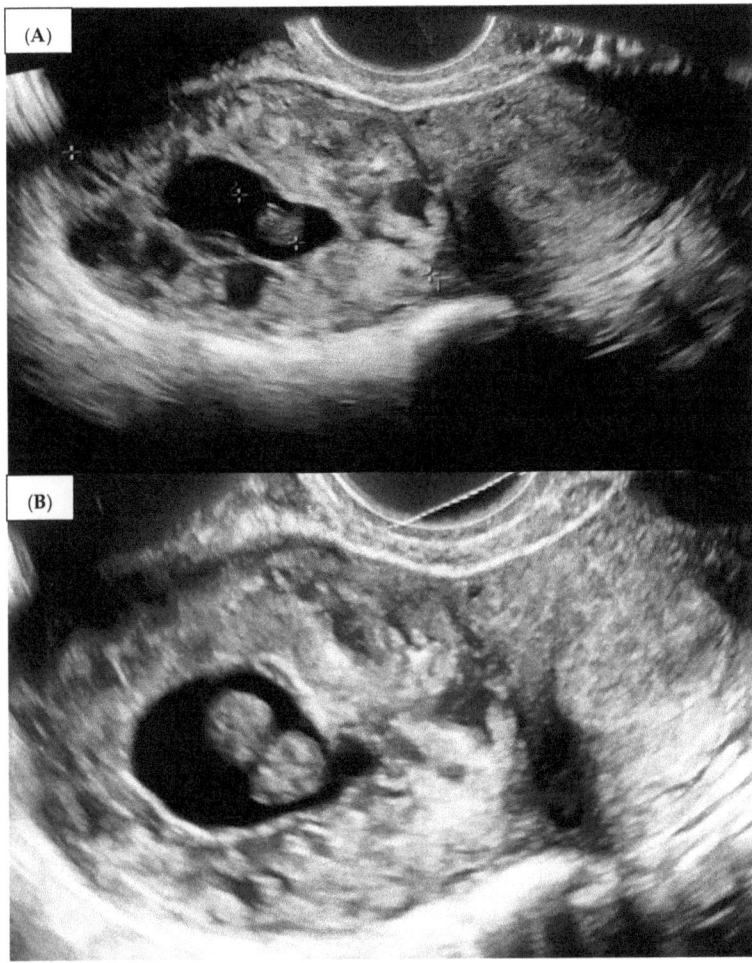

Figure 1. (**A,B**)—Patient A—a 2D transvaginal ultrasound of an interstitial ectopic pregnancy within the right uterine horn in different dimensions.

Following clinical assessment and based on the wishes expressed by the patient and her legal guardian, pharmacological treatment with methotrexate and leucovorin was started, in line with current guidelines. Methotrexate (100 mg) was administered on 2 August 2019, 5 August 2019, 8 August 2019, and 11 August 2019, followed by oral leucovorin 15 mg. The β-HCG levels were determined accordingly, and the results are shown in Table 1.

Table 1. Serum β-HCG levels in the patient A, July/August 2019.

Date	31 July	5 August	8 August	9 August	14 August	16 August
β-HCG (mIU/mL)	22,344	29,502	15,735	17,138	13,171	6463

The follow-up ultrasound on 8 August 2019 confirmed the embryo demise within the right uterine horn. Despite receiving a satisfactory response to the systemic treatment with methotrexate, a surgical intervention followed, due to signs of intra-abdominal bleeding found on ultrasound and increasing abdominal pain. On 16 August 2019, the patient underwent a laparoscopy. Intraoperative findings included an enlarged right uterine horn which was approx. 3 cm in diameter. It contained the ectopic gestational sac and, as a result, was significantly hyperemic and swollen. Right salpingectomy was performed, followed by bipolar cautery along the margin of the ectopic gestational sac, and right cornual resection was performed (with morcellation). The stages of the surgery are shown in Figure 2A,B.

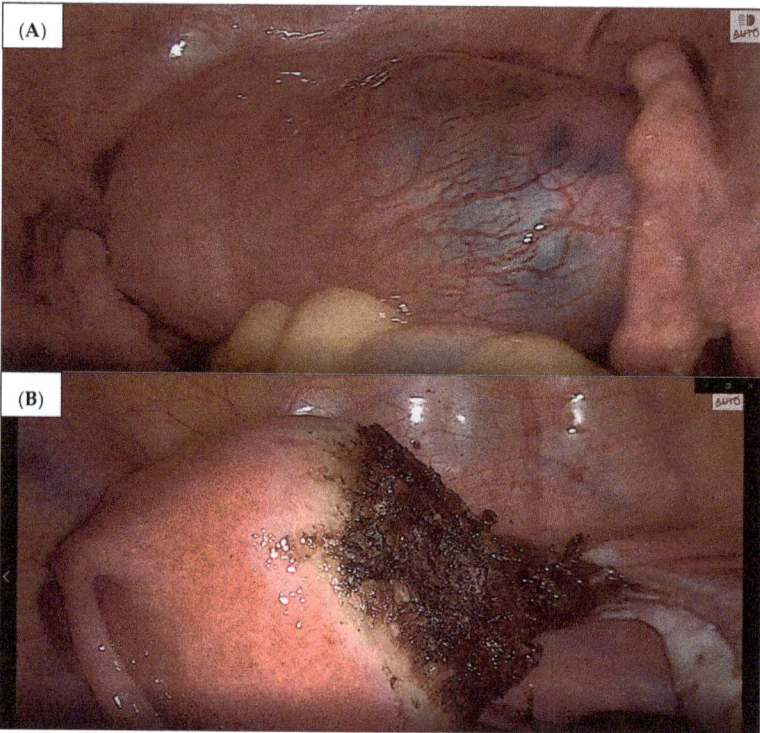

Figure 2. (**A**) Patient A—interstitial ectopic pregnancy within the right uterine horn, viewed from the abdominal cavity. (**B**)—Patient A—Postoperative view following the cornual resection due to interstitial pregnancy. Hemostatic effect after the minimally invasive surgery.

The serum β-HCG level on 19 August 2019 was 232 mIU/mL. The postoperative course was uneventful. The patient was discharged home in a stable condition and with recommendations of combined hormonal contraception.

2.2. Case 2 (Patient B)

Patient B, a 33-year-old woman (G1P0A1) presenting with a 7-week interstitial, ectopic pregnancy located in the left uterine horn was admitted to the Department of Maternal and Child Health, Obstetrics and Gynecology University Hospital, Poznan University of Medical Sciences on 8 December 2020. She had undergone laparotomic right salpingo-oophorectomy in 2006 due to mature teratoma of the right ovary. Her last menstruation was on 20 October 2020. The β-HCG level on admission was 5632 mIU/mL. The patient was asymptomatic. The vaginal examination confirmed a small ectocervix, clear and smooth with a punctuate os, normal vaginal discharge, anteroflexed uterine body, normal in size and mobility, left ovary and Fallopian tube normal on palpation, no pelvic masses, and negative peritoneal signs. A transvaginal ultrasound revealed a live intramural pregnancy within the interstitial part of the left Fallopian tube in the left uterine horn, interstitial line sign, myometrial layer surrounding the gestational sac in all projections, cornual bulge, and moderately severe edema where the trophoblast invaded the myometrium. There was also quite significant vascular proliferation within the enlarged uterine horn. A pseudogestational sac, 3 mm in diameter, was found within the uterine cavity. The mass of a total size of 11 mm presented with a detectable fetal heart rate and CRL of 2 mm. Its interstitial location was confirmed. The 6 mm wide chorionic ring containing the yolk sac was imaged. The ovaries appeared normal. There was no free fluid within the cul-de-sac (Figure 3).

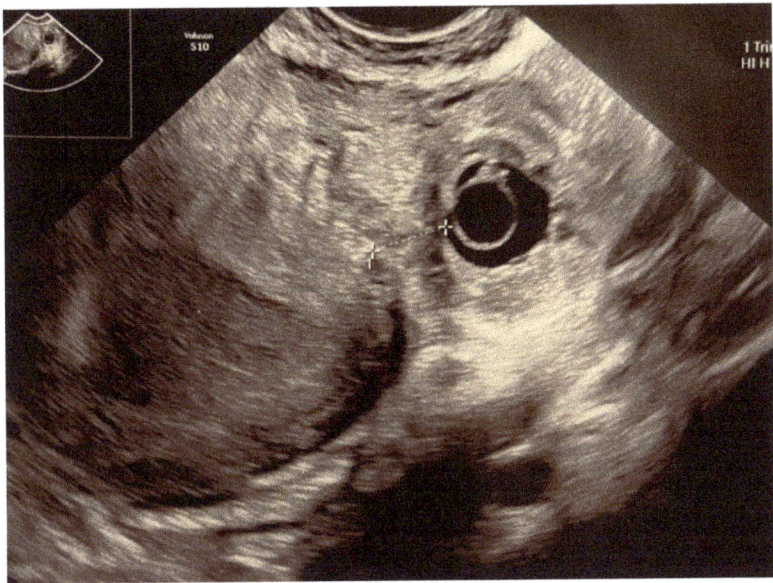

Figure 3. Patient B—2D transvaginal ultrasound of IP within the left uterine horn, cornual bulge.

Following clinical assessment and a case manifestation, based on the patient's wishes, pharmacological treatment with MTX and leucovorin was started, in line with current guidelines. MTX (100 mg) was administered on 8 December 2020 and 11 December 2020, followed by oral leucovorin 15 mg. The β-HCG levels were determined accordingly, and the results are shown in Table 2.

Table 2. Serum β-HCG levels in the patient B, December 2020.

Date	8 December	11 December	14 December
β-HCG (mIU/mL)	5632	5927	5739

The follow-up ultrasound on 14 December 2019 confirmed the embryo demise within the left uterine horn. Due to an unsatisfactory response to pharmacological treatment, a surgery was offered, and the patient consented. On 15 December 2020, laparoscopy was carried out. The procedure revealed a left uterine horn with a tubal fragment preserved after the previous surgery, with tumor-like appearance, 4 cm in diameter, with a soft and heavily vascularized structure. The gestational sac with the fragment of the uterine horn and tubal stump were dissected from the uterine body and resected. Hemostasis was achieved by cautery. The postoperative course was uneventful.

The patient was discharged home on 17 December 2020 in a stable condition with the recommendation of using combined hormonal contraception.

3. Discussion

IP may cause life-threatening complications, as a rare and highly dangerous form of ectopic pregnancy, with its lack of specific manifestations, and so its early diagnosis is crucial. Traditionally, the treatment of IP has been surgical and may include hysterectomy or cornual resection by laparotomy or laparoscopy [1,4,9,12,18–20].

The advances in minimally invasive surgery have provided more therapeutic options for the treatment of ectopic pregnancies, including the combination of systemic and local hysteroscopic administration of MTX [9,14,20–24]. This is an interesting and promising approach, but this type of treatment requires both implementation in the clinics (including the equipment) and skilled gynecologists to be carried out safely.

Surgical laparotomy is the only appropriate route in the case of unstable hemodynamic women with a suspicion of rupture or recurrent IP [24]. More conservative surgical approaches have been proposed, and currently laparoscopy is the most commonly adopted technique of elective surgery [12]. In the case of Patient A, the decision for surgical management, mentioned as one of the treatment options, was made based on intra-abdominal bleeding exponents shown on ultrasound imaging and peritoneal symptoms. Despite the implementation of systemic MTX treatment, with βhCG showing a decreasing trend, there were symptoms of IP rupture and incipient hypovolemic shock.

Cornual or minicornual resection can be performed in the case of a viable IP with a history of failed therapeutic strategy [25] instead of a cornuostomy that could be adopted with an IP of less than 4 cm in diameter [26]. In the last few years, more conservative surgical alternatives, such as cornuostomy rather than cornuectomy, have been introduced to better preserve uterine integrity for future fertility [25,26].

Some cases of laparoscopic cornuostomy have been reported in the literature [2,3,6,27]. However, patients with a history of ipsilateral salpingectomy should be cautioned regarding the possibility of IP. Laparoscopic cornuostomy appears to be an appropriate treatment for IP in patients wishing to preserve fertility, and the use of concomitant prophylactic MTX may reduce the risk of persistent ectopic pregnancy, especially among patients with ruptured masses and high β-HCG levels [28]. Po et al. [17] stated that clinicians may perform either laparoscopic cornuotomy or cornual wedge resection because both procedures have comparable results, but this summary statement was rated as conditional and low in the GRADE evidence quality.

The treatment should be personalized in a way that considers the obstetric history of the patients, the gestational age at the diagnosis, and their desire for future pregnancies [9,14]. Stabile et al. [14] proposed a multidose MTX intramuscular regimen, combined with mifepristone (600 mg orally), in asymptomatic women with low serum levels of β-HCG at an early gestational age. It can be also considered in asymptomatic women with a strong motivation for future conceptions, although in the case of high serum levels of β-HCG, additional dose(s) of MTX may be necessary. The overall efficacy of a single MTX dose is estimated to be 65–95%, and such a variability is due to several factors: the baseline level of β-HCG (the lower the level, the higher the efficacy of the treatment), the rate of serum β-HCG growth over 48 h prior to MTX administration, the visibility of specific elements of the fetal egg on ultrasound, and the rate of decrease in β-HCG levels after the implementation of the pharmacological treatment [29]. Our patient described as a B, despite of the implementation of MTX treatment and leucovorin, presented a non-satisfactory response to drug treatment (β-HCG serum level decreased <15% of the initial level). After discussing possible management routes, the patient consented for a laparoscopic surgery.

Tulandi and Al-Jaroudi [30] discussed the management of 32 interstitial pregnancy cases. Eight women were treated with MTX either systemically (n = 4), locally under ultrasonographic guidance (n = 2), or under laparoscopic guidance (n = 2). Eleven patients were treated by laparoscopy and 13 by laparotomy. Systemic MTX treatment failed in three patients, and they required surgery. Persistently elevated serum β-HCG levels were found in one patient after laparoscopic cornual excision, and she was successfully treated with MTX. Subsequent pregnancy was achieved in 10 patients. No uterine rupture was encountered during pregnancy or labor [30].

Alagbe et al. [31] reported a case of a right interstitial ectopic pregnancy diagnosed in a 39-year-old woman. The gestational sac diameter was 2.7 cm, equivalent to 7 weeks of gestation. The patient was admitted for medical management (using intramuscular MTX 75 mg) and serial ultrasound monitoring. The ultrasound revealed a persistent gestational sac on the 8th day, following MTX injection. On day 10, however, the gestational sac completely disappeared [31].

Dagar et al. [1] retrospectively analyzed three cases of interstitial pregnancy. In the third case they combined both modalities, local and systemic MTX administration, along with local KCl injection. This was one of the few case reports of such an approach.

The combined method, described as hysteroscopy-assisted laparoscopy, was described by some authors as an alternative minimally invasive approach that could be appropriate in some patients with IP. The prerequisites included early recognition of the abnormality and the woman's hemodynamically stable condition [32,33]. Katz et al. [32] presented two cases of patients with diagnosed IP who were successfully treated with laparoscopic-assisted hysteroscopy. The evacuation of the gestational sac was carried out transvaginally under laparoscopic supervision. Similarly, Feng et al. [33] described a case of a patient diagnosed with IP. They were initially unsuccessfully treated with MTX, and then subsequently with laparoscopic-assisted hysteroscopy [33]. In all the cases presented, cornual resection was not necessary, which is undoubtedly an advantage of this method [32,33].

Kahramanoglu et al. [34] presented four cases of patients with IP. In that series, each patient needed a different treatment modality—a single dose of MTX, laparotomy, hysteroscopy followed by vacuum aspiration, and vacuum aspiration under laparoscopic control. The treatments depended on the patients' presenting symptoms, β-HCG levels, and ultrasound images. This article perfectly illustrates the complexity of the IP [34].

In 2021, Marchand et al., presented a comprehensive systematic review [35] and a meta-analysis [36] of the patients diagnosed with IP in which they compared the outcomes of the laparoscopic surgery versus laparotomy treatment. The first paper included one case series study, one cross-sectional study, and four retrospective cohort studies with 70 cases of IP in the laparoscopic surgery group and 83 cases in the laparotomy surgery group [35]. The authors concluded that laparoscopic management was associated with a shorter postoperative hospital stay.

In the mentioned meta-analysis [36] and the review [35], the authors compared the effects of laparoscopic versus laparotomy treatment in 855 women with IP. They included 65 case reports, 23 cohort studies, 6 case series, and 2 case–control studies, meeting the search criteria. They found that 723 women underwent laparoscopy, while 132 were treated with laparotomy [35]. The analysis demonstrated more favorable outcomes of laparoscopy vs. laparotomy, i.e., less bleeding during surgery, shorter duration of the procedure and the hospital stay, and a higher risk of rupture of ectopic pregnancy when laparotomy was performed. In conclusion, the authors suggested laparoscopy as the first-choice method when a surgical approach is necessary in patients diagnosed with IP [35].

The condition of ectopic pregnancy can develop rapidly, leading to hemodynamic instability and death. Thus, it is important to promptly recognize the classic ultrasound presentation. The awareness of appropriate diagnostic approaches, differential diagnoses as well as conservative and surgical treatment methods are equally vital [1,9,14–18,29,32–36].

It is difficult to identify a single management method of uterine horn pregnancy due to the highly variable response to treatment and the dynamics of the development of symptoms, which can threaten the health and life of patients. In the literature, particular management approaches have been proposed, but the level of evidence for them was low [15,17].

4. Conclusions

The effectiveness of pharmacological treatment depends on a variety of factors, and the patient should remain under careful observation until a treatment course is completed. The dynamic development of endoscopic surgery in recent years has made the laparoscopic techniques the treatment of choice in IP. The development of minimally invasive techniques allows for less burdensome treatment of patients with IP, but requires experience in the use of this technique in order to treat the ectopic pregnancy.

Author Contributions: Conceptualization, M.K., K.C.-W. and M.W.; methodology, M.K.; formal analysis, M.K.; K.C.-W. and M.W., investigation, M.K.; resources, M.K., K.C.-W. and M.W.; data curation, M.K., K.C.-W. and M.W. writing—original draft preparation, M.K.; writing—review and editing, K.C.-W., M.W. and K.W.; visualization, M.K.; supervision, M.W. All authors have read and agreed to the published version of the manuscript.

Funding: This research received no external funding.

Institutional Review Board Statement: Not applicable—patient's treatment was not an experiment. The standard treatment was described.

Informed Consent Statement: Patient consent was waived due to the anonymous presentation of both cases. There is no possibility to identify the patients described in this article.

Data Availability Statement: Not applicable.

Conflicts of Interest: The authors declare no conflict of interest.

References

1. Dagar, M.; Srivastava, M.; Ganguli, I.; Bhardwaj, P.; Sharma, N.; Chwala, D. Interstitial and Cornual Ectopic Pregnancy: Conservative Surgical and Medical Management. *J. Obs. Gynaecol. India* **2018**, *68*, 471–476. [CrossRef] [PubMed]
2. Ilea, C.; Ilie, O.-D.; Marcu, O.-A.; Stoian, I.; Doroftei, B. The Very First Romanian Unruptured 13-Weeks Gestation Tubal Ectopic Pregnancy. *Medicina* **2022**, *58*, 1160. [CrossRef]
3. Stabile, G.; Romano, F.; Zinicola, G.; Topouzova, G.A.; Di Lorenzo, G.; Mangino, F.P.; Ricci, G. Interstitial Ectopic Pregnancy: The Role of Mifepristone in the Medical Treatment. *Int. J. Environ. Res. Public Health* **2021**, *18*, 9781. [CrossRef]
4. Brewer, H.; Gefroh, S.; Bork, M.; Munkarah, A.; Hawkins, R.; Redman, M. Asymptomatic rupture of a cornual ectopic in the third trimester. *J. Reprod. Med.* **2005**, *50*, 715–718.
5. Durand, Y.G.; Capoccia-Brugger, R.; Vial, Y.; Balaya, V. Diagnostic dilemma between angular and interstitial ectopic pregnancy: 3D ultrasound features. *J. Ultrasound* **2022**, *25*, 989–994. [CrossRef]
6. Piecha, D.; Pluta, D.; Pas, P.; Plonka, J.; Kowalczyk, K. Interstitial ectopic pregnancy following ipsilateral salpingectomy. *Ginekol. Pol.* **2020**, *91*, 478–479. [CrossRef]
7. Saichandran, S.; Samal, S. Asymptomatic rupture of cornual gestation presented as abdominal mass. *Int. J. Reprod. Contracept. Obstet. Gynecol.* **2016**, *2*, 746–748. [CrossRef]
8. Eyvazzadeh, A.D.; Levine, D. Imaging of Pelvic Pain in the First Trimester of Pregnancy. *Radiol. Clin. N. Am.* **2006**, *44*, 863–877. [CrossRef] [PubMed]
9. Hamon, N.G.; Peng, N.G.; Sharon, L. Laparoscopic Treatment of an Interstitial Pregnancy. *Gynecol. Obs.* **2014**, *4*, 8. [CrossRef]
10. Brincat, M.; Bryant-Smith, A.; Holland, T.K. The diagnosis and management of interstitial ectopic pregnancies: A review. *Gynecol. Surg.* **2019**, *16*, 2. [CrossRef]
11. Chan, L.Y.; Yuen, P.M. Successful treatment of ruptured interstitial pregnancy with laparoscopic surgery. A report of 2 cases. *J. Reprod. Med.* **2003**, *48*, 569–571. [PubMed]
12. Faraj, R.; Steel, M. Management of cornual (interstitial) pregnancy. *Obs. Gynaecol.* **2007**, *9*, 249–255. [CrossRef]
13. Garavaglia, E.; Quaranta, L.; Redaelli, A.; Colombo, G.; Pasi, F.; Candiani, M. Interstitial Pregnancy after In Vitro Fertilization and Embryo Transfer Following Bilateral Salpingectomy: Report of Two Cases and Literature Review. *Int. J. Fertil. Steril.* **2012**, *6*, 131–134. [PubMed]
14. Stabile, G.; Romano, F.; Buonomo, F.; Zinicola, G.; Ricci, G. Conservative Treatment of Interstitial Ectopic Pregnancy with the Combination of Mifepristone and Methotrexate: Our Experience and Review of the Literature. *Biomed. Res. Int.* **2020**, *2020*, 8703496. [CrossRef]
15. Elson, C.J.; Salim, R.; Potdar, N.; Chetty, M.; Ross, J.A.; Kirk, E.J.; on behalf of the Royal College of Obstetricians and Gynaecologists. Diagnosis and management of ectopic pregnancy. *BJOG* **2016**, *123*, e15–e55.
16. Panelli, D.M.; Phillips, C.H.; Brady, P.C. Incidence, diagnosis and management of tubal and nontubal ectopic pregnancies: A review. *Fertil. Res. Pract.* **2015**, *1*, 15. [CrossRef]

17. Po, L.; Thomas, J.; Mills, K.; Zakhari, A.; Tulandi, T.; Shuman, M.; Page, A. Guideline No. 414: Management of Pregnancy of Unknown Location and Tubal and Nontubal Ectopic Pregnancies. *J. Obs. Gynaecol. Can.* **2021**, *43*, 614–630.e1. [CrossRef]
18. Casadio, P.; Arena, A.; Verrelli, L.; Ambrosio, M.; Fabbri, M.; Giovannico, K.; Magnarelli, G.; Seracchioli, R. Methotrexate injection for interstitial pregnancy: Hysteroscopic conservative mini-invasive approach. *Facts Views Vis. Obgyn.* **2021**, *13*, 73–76. [CrossRef]
19. Santos, L.T.R.; Oliveira, S.C.S.; Rocha, L.G.A.; Sousa, N.D.S.; Figueiredo, R.S. Interstitial Pregnancy: Case Report of Atypical Ectopic Pregnancy. *Cureus* **2020**, *13*, e8081. [CrossRef] [PubMed]
20. Lau, S.; Tulandi, T. Conservative medical and surgical management of interstitial ectopic pregnancy. *Fertil. Steril.* **1999**, *72*, 9. [CrossRef]
21. Mangino, F.P.; Romano, F.; Di Lorenzo, G.; Buonomo, F.; De Santo, D.; Scrimin, F.; Ricci, G. Total hysteroscopic treatment of cervical pregnancy: The 2-step technique. *J. Minim. Invasive Gynecol.* **2019**, *26*, 1011–1012. [CrossRef] [PubMed]
22. Tantchev, L.; Kotzev, A.; Yordanov, A.A. Disturbed interstitial pregnancy: A first case of successful treatment using a mini-laparoscopic approach. *Medicina* **2019**, *55*, 215. [CrossRef]
23. Warda, H.; Mamik, M.M.; Ashraf, M.; Abuzeid, M.I. Interstitial Ectopic Pregnancy: Conservative Surgical Management. *J. Soc. Laparoendosc. Surg.* **2014**, *18*, 197–203. [CrossRef]
24. Moawad, N.S.; Mahajan, S.T.; Moniz, M.H.; Taylor, S.E.; Hurd, W.W. Current diagnosis and treatment of interstitial pregnancy. *Am. J. Obstet. Gynecol.* **2010**, *202*, 15–29. [CrossRef]
25. Moawad, N.S.; Dayaratna, S.; Mahajan, S.T. Mini-cornual excision: A simple stepwise laparoscopic technique for the treatment of cornual pregnancy. *J. Soc. Laparoendosc. Surg.* **2009**, *13*, 87–91. [CrossRef]
26. Bremner, T.; Cela, V.; Luciano, A.A. Surgical management of interstitial pregnancy. *J. Am. Assoc. Gynecol. Laparosc.* **2000**, *7*, 387–389. [CrossRef]
27. Moon, H.S.; Choi, Y.J.; Park, Y.H.; Kim, S.G. New simple endoscopic operations for interstitial pregnancies. *Am. J. Obs. Gynecol.* **2000**, *182*, 114–121. [CrossRef]
28. Gao, M.Y.; Zhu, H.; Zheng, F.Y. Interstitial Pregnancy after Ipsilateral Salpingectomy: Analysis of 46 Cases and a Literature Review. *J. Minim. Invasive Gynecol.* **2020**, *27*, 613–617. [CrossRef]
29. Haestier, A. Guideline for the Medical Management of Ectopic Pregnancy with Methotrexate, Version 5. Norfolk and Norwich University Hospitals. NHS Foundation Trust. Date Approved: 17 July 2020. Available online: https://www.google.com/url?sa=t&rct=j&q=&esrc=s&source=web&cd=&cad=rja&uact=8&ved=2ahUKEwiI1euUjJ_7AhVii8MKHertBL4QFnoECAoQAQ&url=https%3A%2F%2Fwww.nnuh.nhs.uk%2Fpublication%2Fdownload%2Fectopic-pregnancy-with-methotrexate-treatment-g27v5%2F&usg=AOvVaw0Kl_UTnnD55Jma5ehZYR_J (accessed on 27 September 2022).
30. Tulandi, T.; Al-Jaroudi, D. Interstitial pregnancy: Results generated from the Society of Reproductive Surgeons' Registry. *Obs. Gynecol.* **2004**, *103*, 47–50. [CrossRef]
31. Alagbe, O.A.; Adeniyi, T.O.; Abayomi, O.A.; Onifade, E.O. Interstitial ectopic pregnancy: A case report. *Pan. Afr. Med. J.* **2017**, *11*, 135. [CrossRef]
32. Katz, D.L.; Barrett, J.P.; Sanfilippo, J.S.; Badway, D.M. Combined hysteroscopy and laparoscopy in the treatment of interstitial pregnancy. *Am. J. Obstet. Gynecol.* **2003**, *188*, 1113–1114, ISSN 0002-9378. [CrossRef]
33. Feng, Q.; Zhong, J.; Liu, Y.; Li, S.T.; Zong, L. Surgical treatment of interstitial pregnancy without cornual resection: A case report. *Medicine* **2022**, *101*, e29730. [CrossRef]
34. Kahramanoglu, I.; Mammadov, Z.; Turan, H.; Urer, A.; Tuten, A. Management options for interstitial ectopic pregnancies: A case series. *Pak. J. Med. Sci.* **2017**, *33*, 476–482. [CrossRef]
35. Marchand, G.; Masoud, A.T.; Sainz, K.; Azadi, A.; Ware, K.; Vallejo, J.; Anderson, S.; King, A.; Osborn, A.; Ruther, S.; et al. A systematic review and meta-analysis of laparotomy compared with laparoscopic management of interstitial pregnancy. *Facts Views Vis. Obgyn.* **2021**, *12*, 299–308. [PubMed]
36. Marchand, G.; Masoud, A.T.; Galitsky, A.; Azadi, A.; Ware, K.; Vallejo, J.; Anderson, S.; King, A.; Ruther, S.; Brazil, G.; et al. Management of interstitial pregnancy in the era of laparoscopy: A meta-analysis of 855 case studies compared with traditional techniques. *Obs. Gynecol. Sci.* **2021**, *64*, 156–173. [CrossRef]

Disclaimer/Publisher's Note: The statements, opinions and data contained in all publications are solely those of the individual author(s) and contributor(s) and not of MDPI and/or the editor(s). MDPI and/or the editor(s) disclaim responsibility for any injury to people or property resulting from any ideas, methods, instructions or products referred to in the content.

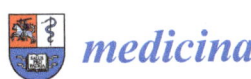

Article

Managing Fetal Ovarian Cysts: Clinical Experience with a Rare Disorder

Alina-Sinziana Melinte-Popescu [1,†], Radu-Florin Popa [2,*,†], Valeriu Harabor [3,†], Aurel Nechita [3], AnaMaria Harabor [3], Ana-Maria Adam [3], Ingrid-Andrada Vasilache [4], Marian Melinte-Popescu [5,†], Cristian Vaduva [6] and Demetra Socolov [4]

1. Department of Mother and Newborn Care, Faculty of Medicine and Biological Sciences, 'Ștefan cel Mare' University, 720229 Suceava, Romania
2. Department of Vascular Surgery, University of Medicine and Pharmacy "Grigore T. Popa", 700111 Iasi, Romania
3. Clinical and Surgical Department, Faculty of Medicine and Pharmacy, 'Dunarea de Jos' University, 800216 Galati, Romania
4. Department of Obstetrics and Gynecology, University of Medicine and Pharmacy "Grigore T. Popa", 700115 Iasi, Romania
5. Department of Internal Medicine, Faculty of Medicine and Biological Sciences, 'Ștefan cel Mare' University, 720229 Suceava, Romania
6. Department of Mother and Child Medicine, Faculty of Medicine, University of Medicine and Pharmacy, 200349 Craiova, Romania
* Correspondence: rfpopa2008@yahoo.com
† These authors contributed equally to this work.

Abstract: *Background and Objectives*: Fetal ovarian cysts (FOCs) are a very rare pathology that can be associated with maternal–fetal and neonatal complications. The aim of this study was to assess the influence of ultrasound characteristics on FOC evolution and therapeutic management. *Materials and Methods*: We included cases admitted to our perinatal tertiary center between August 2016 and December 2022 with a prenatal or postnatal ultrasound evaluation indicative of FOC. We retrospectively analyzed the pre- and postnatal medical records, sonographic findings, operation protocols, and pathology reports. *Results*: This study investigated 20 cases of FOCs, of which 17 (85%) were diagnosed prenatally and 3 (15%) postnatally. The mean size of prenatally diagnosed ovarian cysts was 34.64 ± 12.53 mm for simple ovarian cysts and 55.16 ± 21.01 mm for complex ovarian cysts ($p = 0.01$). The simple FOCs ≤ 4 cm underwent resorption (n = 7, 70%) or size reduction (n = 3, 30%) without complications. Only 1 simple FOC greater than 4 cm reduced its size during follow-up, while 2 cases (66.6%) were complicated with ovarian torsion. Complex ovarian cysts diagnosed prenatally underwent resorption in only 1 case (25%), reduced in size in 1 case (25%), and were complicated with ovarian torsion in 2 cases (50%). Moreover, 2 simple (66.6%) and 1 complex (33.3%) fetal ovarian cysts were postnatally diagnosed. All of these simple ovarian cysts had a maximum diameter of ≤ 4 cm, and all of them underwent size reduction. The complex ovarian cyst of 4 cm underwent resorption during follow-up. *Conclusions*: Symptomatic neonatal ovarian cysts, as well as those that grow in size during sonographic follow-up, are in danger of ovarian torsion and should be operated on. Complex cysts and large cysts (with >4 cm diameter) could be followed up unless they become symptomatic or increase in dimensions during serial ultrasounds.

Keywords: fetal ovarian cysts; ultrasound evaluation; complicated cysts; therapeutic approach

Citation: Melinte-Popescu, A.-S.; Popa, R.-F.; Harabor, V.; Nechita, A.; Harabor, A.; Adam, A.-M.; Vasilache, I.-A.; Melinte-Popescu, M.; Vaduva, C.; Socolov, D. Managing Fetal Ovarian Cysts: Clinical Experience with a Rare Disorder. *Medicina* 2023, 59, 715. https://doi.org/10.3390/medicina59040715

Academic Editors: Marius L. Craina, Elena Bernad and Simone Ferrero

Received: 20 March 2023
Accepted: 4 April 2023
Published: 6 April 2023

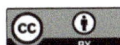

Copyright: © 2023 by the authors. Licensee MDPI, Basel, Switzerland. This article is an open access article distributed under the terms and conditions of the Creative Commons Attribution (CC BY) license (https://creativecommons.org/licenses/by/4.0/).

1. Introduction

Ovarian cysts are one of the rarest gynecological disorders that develop during fetal life and could have important consequences both in utero and after birth. The estimated incidence of fetal ovarian cysts (FOCs) is cited in the literature as 1 in every 2500 live births [1]. FOCs typically manifest as functional or benign cysts, with the prevailing hypothesis regarding their etiology attributing their development to augmented levels of maternal estrogens, fetal gonadotropins, and placental human chorionic gonadotropin (HCG) in the fetus [2]. Newborn ovarian neoplasms, including cystadenomas, teratomas, and granulosa cell tumors, are rare occurrences [3].

A typical ultrasonographic presentation of a fetal ovarian cyst is that of an abdominal, usually anechoic, and thin-walled cyst, located superiorly and parasagittally to the bladder in a female fetus [4]. However, it is important to consider various differential diagnoses for FOC such as urachal cyst, mesenteric cyst, intestinal duplication anomalies, intestinal obstruction, and lymphangioma [5]. In rare cases, the identification of a "daughter cyst" serves as a distinctive sign of ovarian cyst presence [4,6].

FOCs are classified into two categories based on ultrasound (US) criteria, as established by Nussbaum: simple and complex [4]. A complex cyst is typically characterized by heterogeneity, the presence of hyperechogenic components, a thickened wall, free-floating material, fluid–fluid levels, and intracystic septations. Conversely, a simple cyst is typically described as an intrapelvic structure that is spherical, thin-walled, anechoic, unilocular, and less than 2 cm in diameter [4].

Fetal ovarian cysts typically exhibit stability throughout gestation and are known to dissolve spontaneously within the first few months following delivery. However, in rare instances, FOCs can lead to complications, such as torsion or bleeding during the prenatal period [7]. A retrospective study by Toker Kurtmen et al., which examined 28 cases of antenatal ovarian torsion, revealed that it can be misdiagnosed as a variety of cystic disorders, including intestinal duplication cyst/mesenteric cyst, complex ovarian cyst, mature cystic teratoma, and simple renal cyst [8]. Ovarian loss is commonly associated with torsion, which is often detected prenatally by alterations in the ultrasound image from a simple to a complex appearance, as well as an increase in size [9].

Following a diagnosis of fetal ovarian cysts, routine serial ultrasound examinations are necessary to monitor for any structural changes or complications such as massive hemorrhage, cyst rupture, or ovarian torsion resulting in infarction [10]. Large cysts may result in complications such as ascites due to the rupture of the cystic wall; mass effect; compression of ureters, inferior vena cava, and large and small intestines; intraabdominal adhesions; respiratory compromise; and ovarian torsion with or without autoamputation of the ovary [11,12]. To prevent such complications, some surgeons recommend prenatal aspiration of large fetal ovarian cysts, particularly for those greater than 4 cm in diameter.

A recent scoping review by Bucuri et al. reported a 34% higher risk of complications in cases of a complex fetal ovarian cyst diagnosis, based on an evaluation of 15 articles published within the last 10 years [13]. In addition, a systematic review and meta-analysis by Bascietto et al., based on 34 studies published up to 2017, showed a higher risk of ovarian torsion for cysts measuring ≥40 mm compared with those measuring less than 40 mm (odds ratio—OR: 30.8; 95% CI: 8.6–110.0) [7]. The authors also reported a recurrence rate of 37.9% (95% CI: 14.8–64.3%) for cases that underwent in utero aspiration, as well as a pooled proportion of 10.8% (95% CI: 4.4–19.7%) for ovarian torsion and 12.8% (95% CI: 3.8–26.0%) for intracystic hemorrhage after birth.

Pre- and postnatal management of fetal ovarian cysts is often a topic of debate among clinicians. Despite clinicians' concerns regarding the safety of fetal cyst aspiration, Bagolan et al. [14] recommended prenatal cyst aspiration if the cyst diameter is greater than 5 cm or if the diameter increases by more than 1 cm per week. On the other hand, some authors suggest that there is no need for postnatal surgical treatment for simple ovarian cysts with the largest diameter of <5 cm or <4 cm [11,15].

Given the heterogeneous therapeutic approaches and rarity of this disorder, there is a need for more descriptive studies on FOC management to establish a comprehensive database for future meta-analyses. Therefore, the aim of this study was to evaluate the impact of ultrasound characteristics on the evolution and therapeutic management of FOCs.

2. Materials and Methods

This retrospective cohort study comprised a population of 20 pregnant women who were assessed at the Clinical Hospital of Obstetrics and Gynecology "Cuza-Voda" in Iasi, Romania, between August 2016 and December 2022, based on prenatal or postnatal ultrasound evaluations indicative of a fetal ovarian cyst. The Institutional Ethics Committee of Hospital "Cuza Voda", Iasi, Romania (No. 790/25.01.2017) provided approval for the study, and all legal guardians of the newborns included in the study provided informed consent. All procedures were conducted in compliance with applicable regulations and guidelines.

We tested two hypotheses in accordance with the existing literature [9,15,16]. The first hypothesis postulates that simple cysts, small cysts (≤ 4 cm), and those that show a tendency to decrease in size during fetal life through regular follow-up, will regress and thus should be monitored in the postnatal period. The second hypothesis suggests that complex cysts, large cysts (>4 cm), or those with an increasing size during follow-up in fetal life, have a propensity for torsion with ovarian amputation, and thus necessitate surgical intervention in postnatal life [9,15,16].

The study included female fetuses with cystic masses in the lower abdomen, either unilateral or bilateral, that exhibited characteristics of simple or complicated ovarian cysts as per the Nussbaum categorization. Complicated ovarian cysts were defined as those having a fluid–debris level indicative of internal hemorrhage, septations with or without internal echoes, calcifications, or a solid component, in accordance with the literature [17]. Patients with urachal cysts, mesenteric cyst, intestinal duplication abnormalities, intestinal obstruction, and lymphangioma were excluded from the study, as well as those with incomplete medical records or whose mothers were unable to provide informed consent.

The present study retrospectively collected data on gestational age at diagnosis, sonographic characteristics of ovarian cystic masses, and pre- and postnatal care from the medical records of the patients. The admission diagnosis was confirmed using an obstetrical ultrasound examination, which was performed using an E8 scanner with a 4.8 MHz transabdominal probe (GE Medical Systems, Milwaukee, WI, USA), and the examination was completed by a vaginal approach using an intravaginal probe of 5–15 MHz when the fetal abdomen was accessible.

Periodic ultrasound scans were carried out until delivery to monitor the evolution of the cystic masses. Only cases with a high degree of confidence in the presumptive ultrasound diagnosis were included in the study, and no ultrasound-guided cyst aspiration was performed during pregnancy.

Postpartum ultrasound examinations were performed by neonatologists within 72 h of birth using a GE machine with a transabdominal 7.5 MHz transabdominal transducer (GE Medical Systems, Milwaukee, WI, USA). All neonates underwent examinations by neonatologists, radiologists, and pediatric surgeons after birth. Patients with simple FOCs that had the largest diameter of 4 cm or less were followed up postnatally with a transabdominal ultrasound examination at 6 months of age. Patients with large ovarian cysts (>4 cm) or complex structures were considered emergencies and referred to the pediatric surgery department for evaluation and surgical treatment.

The study recorded the ultrasound features and size of ovarian masses in neonates, with subsequent management consisting of sonographic follow-up or surgical intervention, including ovariectomy, cystectomy, or removal of an autoamputated ovary. No laparoscopic or ultrasound-guided aspiration was performed on neonates. Postnatal final diagnoses and outcomes were also documented. A perspective on the evolution of FOCs in our cohort of patients is presented in Figure 1.

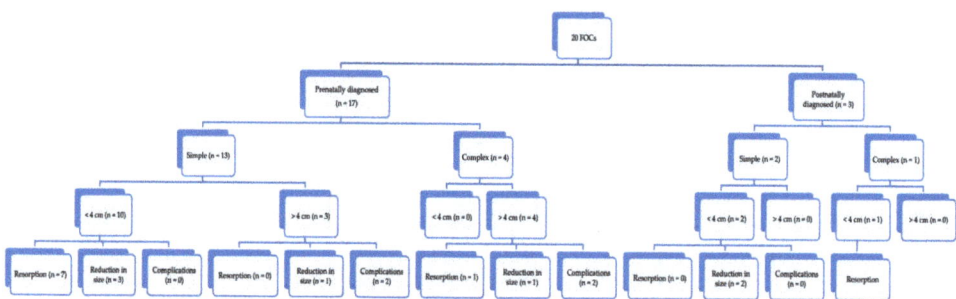

Figure 1. Flowchart of the evolution of FOCs in our cohort of patients.

The data were compiled into a database using SPSS software (version 28.0.1, IBM Corporation, Armonk, NY, USA), and the results were analyzed using descriptive statistics. Continuous data were expressed as means and standard deviations, while categorical data were reported as numbers and percentages. Each variable was evaluated with chi-squared and Fisher's exact tests for categorical variables, and with t-tests for continuous variables.

3. Results

The present study investigated 20 cases of fetal ovarian cysts, with 17 cases (85%) being diagnosed prenatally and 3 cases (15%) postnatally. The prenatally diagnosed fetal ovarian cysts (FOCs) were classified as simple in 13 cases (76.48%) based on their ultrasound appearance, whereas 4 cases (23.52%) were deemed complex. Among the simple FOCs diagnosed prenatally, the majority (n = 10, 76.92%) had a maximum diameter of 4 cm or less, while only 3 cases (23.08%) had a larger diameter. Conversely, all complex FOCs (n = 4, 100%) diagnosed prenatally had a maximum diameter larger than 4 cm.

The mean gestational age at prenatal diagnosis and standard deviation were 26 ± 2.02 weeks for simple ovarian cysts and 32 ± 1.06 weeks for complex ovarian cysts. In terms of the size of prenatally diagnosed ovarian cysts, the mean size was 34.64 ± 12.53 mm for simple ovarian cysts and 55.16 ± 21.01 mm for complex ovarian cysts, achieving statistical significance ($p = 0.01$).

Regarding fetal ovarian cyst management, the simple FOCs with a maximum diameter of 4 cm or less, identified during prenatal and/or postnatal examinations, underwent resorption (n = 7, 70%) or size reduction (n = 3, 30%) without complications. However, only 1 simple FOC greater than 4 cm reduced in size during follow-up, while 2 cases (66.6%) were complicated with ovarian torsion. Complex ovarian cysts diagnosed prenatally underwent resorption in only 1 case (25%), reduced in size in 1 case (25%), and were complicated with ovarian torsion in 2 cases (50%).

No other fetal intra-abdominal malformations were identified during serial ultrasound evaluations, but two cases of ovarian cysts were associated with polyhydramnios. More images corresponding to the described cases can be found in the Supplementary Materials (Figures S1–S5). Only one case with a bilateral ovarian cyst was diagnosed and had a simple echogenic structure.

Moreover, 2 simple (66.6%) and 1 complex (33.3%) fetal ovarian cysts were postnatally diagnosed. All of these simple ovarian cysts had a maximum diameter of 4 cm or less, and all of them underwent a reduction in size. The mean diameter and standard deviation of the simple cysts diagnosed in the postpartum period (in the first 72 h of life) were 29.4 ± 10.5 mm. The complex ovarian cyst of 4 cm underwent resorption during follow-up.

Taken together, our cohort of patients comprised 15 simple (75%) and 5 complex (25%) FOCs. The demographic characteristics of the pregnant patients, fetal ovarian cysts' location, and pregnancy outcomes are included in Table 1.

Patients diagnosed with simple fetal ovarian cysts were born from significantly younger mothers compared with those diagnosed with complex fetal ovarian cysts ($p < 0.001$). The majority of patients were born by cesarean section in both groups, but no statistically significant difference could be found between them regarding the type of birth.

The birthweight of newborns with complex ovarian cysts was significantly lower than the birthweight of those with simple FOCs ($p = 0.01$). However, we could not find any statistically significant difference between groups regarding their Apgar score at 1 min ($p = 0.14$) or the rate of preterm birth ($p = 0.07$).

Table 1. Clinical characteristics and ultrasound findings of FOC.

Parameter	Simple Cyst n = 15	Complex Cyst n = 5	p Value
Mother's age (years)	26.1 ± 2.7	34 ± 2.1	<0.001
Gestation	1.9 ± 0.5	1.6 ± 1.1	0.40
Nulliparity (%)	Yes = 6 (40%)	Yes = 3 (60%)	0.43
GA at birth (weeks)	39 ± 0.36	37.2 ± 4.33	0.10
Type of birth (n/%)	Cesarean: 11 (73.3%) Vaginal: 4 (26.7%)	Cesarean: 3 (60%) Vaginal: 2 (40%)	0.57
Birthweight (g)	3374.54 ± 212.99	3080 ± 141.76	0.01
Apgar score at 1 min (mean ± SD)	8.64 ± 1.68	8.19 ± 1.93	0.14
Preterm birth (n/%)	Yes = 0%	Yes = 1 (20%)	0.07
Cyst location	Right: n = 10 (66.7%) Left: n = 4 (26.7%) Bilateral: n = 1 (6.7%)	Right: n = 4 (80%) Left: n = 1 (20%) Bilateral: n = 0 (0%)	0.78

Table legend: GA: gestational age; US: ultrasound.

After birth, patients with simple cysts <4 cm in diameter (5 cases, 25%) were referred for an ultrasound follow-up at 6 months. All simple cysts were reduced in size at the 6-month follow-up, with a mean diameter and standard deviation of 22.16 ± 0.98 mm. No other complications occurred. Meanwhile, patients with cysts with a diameter of >4 cm or with a complex structure (n = 4, 20%) were sent to surgery. Another two cases of FOC, which had an indication for surgery, underwent a conservative approach. The parents of 1 patient, with US features suggesting a fetal teratoma, opted for follow-up every 6 months, and during 3 follow-ups the cyst reduced its size to 4 cm. This patient underwent an MRI examination both prenatally and postnatally which confirmed the diagnosis of teratoma. Another patient had a complex cyst, but because of prematurity (delivery at 31 weeks), the surgical procedure was postponed, and the cyst disappeared in the next 4 months.

Two ovariectomies, one cystectomy, and a laparoscopic adnexectomy for the removal of an autoamputated ovary were performed on four patients with suspicion of ovarian torsion, which was further confirmed through surgery. During follow-up, all of these individuals were either symptomatic or had significant ovarian cyst growth. All surgical interventions were performed in the first weeks of life, and no complications occurred during or after surgery. Pathology reports indicated four hemorrhagic cysts.

4. Discussion

The aim of this study was to assess the influence of ultrasound characteristics on FOC evolution and therapeutic management. Our findings are consistent with previous studies examining various aspects related to FOC, thereby confirming our initial hypothesis.

The diagnosis of FOC is based on two non-specific ultrasound criteria: positive criteria, which involve the identification of a fluid-filled mass located in the lower and lateral region of the abdomen, above the bladder of a female fetus, and negative criteria, which involve a sonographic examination to confirm the integrity of the urinary and gastrointestinal tracts [18].

A pathognomonic sign for ovarian fetal cysts is the 'Daughter Cyst Sign', with a reported 82% sensitivity and 100% specificity [6]. It is a small, round, anechoic structure within a cyst, attached to its wall, and pathological studies demonstrated it was a follicle inside an ovarian cyst [6]. In our series, we observed this sign in 5 out of 17 cases diagnosed during prenatal sonographic examination.

Differential diagnosis is an important step in the prenatal and postnatal evaluation of fetal ovarian cysts, as many other abdominal or pelvic masses can mimic this pathology [19,20], and serological markers could be helpful in the postnatal differentiation of various types of masses [21,22]. Thus, we included only cases with highly suggestive ultrasound appearances of FOC in our study. The four surgeries performed in the postpartum period confirmed the cystic structures as belonging to the ovaries. No other associated structural abnormalities of the urinary or gastrointestinal tract were encountered during ultrasound examinations or during laparoscopic procedures.

Most fetal ovarian cysts are diagnosed during the third trimester. Chen et al. reported that 87.2% of fetal ovarian cysts were diagnosed after 28 weeks of gestation [9]. Moreover, Rotar et al. indicated in an observational study a mean gestational age of 31.28 weeks for the initial diagnosis of fetal ovarian cysts [23]. In our series, 8 cases (40%) were diagnosed during the second trimester, at the time of morphological ultrasound; 9 cases (45%) were diagnosed during the third trimester; and the remaining 3 cases (15%) were diagnosed after delivery, when an abdominal US was performed for clinical symptoms: abdominal enlargement in all cases, and tachycardia and vomiting in 2 cases.

The effectiveness of MRI in the diagnosis of prenatal and neonatal cysts is controversial. In contrast to the major contribution of MR imaging in fetal neoplasms, the clinical influence of MRI on the perinatal management of ovarian cysts may be limited [24]. Furthermore, when compared with the imaging of ovarian masses in pediatric and adult cohorts, where MRI can provide crucial information in confirming the diagnosis and selecting treatment, the importance of MRI in prenatal ovarian cyst management is minor [24]. In our series, an MRI was performed both prenatally and postnatally for a single case of complex neonatal cyst, suggesting a teratoma, because despite the physician's recommendation of surgery, the parents opted for a follow-up, so we needed a second opinion regarding the diagnosis.

Most fetal ovarian cysts spontaneously regress during fetal life or during the neonatal period [25]. Others persist, and even increase in size, with a higher risk of complications such as ovarian torsion with the risk of autoamputation, intracystic hemorrhage, bowel obstruction, mass effect, or rupture, thus increasing the risk of surgical intervention, sometimes resulting in the loss of the gonad [26]. In our series, we had spontaneous resorption of FOC in 9 cases, the majority of whom (7 cases, 35%) were simple and had the largest diameter of 4 cm or less.

Regarding the prediction of complications and surgical need in FOC, considering cyst size, many authors support the following determinants of the neonatal outcome: a 4 cm cutoff, the US appearance (simple or complex), and the progression of the cysts during follow-up [7,27,28]. Small, unilocular cysts appear more likely to spontaneously resolve, whereas larger, complex cysts are at higher risk of persistence, complications, and surgical interventions [15].

Other authors recommend a cutoff of 50 mm for the cystic diameter to differentiate between cysts that spontaneously disappear and those at risk of complications [14,29]. In Bagolan's statistics, 85% of ovarian cysts in neonates with a diameter of >50 mm required ovariectomy [14]. On the other hand, cysts less than 2 cm, and also very large cysts which, due to their volume, cannot be mobilized to twist, are almost never complicated by torsion.

In our series, all 4 cysts operated on for ovarian torsion had a diameter of > 4 cm. It is important to note that simple cysts, after torsion, increase in size and become complex in structure [30]. Moreover, the fluid–debris level seems to be a significant hallmark for ovarian torsion on ultrasound examination [17]. In our study, only two out of four cases of ovarian torsion were determined to be complex cysts. On the other hand, all cysts that suffered torsion increased in volume at serial US follow-ups.

Therapeutic approaches for ovarian fetal and neonatal cysts are still controversial. A recent study has shown that simple cysts smaller than 50 mm on postnatal imaging will likely spontaneously resolve and can be monitored using serial ultrasound examinations [29]. Due to the risk of bleeding, rupture, or intestinal blockage, several studies have recommended that neonatal cysts with complex characteristics be operated on as soon as possible [31–33]. Other publications, on the other hand, indicate a high rate of spontaneous remission of complicated cysts without complications, which we also found in our research [34,35].

Papic et al. found that postnatal torsion during observation is uncommon and that observation has no negative impact on the rate of ovarian preservation [29]. Given these findings, all asymptomatic neonatal ovarian cysts should be treated with surveillance. If surgery is required, an ovarian-preserving strategy should be used for all cysts, regardless of size, complexity, or the presence of prenatal or postnatal torsion, wherever possible [36].

We did not perform prenatal aspiration of the fetal cyst, which some authors have advocated because of the risks of preterm labor, chorioamnionitis, fetal injury, and fetal pain, as cited in the literature [36,37]. Furthermore, recurrence may occur due to persistent fetal exposure to hormonal stimulation after the procedure until birth [38]. The effectiveness of prenatal intrauterine aspiration in preventing neonatal surgery was compared with expectant treatment in a randomized open trial conducted by Diguisto et al. on 61 pregnant women whose fetuses were diagnosed with an anechoic ovarian cyst mass [36]. The authors reported that this procedure was associated with higher rates of in utero involution of cysts (47.1%; relative risk—RR: 2.54, 95%CI: 1.07–6.05), as well as reduced rates of oophorectomy after birth (3.0%; RR: 0.13, 95%CI: 0.02–1.03).

Our results support the conclusions of Dimitriaki et al. [39], suggesting that symptomatic neonatal ovarian cysts and those with increasing size at serial US follow-ups are at risk of torsion and must be operated on. For all ovarian cysts suspected of torsion, the diagnosis was confirmed intraoperatively, and one of the ovaries had already self-amputated at the time of surgery. Although all the cysts that became torsioned had a diameter of >4 cm, smaller dimensions than 4 cm cannot be considered a resorption criterion.

A multicentric retrospective study by Tyraskis et al. evaluated the risk of ovarian torsion in relationship to FOC size [40]. Their results showed that the rate of ovarian torsion increased from 0% in cysts measuring less than 20 mm to 33% in cysts measuring more than 50 mm, but they failed to demonstrate a statistically significant difference in this overall trend.

Our study has several limitations. First of all, this study has a retrospective design and includes a small number of patients. Furthermore, prenatal sonographic data on the size and changes in the appearance of the cyst throughout pregnancy were lacking for certain individuals, resulting in the diagnosis being made after birth in three patients.

Additionally, even if ultrasound imaging of the ovaries in the neonatal period can rule out autoamputation, the ovarian origin of the cyst, and even the diagnosis of hemorrhagic cyst without torsion, cannot be supported in cases where the cysts have been resorbed without surgical confirmation.

The strength of this study is the fact that it assessed the pre- and postnatal management of fetal ovarian cysts, which is a rare gynecological disorder, and our results could represent a base, along with other descriptive studies, for future meta-analysis that could offer clinicians a better assessment of the therapeutic strategies' utility.

5. Conclusions

In conclusion, symptomatic neonatal ovarian cysts and those with increasing size at serial US follow-up are at risk of torsion and should be operated on. Complex cysts and large cysts (with a >4 cm diameter) could be followed up, unless they become symptomatic or increase in dimensions during serial ultrasounds.

The most important complication of fetal ovarian cysts is ovarian torsion, which represents a surgical emergency, and clinicians should be aware of this clinical scenario in the presence of large ovarian cysts with a complex ultrasound appearance and specific symptomatology.

FOCs can also have a malignant nature and should be carefully examined by a multi-disciplinary team for specific symptoms, imaging features, and clinical risk factors in order to provide the best therapeutic management.

Supplementary Materials: The following supporting information can be downloaded at: https://www.mdpi.com/article/10.3390/medicina59040715/s1, Figure S1: Ultrasound aspect of a simple fetal ovarian cyst. Figure S2: Bilateral simple fetal ovarian cysts. Figure S3: Complicated simple serous cyst. Figure S4: Fetal teratoma. Figure S5: Large fetal ovarian cyst.

Author Contributions: Conceptualization, A.-S.M.-P., R.-F.P., V.H., A.-M.A., M.M.-P. and D.S.; methodology, A.N., I.-A.V. and A.H.; software C.V.; validation, C.V.; formal analysis, A.N., I.-A.V. and A.H.; investigation, A.-S.M.-P., R.-F.P., V.H., A.-M.A., M.M.-P. and D.S.; resources, C.V.; data curation, A.N., I.-A.V. and A.H.; writing—original draft preparation, A.-S.M.-P., R.-F.P., V.H., A.-M.A., M.M.-P. and D.S.; writing—review and editing, A.-S.M.-P., R.-F.P., V.H., A.-M.A., M.M.-P. and D.S.; visualization, C.V.; supervision, D.S.; project administration, D.S. All authors have read and agreed to the published version of the manuscript.

Funding: This research received no external funding.

Institutional Review Board Statement: The study was conducted according to the guidelines of the Declaration of Helsinki and approved by the Institutional Ethics Committee of Hospital "Cuza Voda"—Iasi, Romania (protocol approval: 790/25.01.2017).

Informed Consent Statement: Informed consent was obtained from all subjects involved in the study.

Data Availability Statement: The data presented in this study are available on request from the corresponding author. The data are not publicly available due to local policies.

Conflicts of Interest: The authors declare no conflict of interest.

References

1. Bryant, A.E.; Laufer, M.R. Fetal ovarian cysts: Incidence, diagnosis and management. *J. Reprod. Med.* **2004**, *49*, 329–337.
2. Brandt, M.L.; Helmrath, M.A. Ovarian cysts in infants and children. *Semin. Pediatr. Surg.* **2005**, *14*, 78–85. [CrossRef] [PubMed]
3. Amies Oelschlager, A.M.; Sawin, R. Teratomas and ovarian lesions in children. *Surg. Clin. N. Am.* **2012**, *92*, 599–613. [CrossRef]
4. Nussbaum, A.R.; Sanders, R.C.; Hartman, D.S.; Dudgeon, D.L.; Parmley, T.H. Neonatal ovarian cysts: Sonographic-pathologic correlation. *Radiology* **1988**, *168*, 817–821. [CrossRef]
5. Trinh, T.W.; Kennedy, A.M. Fetal ovarian cysts: Review of imaging spectrum, differential diagnosis, management, and outcome. *Radiographics* **2015**, *35*, 621–635. [CrossRef] [PubMed]
6. Quarello, E.; Gorincour, G.; Merrot, T.; Boubli, L.; D'Ercole, C. The 'daughter cyst sign': A sonographic clue to the diagnosis of fetal ovarian cyst. *Ultrasound Obstet. Gynecol.* **2003**, *22*, 433–434. [CrossRef] [PubMed]
7. Bascietto, F.; Liberati, M.; Marrone, L.; Khalil, A.; Pagani, G.; Gustapane, S.; Leombroni, M.; Buca, D.; Flacco, M.E.; Rizzo, G.; et al. Outcome of fetal ovarian cysts diagnosed on prenatal ultrasound examination: Systematic review and meta-analysis. *Ultrasound Obstet. Gynecol.* **2017**, *50*, 20–31. [CrossRef]
8. Toker Kurtmen, B.; Divarci, E.; Ergun, O.; Ozok, G.; Celik, A. The Role of Surgery in Antenatal Ovarian Torsion: Retrospective Evaluation of 28 Cases and Review of the Literature. *J. Pediatr. Adolesc. Gynecol.* **2022**, *35*, 18–22. [CrossRef]
9. Chen, L.; Hu, Y.; Hu, C.; Wen, H. Prenatal evaluation and postnatal outcomes of fetal ovarian cysts. *Prenat. Diagn.* **2020**, *40*, 1258–1264. [CrossRef] [PubMed]
10. Akın, M.A.; Akın, L.; Özbek, S.; Tireli, G.; Kavuncuoğlu, S.; Sander, S.; Akçakuş, M.; Güneş, T.; Öztürk, M.A.; Kurtoğlu, S. Fetal-neonatal ovarian cysts–their monitoring and management: Retrospective evaluation of 20 cases and review of the literature. *J. Clin. Res. Pediatr. Endocrinol.* **2010**, *2*, 28–33. [CrossRef]
11. Jeanty, C.; Frayer, E.A.; Page, R.; Langenburg, S. Neonatal ovarian torsion complicated by intestinal obstruction and perforation, and review of the literature. *J. Pediatr. Surg.* **2010**, *45*, e5–e9. [CrossRef] [PubMed]
12. Cass, D.L. Fetal abdominal tumors and cysts. *Transl. Pediatr.* **2021**, *10*, 1530–1541. [CrossRef] [PubMed]
13. Bucuri, C.; Mihu, D.; Malutan, A.; Oprea, V.; Berceanu, C.; Nati, I.; Rada, M.; Ormindean, C.; Blaga, L.; Ciortea, R. Fetal Ovarian Cyst-A Scoping Review of the Data from the Last 10 Years. *Medicina* **2023**, *59*, 186. [CrossRef]
14. Bagolan, P.; Giorlandino, C.; Nahom, A.; Bilancioni, E.; Trucchi, A.; Gatti, C.; Aleandri, V.; Spina, V. The management of fetal ovarian cysts. *J. Pediatr. Surg.* **2002**, *37*, 25–30. [CrossRef]
15. Akalin, M.; Demirci, O.; Dayan, E.; Odacilar, A.S.; Ocal, A.; Celayir, A. Natural history of fetal ovarian cysts in the prenatal and postnatal periods. *J. Clin. Ultrasound.* **2021**, *49*, 822–827. [CrossRef]

16. Lewis, S.; Walker, J.; McHoney, M. Antenatally detected abdominal cyst: Does cyst size and nature determine postnatal symptoms and outcome? *Early Hum. Dev.* **2020**, *147*, 105102. [CrossRef] [PubMed]
17. Ozcan, H.N.; Balci, S.; Ekinci, S.; Gunes, A.; Oguz, B.; Ciftci, A.O.; Haliloglu, M. Imaging Findings of Fetal-Neonatal Ovarian Cysts Complicated with Ovarian Torsion and Autoamputation. *AJR Am. J. Roentgenol.* **2015**, *205*, 185–189. [CrossRef]
18. Zampieri, N.; Borruto, F.; Zamboni, C.; Camoglio, F.S. Foetal and neonatal ovarian cysts: A 5-year experience. *Arch. Gynecol. Obstet.* **2008**, *277*, 303–306. [CrossRef] [PubMed]
19. Souganidis, E.; Chen, A.; Friedlaender, E. Symptomatic Persistent Fetal Ovarian Cysts. *Pediatr. Emerg. Care.* **2021**, *37*, e672–e674. [CrossRef]
20. Cheng, Y. Ovarian cysts. *Am. J. Obstet. Gynecol.* **2021**, *225*, B23–B25. [CrossRef]
21. Filip, C.; Socolov, D.G.; Albu, E.; Filip, C.; Serban, R.; Popa, R.F. Serological Parameters and Vascular Investigation for a Better Assessment in DVT during Pregnancy—A Systematic Review. *Medicina* **2021**, *57*, 160. [CrossRef] [PubMed]
22. Lawrence, A.E.; Fallat, M.E.; Hewitt, G.; Hertweck, P.; Onwuka, A.; Afrazi, A.; Bence, C.; Burns, R.C.; Corkum, K.S.; Dillon, P.A.; et al. Understanding the Value of Tumor Markers in Pediatric Ovarian Neoplasms. *J. Pediatr. Surg.* **2020**, *55*, 122–125. [CrossRef] [PubMed]
23. Rotar, I.C.; Tudorache, S.; Staicu, A.; Popa-Stanila, R.; Constantin, R.; Surcel, M.; Zaharie, G.C.; Mureşan, D. Fetal Ovarian Cysts: Prenatal Diagnosis Using Ultrasound and MRI, Management and Postnatal Outcome-Our Centers Experience. *Diagnostics* **2021**, *12*, 89. [CrossRef]
24. Nemec, U.; Nemec, S.F.; Bettelheim, D.; Brugger, P.C.; Horcher, E.; Schöpf, V.; Graham, J.M., Jr.; Rimoin, D.L.; Weber, M.; Prayer, D. Ovarian cysts on prenatal MRI. *Eur. J. Radiol.* **2012**, *81*, 1937–1944. [CrossRef]
25. Norton, M.E.; Cheng, Y.; Chetty, S.; Chyu, J.K.; Connolly, K.; Ghaffari, N.; Hopkins, L.M.; Jelin, A.; Mardy, A.; Osmundson, S.S.; et al. SMFM Fetal Anomalies Consult Series #4: Genitourinary anomalies. *Am. J. Obstet. Gynecol.* **2021**, *225*, B2–B35. [PubMed]
26. Hara, T.; Mimura, K.; Endo, M.; Fujii, M.; Matsuyama, T.; Yagi, K.; Kawanishi, Y.; Tomimatsu, T.; Kimura, T. Diagnosis, Management, and Therapy of Fetal Ovarian Cysts Detected by Prenatal Ultrasonography: A Report of 36 Cases and Literature Review. *Diagnostics* **2021**, *11*, 2224. [CrossRef] [PubMed]
27. Słodki, M.; Respondek-Liberska, M. Fetal ovarian cysts—420 cases from literature—Metaanalysis 1984–2005. *Ginekol. Pol.* **2007**, *78*, 324–328. [PubMed]
28. Senarath, S.; Ades, A.; Nanayakkara, P. Ovarian cysts in pregnancy: A narrative review. *J. Obstet. Gynaecol.* **2021**, *41*, 169–175. [CrossRef]
29. Papic, J.C.; Billmire, D.F.; Rescorla, F.J.; Finnell, S.M.; Leys, C.M. Management of neonatal ovarian cysts and its effect on ovarian preservation. *J. Pediatr. Surg.* **2014**, *49*, 990–993; discussion 993–994. [CrossRef] [PubMed]
30. Aziz, M.A.; Zahra, F.; Razianti Zb, C.; Kharismawati, N.; Sutjighassani, T.; Almira, N.L.; Tjandraprawira, K.D. Challenges in prenatal diagnosis of foetal anorectal malformation and hydrocolpos—Case report. *Ann. Med. Surg.* **2022**, *84*, 104949. [CrossRef]
31. Dolgin, S.E. Ovarian masses in the newborn. *Semin. Pediatr. Surg.* **2000**, *9*, 121–127. [CrossRef]
32. Croitoru, D.P.; Aaron, L.E.; Laberge, J.M.; Neilson, I.R.; Guttman, F.M. Management of complex ovarian cysts presenting in the first year of life. *J. Pediatr. Surg.* **1991**, *26*, 1366–1368. [CrossRef]
33. Strickland, J.L. Ovarian cysts in neonates, children and adolescents. *Curr. Opin. Obstet. Gynecol.* **2002**, *14*, 459–465. [CrossRef] [PubMed]
34. Luzzatto, C.; Midrio, P.; Toffolutti, T.; Suma, V. Neonatal ovarian cysts: Management and follow-up. *Pediatr. Surg. Int.* **2000**, *16*, 56–59. [CrossRef] [PubMed]
35. Enríquez, G.; Durán, C.; Torán, N.; Piqueras, J.; Gratacós, E.; Aso, C.; Lloret, J.; Castellote, A.; Lucaya, J. Conservative versus surgical treatment for complex neonatal ovarian cysts: Outcomes study. *AJR Am. J. Roentgenol.* **2005**, *185*, 501–508. [CrossRef] [PubMed]
36. Diguisto, C.; Winer, N.; Benoist, G.; Laurichesse-Delmas, H.; Potin, J.; Binet, A.; Lardy, H.; Morel, B.; Perrotin, F. In-utero aspiration vs expectant management of anechoic fetal ovarian cysts: Open randomized controlled trial. *Ultrasound Obstet. Gynecol.* **2018**, *52*, 159–164. [CrossRef] [PubMed]
37. Tyraskis, A.; Bakalis, S.; David, A.L.; Eaton, S.; De Coppi, P. A systematic review and meta-analysis on fetal ovarian cysts: Impact of size, appearance and prenatal aspiration. *Prenat. Diagn.* **2017**, *37*, 951–958. [CrossRef] [PubMed]
38. Heling, K.S.; Chaoui, R.; Kirchmair, F.; Stadie, S.; Bollmann, R. Fetal ovarian cysts: Prenatal diagnosis, management and postnatal outcome. *Ultrasound Obstet. Gynecol.* **2002**, *20*, 47–50. [CrossRef]
39. Dimitraki, M.; Koutlaki, N.; Nikas, I.; Mandratzi, T.; Gourovanidis, V.; Kontomanolis, E.; Zervoudis, S.; Galazios, G.; Liberis, V. Fetal ovarian cysts. Our clinical experience over 16 cases and review of the literature. *J. Matern Fetal Neonatal. Med.* **2012**, *25*, 222–225. [CrossRef]
40. Tyraskis, A.; Bakalis, S.; Scala, C.; Syngelaki, A.; Giuliani, S.; Davenport, M.; David, A.L.; Nicolaides, K.; Eaton, S.; De Coppi, P. A retrospective multicenter study of the natural history of fetal ovarian cysts. *J. Pediatr. Surg.* **2018**, *53*, 2019–2022. [CrossRef]

Disclaimer/Publisher's Note: The statements, opinions and data contained in all publications are solely those of the individual author(s) and contributor(s) and not of MDPI and/or the editor(s). MDPI and/or the editor(s) disclaim responsibility for any injury to people or property resulting from any ideas, methods, instructions or products referred to in the content.

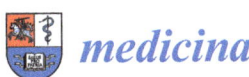

Case Report

Extremely Rare Case of Fetal Anemia Due to Mitochondrial Disease Managed with Intrauterine Transfusion

Jinha Chung, Mi-Young Lee, Jin-Hoon Chung and Hye-Sung Won *

Department of Obstetrics and Gynecology, Asan Medical Center, University of Ulsan College of Medicine, 88, Olympic-ro 43-gil, Songpa-gu, Seoul 05505, Korea; waterlilyv@naver.com (J.C.); poptwinkle@hanmail.net (M.-Y.L.); sabi0515@hanmail.net (J.-H.C.)
* Correspondence: hswon@amc.seoul.kr

Abstract: This report describes a rare case of fetal anemia, confirmed as a mitochondrial disease after birth, treated with intrauterine transfusion (IUT). Although mitochondrial diseases have been described in newborns, research on their prenatal features is lacking. A patient was referred to our institution at 32 gestational weeks owing to fetal hydrops. Fetal anemia was confirmed by cordocentesis. After IUT had been performed three times, the anemia and associated fetal hydrops showed improvement. However, after birth, the neonate had recurrent pancytopenia and lactic acidosis. He was eventually diagnosed with Pearson syndrome and died 2 months after birth. This is the first case report of fetal anemia associated with mitochondrial disease managed with IUT.

Keywords: anemia; blood transfusion; case report; hydrops fetalis; mitochondrial diseases; Pearson syndrome

1. Introduction

Fetal anemia is a rare condition that can cause fetal hydrops, fetal distress, and eventually fetal death if left untreated. Fetal anemia has many causes. However, the leading cause is an alloimmune disease, and the incidence has been rapidly decreasing owing to the use of immunoglobulins [1]. Nonimmune-related causes include parvovirus B19 infection, fetomaternal hemorrhage, monochorionic pregnancy complications, and other rare diseases [2]. Intrauterine transfusion (IUT) effectively treats fetal alloimmune anemia and nonimmune-related diseases [3]. However, to date, few reports have been published regarding the outcomes of rare diseases that cause fetal anemia. Herein, we report an extremely rare case of fetal anemia associated with Pearson syndrome. Although there was a limit to prenatal diagnosis, this rare mitochondrial disease can cause fetal anemia [4]. This is the first report on fetal anemia caused by mitochondrial disease managed with IUT.

2. Case Presentation

A 38-year-old, high-risk pregnant primiparous woman visited our hospital at 32 gestational weeks owing to fetal hydrops and oligohydramnios observed on ultrasonography. She had no remarkable medical or family history. Antenatal examination conducted at another hospital 3 weeks before her first visit to our hospital revealed no abnormal findings. The fetus was hydropic with generalized skin edema, ascites, pericardial effusion, cardiomegaly, and bilateral hydrocele (Figure 1A,B). The estimated fetal weight was 1873 g (50th percentile), which might have been overestimated owing to fetal ascites. No other structural abnormalities were noted.

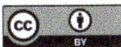

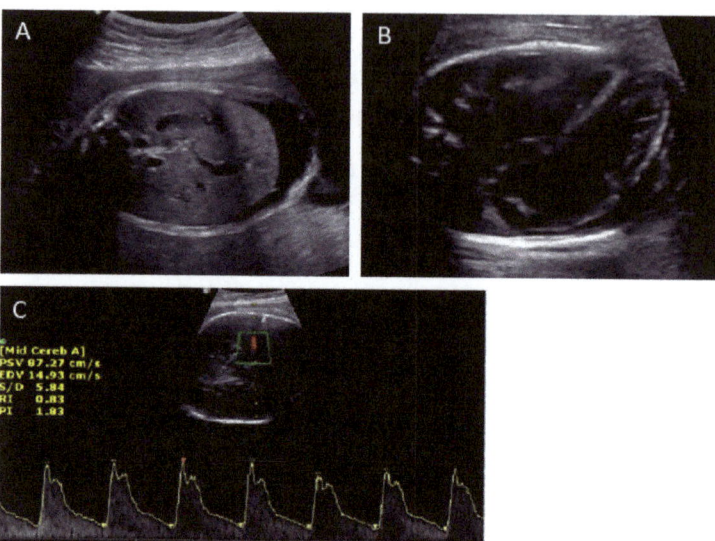

Figure 1. Initial ultrasonographic findings show fetal ascites (**A**) and pericardial effusion with cardiomegaly (**B**). Middle cerebral artery peak systolic velocity on Doppler ultrasonography before intrauterine transfusion was 87 cm/s (1.95 MoM) (**C**).

Doppler ultrasonography revealed that the middle cerebral artery peak systolic velocity (MCA-PSV) was 87 cm/s (1.95 MoM) [5], indicating fetal anemia (Figure 1C). Cordocentesis confirmed severe anemia with a hemoglobin level of 1.4 g/dL. To prevent abrupt changes in the fetal cardiovascular system and to improve fetal anemia, IUT was performed three times at 32.0, 32.1, and 32.4 gestational weeks with transfused volumes of 34, 50, and 48 cm^3, respectively. After the IUTs, the MCA-PSV and hemoglobin levels improved to 56 cm/s (1.3 MoM) and 9.8 g/dL, respectively. The toxoplasmosis, rubella, cytomegalovirus, and herpes simplex virus (TORCH) panel test and parvovirus B19 test from the maternal blood and amniotic fluid were negative. Fetal karyotyping from the amniotic fluid revealed normal findings. Maternal ABO/Rh typing and antibody screening tests revealed O, Rh+ and negative antibodies to rule out alloimmune fetal anemia. In addition, the blood type of the fetus examined with cordocentesis was O, Rh+.

The patient was followed up weekly. The fetal hydropic features, generalized skin edema, ascites, pericardial effusion, cardiomegaly, and bilateral hydrocele were fully resolved two weeks after IUT, and the umbilical artery and ductus venosus Doppler ultrasonography findings were normal. The MCA-PSV was 54.19 cm/s (1–1.3 MoM); thus, no additional IUT was required. The patient underwent elective cesarean delivery at 39.0 gestational weeks and gave birth to a 2110 g male neonate, with 1 and 5 min Apgar scores of 6 and 7, respectively. The neonate's birth weight was below the third percentile. No gross anomalies were noted.

The neonate was admitted to the neonatal intensive care unit for further evaluation. Initial abdomen ultrasonography showed diffuse dense calcifications in the bilateral adrenal glands. Brain ultrasonography and echocardiography revealed no structural abnormalities. The neonate's blood type was O, Rh+, and antibody screening was negative. In addition, the TORCH study and direct Coombs' test were negative. However, initial white blood cell (WBC), hemoglobin (Hb), and platelet (Plt) levels were 3400/μL, 6.5 g/dL, and 156,000/μL, respectively. The initial lactic acid level was 8.0 mmol/L. Peripheral blood smear revealed sideroblastic anemia. Laboratory examinations responded only temporarily to blood transfusion and revealed recurrent pancytopenia and lactic acidosis within a few days. The patient was discharged after repeated blood transfusions. When the patient was rehospitalized due to pancytopenia, his WBC, Hb, and Plt levels were 2500/μL, 6.1 g/dL, and 25,000/μL, respectively. Wolman disease or mitochondrial disease was most likely. His triglycerides, cholesterol, and cortisol levels were normal; thus, the likelihood of Wolman disease was low. Whole exome sequencing for lysosomal acid lipase enzyme gene, mitochondrial deoxyribonucleic acid (DNA) gene mutation, urine organic acid analysis, and acylcarnitine profiling were performed on the 10th day after birth. Mitochondrial gene mutation (m.9424_14840del of the mitochondrial genome) was observed by polymerase chain reaction sequencing using peripheral blood with normal findings of the other studies. The neonate was diagnosed with Pearson syndrome, a mitochondrial disease. Having pancytopenia, the neonate was prone to infection. He died of sepsis secondary to a hospital-acquired *Klebsiella pneumoniae* infection at two months.

3. Discussion

Owing to the advances in diagnosis and treatment in the last 20 years, the survival rate of patients with fetal anemia has improved. For decades, fetal anemia had been diagnosed using invasive techniques such as amniocentesis and cordocentesis. In 2000, MCA-PSV Doppler assessment was introduced to predict fetal anemia. However, it has a 10–18% false positivity rate, requiring cordocentesis for confirmation [6]. Nonetheless, it is still widely used as a noninvasive technique for screening fetal anemia [5].

Known causes of fetal anemia include alloimmune anemia, congenital infection, hemorrhage, monochorionic pregnancy complications, and fetal or placental tumors [2,7]. However, only a few reports have described rare causes of fetal anemia. For example, Amann et al. [7] reported 15 cases of fetal anemia, the causes of which were determined after birth. Among the causes were Blackfan–Diamond anemia, elliptocytosis, hemochromatosis, and mucopolysaccharidosis type VII.

Mitochondrial diseases are rare, with a prevalence of 1 in 10,000 births [8], and can be caused by mitochondrial or DNA mutations. The incidence of mitochondrial DNA (mtDNA) deletion disorder does not increase with maternal age [9]. These diseases present a complexity of clinical features and genetic factors, and various features can be exhibited in different organs. Before 4 years of age, the fatality rate is reportedly 57% [10]. The presented case is the first report on a fetus with mitochondrial disease managed with IUT. The fetus showed antenatal features of mitochondrial disease such as fetal growth restriction, oligohydramnios, and fetal anemia [4].

Pearson syndrome, a mitochondrial disease, occurs due to a single, large-scale mtDNA deletion gene defect. The main clinical features of Pearson syndrome are sideroblastic anemia, lactic acidosis, and pancreatic exocrine disorder [11]. Sideroblastic anemia is transfusion-dependent anemia, which might explain why IUT resolved the fetal anemia-associated hydrops in this case. However, studies on the perinatal outcomes of Pearson syndrome with severe fetal anemia are lacking.

4. Conclusions

Although extremely rare, mitochondrial disease may cause severe fetal anemia, which can be treated with IUT. However, congenital genetic disorders or hematologic diseases might have a worse prognosis after birth. Therefore, the findings in this report are meaningful in counseling parents about the need for postnatal evaluation and the possibility of fatal prognosis, depending on the diagnosed or suspected cause of fetal anemia.

Author Contributions: Conceptualization, H.-S.W. and M.-Y.L.; investigation, J.C.; resources, H.-S.W.; data curation, J.C.; writing—original draft preparation, J.C.; writing—review and editing, J.-H.C. and M.-Y.L.; supervision, H.-S.W.; All authors have read and agreed to the published version of the manuscript.

Funding: This research received no external funding.

Institutional Review Board Statement: Ethical review and approval were waived for this study because of the retrospective nature of the study.

Informed Consent Statement: Informed consent was obtained from the patient directly.

Data Availability Statement: The data are available upon request.

Conflicts of Interest: The authors declare no conflict of interest.

References

1. Ruma, M.S.; Moise, K.J., Jr.; Kim, E.; Murtha, A.P.; Prutsman, W.J.; Hassan, S.S.; Lubarsky, S.L. Combined plasmapheresis and intravenous immune globulin for the treatment of severe maternal red cell alloimmunization. *Am. J. Obstet. Gynecol.* **2007**, *196*, 138.e1–138.e6. [CrossRef]
2. Mizuuchi, M.; Murotsuki, J.; Ishii, K.; Yamamoto, R.; Sasahara, J.; Wada, S.; Takahashi, Y.; Nakata, M.; Murakoshi, T.; Sago, H. Nationwide survey of intrauterine blood transfusion for fetal anemia in Japan. *J. Obstet. Gynaecol. Res.* **2021**, *47*, 2076–2091. [CrossRef] [PubMed]
3. Lindenburg, I.T.; van Kamp, I.L.; Oepkes, D. Intrauterine blood transfusion: Current indications and associated risks. *Fetal Diagn. Ther.* **2014**, *36*, 263–271. [CrossRef] [PubMed]
4. Tavares, M.V.; Santos, M.J.; Domingues, A.P.; Pratas, J.; Mendes, C.; Simoes, M.; Moura, P.; Diogo, L.; Grazina, M. Antenatal manifestations of mitochondrial disorders. *J. Inherit. Metab. Dis.* **2013**, *36*, 805–811. [CrossRef] [PubMed]
5. Mari, G.; Deter, R.L.; Carpenter, R.L.; Rahman, F.; Zimmerman, R.; Moise, K.J., Jr.; Dorman, K.F.; Ludomirsky, A.; Gonzalez, R.; Gomez, R.; et al. Noninvasive diagnosis by Doppler ultrasonography of fetal anemia due to maternal red-cell alloimmunization. Collaborative Group for Doppler Assessment of the Blood Velocity in Anemic Fetuses. *N. Engl. J. Med.* **2000**, *342*, 9–14. [CrossRef] [PubMed]
6. Oepkes, D.; Seaward, P.G.; Vandenbussche, F.P.; Windrim, R.; Kingdom, J.; Beyene, J.; Kanhai, H.H.; Ohlsson, A.; Ryan, G.; Group, D.S. Doppler ultrasonography versus amniocentesis to predict fetal anemia. *N. Engl. J. Med.* **2006**, *355*, 156–164. [CrossRef] [PubMed]
7. Amann, C.; Geipel, A.; Muller, A.; Heep, A.; Ritgen, J.; Stressig, R.; Kozlowski, P.; Gembruch, U.; Berg, C. Fetal anemia of unknown cause—A diagnostic challenge. *Ultraschall Med.* **2011**, *32* (Suppl. S2), E134–E140. [CrossRef] [PubMed]
8. van den Heuvel, L.; Smeitink, J. The oxidative phosphorylation (OXPHOS) system: Nuclear genes and human genetic diseases. *Bioessays* **2001**, *23*, 518–525. [CrossRef] [PubMed]
9. Chinnery, P.F.; DiMauro, S.; Shanske, S.; Schon, E.A.; Zeviani, M.; Mariotti, C.; Carrara, F.; Lombes, A.; Laforet, P.; Ogier, H.; et al. Risk of developing a mitochondrial DNA deletion disorder. *Lancet* **2004**, *364*, 592–596. [CrossRef]
10. Rotig, A.; Bourgeron, T.; Chretien, D.; Rustin, P.; Munnich, A. Spectrum of mitochondrial DNA rearrangements in the Pearson marrow-pancreas syndrome. *Human Mol. Genet.* **1995**, *4*, 1327–1330. [CrossRef] [PubMed]
11. Rahman, S. Mitochondrial disease in children. *J. Intern. Med.* **2020**, *287*, 609–633. [CrossRef] [PubMed]

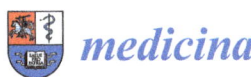

Case Report

Endocrine Disorders in a Newborn with Heterozygous Galactosemia, Down Syndrome and Complex Cardiac Malformation: Case Report

Ioana Rosca [1,2], Alina Turenschi [3], Alin Nicolescu [4], Andreea Teodora Constantin [5,6], Adina Maria Canciu [3], Alice Denisa Dica [7], Elvira Bratila [5,8], Ciprian Andrei Coroleuca [5,8,*] and Leonard Nastase [5,9]

1. Neonatology Department, Clinical Hospital of Obstetrics and Gynecology "Prof. Dr. P.Sirbu", 060251 Bucharest, Romania
2. Faculty of Midwifery and Nursery, University of Medicine and Pharmacy "Carol Davila", 020021 Bucharest, Romania
3. Emergency Clinical Hospital for Children "Grigore Alexandrescu", 011743 Bucharest, Romania
4. Cardiology Department, Emergency Clinical Hospital for Children "M.S. Curie", 41451 Bucharest, Romania
5. Faculty of Medicine, University of Medicine and Pharmacy "Carol Davila", 020021 Bucharest, Romania
6. Pediatrics Department, National Institute for Mother and Child Health "Alessandrescu-Rusescu", 020395 Bucharest, Romania
7. Pediatric Neurology Department, Clinical Psychiatric Hospital "Al. Obregia", 041914 Bucharest, Romania
8. Obstetrics and Gynecology Department, Clinical Hospital of Obstetrics and Gynecology "Prof. Dr. P.Sirbu", 060251 Bucharest, Romania
9. Neonatology Department, National Institute for Mother and Child Health "Alessandrescu-Rusescu", 011061 Bucharest, Romania
* Correspondence: ciprian.coroleuca@umfcd.ro

Abstract: Down syndrome is the most common chromosomal abnormality diagnosed in newborn babies. Infants with Down syndrome have characteristic dysmorphic features and can have neuropsychiatric disorders, cardiovascular diseases, gastrointestinal abnormalities, eye problems, hearing loss, endocrine and hematologic disorders, and many other health issues. We present the case of a newborn with Down syndrome. The infant was a female, born at term through c-section. She was diagnosed before birth with a complex congenital malformation. In the first few days of life, the newborn was stable. In her 10th day of life, she started to show respiratory distress, persistent respiratory acidosis, and persistent severe hyponatremia, and required intubation and mechanical ventilation. Due to her rapid deterioration our team decided to do a screening for metabolic disorders. The screening was positive for heterozygous Duarte variant galactosemia. Further testing on possible metabolic and endocrinologic issues that can be associated with Down syndrome was performed, leading to hypoaldosteronism and hypothyroidism diagnoses. The case was challenging for our team because the infant also had multiple metabolic and hormonal deficiencies. Newborns with Down syndrome often require a multidisciplinary team, as besides congenital cardiac malformations they can have metabolic and hormonal deficiencies that can negatively impact their short- and long-term prognosis.

Keywords: Down syndrome; newborn; galactosemia; hypothyroidism; hypoaldosteronism; multidisciplinary team

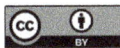

1. Introduction

Down syndrome is one of the most frequent chromosomal abnormalities diagnosed in newborn babies. It is also called Trisomy 21, because it is determined by the presence of an extra 21st chromosome [1–4]. A recent study [5] estimated that, in Europe in 2015, there were 419,000 people with Down syndrome. Patients affected by this syndrome can have multiple medical issues that can range from intellectual disability to congenital heart malformations, celiac disease, and endocrine disorders [3,6,7].

Studies report that the incidence of congenital cardiac malformations associated with Down syndrome is around 45–50% of the individuals affected by this syndrome [8]. The most common cardiac defects identified prenatally in fetuses with Down syndrome are atrioventricular septal defects, ventricular septal defects, secundum atrial septal defects, and persistent arterial ducts [9–11].

Patients with Down syndrome also have higher rates of endocrine disorders such as obesity, diabetes mellitus, short stature, vitamin D deficiency, and thyroid dysfunction [12–14].

Life expectancy in patients with Down syndrome has improved significantly. In United States of America in the 1950s, the median life expectancy age was 4 years; in 2010, it was as high as 58 years [15].

The medical management of newborn babies diagnosed with Down syndrome requires a multidisciplinary team. The long- and short-term prognosis of these patients is improved by reliable screening programs that help identify associated malformations as soon as possible.

2. Case Report

We present the case of a newborn baby, a girl, born at term. Her birth weight was 3990 g, and she was born at the gestational age of 38–39 weeks (postmenstrual gestational age). The pregnancy was surveyed by a Gynecology and Obstetrics specialist. It was considered a high-risk pregnancy, due to the facts that her mother had had a previous cesarean-section and the fetus was diagnosed in utero with a cardiac malformation. She was born through cesarean-section, and her APGAR score was 8 at one minute.

Right after birth, the newborn had a satisfactory general appearance; she had facial features characteristic for Down syndrome, no heart murmurs, and no other noticeable distress signs. Due to the fact that the medical team knew this infant had a congenital cardiac malformation, she was admitted to the Neonatal Intensive Care Unit (NICU).

The cardiology consultant diagnosed the patient with a complete atrioventricular canal defect with a large atrial septal defect (type C according to the Rastelli classification [16]), grade II left and right atrioventricular valve regurgitation, and small functional atria (Figure 1). Medical treatment with furosemide, spironolactone, and captopril was recommended and started with good tolerance and evolution. In her second day of life, a systolic murmur of grade II/VI could be heard on cardiac auscultation.

For the first seven days of life the newborn baby continued to be stable, with a good general appearance, some jaundice, and stable respiration with a SpO_2 of 96% in atmospheric air. The neonatology medical team was able to start enteral nutrition with good digestive tolerance. She was bottle fed with milk formula (partially hydrolyzed milk formula). She had a 10% body weight loss. Blood tests, as well as abdominal and transfontanellar ultrasound, were within normal range.

In the 9th day of life, her general appearance changed; the jaundice suddenly accentuated (transcutaneous bilirubin 13.8 mg/dL), the systolic murmur accentuated (grade III/VI), and her body weight decreased. She started to require fraction of inspired oxygen (FiO_2) of 40% to keep her SpO_2 over 95% and she also developed signs of respiratory distress (intercostal, subcostal retractions, polypnea with approximately 70 respirations/minute, bradycardia with ventricular rate of 90–100 bpm). From this moment forward, she required continuous oxygen supplementation (both invasive and noninvasive respiratory support) as well as respiratory stimulation (kinesiotherapy).

Because of the rapid and sudden deterioration, the medical team decided to ask for a metabolic diseases panel. The results showed increased levels of galactose. Investigations continued in this direction with dosing of Galactose-1-phosphate uridylyl transferase, which confirmed the diagnosis of heterozygote galactosemia or homozygous Duarte 2 variant. The patient was started on a specific galactosemia milk formula (soy based), and 24 h later we were able to wean her off the ventilator, since her respiratory function had improved significantly.

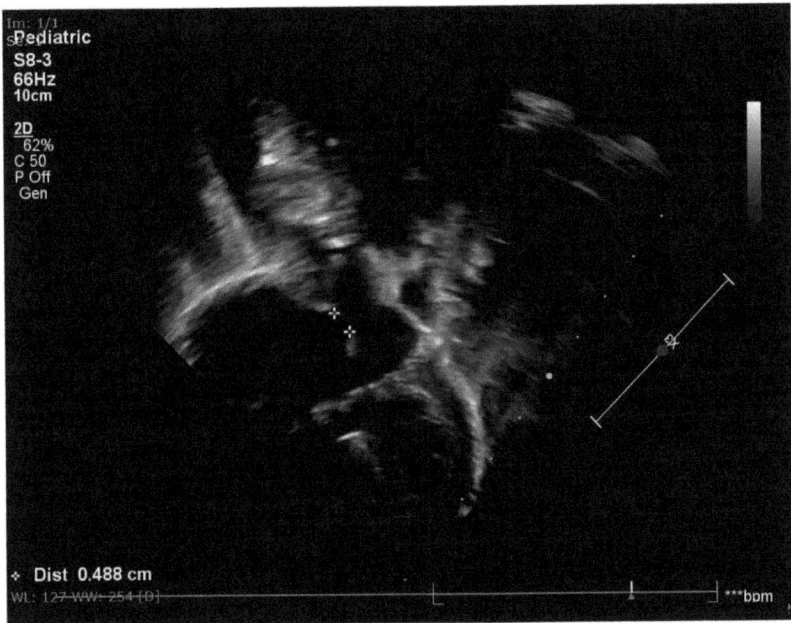

Figure 1. Echocardiography of the patient showing atrial septal defect, inlet type ventricular septal defect, one atrioventricular valve and balanced ventricles.

During her entire hospitalization time, the infant had hyponatremia (dropping as low as 130 mmol/L). Therefore, the suspicion of hypoaldosteronism was raised and subsequently confirmed through aldosterone dosing. Treatment with Fludrocortisone was initiated, with a dose of 0.1 mg/day with good tolerance and favorable evolution (normalization of serum sodium level).

Screening for other possible endocrinological issues was in order at this time, and this showed hypothyroidism, thus adding to her medication Levothyroxine in a dose of 25 µg/day.

This patient spent a total of 80 days in our hospital. Her evolution was uncertain, with ups and downs, including respiratory distress syndrome of varying severity, and blood gas analysis showing high pCO_2 values (as high as 60–70 mmHg) and low pO_2 values. She repeatedly needed mechanical respiratory support through orotracheal intubation. Despite maximal medical treatment and the extensive efforts of a multidisciplinary medical team, she had multiple episodes of severe bradycardia and desaturation which were ultimately unresponsive to resuscitation maneuvers.

Newborn babies born with complete atrioventricular canal defect (CAVC) can present at birth with slight cyanosis due to high vascular pulmonary resistance. Cardiac insufficiency signs usually appear in the first month of life, as pulmonary neonatal vascular resistance decreases physiologically and the shunt flow increases [17,18]. In our patient, cardiac failure signs were early, at one week postnatal age. The newborn had tachypnea, needed oxygen supplementation, and had feeding difficulties and growth failure, making her congenital cardiac malformation the main cause for her respiratory distress.

Another cause for respiratory distress in newborn babies is infection. Patients with cardiac failure can have recurrent respiratory infections [17,18]. Ventilation pneumonia is a common occurrence in infants that require intubation and mechanical ventilation for a large amount of time. It is usually considered a nosocomial infection and definitive diagnosis criteria include: more than 48 h of mechanical ventilation; changes in blood gases; a need to increase ventilation parameters; temperature instability; tachypnea, wheezing, cough, or abundant secretions; changes in cardiac rhythm; and leukocytosis. Three signs or symptoms from those listed above are necessary to diagnose ventilation pneumonia [19]. Our patient had clinical criteria for ventilation pneumonia and needed prolonged mechanical ventilation.

In patients with CAVC and Down syndrome, pulmonary hypertension appears earlier and has increased severity due to genetic factors, pulmonary hypoplasia, and associated chronic hypoventilation [17,20]. Among the causes of pulmonary hypertension in newborn babies, there is alveolar hypoxia due to respiratory failure, alveolar hypoventilation due to abnormalities of the central nervous system, and acidosis and shock due to left ventricular dysfunction [18]. Our patient met these criteria. The X-ray (Figure 2) had non-specific findings: cardiac enlargement with signs of overload on pulmonary circulation and dilatation of the pulmonary artery [17]. In our case, the X-ray showed these suggestive findings.

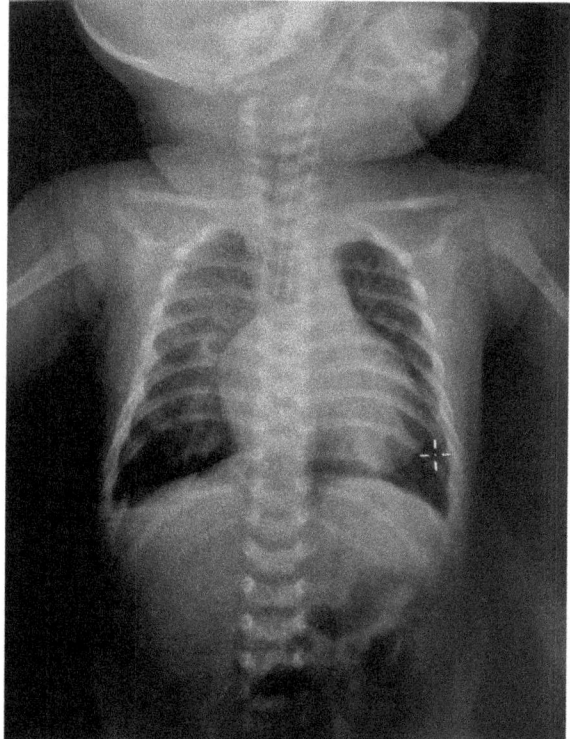

Figure 2. X-ray for the patient at approximately one month age. The patient was intubated and mechanically ventilated. We noticed the enlarged cardio-thoracic index (>0.6), pulmonary hypoventilation, and accentuation of pulmonary hilum.

We took into consideration other causes for respiratory failure—narrow respiratory airway, laryngomalacia, hypotonia—that are specific to a patient with Down syndrome. Prolonged endotracheal intubation can be associated with subglottic stenosis, tracheobronchomalacia, and chronic lung disease. We did take all these possible diagnoses into consideration for our patient. The ENT specialist was able to exclude laryngomalacia and congenital obstruction of upper respiratory airways.

3. Discussion

Down syndrome, besides being the most frequently identified chromosomal abnormality, is also one of the most studied in the last 150 years. The most frequent malformations associated with Down syndrome are cardiac, gastrointestinal, musculoskeletal, urinary, and endocrine [7,11,21,22]. In the presented case, the congenital cardiac malformation was diagnosed before birth, which required the patient to be taken in charge in a level III maternity ward with an advanced NICU and a multidisciplinary team.

As we previously mentioned, this patient presented with respiratory distress almost throughout her entire hospitalization. This led the medical team to multiple differential diagnoses, such as pneumonia, pulmonary edema, and ear, nose and throat (ENT) pathology. Confirming the cardiac malformation in the first 24 h of life allowed the medical team to initiate specific treatment as soon as possible and to initiate advanced monitoring. There were multiple causes for her respiratory distress, starting with her complex cardiac malformation, pulmonary hypertension secondary to the cardiac malformation, a narrow upper respiratory tract that is specific to Down syndrome, gastrointestinal reflux, and her metabolic and endocrine associated disorders (hypoaldosteronism, hypothyroidism, galactosemia).

Galactosemia is an inborn error of metabolism that affects carbohydrate metabolism. Severe galactose-1-phosphate uridylyl transferase (GALT) deficiency and classic galactosemia can be deadly for newborns [23–25]. There are certain variants of galactosemia. The Duarte variant is characterized by GALT activity of about 50% in the red blood cells (if homozygotes). Heterozygotes for the Duarte variant have about 75% GALT activity [26]. Although classic galactosemia is considered to be a medical emergency, the Duarte variant is considered to be asymptomatic and usually does not necessitate a galactose restricted diet [27,28]. Our patient had no digestive symptoms specific to classic galactosemia (she had good digestive tolerance, no loose stools, no emesis). Her blood work did not show metabolic acidosis but respiratory acidosis, which is atypical for galactosemia. However, the respiratory distress and respiratory acidosis improved significantly when a galactose-restrictive diet with a soy-based formula was initiated.

Hypoaldosteronism is an endocrine disorder characterized by aldosterone deficiency or defective aldosterone activity on the tissue level. The severity is usually inversely related to age [29]. The most frequent clinical findings are hyperkaliemia, hyponatremia associated with hypovolemia, and metabolic acidosis [30]. In our patient, what raised the suspicion was persistent hyponatremia, despite appropriate intravenous correction. We decided to verify the serum cortisol level (which was within normal range) and serum aldosterone level (low level). Thus, oral treatment with fludrocortisone was initiated.

When compared to the general population, patients with Down syndrome are 25–38-fold more likely to have thyroid dysfunction [31,32]. In patients with Down syndrome, screening for thyroid using thyroid-stimulating hormone (TSH), free T4, and free T4 should be started at birth and repeated at 6 months, 12 months, and annually thereafter [33–35]. This recommendation is supported by the fact that, in our patient, the initial newborn screening was negative for hypothyroidism. The medical team decided to repeat thyroid functional tests and could diagnose hypothyroidism and initiate appropriate treatment with Levothyroxine.

The decision to start feeding our patient with hydrolyzed milk was made for the prevention of necrotizing enterocolitis (NEC), as the newborn was diagnosed with severe heart disease. NEC is an ischemic and inflammatory necrosis of the bowel, primarily affecting premature neonates after the initiation of enteral feeding, but 10% of all cases of NEC occur in term infants [36]. Risk factors for this group of term neonates include congenital heart disease with presumed low intestinal perfusion [20]. The pathogenesis of NEC is multifactorial, and additional risk factors for this pathology include ischemia, intestinal dysbiosis, and formula feedings; almost all newborns with NEC received enteral nutrition before the onset of the disease [20,36]. Infants with congenital heart disease may have compromised bowel perfusion, making them susceptible to ischemic injury; hypoxic/ischemic events play a greater role in the pathogenesis of NEC [36]. For the prevention of NEC, several strategies are needed, including the exclusive use of breast milk and minimizing exposure to empiric antibiotic therapy [20]. Enteral feeding provides a necessary substrate for the proliferation of enteric pathogens. Hyperosmolar formulas or medications may alter mucosal permeability and cause mucosal damage. Human milk, with the benefit of providing immunoprotective as well as local growth promoting factors, significantly lowers the risk of NEC [36,37]. Moreover, enteral immunoglobulin A-immunoglobulin G (IgA-IgG) feeding also decreased the risk for NEC in preliminary clinical studies [36]. Our patient could not be fed with breast milk because the mothers' lactate secretion was installed late after the cesarean section; she initially had hypogalactia and later was discharged from our hospital unit. In our unit, there is no breast milk bank, and in this situation, we chose to feed the newborn with hydrolyzed milk, the most appropriate formula in this case with risk factors for NEC. Another risk factor for NEC is bacterial colonization; bacteria including Escherichia coli, Klebsiella species, Clostridia species, and Staphylococcus epidermidis are implicated in NEC [36].

This case is unique because of the coexistent conditions of our patient. In patients with Down syndrome, congenital cardiac malformations are quite frequent, ranging from 20 to 57.9% depending on the study [38]. Most studies report atrioventricular septal defect as being one of the most frequent congenital heart diseases associated with Down syndrome [39–41]. Although our patient had one of the most frequent congenital heart defects associated with Down syndrome, it was not isolated, being associated with other defects, thus being life threatening and requiring medical treatment. Hypothyroidism is known to be frequently associated with Down syndrome [42]. We did not find reports of other cases of Down syndrome associated with galactosemia, but there are recent studies and theories about different metabolic deficiencies associated with Down syndrome [43]. Although not unexpected, the association of Down syndrome, congenital heart disease, and hypothyroidism, with the addition of Duarte galactosemia, is of interest due to the challenges multiple-pathology cases imply for the medical team. The sudden deterioration of this patient had multiple etiological factors: pulmonary, cardiac, neurological, metabolic, and hormonal, and the management was complex.

Communication with the parents of the child with Down syndrome is very important in the diagnosis, treatment, and follow-up of such patients. Their families have complex needs and lives. It is important for them to understand the importance of a multidisciplinary team and have a good collaboration with such a team [44].

Limitations in our approach to this case arises from the fact that all interdisciplinary consultations occurred in other medical units (cardiology, ENT, endocrinology, pediatric neurology, genetics) and required the newborn baby being transported to those hospitals, involving additional stress for the patient.

Although not unexpected, the association of Down syndrome, congenital heart disease, and hypothyroidism, with the addition of Duarte galactosemia, is of interest due to the challenges multiple-pathology cases imply for the medical team. The sudden deterioration of this patient had multiple etiological factors: pulmonary, cardiac, neurological, metabolic, and hormonal, and the management was complex.

In the medical field, maybe more than anywhere else, it is important to keep an open mind and think outside of the box when searching for the right diagnosis and treatment.

Even if there are known associations, such as Down syndrome with congenital cardiac malformations and hypothyroidism, we should always take into consideration other possible diagnoses.

Any newborn baby can have congenital metabolic disease that are clinically difficult to diagnose.

The newborn screening national program should include as many metabolic disorders as possible.

4. Conclusions

In conclusion, the case we presented emphasizes the need for a multidisciplinary team in the management of such a complex case. Endocrine dysfunction had an important impact on the evolution of this patient, thus adding to the importance of screening for endocrine disorders in patients with Down syndrome, even if the initial evaluation is normal.

Regardless of the severity of the disease and the prognosis, any newborn has the right to advanced medical assistance. The parents of this newborn were aware of the severity of the disease before she was born, decided to continue with the pregnancy, and did not regret their decision as far as we know.

Author Contributions: Conceptualization, I.R. and C.A.C.; investigation, A.M.C. and A.T.; resources, L.N., C.A.C., A.N., E.B. and A.D.D.; writing—original draft preparation, A.T.C. and E.B.; writing—review and editing, I.R. and A.T.; visualization, C.A.C.; supervision, I.R. All authors have read and agreed to the published version of the manuscript.

Funding: This research received no external funding.

Institutional Review Board Statement: The study was conducted in accordance with the Declaration of Helsinki, and approved by the Ethics Committee of Clinical Hospital of Obstetrics and Gynecology "Prof. Dr. P.Sirbu" (approval code 4579, approval date 24 April 2023).

Informed Consent Statement: Written informed consent has been obtained from the patient(s) to publish this paper.

Data Availability Statement: Data sharing not applicable.

Conflicts of Interest: The authors declare no conflict of interest.

References

1. Ranweiler, R. Assessment and Care of the Newborn with Down Syndrome. *Adv. Neonatal Care Off. J. Natl. Assoc. Neonatal Nurses* **2009**, *9*, 16–17. [CrossRef] [PubMed]
2. Antonarakis, S.E.; Skotko, B.G.; Rafii, M.S.; Strydom, A.; Pape, S.E.; Bianchi, D.W.; Sherman, S.L.; Reeves, R.H. Down Syndrome. *Nat. Rev. Dis. Prim.* **2020**, *6*, 9. [CrossRef] [PubMed]
3. Bull, M.J. Down Syndrome. *N. Engl. J. Med.* **2020**, *382*, 2344–2352. [CrossRef] [PubMed]
4. Agarwal Gupta, N.; Kabra, M. Diagnosis and Management of Down Syndrome. *Indian J. Pediatr.* **2014**, *81*, 560–567. [CrossRef]
5. de Graaf, G.; Buckley, F.; Skotko, B.G. Estimation of the Number of People with Down Syndrome in Europe. *Eur. J. Hum. Genet.* **2021**, *29*, 402–410. [CrossRef]
6. Whooten, R.; Schmitt, J.; Schwartz, A. Endocrine Manifestations of Down Syndrome. *Curr. Opin. Endocrinol. Diabetes. Obes.* **2018**, *25*, 61–66. [CrossRef]
7. Asim, A.; Kumar, A.; Muthuswamy, S.; Jain, S.; Agarwal, S. Down Syndrome: An Insight of the Disease. *J. Biomed. Sci.* **2015**, *22*, 41. [CrossRef]
8. Venegas-Zamora, L.; Bravo-Acuña, F.; Sigcho, F.; Gomez, W.; Bustamante-Salazar, J.; Pedrozo, Z.; Parra, V. New Molecular and Organelle Alterations Linked to Down Syndrome Heart Disease. *Front. Genet.* **2022**, *12*, 2734. [CrossRef]
9. De Rubens Figueroa, J.; del Pozzo Magaña, B.; Pablos Hach, J.L.; Calderón Jiménez, C.; Castrejón Urbina, R. Heart malformations in children with Down syndrome. *Rev. Esp. Cardiol.* **2003**, *56*, 894–899. [CrossRef] [PubMed]
10. Mogra, R.; Zidere, V.; Allan, L.D. Prenatally Detectable Congenital Heart Defects in Fetuses with Down Syndrome. *Ultrasound Obstet. Gynecol.* **2011**, *38*, 320–324. [CrossRef] [PubMed]
11. Stoll, C.; Dott, B.; Alembik, Y.; Roth, M.-P. Associated Congenital Anomalies among Cases with Down Syndrome. *Eur. J. Med. Genet.* **2015**, *58*, 674–680. [CrossRef] [PubMed]
12. Metwalley, K.A.; Farghaly, H.S. Endocrinal Dysfunction in Children with Down Syndrome. *Ann. Pediatr. Endocrinol. Metab.* **2022**, *27*, 15–21. [CrossRef]
13. Lagan, N.; Huggard, D.; McGrane, F.; Leahy, T.R.; Franklin, O.; Roche, E.; Webb, D.; O'Marcaigh, A.; Cox, D.; El-Khuffash, A.; et al. Multiorgan Involvement and Management in Children with Down Syndrome. *Acta Paediatr.* **2020**, *109*, 1096–1111. [CrossRef]
14. Guaraldi, F.; Rossetto Giaccherino, R.; Lanfranco, F.; Motta, G.; Gori, D.; Arvat, E.; Ghigo, E.; Giordano, R. Endocrine Autoimmunity in Down's Syndrome. *Front. Horm. Res.* **2017**, *48*, 133–146. [CrossRef] [PubMed]
15. de Graaf, G.; Buckley, F.; Skotko, B.G. Estimation of the Number of People with Down Syndrome in the United States. *Genet. Med. Off. J. Am. Coll. Med. Genet.* **2017**, *19*, 439–447. [CrossRef]
16. Calabrò, R.; Limongelli, G. Complete Atrioventricular Canal. *Orphanet J. Rare Dis.* **2006**, *1*, 8. [CrossRef]
17. Nicolescu, A.; Cinteză, E. *Esențialul În Cardiologia Pediatrica*; Amaltea: Bucharest, Romania, 2022; ISBN 9789731622255.
18. Maria, S.; Andreea-Luciana, A. *Urgențe Neonatale*; Tehnopress: Iasi, Romania, 2018; ISBN 978-606-687-363-5.
19. Florea, I. *Tratat de Pediatrie*; ALL: Bucharest, Romania, 2019; ISBN 978-606-587-550-0.
20. Eichenwald, E.C.; Hansen, R.A.; Martin, C.R.; Stark, A.R. *Cloherty and Stark's Manual of Neonatal Care*; Wolters Kluwer: Mumbai, India, 2021; Volume 8, ISBN 9788194864554.
21. Colvin, K.L.; Yeager, M.E. What People with Down Syndrome Can Teach Us about Cardiopulmonary Disease. *Eur. Respir. Rev.* **2017**, *26*, 160098. [CrossRef]

22. Santoro, J.D.; Pagarkar, D.; Chu, D.T.; Rosso, M.; Paulsen, K.C.; Levitt, P.; Rafii, M.S. Neurologic Complications of Down Syndrome: A Systematic Review. *J. Neurol.* **2021**, *268*, 4495–4509. [CrossRef] [PubMed]
23. Demirbas, D.; Coelho, A.I.; Rubio-Gozalbo, M.E.; Berry, G.T. Hereditary Galactosemia. *Metabolism* **2018**, *83*, 188–196. [CrossRef]
24. Rubio-Gozalbo, M.E.; Haskovic, M.; Bosch, A.M.; Burnyte, B.; Coelho, A.I.; Cassiman, D.; Couce, M.L.; Dawson, C.; Demirbas, D.; Derks, T.; et al. The Natural History of Classic Galactosemia: Lessons from the GalNet Registry. *Orphanet J. Rare Dis.* **2019**, *14*, 86. [CrossRef]
25. Succoio, M.; Sacchettini, R.; Rossi, A.; Parenti, G.; Ruoppolo, M. Galactosemia: Biochemistry, Molecular Genetics, Newborn Screening, and Treatment. *Biomolecules* **2022**, *12*, 968. [CrossRef] [PubMed]
26. Coelho, A.I.; Rubio-Gozalbo, M.E.; Vicente, J.B.; Rivera, I. Sweet and Sour: An Update on Classic Galactosemia. *J. Inherit. Metab. Dis.* **2017**, *40*, 325–342. [CrossRef]
27. Waisbren, S.E.; Tran, C.; Demirbas, D.; Gubbels, C.S.; Hsiao, M.; Daesety, V.; Berry, G.T. Transient Developmental Delays in Infants with Duarte-2 Variant Galactosemia. *Mol. Genet. Metab.* **2021**, *134*, 132–138. [CrossRef]
28. Carlock, G.; Fischer, S.T.; Lynch, M.E.; Potter, N.L.; Coles, C.D.; Epstein, M.P.; Mulle, J.G.; Kable, J.A.; Barrett, C.E.; Edwards, S.M.; et al. Developmental Outcomes in Duarte Galactosemia. *Pediatrics* **2019**, *143*, e20182516. [CrossRef]
29. Vlachopapadopoulou, E.-A.; Bonataki, M. Diagnosis of Hypoaldosteronism in Infancy. In *Renin-Angiotensin Aldosterone System*; McFarlane, S.I., Ed.; IntechOpen: Rijeka, Croatia, 2021.
30. Rivelli, A.; Fitzpatrick, V.; Wales, D.; Chicoine, L.; Jia, G.; Rzhetsky, A.; Chicoine, B. Prevalence of Endocrine Disorders Among 6078 Individuals With Down Syndrome in the United States. *J. Patient-Cent. Res. Rev.* **2022**, *9*, 70–74. [CrossRef]
31. Graber, E.; Chacko, E.; Regelmann, M.O.; Costin, G.; Rapaport, R. Down Syndrome and Thyroid Function. *Endocrinol. Metab. Clin. N. Am.* **2012**, *41*, 735–745. [CrossRef] [PubMed]
32. Fort, P.; Lifshitz, F.; Bellisario, R.; Davis, J.; Lanes, R.; Pugliese, M.; Richman, R.; Post, E.M.; David, R. Abnormalities of Thyroid Function in Infants with Down Syndrome. *J. Pediatr.* **1984**, *104*, 545–549. [CrossRef]
33. Bull, M.J. Health Supervision for Children with Down Syndrome. *Pediatrics* **2011**, *128*, 393–406. [CrossRef]
34. Karlsson, B.; Gustafsson, J.; Hedov, G.; Ivarsson, S.A.; Annerén, G. Thyroid Dysfunction in Down's Syndrome: Relation to Age and Thyroid Autoimmunity. *Arch. Dis. Child.* **1998**, *79*, 242–245. [CrossRef] [PubMed]
35. Van Cleve, S.N.; Cohen, W.I. Part I: Clinical Practice Guidelines for Children with Down Syndrome from Birth to 12 Years. *J. Pediatr. Health Care Off. Publ. Natl. Assoc. Pediatr. Nurse Assoc. Pract.* **2006**, *20*, 47–54. [CrossRef] [PubMed]
36. Gomella, T.L.; Cunningham, M.D.; Eyal, F.G.; Tuttle, D. *Neonatology: Management, Procedures, on-Call Problems, Diseases, and Drugs*, 7th ed.; Fried, A.K., Lebowitz, H., Eds.; McGraw-Hill: New York, NY, USA, 2013; ISBN 978-1-259-64481-8.
37. Maria, S. *Aspecte Practice in Nutritia Neonatala*, 1st ed.; Editura Universitară: Carol Davila, Romania, 2013.
38. Santoro, S.L.; Steffensen, E.H. Congenital Heart Disease in Down Syndrome—A Review of Temporal Changes. *J. Congenit. Cardiol.* **2021**, *5*, 1. [CrossRef]
39. Ujuanbi Amenawon, S.; Onyeka Adaeze, C. Prevalence and Pattern of Congenital Heart Disease among Children with Down Syndrome Seen in a Federal Medical Centre in the Niger Delta Region, Nigeria. *J. Cardiol. Cardiovasc. Med.* **2022**, *7*, 030–035. [CrossRef]
40. Ko, J.M. Genetic Syndromes Associated with Congenital Heart Disease. *Korean Circ. J.* **2015**, *45*, 357–361. [CrossRef]
41. Benhaourech, S.; Drighil, A.; Hammiri, A. El Congenital Heart Disease and Down Syndrome: Various Aspects of a Confirmed Association. *Cardiovasc. J. Afr.* **2016**, *27*, 287–290. [CrossRef] [PubMed]
42. Amr, N.H. Thyroid Disorders in Subjects with Down Syndrome: An Update. *Acta Biomed.* **2018**, *89*, 132–139. [CrossRef]
43. Caracausi, M.; Ghini, V.; Locatelli, C.; Mericio, M.; Piovesan, A.; Antonaros, F.; Pelleri, M.C.; Vitale, L.; Vacca, R.A.; Bedetti, F.; et al. Plasma and Urinary Metabolomic Profiles of Down Syndrome Correlate with Alteration of Mitochondrial Metabolism. *Sci. Rep.* **2018**, *8*, 2977. [CrossRef] [PubMed]
44. Cooke, E.; Coles, L.; Staton, S.; Thorpe, K.; Chawla, J. Communicating the Complex Lives of Families That Include a Child with Down Syndrome. *Health Sociol. Rev. J. Health Sect. Aust. Sociol. Assoc.* **2023**, *32*, 1–23. [CrossRef] [PubMed]

Disclaimer/Publisher's Note: The statements, opinions and data contained in all publications are solely those of the individual author(s) and contributor(s) and not of MDPI and/or the editor(s). MDPI and/or the editor(s) disclaim responsibility for any injury to people or property resulting from any ideas, methods, instructions or products referred to in the content.

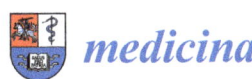

Case Report

Diagnosis and Management of Fetal and Neonatal Thyrotoxicosis

Roxana-Elena Bohîlțea [1,2], Bianca-Margareta Mihai [2,3,*], Elena Szini [4], Ileana-Alina Șucaliuc [5] and Corin Badiu [5,6]

1. Department of Obstetrics and Gynecology, 'Carol Davila' University of Medicine and Pharmacy, 020021 Bucharest, Romania
2. Department of Obstetrics and Gynecology, Filantropia Clinical Hospital, 011132 Bucharest, Romania
3. Doctoral School, 'Carol Davila' University of Medicine and Pharmacy, 020021 Bucharest, Romania
4. Department of Neonatology, University Emergency Hospital, 050098 Bucharest, Romania
5. Department of Thyroid Disorders, 'C.I. Parhon' National Institute of Endocrinology, 011863 Bucharest, Romania
6. Department of Endocrinology, 'Carol Davila' University of Medicine and Pharmacy, 020021 Bucharest, Romania
* Correspondence: bmmihai@gmail.com

Abstract: *Background and Objectives*: Clinical fetal thyrotoxicosis is a rare disorder occurring in 1–5% of pregnancies with Graves' disease. Although transplacental passage of maternal TSH receptor stimulating autoantibodies (TRAb) to the fetus occurs early in gestation, their concentration in the fetus is reduced until the late second trimester, and reaches maternal levels in the last period of pregnancy. The mortality of fetal thyrotoxicosis is 12–20%, mainly due to heart failure. *Case report*: We present a case of fetal and neonatal thyrotoxicosis with favorable evolution under proper treatment in a 37-year-old woman. From her surgical history, we noted a thyroidectomy performed 12 years ago for Graves' disease with orbitopathy and ophthalmopathy; the patient was hormonally balanced under substitution treatment for post-surgical hypothyroidism and hypoparathyroidism. From her obstetrical history, we remarked a untreated pregnancy complicated with fetal anasarca, premature birth, and neonatal death. The current pregnancy began with maternal euthyroid status and persistently increased TRAb, the value of which reached 101 IU/L at 20 weeks gestational age and decreased rapidly within 1 month to 7.5 IU/L, probably due to the placental passage, and occurred simultaneously with the development of fetal tachycardia, without any other fetal thyrotoxicosis signs. In order to treat fetal thyrotoxicosis, the patient was administered methimazole, in addition to her routine substitution of 137.5 ug L-Thyroxine daily, with good control of thyroid function in both mother and fetus. *Conclusions*: Monitoring for fetal thyrotoxicosis signs and maternal TRAb concentration may successfully guide the course of a pregnancy associated with Graves' disease. An experienced team should be involved in the management.

Keywords: fetal thyrotoxicosis; Graves' disease; TSH receptor stimulating antibodies; fetal tachycardia

1. Introduction

Fetal thyrotoxicosis represents a rare disorder that complicates 1 out of 4000–50,000 pregnancies. The most important etiology of fetal thyrotoxicosis is represented by Graves' disease [1]. Other rare involved etiologies are thyrotropin-receptor activating mutations [2,3] and an alpha subunit G protein-activating mutation, known as McCune–Albright syndrome [4]. In pregnant patients suffering from Graves' disease, 1 out of 70 pregnancies will develop fetal thyrotoxicosis, while pregnant patients requiring antithyroid treatment in the last trimester have a 22% chance of delivering a baby with neonatal thyrotoxicosis [5]. Thyroid stimulating hormone (TSH) is synthesized beginning at the 10th–12th gestational week, when the fetal thyroid begins to concentrate iodine and has the ability to produce iodothyronines. The hormone production is quantitatively reduced until the 18th–20th week of gestation, after which it intensifies gradually [6]. In the first trimester, the maternal thyroid hormones are fundamental

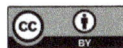

for the normal development of the fetus in the absence of a functional fetal thyroid. The placental passage of maternal thyroid hormones has been demonstrated in newborns with congenital absence of the thyroid, where cord serum concentrations of thyroid hormones were between 20 and 50% of those of euthyroid newborns [7]. Fetal, followed by neonatal, thyrotoxicosis occurs when transplacental passage of the TSH receptor antibodies (TRAb) reaches a high serum concentration, and it is increased in the second half of the pregnancy, when the placental permeability reaches a maximum capacity [8]. TRAb could either stimulate the fetal thyroid, resulting in thyrotoxicosis, or have an inhibiting effect, inducing fetal hypothyroidism [9]. Fetal thyrotoxicosis is considered to be a rare disease due to the fact that maternal immunity in pregnancy is modulated, and, therefore, the TRAb serum concentration should diminish [10]. Maternal medical history of Graves' disease, despite being euthyroid under anti-thyroid therapy or in substitution treatment after radioiodine treatment or thyroidectomy, is of the utmost importance considering the potentially elevated TRAb serum levels [11]. Studies have shown that fetal and neonatal thyrotoxicosis occurs only in women with three to five times the normal serum concentrations of stimulating TRAb [9]. Regarding the neonatal prognosis, the majority of newborns from mothers suffering from Graves' disease has goiter. Newborns with manifest thyrotoxicosis are recognized by restlessness, jitteriness, irritability, tachycardia, arrhythmias, systemic and pulmonary hypertension, cardiac failure, periorbital edema, exophthalmia, lid retraction, insatiable appetite, diarrhea, weight loss, sweating, flushing, hepatosplenomegaly, thymic enlargement, persisting acrocyanosis, lymphadenopathy, advanced bone age, microcephaly or craniosynostosis [12]. Neonatal improvement is strongly associated with the moment of maternal TRAb disappearance from fetal circulation [12]. The fetal prognosis is mostly favorable with the optimum therapy promptly instituted. Unfortunately, however, some infants have low intelligence quotients despite being treated for neonatal thyrotoxicosis, suggesting the complexity of fetal or neonatal hyperthyroidism's effect on the developing central nervous system. Other long-term complications of neonatal thyrotoxicosis are craniosynostosis, growth retardment, hyperactivity and behavioral issues [13]. Rarely, neonatal Graves' disease may convert into central hypothyroidism with decreased TSH secretion, due to intrauterine exposure to elevated serum thyroid hormone concentrations during a vital phase of development [14].

We present the case of fetal, followed by neonatal, thyrotoxicosis with good neonatal evolution under substitution therapy combined with thioamides in a pregnant woman with prior thyroidectomy, with elevated TRAb serum concentration from the beginning of the pregnancy.

2. Case Presentation

A 37-year-old pregnant Caucasian female, 170 cm and 65 kg, presented in our medical unit for pregnancy monitoring. She was known to have Graves' disease and orbitopathy, being euthyroid in substitution treatment with Levothyroxine 112.5 µg, 1 g calcium carbonate in association with 1 µg alfacalcidol daily, for postoperative hypothyroidism and hypoparathyroidism after a thyroidectomy performed 12 years prior. From the patient's obstetrical history, we noted a miscarriage and an iatrogenic premature delivery, which occurred at the age of 29 by emergency Cesarean section at 31 gestational weeks, of a 1400 g newborn with cardiac insufficiency due to manifest fetal hyperthyroidism with goiter, tachycardia, hydrops and associating fetal cerebral ventriculomegaly, gradually progressing to postpartum hydrocephaly. The newborn deceased at 21 days postpartum due to bronchopulmonary complications. The evolution of this previous pregnancy was marked by a massive increase of the TRAb serum concentration, with no treatment for the fetal hyperthyroidism.

The actual pregnancy started under neural tube defect protection with 400 µg folic acid and 400 µg calcium L-methylfolate, 400 IU vitamin E, enoxaparin 4000 IU and 150 mg aspirin daily for the thromboembolic disease prophylaxis in the context of the existing 1691G>A heterozygote Factor V Leiden mutation. The levothyroxine dose was increased to 150 µg daily. A non-invasive prenatal DNA screening test was performed for the entire genome at 12 gestational weeks. A fetal fraction of 7.83% was tested and it revealed low risk for the trisomies 21, 18, 13, 9, 16 and 22; aneuploidies XO, XXX, XXY and XYY; and for the microdeletion or duplication syndromes.

The normal course of the pregnancy was disturbed at 23 gestational weeks, when the fetal heart rate began to increase up to 180 bpm and we observed a fetal hyperdynamic status. At that moment, there were no fetal signs of cardiac failure or goiter. One week later, the levothyroxine dose was decreased to 137.5 µg daily. As there was no improvement in the fetal heart rate (Figure 1), in collaboration with the endocrinologist, a dose of 10 mg methimazole daily was introduced into the patient's treatment in the 26th gestational week.

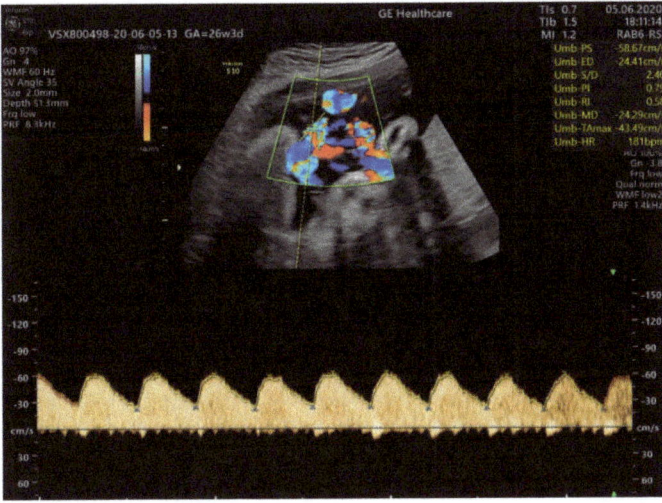

Figure 1. Fetal tachycardia at 26 weeks of gestation despite reducing the daily Levothyroxine dose.

During the 30th gestational week, the patient was administered four doses of 8 mg dexamethasone to aid in the acceleration of fetal lung maturity. The pregnancy was closely monitored using ultrasound markers. We examined the early signs of fetal cardiac failure, the size and vascularization of the fetal thyroid, the fetal heart rate, the maternal TRAb serum concentration and the thyroid function tests (Figure 2). The methimazole dose was gradually increased, as our patient, at 31st gestational weeks, received 30 mg methimazole daily, divided into three doses (Figure 3).

We monitored the fetal thyroid vascularization and dimensions, which were in the normal range according to the gestational age (Figure 4).

Due to fetal status deterioration, which was suspected at the ultrasound evaluation of the Doppler parameters and the fetal biophysical profile, an emergency Cesarean section was performed at 35 weeks of gestation, and a male fetus weighing 2530 g and 50 cm in length was delivered, with an APGAR score of 6 at 1 min and 8 at 5 min. Mild perinatal hypoxia, a tight double nuchal cord and the presence of meconium in the amniotic fluid were noticed. The patient received ablactation treatment with cabergoline to decrease the risk of further TRAb passage to the fetus. The newborn had a 32 cm fronto-occipital head circumference, a 30 cm chest circumference, mild exophthalmia, moderate congenital ventriculomegaly (occipital horns of the lateral ventricles of 14 mm and, respectively, 16 mm), no clinical or ultrasound heart abnormalities and normal heart rate. The fetal thyroid function tests were performed at birth from the cord blood, confirming the fetal thyrotoxicosis with fT4 > 100 pmol/L, T3 = 8.4 nmol/L (N = 1.23–4.22 nmol/L) and TRAb 39.74 UI/L, and were also performed at 48 h and 72 h after delivery. After that, the newborn was closely monitored and administered thiamazole at 0.5–2 mg/kg bodyweight daily, beginning with the second day of life, with dose adjustment depending on the thyroid hormone values and with liver function under close monitoring. Propranolol was also administered at a dose of 2 mg/kg bodyweight daily in order to control the fetal tachycardia. The medication was decreased gradually as the newborn's clinical status improved and the TRAb serum concentration declined. At 2 months, the baby had a significant decrease in TRAb serum concentration (2.45 UI/L) with subclinical hyperthyroidism (TSH < 0.005, fT4 9.8 pmol/L), and presented a normal development.

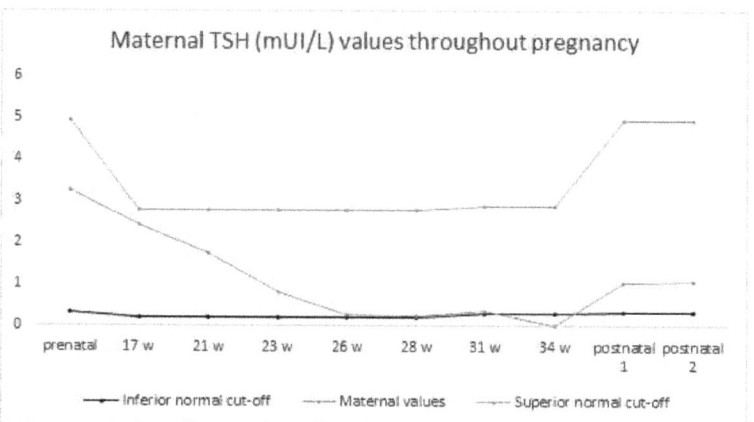

Figure 2. Maternal TSH values before pregnancy, throughout pregnancy and postnatally as compared to normal TSH values in pregnant and non-pregnant women The maternal TSH values were monitored before and during the pregnancy, with a monthly frequency at the beginning of the second trimester; further, with the appearance of the ultrasonographic signs of fetal thyrotoxicosis, the monitoring frequency increased. The TSH values had a descending tendency with the advancing pregnancy.

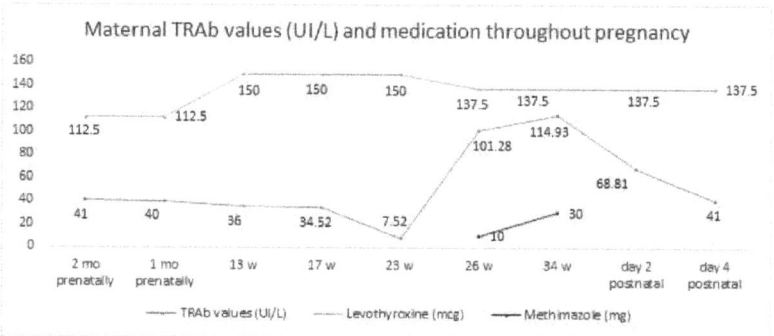

Figure 3. Maternal TRAb levels before pregnancy, throughout pregnancy and postnatally. The decrease of TRAb values in the 23rd gestational week corresponded to the appearance of fetal thyrotoxicosis ultrasonographic signs. The Levothyroxine was increased in the first trimester, with a decrease in the 23rd gestational week. Methimazole was introduced in the 26th gestational week.

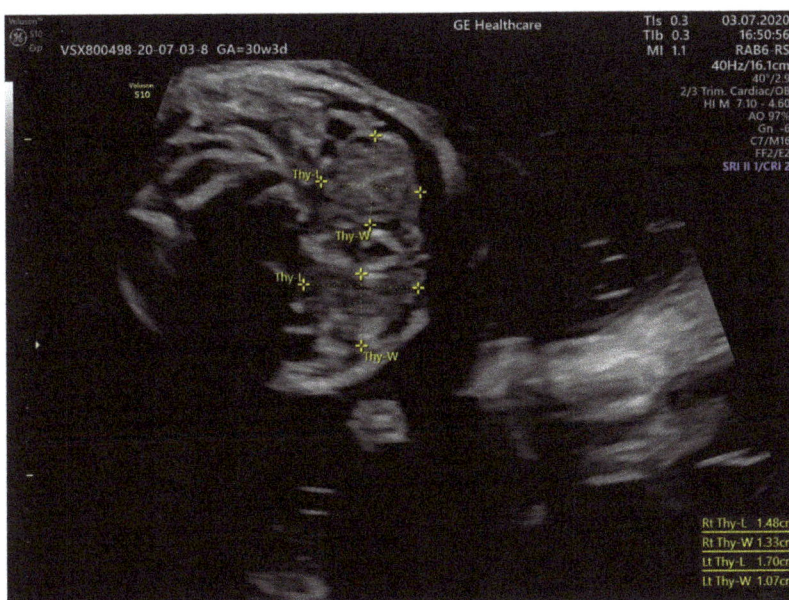

Figure 4. 2-D Ultrasonographic measurements of the fetal thyroid at 30 weeks and 3 days of gestation: right thyroid lobe measures 1.48/1.33 cm and the left thyroid lobe measures 1.70/1.07 cm.

3. Discussion

The particularity of this case consists of a pregnant patient who had very high TRAb serum levels from the beginning of the pregnancy, after 12 years since the thyroidectomy, with the initiation of the thioamide treatment in the second trimester with good fetal and neonatal prognosis.

The 2017 American Thyroid Association (ATA) Guidelines for the Diagnosis and Management of Thyroid Disease during Pregnancy [15] and the Postpartum, as well as the 2018 European Thyroid Association (ETA) Guideline for the Management of Graves' Hyperthyroidism [16], are against iodine ablative therapy for Graves' disease treatment during pregnancy. A future pregnancy should be postponed for 6 months until the patient is euthyroid, after iodine ablative therapy and after introducing levothyroxine substitution treatment. In addition, ETA does not recommend iodine ablative therapy while breast-feeding [16]. ATA recommends surgical treatment in cases of thyrotoxicosis resistant to high doses of thioamides, and the timing of the intervention should be in the second trimester [17]. ETA recommends thyroidectomy in cases of allergy or contraindications to thioamides [16]. Besides the risk of infection or bleeding, the risk of parathyroid glands injuries is not negligible, so it is fundamental to evaluate the need for active vitamin D supplementing in order to avoid additional fetal and neonatal adverse outcomes [18].

Regarding thioamide drugs (propylthiouracil, methimazole and carbimazole), both propylthiouracil (PTU) and methimazole (MMI) are associated with the risk of birth defects: MMI has a risk of 3–4% [19] and PTU 2–3%, but less severe [20]. ATA and ETA recommend avoiding antithyroid drugs in the first trimester, but if the case imposes immediate treatment, PTU is preferred for this gestational period [16,21]. After 16 gestational weeks, ETA recommends switching PTU to MMI if medical treatment is required, as well as measuring the maternal FT4 and TSH every two weeks after treatment initiation [16]. Thioamides inhibit the production of thyroid hormones. The main side effects occurring in the mother are allergic reactions, agranulocytosis (0.15%) and liver failure (<0.1%) [22,23]. When recommending PTU therapy, it is advisable to monitor hepatic enzymes for the risk of liver failure. Besides having teratogenic effects, thioamides have been associated with certain birth defects. MMI carries the risk of aplasia cutis, dysmorphic facies, choanal or esophageal atresia, abdominal wall defects (omphalocele), ventricular sept defects and eye and urinary system abnormalities [19,24,25]. PTU is linked with fetal face and neck cysts, as well as with urinary tract anomalies occurring in males [15]. In our case, we delayed the thioamide treatment and introduced thiamazole in the 26th gestational week, after excluding a possible iatrogenic thyrotoxic effect of levothyroxine on the fetus and, thus, avoiding the risk of fetal malformations due to thioamides in the first trimester.

In the literature, the possibility of performing a scintigraphy to assess the remnant tissue of the thyroid gland after thyroidectomy, or an ectopic localization of thyroid tissue in order to evaluate the best candidates for radioiodine ablation therapy for Graves' orbitopathy, have been described [26,27]. In our case, the patient did not benefit from this type of investigation prior to the pregnancy.

An article published by Batra et al. in 2015 [28] describes the difficulties encountered while managing two cases of severe thyrotoxicosis during pregnancy, with fetal and subsequent neonatal thyrotoxicosis in a woman with subtotal thyroidectomy for recurrent thyrotoxicosis, followed by hypothyroidism. the authors concluded that early diagnosis and proper treatment may improve fetal morbidity and mortality. Moreover, another case report, published by Sato et al. in 2014 [29], communicates the positive effect of thioamides, more specifically of methimazole, when administered to a pregnant woman who received radical treatment 7 years prior to pregnancy and who presented with oligohydramnios, fetal tachycardia, fetal goiter and accelerated bone maturation in the early third trimester of pregnancy. After 2 weeks of treatment, the fetal heart rate and amniotic fluid index were normal for the gestational age, and after 4 weeks, the fetal thyroid had a normal circumference.

ATA and ETA recommend testing TRAb serum concentration in early pregnancy, along with a laboratory assessment of the TF in patients presenting a history of Graves' disease treated with ablation, either surgically or with radioiodine. In case of a high maternal TRAb serum concentration, the testing should be repeated between 18–22 gestational weeks [16,30]. If a high TRAb serum concentration is detected (more than three times the upper normal maternal limit or more than 5 IU/L), according to ATA, the mother is counseled to receive thioamides in the third trimester, and further TRAb testing should be conducted between 30–34 gestational weeks in order to estimate the need for the newborn to be monitored and, if necessary, to receive treatment [30]. Besides monitoring the maternal hormones, our monthly maternal TRAb serum concentration monitoring plan was extremely helpful in observing the dynamics of the antibodies and in identifying the moment of the placental TRAb passage to the fetus. This corresponded with the appearance of the early fetal thyrotoxicosis signs, namely fetal tachycardia and fetal hyperdynamic status.

Another particularity is represented by the fact that, even though most newborns from mothers with Graves' disease present a goiter, in our case, despite the presence of the manifest neonatal hyperthyroidism, the newborn did not have a goiter.

Finally, Graves' disease being an autoimmune disease, despite the fact that our patient received radical treatment, the autoimmune disease remained active and could endanger each and every future pregnancy. Thus, it is important to monitor the maternal TRAb and the hormonal status of the mother, considering the transplacental passage that is currently incompletely discovered and explained in the current literature, and which occurs in every pregnancy (Figure 5).

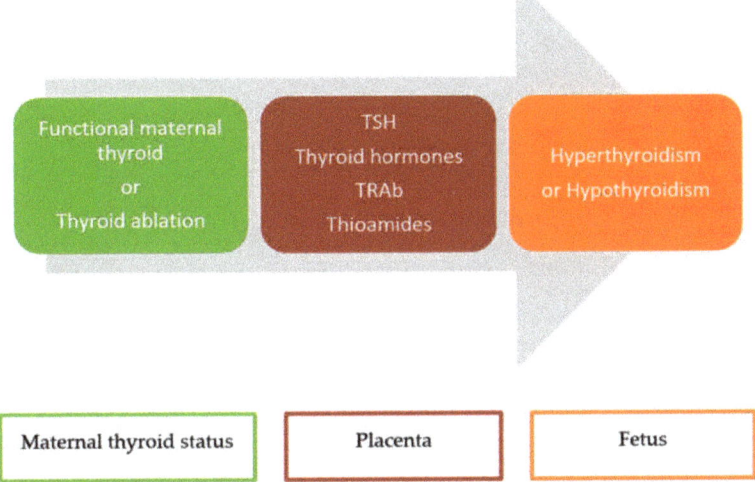

Figure 5. Transplacental passage of maternal hormones, medication and antibodies during pregnancy in women with or without thyroidectomy; TSH = thyroid stimulating hormone; TRAb = TSH receptor antibodies.

4. Conclusions

The first signs of fetal thyrotoxicosis are fetal tachycardia and fetal hyperdynamic status. We consider it fundamental to monitor the maternal TRAb and thyroid function monthly in order to detect the passage of transplacental antibodies to the fetus, and to establish the optimum treatment so that the mother and fetus have the chance for a normal life. A substitution therapy combined with thioamides could be recommended in cases of pregnant women with postprocedural hypothyroidism and active autoimmune disease.

Author Contributions: Conceptualization, R.-E.B. and B.-M.M.; methodology, E.S.; software, C.B.; validation, R.-E.B., B.-M.M., I.-A.Ș. and C.B.; formal analysis, E.S.; investigation, B.-M.M. and I.-A.Ș.; resources, R.-E.B.; data curation, I.-A.Ș. and C.B.; writing—original draft preparation, B.-M.M.; writing—review and editing, R.-E.B.; visualization, E.S.; supervision, R.-E.B.; project administration, C.B.; funding acquisition, R.-E.B. All authors have read and agreed to the published version of the manuscript.

Funding: This research received no external funding.

Institutional Review Board Statement: Not applicable.

Informed Consent Statement: Written informed consent has been obtained from the patient(s) to publish this paper.

Data Availability Statement: The datasets used and/or analyzed during the current study are available from the corresponding author upon reasonable request.

Conflicts of Interest: The authors declare no conflict of interest.

References

1. Polak, M.; Legac, I.; Vuillard, E.; Guibourdenche, J.; Castanet, M.; Luton, D. Congenital Hyperthyroidism: The Fetus as a Patient. *Horm. Res. Paediatr.* **2006**, *65*, 235–242. [CrossRef] [PubMed]
2. Duprez, L.; Parma, J.; Van Sande, J.; Allgeier, A.; Leclère, J.; Schvartz, C.; Delisle, M.J.; Decoulx, M.; Orgiazzi, J.; Dumont, J.; et al. Germline mutations in the thyrotropin receptor gene cause non–autoimmune autosomal dominant hyperthyroidism. *Nat. Genet.* **1994**, *7*, 396–401. [CrossRef] [PubMed]
3. Holzapfel, H.-P.; Wonerow, P.; Von Petrykowski, W.; Henschen, M.; Scherbaum, W.A.; Paschke, R. Sporadic Congenital Hyperthyroidism due to a Spontaneous Germline Mutation in the Thyrotropin Receptor Gene. *J. Clin. Endocrinol. Metab.* **1997**, *82*, 3879–3884. [CrossRef] [PubMed]

4. Mastorakos, G.; Mitsiades, N.S.; Doufas, A.G.; Koutras, D.A. Hyperthyroidism in McCune-Albright Syndrome with a Review of Thyroid Abnormalities Sixty Years After the First Report. *Thyroid* **1997**, *7*, 433–439. [CrossRef] [PubMed]
5. Ogilvy-Stuart, A.L. Neonatal thyroid disorders. *Arch. Dis. Child.—Fetal Neonatal Ed.* **2002**, *87*, 165F–171F. [CrossRef]
6. Epstein, F.H.; Burrow, G.N.; Fisher, D.A.; Larsen, P.R. Maternal and Fetal Thyroid Function. *N. Engl. J. Med.* **1994**, *331*, 1072–1078. [CrossRef]
7. Vulsma, T.; Gons, M.H.; de Vijlder, J.J. Maternal-Fetal Transfer of Thyroxine in Congenital Hypothyroidism Due to a Total Organification Defect or Thyroid Agenesis. *N. Engl. J. Med.* **1989**, *321*, 13–16. [CrossRef]
8. Chan, G.W.; Mandel, S.J. Therapy Insight: Management of Graves' disease during pregnancy. *Nat. Clin. Pract. Endocrinol. Metab.* **2007**, *3*, 470–478. [CrossRef]
9. Barbesino, G.; Tomer, Y. Clinical Utility of TSH Receptor Antibodies. *J. Clin. Endocrinol. Metab.* **2013**, *98*, 2247–2255. [CrossRef]
10. González-Jiménez, A.; Fernández-Soto, M.L.; Escobar-Jiménez, F.; Glinoer, D.; Navarrete, L. Thyroid function parameters and TSH-receptor antibodies in healthy subjects and Graves' disease patients: A sequential study before, during and after pregnancy. *Thyroidology* **1993**, *5*, 13–20.
11. Laurberg, P.; Wallin, G.; Tallstedt, L.; Abraham-Nordling, M.; Lundell, G.; Tørring, O. TSH-receptor autoimmunity in Graves' disease after therapy with anti-thyroid drugs, surgery, or radioiodine: A 5-year prospective randomized study. *Eur. J. Endocrinol.* **2008**, *158*, 69–75. [CrossRef]
12. Batra, C.M. Fetal and neonatal thyrotoxicosis. *Indian J. Endocrinol. Metab.* **2013**, *17*, 50–54. [CrossRef]
13. Daneman, D.; Howard, N.J. Neonatal thyrotoxicosis: Intellectual impairment and craniosynostosis in later years. *J. Pediatr.* **1980**, *97*, 257–259. [CrossRef]
14. Kempers, M.J.E.; Van Tijn, D.A.; Van Trotsenburg, A.S.P.; De Vijlder, J.J.M.; Wiedijk, B.M.; Vulsma, T. Central Congenital Hypothyroidism due to Gestational Hyperthyroidism: Detection Where Prevention Failed. *J. Clin. Endocrinol. Metab.* **2003**, *88*, 5851–5857. [CrossRef]
15. Alexander, E.K.; Pearce, E.N.; Brent, G.A.; Brown, R.S.; Chen, H.; Dosiou, C.; Grobman, W.A.; Laurberg, P.; Lazarus, J.H.; Mandel, S.J.; et al. 2017 Guidelines of the American Thyroid Association for the Diagnosis and Management of Thyroid Disease During Pregnancy and the Postpartum. *Thyroid* **2017**, *27*, 315–389. [CrossRef]
16. Kahaly, G.J.; Bartalena, L.; Hegedüs, L.; Leenhardt, L.; Poppe, K.; Pearce, S.H. 2018 European Thyroid Association Guideline for the Management of Graves' Hyperthyroidism. *Eur. Thyroid J.* **2018**, *7*, 167–186. [CrossRef]
17. Laurberg, P.; Bournaud, C.; Karmisholt, J.; Orgiazzi, J. Management of Graves' hyperthyroidism in pregnancy: Focus on both maternal and foetal thyroid function, and caution against surgical thyroidectomy in pregnancy. *Eur. J. Endocrinol.* **2009**, *160*, 1–8. [CrossRef]
18. Bohiltea, R.E.; Zugravu, C.-A.; Neacsu, A.; Navolan, D.; Berceanu, C.; Nemescu, D.; Bodean, O.; Turcan, N.; Baros, A.; Cirstoiu, M.M. The Prevalence of Vitamin D Deficiency and its Obstetrical Effects. A prospective study on Romanian patients. *Rev. Chim.* **2019**, *70*, 1228–1233. [CrossRef]
19. Yoshihara, A.; Noh, J.; Yamaguchi, T.; Ohye, H.; Sato, S.; Sekiya, K.; Kosuga, Y.; Suzuki, M.; Matsumoto, M.; Kunii, Y.; et al. Treatment of Graves' Disease with Antithyroid Drugs in the First Trimester of Pregnancy and the Prevalence of Congenital Malformation. *J. Clin. Endocrinol. Metab.* **2012**, *97*, 2396–2403. [CrossRef]
20. Andersen, S.L.; Olsen, J.; Wu, C.S.; Laurberg, P. Birth Defects After Early Pregnancy Use of Antithyroid Drugs: A Danish Nationwide Study. *J. Clin. Endocrinol. Metab.* **2013**, *98*, 4373–4381. [CrossRef]
21. Bahn, R.S.; Burch, H.S.; Cooper, D.S.; Garber, J.R.; Greenlee, C.M.; Klein, I.L.; Laurberg, P.; McDougall, I.R.; Rivkees, S.A.; Ross, D.; et al. The Role of Propylthiouracil in the Management of Graves' Disease in Adults: Report of a Meeting Jointly Sponsored by the American Thyroid Association and the Food and Drug Administration. *Thyroid* **2009**, *19*, 673–674. [CrossRef] [PubMed]
22. Watanabe, N.; Narimatsu, H.; Noh, J.Y.; Yamaguchi, T.; Kobayashi, K.; Kami, M.; Kunii, Y.; Mukasa, K.; Ito, K. Antithyroid drug-induced hematopoietic damage: A retrospective cohort study of agranulocytosis and pancytopenia involving 50, 385 patients with Graves' disease. *J. Clin. Endocrinol. Metab.* **2012**, *97*, E49–E53. [CrossRef]
23. Mandel, S.J.; Cooper, D.S. The Use of Antithyroid Drugs in Pregnancy and Lactation. *J. Clin. Endocrinol. Metab.* **2001**, *86*, 2354–2359. [CrossRef] [PubMed]
24. Milham, S.J.; Elledge, W. Maternal methimazole and congenital defects in children. *Teratology* **1972**, *5*, 125–126. [CrossRef]
25. Clementi, M.; Di Gianantonio, E.; Cassina, M.; Leoncini, E.; Botto, L.D.; Mastroiacovo, P.; SAFE-Med Study Group. Treatment of Hyperthyroidism in Pregnancy and Birth Defects. *J. Clin. Endocrinol. Metab.* **2010**, *95*, E337–E341. [CrossRef]
26. Oeverhaus, M.; Koenen, J.; Bechrakis, N.; Stöhr, M.; Herrmann, K.; Fendler, W.P.; Eckstein, A.; Weber, M. Radioiodine ablation of thyroid remnants in patients with Graves' orbitopathy. *J. Nucl. Med.* **2022**, *63*, jnumed.122.264660. [CrossRef]
27. Moleti, M.; Violi, M.A.; Montanini, D.; Trombetta, C.; Di Bella, B.; Sturniolo, G.; Presti, S.; Alibrandi, A.; Campennì, A.; Baldari, S.; et al. Radioiodine Ablation of Postsurgical Thyroid Remnants After Treatment with Recombinant Human TSH (rhTSH) in Patients with Moderate-to-Severe Graves' Orbitopathy (GO): A Prospective, Randomized, Single-Blind Clinical Trial. *J. Clin. Endocrinol. Metab.* **2014**, *99*, 1783–1789. [CrossRef]
28. Batra, C.M.; Gupta, V.; Gupta, N.; Menon, P.S.N. Fetal Hyperthyroidism: Intrauterine Treatment with Carbimazole in Two Siblings. *Indian J. Pediatr.* **2015**, *82*, 962–964. [CrossRef]

29. Sato, Y.; Murata, M.; Sasahara, J.; Hayashi, S.; Ishii, K.; Mitsuda, N. A case of fetal hyperthyroidism treated with maternal administration of methimazole. *J. Perinatol.* **2014**, *34*, 945–947. [CrossRef]
30. Andersen, S.L.; Olsen, J.; Wu, C.S.; Laurberg, P. Severity of Birth Defects After Propylthiouracil Exposure in Early Pregnancy. *Thyroid* **2014**, *24*, 1533–1540. [CrossRef]

Disclaimer/Publisher's Note: The statements, opinions and data contained in all publications are solely those of the individual author(s) and contributor(s) and not of MDPI and/or the editor(s). MDPI and/or the editor(s) disclaim responsibility for any injury to people or property resulting from any ideas, methods, instructions or products referred to in the content.

MDPI
St. Alban-Anlage 66
4052 Basel
Switzerland
www.mdpi.com

Medicina Editorial Office
E-mail: medicina@mdpi.com
www.mdpi.com/journal/medicina

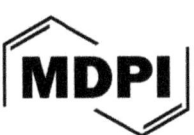

Disclaimer/Publisher's Note: The statements, opinions and data contained in all publications are solely those of the individual author(s) and contributor(s) and not of MDPI and/or the editor(s). MDPI and/or the editor(s) disclaim responsibility for any injury to people or property resulting from any ideas, methods, instructions or products referred to in the content.

www.ingramcontent.com/pod-product-compliance
Lightning Source LLC
LaVergne TN
LVHW070223100526
838202LV00015B/2079